Oxygen and the Brain
The Journey of Our Lifetime

Philip B. James

Contents

Every effort has been made to obtain permissions to reproduce figures and images but, as the material has been collected over a period of 30 years, this has unfortunately not been possible. My apologies to all those concerned.

P.B. James

Preface

The second title of this book is *The Journey of Our Lifetime;* I have been privileged to follow the lifetime of a very remarkable man from Scotland, John Scott Haldane. Born into an aristocratic family, Haldane was comfortable in every human situation, from sampling the air in the slums of Dundee, to working in the rarefied atmosphere of New College, Oxford. His investigations brought him into contact with miners, divers, munitions workers, soldiers, engineers, scientists, politicians, and royalty. He counted Einstein among his friends and shared with him the distinction of being awarded the oldest prize in science, the Copley Medal of the Royal Society of London. Uncomfortable with the constraints of academic life, he established a laboratory at his home in Oxford. His colleagues were known as "partners" and he would readily discuss his research with anyone who would listen.

Haldane was truly a polymath, readily crossing disciplinary boundaries in the investigation of a multitude of human conditions. His clarity of thought produced solutions to medical problems that many still allege to be unresolved today, despite astonishing advances in medical technology. In his famous book *Respiration*, published by Yale University Press in 1922, he explains the importance of breathing, not just to gain sufficient oxygen to sustain life and health, but to ensure healing from illness and injury.

It has been the interface between engineering and medicine that proved an irresistible fascination for me and it led to a career in industrial medicine. Immersion in thousands of papers across many disciplines, decades of treating deep sea divers and hospital patients with high levels of oxygen in pressure chambers has amply confirmed Haldane's contention that the oxygen in air is often not enough. Giving more oxygen, possible with a modest increase in the pressure around us, can greatly extend the envelope of natural recovery.

The developing use of oxygen treatment in medicine was sidelined after WW2 by the spectacular growth of the multinational pharmaceutical industry. But, as Haldane would surely have pointed out, it is obvious that all recovery, whether natural, assisted by drugs, or induced by a placebo effect, is only possible when there is sufficient oxygen present and, moreover, *there is NO substitute*. He would have been astonished, although probably not surprised, by the pivotal discovery that oxygen actually is the controller of our most important genes. The implications of this research can be distilled down to a simple statement: We need to use more oxygen in medical practice and, especially, in the treatment of disorders of the brain. The allegation that giving more oxygen is "alternative" medicine is unscientific and absurd: Illness and injury always reduce the oxygen available to cells and healing only occurs when adequate levels are restored. It is drugs that are alternative.

I hope that others will share my excitement over the latest discoveries about the molecule of life and also gain the satisfaction that comes from using oxygen in treatment. There is so much more to do: To quote Winston Churchill after the pivotal victory of WW2 at El Alamein: "Now this is not the end. It is not even the beginning of the end, but it is, perhaps, the end of the beginning."

Philip B. James
January 2014

Acknowledgements

This book has taken many years to complete and distils the work of many hundreds of physicians and scientists dating back to the 1600s. It would not have been possible without the help of my partner Petra Kliempt, who has patiently read the manuscript and continued entries in my database, which now contains nearly 7,000 papers. My family, Barbara, Adrian, Elliot, my sister Joan, and her husband Brian have been constantly supportive through difficult times. Sadly, my brother Ivan has not lived to see the book finished.

My thanks are due to friends who have contributed in a special way over the years, discussing concepts, sending information, and commenting on endless manuscripts; Yehuda Melamed, Duncan Black, Vance Spence, Paul Harch, Pierre Marois, Cyril Lafferty, David Downie, George Arnoux, and the late Richard Neubauer. I am also grateful to John Peters, Jennifer Calabro, and Cyndi Chong of Best Publishing Company; without their efforts this book would not have been published. Jim Joiner and Liz Bestic have also given helpful editorial assistance. My thanks to John Cooper who created my database which has proven invaluable. The biography of J.S. Haldane by Martin Goodman and the books of Nick Lane, especially *Oxygen: The Molecule that Made the World*, have been an inspiration. I also thank Sir David and Sir Frederick Barclay for their continued support and helping to fund the hyperbaric facilities still in use in Ninewells Hospital and Medical School, Dundee. The late Lord Whaddon deserves special mention for his support of the MS Therapy Centres in the corridors of power. I am indebted to my Alma Mater, the University of Liverpool, for the first class teaching I received in the Medical School and the University of Dundee also deserves my thanks for providing my academic home for over 30 years.

I am especially grateful to everyone who has been involved in the MS Therapy Centre movement over its three decades, especially the patients and carers; they have broken through the glass ceiling and shown that hyperbaric oxygen treatment can easily and safely provided by lay people in the community.

This list of others who have been of particular help is simply alphabetical based on first names. So many have helped that it is impossible to acknowledge everyone. I can only apologise in advance to those who feel they should have been included.

Alan Vardy, Anna Bublitz, Arun Mukherjee, Bernd Sostawa, Bill Maxfield, Bob Gardiner, Brian Paterson, Carol Henricks, Christine and Roddie Cameron, Christine Kinnear, Christopher Fox Walker, Claudine Lanoix, Colin Webster, Dan Walker, David Annis, David Freels, David Pullar, David Stirling, Derek Murphy, Douglas Fulton, Elizabeth Hughes, Eugene Levich, James Pratts, Jane Dean, Jane Orient, Jill Milne, John Clark, John Ellis, John Simkins, Karen and John Darcy, Ken Stoller, Knut Kliempt, Linda Scotson, Max Volino, Mike Allen, Nick Lane, Norma Philip, Peter McCann, Phil Connolly, Ray Cralle, Raymond Galloway, Richard Haldane, Richard Price, Sheldon Gottlieb, Stuart Bain, Tom Mills, Tom Fox, Valerie and Rex Woods, Winkie Neubauer.

Introduction

This book is about the importance of oxygen to the brain, not only to its function, but also to its recovery from the many conditions that may affect us. The story takes us from the first conquest of the skies by the balloonists, to the deepest dives made in the ocean. The science underpinning these exploits was used to put men on the moon and it now allows thousands of us to jet around the world every day. The technology is set to impact on mainstream medicine because scientists have discovered a dramatic new dimension to the role of oxygen in the body; far from simply providing energy, this vital gas actually controls many of our most important genes.

Despite the astonishing advances made in medicine, from the discovery of penicillin to heart transplant surgery, something has been overlooked, something so fundamental that it defies belief; it is simply how oxygen can be used as a treatment. We have forgotten that the oxygen we gain from breathing not only allows us to function, it is the key to our recovery from injury or disease. For the most part, breathing is silent; moving an invisible gas in and out of the lungs usually goes unnoticed in our daily lives, although we can generate plenty of noise when we speak! But there are times when the oxygen in the air is simply not enough and, even after a delay of years, breathing more may restart a stalled recovery. This was, perhaps, anticipated by William Shakespeare in Act 3 of *King Lear* when he wrote, "Here is better than the open air, take it thankfully."

As an element, oxygen is unique and, as stated, there is no substitute; water and glucose are also unique, but they are compounds and the body can make them from food; we must breathe to gain oxygen molecules from the air of the atmosphere. This layer of gas extends from the surface of the earth to the edge of space about 140 miles above us. Although the discovery of oxygen and its importance to most living things dates from the seventeenth century, only a handful of doctors in the world have become aware of the immense power of using high levels of the gas to extend the ability of the body to heal. There is, however, an obvious stumbling block for most of the medical profession; it is simply, why giving a large dose of oxygen for just one hour in the 24 hours of a day can mean that wounds begin to heal, even after a delay of many years. The science is now in place, but giving oxygen has yet to be recognised as a treatment in medicine and is even viewed as "alternative" or "complementary" therapy, when it is actually impossible for healing to take place in its absence. This is partly because medicine has been fractured by the creation of specialities, largely based on our organs, the "ologies," as for example, cardiology, dermatology, and neurology etc. However, all of our organs are linked by blood vessels and blood, and their prime function is to transport oxygen. Unfortunately today the central importance of oxygen, and the hydraulics of blood flow, barely rate a mention in the curricula of our medical schools; medicine has moved on to molecules and drugs. This reflects the fact that many who teach in our institutions think that oxygen is understood and "old hat"; being involved in the latest research, they do not have time to revisit well-travelled paths. Most of the research into the physiology of breathing was done more than 50 years ago, well before the sophisticated technologies available today were developed. Our investment in understanding life is dwarfed by the vast amounts of money spent in exotic particle physics, constructing machines like the Large Hadron Collider in Geneva, just to collide protons, when the complexities involved are dwarfed by the processes that take place in a single living cell. Ironically, it is "proton pumping" in our cells that generates the energy we need to live!

No one can seriously doubt the importance of oxygen to the brain; if we stop breathing, consciousness, the window that allows us to be aware of our surroundings, rapidly fades. The most critical function of the "machinery" of the body is to maintain our consciousness but, isolated in the bony skull, the brain cannot alert us to its own problems. The brain has no pain receptors and so cannot feel pain when it is injured; it can only experience the pain produced by damage to other tissues. This is not to discount the emotional distress of the many life events that may affect us, but to retain our sanity, it is important to recognise that no greater pain can exist than is felt by the consciousness that resides in just a single brain. And consciousness cannot be shared, every man is indeed an island; each of us has our own and unique view of the world. It is unfortunate that the incessant global media coverage of disasters makes it seem that the pain we each feel is somehow added together.

It is universally recognised that deprivation of oxygen soon causes brain damage, although this may be prevented if the deficit is corrected quickly, the timing is critical. Based on textbook accounts, most would say this is measured in minutes, but this is certainly wrong; the uncomfortable evidence, which will be discussed later, is that after the heart has stopped, the cells of the brain may remain alive for several hours.[1] But, to take matters a step further, will giving more oxygen to patients with brain injuries help them to recover? The purpose of this text is to show that it can and why. In 1981[2] three eminent neurologists introduced the concept of the "idling neuron," recognising that, after an injury, brain cells may be not dead, but sleeping. Although this still awaits acceptance by many leading scientists involved in brain research, there is overwhelming evidence to indicate that it is correct. This quote, attributed to a neuroscientist in a 2010 *Daily Telegraph* article, illustrates the popular view that brain cells are simply either alive, or dead.

When we have a stroke, our brain is starved of oxygen, causing the catastrophic death of those nerve cells and leaving us paralysed and unable to speak. Yet within days, the same patients start to regain movement and the ability to speak. This is not a sign of nerves coming back to life, but the brain rebuilding itself, creating new nerve connections and bypassing the damaged areas.

It is most unlikely that new connections can actually form within days. However, brain imaging has shown that nerve cells may become dormant and can be revived after injury, but it depends on sufficient oxygen being available. There has been a second important discovery relating to brain repair; the stem cells that form the brain as we grow in the womb are still present in our brains as adults and they retain the ability to grow new nerve cells.[3] Astonishing studies of patients who have received bone marrow or heart transplants from a donor of the opposite sex have shown that stem cells produced by the donated bone marrow can migrate into the recipient's brain.[4] They have been identified after death by their sex chromosomes and the phenomenon has been termed chimerism. This has shown that, rather ironically, the sex chromosomes are not a factor in the rejection that often effects transplanted organs. Not only are the primary cells added, for example, muscle cells in the heart,[5] or neurons in the brain, new blood vessels are constantly formed. So, the brain, like other tissues, is constantly rebuilding itself using stem cells, which suggests that aging occurs when our ability to repair damage fails.

Unfortunately, because oxygen has not been given its rightful place in treatment, medicine remains in the "Dark Ages" in managing disorders of the brain; drugs have been the rallying point for medical effort, often generating huge profits for investors before being discarded. The mistaken belief that everything will eventually be cured by a pill is a delusion no longer shared by the executives of pharmaceutical companies. It was reported on the BBC Radio 4 programme *Today* in February 2011, by Professors David Nutt and Douglas Kell, that the giant multinational drug companies Pfizer, Glaxo Smith Kline, and Astra Zeneca had closed their neuroscience divisions. Ironically, they referred to it as "the last nail in the coffin."

Despite the universal acknowledgement of the importance of oxygen to life, it will come as a surprise to many that using oxygen as a treatment, rather than just a supplement, is often dismissed by otherwise knowledgeable doctors. Today, with few exceptions, additional oxygen is given to patients simply to ensure that their blood is carrying a normal quantity; that it is as red as possible, but not to ensure that sufficient oxygen is available to the cells of our tissues. Ironically, blood is the one tissue little affected by lack of oxygen. The failure to consider the transport of oxygen to the tissues is apparent in a 2008 UK guideline on the emergency use of oxygen in adult patients,[6] which advocates "target" oxygen saturations in blood based on the so-called "saturation" of the carrier molecule haemoglobin in forming oxyhaemoglobin. This is the molecule containing iron, which is responsible for the redness of blood. But oxyhaemoglobin is a compound which contains oxygen, just as water contains oxygen bound to hydrogen and, in both cases, the oxygen is part of the molecule and is not free to be used. Only when oxygen is free and dissolved in the watery liquid of plasma can it enter tissues and cells. It is tragic that, despite the certain science involved, this fact is constantly overlooked in medical practice.

This failure has historical roots that need to be explored, especially because some believe that oxygen is poisonous and that giving more may be harmful. Too much of even essential nutrients can be harmful, even water and glucose. But there is ample evidence, which will be discussed in detail later, that the phenomena described as the "toxic" effects of oxygen on the lungs and the brain are extensions of the normal physiological actions of the gas. Here the unique knowledge gained from the fields of aviation, space exploration, and diving is desperately needed to change opinions firmly held in mainstream medicine. As will be seen, the body is able to cope with short periods of breathing oxygen levels vastly in excess of the concentration we normally breathe in air. In contrast, it is painfully obvious that lack of oxygen is much more dangerous; indeed we all ultimately die from it. Significant progress in the treatment of many disorders of the brain will not be possible until the fears relating to the use of oxygen, embedded in the minds of the medical profession, have been allayed. There will, inevitably, be resistance; suggesting that doctors do not understand how to use oxygen is a full frontal assault on their professional competence. The critical question, given that doctors are constantly bombarded with multimillion dollar advertising to adopt new drugs is: How can this truly monumental change be achieved when there is no financial incentive? Based on the experience of the author over many years, it can only be achieved by giving the facts to patients, their relatives, and carers; it is painfully obvious that they have the greatest motivation to promote recovery. Doctors can, of course, also be patients and it is a constant surprise to discover that their opinions about oxygen treatment change.

This text brings together the work of many thousands who have been involved in oxygen-related research since science began to influence the practice of medicine about 150 years ago. No claims for priority are made; it is obvious that the enormous growth of knowledge in every field of human activity makes it impossible for any single individual to be expert in more than a small area, and our lifespan is the ultimate biological limitation. Although we have developed many ways to increase our productivity, we still need leisure, as well as work, and we spend about a quarter of our lives asleep. Also, the problem of information overload has spawned a new discipline called "complexity science," which aims to determine unifying principles and is the approach used in this book. We now live under a veritable Tower of Babel, with millions of new papers published in medicine every year. Incredibly, it is becoming common to cite only papers published in the last 10 years; few are now aware of the work of the early pioneers. Sadly, the unfettered clarity of thought they were able to bring to medicine is now rarely possible. Unfortunately, attempts to generalise often upset experts, but this risk must be taken so that sense can be made of the vast amount of data that has been accumulated about oxygen. The biochemist Dr. Nick Lane grasped this nettle in writing his scholarly text, *Oxygen: The Molecule that Made the World*. Published by Oxford University Press in 2002, it brings together key information about the central role of oxygen in the development of life on our planet. Unfortunately, it repeats much of the current misinformation about the use of oxygen in medicine. Nevertheless, the author is pleased to take this opportunity to acknowledge helpful discussions with Dr. Lane and the stimulus given by this and his subsequent books.[7,8]

Most of us are content to accept the advances that science has made possible; they allow us to live longer, communicate more freely, travel further, and certainly play more than our forbears; not having to worry about keeping a roof over our heads, or finding food every day, we have the time. Nevertheless, many people do not want to know what happens inside us, not least because it reminds us of our vulnerability and mortality. It also brings us face to face with our origins; it is now well established that we share more than 98% of our genes with chimpanzees. No doubt, if they could understand this, they would actually be much more uncomfortable with the fact than we are; we are far more terrible than any other species on our planet. Other facts should also make us feel awkward; we rely on other members of the animal kingdom not just to work for us, but for experimental models of our diseases, to test our drugs, and to develop surgical techniques. There can be little doubt that it is easier to leave these uncomfortable matters in the hands of professionals, but today, this is simply not good enough. When we are children we have no choice but to trust others, but it is part of growing up to recognise that we live in an imperfect world and must take some responsibility for the actions taken by our societies.

Some may question why this book is necessary; surely, doctors are kept aware of the latest research? Unfortunately, we are all children of our time, the pressures of medical practice mean that doctors have little time to read journals and increasingly rely on other agencies and drug companies for information. As more than $1 billion may be spent on the marketing of a single drug,[9] an ambience has been created in medicine where, unless this level of effort is seen to be expended, a treatment does not appear to be worthwhile. Obviously, oxygen cannot be patented, and it is a rule of business that there can be "no promotion without protection" of a financial investment.

Suggesting more oxygen should be used in treatment is regarded today as "controversial," despite the end point being to restore normal values in our tissues. It would be difficult to imagine a more sensible, indeed a more scientific objective! We are entering an exciting era and remarkable new information can dispel the myths surrounding oxygen that are impeding progress. Although at times this book may be a disturbing read, to be in control of our lives the information is needed in the public domain. A comprehensive list of references is provided for each chapter at the end of the book, so that readers can access the primary sources of the information. Chapter 1 sets the scene.

CHAPTER 1
Setting the Scene

The presence of oxygen in a planetary atmosphere is the litmus test of life: Water signals the potential for life, but oxygen is the sign of its fulfilment.

Oxygen: The Molecule that Made the World. Nick Lane, 2002.

There can be no doubt that the human brain represents the pinnacle of development in our solar system, making any of our own creations in comparison, even the most sophisticated supercomputers, appear primitive. We are capable of astonishing genius; over the last few thousand years we have dominated the planet, making our mark in even the most inhospitable places, and building giant structures clearly visible from space. At night, satellite images show myriad centres of population glowing—stark evidence of our contribution to global warming (see http://visibleearth.nasa.gov/). As far as we can tell, we are on our own in the galaxy known as the Milky Way, and it will not be possible to travel to other stars with planetary systems because it would take far too many lifetimes. The adult human brain typically weighs just over three pounds, about 1,350 grams, and all of the complex apparatus of the body has the sole purpose of supporting the astronomic number of 100 billion cells it is said to contain. There is also one certainty; its development would not have been possible without the oxygen present in the earth's atmosphere.

It appears that a single event several billion years ago led to the development of organisms containing multiple cells, and prepared the way for the complexity of the human brain. The most likely explanation is that a single-celled animal, rather like an amoeba, engulfed a purple bacterium, encapsulating it within the confines of its cell membrane.[1] However, the bacterium was not destroyed; it survived to form a partnership with the cell. Ironically, a similar event takes place daily in every one of us and can be seen by viewing a sample of fresh blood under a microscope. Neutrophils, one of our white blood cells—also known as *phagocytes*, continually engulf bacteria in our blood to destroy them before they do us harm. They are also capable of capturing other particles and the sequence in which human neutrophils ingest latex granules over just a few minutes has been filmed.[2] After contact with the latex spheres, the phagocyte sends out projections which surround them and they are then incorporated within the cell membrane.

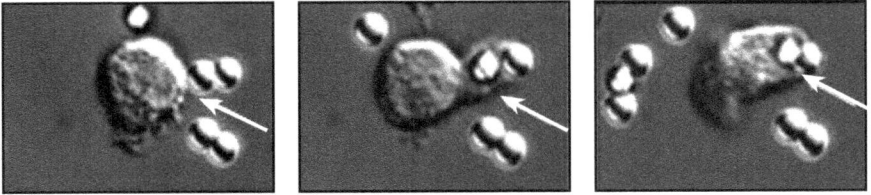

Figure 1.1: A neutrophil ingesting latex microspheres.
Frame two is after 1 minute and frame three is after 3.5 minutes.
(Courtesy of Dr. W.L. Lee.)

The coming together of a single-celled organism with a purple bacterium billions of years ago was to benefit both. The bacterium found a safe haven, and the cell was given a way to generate vastly more energy from the glucose molecule—enough to eventually allow the development of organisms with many billions of cells, including the species we have called ourselves, *Homo sapiens*. The purple bacterium was the ancestor of the hundreds of tiny structures within our cells called mitochondria, which are responsible for the production of most of our energy. They are one of a number of structures within the cytoplasm of our cells outside the cell nucleus, known as *organelles*. The purple bacterium had its own DNA containing about 1,500 genes, although it did not possess a nucleus. After the bacterium was incorporated into the cytoplasm of the engulfing cell, most of its genes transferred to the nucleus of the host cell, leaving only about a hundred or so behind in the mitochondrium. The genes retained within mitochondria allow them a degree of independence, for they are actually capable of reproducing within our cells. Fragments of the DNA released from mitochondria when cells are ruptured are now used for identifying tissue from victims of disasters, as they were following the destruction of the Twin Towers in the 9/11 attack in 2001. They can also be detected in the circulating blood of patients after injury, and may be responsible for the generalised inflammation seen in severely injured patients known as SIRS—short for systemic inflammatory response syndrome, which is a leading cause of death after trauma.[3]

The chemical apparatus that mitochondria donate to our cells allows access to the energy locked in the glucose molecule by removing its electrons. It is the unique structure of molecular oxygen that renders it capable of accepting electrons—a process that is known as *oxidation*. The energy gained by stripping the electrons from glucose is used to create the molecule central to life known as adenosine triphosphate (ATP). It is now accepted that the production of energy from ATP actually involves pumping protons and osmotic forces, and it was termed chemiosmosis by its discoverer Sir Peter Mitchell[4] (1920–1992). Although his work was fiercely contested for many years, he was eventually awarded the Nobel Prize in 1978. The efficiency of oxidation in mitochondria has been critical to the development of multi-cellular organisms, especially those, like us, with large, complex, energy-demanding brains. All living things on earth, with the exception of some species of microbe and, apparently, one nematode worm living at the bottom of the Black Sea,[5] can only function if there is sufficient oxygen available to release the energy contained in the glucose molecule.

Everyone knows that the primary reason we breathe is to get oxygen from the air, but most remain unaware that, because it is a gas, the amount of oxygen we take in by breathing is determined by pressure—the atmospheric or *barometric* pressure that surrounds us. This pressure is exerted by *gravity* acting on the gases in the atmosphere of our planet, constantly pulling them down towards the ground. The clouds suspended above us are a constant reminder of the presence of the atmosphere, which is clearly visible as a thin blue haze around earth on this photograph taken on an Apollo mission.

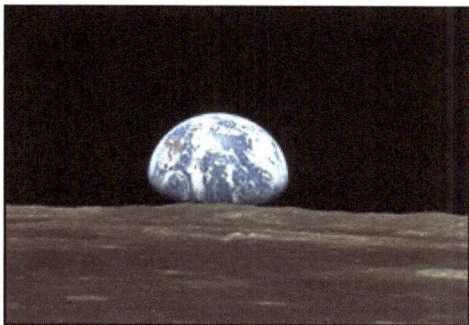

Figure 1.2:
The earth photographed from the moon.
(Courtesy of NASA.)

We all live *under pressure*, the atmosphere of our planet being effectively an enormous pressure chamber without walls, maintained by the force of gravity. Continue to lie in a bath when letting the water out quickly, and the effect of gravity becomes very obvious. We owe our lives to the concentration of oxygen in the atmosphere, and it is all down to gravity.

It is now more than 40 years since the late Neil Armstrong and Buzz Aldrin first walked on the moon, in what was probably the most complex project ever undertaken. Its success is in stark contrast to the failure of the initiative launched by President Richard Nixon to solve the riddle of cancer. The reason is simple: The biological issues involved in cancer are much more complex than rocket science. Space missions, of course, require a detailed understanding of the effects of gravity, pressure, and oxygen. Because the moon has no atmosphere, astronauts have to wear a *pressure suit*; without a suit, the water in the body would actually boil in the vacuum of space. A fasci-

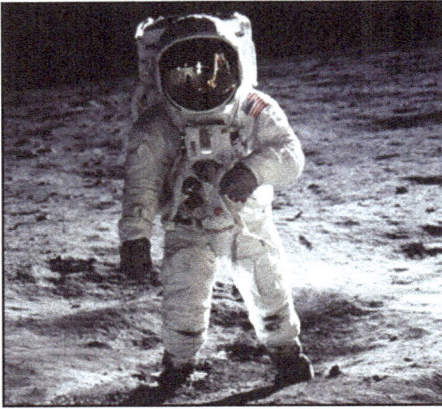

Figure 1.3:
Buzz Aldrin, photographed by Neil Armstrong on the Apollo 11 mission in 1969.
(Courtesy of NASA.)

nating book by Nicholas de Monchaux details the development of the Apollo suit by the International Latex Corporation in the face of determined opposition from defence contractors.[6] Space suits are personal high-pressure (hyperbaric) chambers, which are pressurised with pure oxygen supplied from cylinders contained in the backpack. The gas is circulated by a fan through a canister of lithium hydroxide to remove the carbon dioxide an astronaut exhales with each breath.

The suit can only be pressurised to about a third of earth's atmospheric pressure at sea level because, at a higher pressure, the glove becomes too rigid for astronauts to be able to bend their fingers. Let no one doubt the risks that astronauts take—loss of suit pressure from a puncture, for example by a meteorite, would be very rapidly fatal.

Today, pressure is a word in constant use, as in the "pressures of life" and the "pressures to conform," etc. Although we may not think much about it, we constantly rely on the pressures exerted by gases and liquids in everyday life, from using the hydraulic pressure controlled by a tap to fill a glass of water, to adjusting the air pressure in our car tyres. As biological machines, we are able to live because of the pressure changes produced by the pneumatic pump which inflates the lungs and the hydraulic pressure produced by the heart to drive the circulation. The primary function of both is to provide oxygen to our trillions of cells. Medical students are taught how to take a patient's blood pressure and its relevance to the circulation of blood, and also about the pressure changes in the chest associated with breathing. But they are *not* taught the importance of atmospheric pressure to the final delivery of oxygen to our cells or, indeed, the critical importance of oxygen to our recovery from illness or injury. Astronomers today are obsessed with black holes—the tragic failure to recognise the importance of giving patients more oxygen to assist their recovery could well be called the "black hole" of medical practice.

We all know from daily weather forecasts that atmospheric, or barometric, pressure varies with the weather. It is more likely to rain on a low-pressure day and be sunny when the pressure is high. We watch the developing low and high pressure systems ringed by the isobars on television weather forecasts, knowing what they bring. Weather systems are so powerful that they even make the planet wobble on its axis. Figure 1.4 shows the isobars defining areas of high and low pressure on a typical Atlantic weather chart. The units are *millibars* (SI unit hectoPascals) and normal atmospheric pressure is regarded as 1,013 millibars.

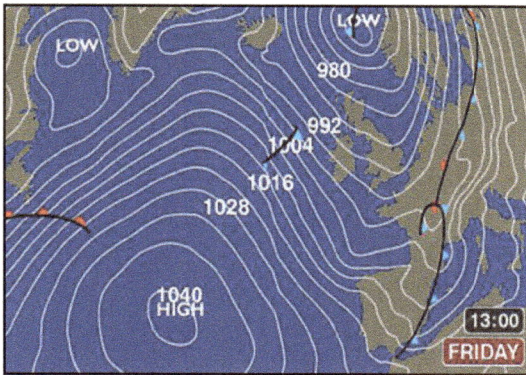

Figure 1.4:
Isobars on an Atlantic weather chart.

The range from the lowest to the highest barometric pressure in the UK is actually *more than 10%*, and it is even greater in some countries. This means that our intake of oxygen varies by the same amount, and it is one reason why we feel better on a high pressure day. When ascending high mountains, climbers become breathless because the air pressure reduces with increasing altitude. But is atmospheric pressure *really* important to our health? It may initially be tempting to say no, especially when it is obvious that changes in pressure are ignored in mainstream medicine; barometers certainly do not feature in our hospitals. In fact, the variation is not important to healthy, normal people but, as we shall see, it may be a matter of life and death to critically ill patients needing intensive care.

As a gas, oxygen obviously must be at pressure and it exerts about 21% of the pressure of the air we breathe, with nitrogen contributing an additional 78%. The remaining 1% is composed of the noble gases, principally argon, together with water vapour and carbon dioxide. It is the pressure exerted by oxygen that determines how much of it dissolves in the blood passing through our lungs. The physics involved is much the same as using pressure to put the carbon dioxide in a drink during manufacture to produce the fizz. The quantity of carbon dioxide that dissolves is directly proportional to the pressure of the gas, so doubling the pressure doubles the amount of the gas dissolved. This relationship was first described by the English chemist William Henry (1775–1836), and so is known as Henry's law. When we breathe in, we create negative pressure within the chest cavity and it is atmospheric pressure that actually drives the air into our lungs. In the lungs, oxygen dissolves in the blood passing through the capillaries next to the air sacs known as alveoli. It is, therefore, the *concentration* of the oxygen dissolved in the plasma of blood that is directly responsible for its final transfer when blood is transported into the tissues of the body to each cell.

Despite being the element most critical to life, oxygen has had bad press in recent years with much loose talk of oxygen free radicals. Indeed, it almost seems that the first word it evokes in the minds of doctors is "toxicity." This has had two unfortunate consequences: a tragic restriction of the use of oxygen for patients, and the lucrative marketing of antioxidants by the health food industry. Administering a higher level of oxygen to patients, whether it is at normal atmospheric pressure or in a hyperbaric chamber, is termed *hyperoxia*. It is common to see the unqualified statement in medical papers that "Hyperoxia produces free radicals." This is, perhaps, not too surprising in view of the paper unfortunately entitled "Oxygen is Toxic!" published in 1977 by the celebrated biochemist, Professor Irwin Fridovich.[7] The author visited him at his laboratory in Duke University in 1991 to discuss the subject, and found that he does not support the view that oxygen itself is toxic; indeed, he has stated emphatically that "Molecular oxygen is surprisingly unreactive" and bases his argument on quantum mechanics:

The modern view holds that oxygen is toxic not in and of itself, but rather because its reduction to water often proceeds by a univalent, stepwise process which creates dangerously reactive intermediates. Oxygen toxicity is, then, due to these intermediates. This point of view has been presented in several reviews.

Molecular oxygen is surprisingly unreactive. Its paramagnetism indicates the presence of two unpaired, parallel, electronic spins. This electronic configuration accounts for its modest reactivity under ordinary conditions. Thus, stable organic substances, which might react with oxygen, contain only pairs of electrons. Direct insertion of a pair of electrons into the half filled orbitals of oxygen would result in two parallel spins in the same orbital. This situation is disallowed by the well-tested rules of quantum mechanics. Specifically, it would violate Pauli's exclusion principle.

Fridovich I. *Bioscience* 1977;27:462-6.

But the desperate confusion about the properties of molecular oxygen is not restricted to medicine; in a Wikipedia entry discussing free radicals, there are conflicting statements on the same page. It states:

The high reactivity of atmospheric oxygen is due to its diradical state.

It is then pointed out that,

> *...the triplet-singlet transition is also spin forbidden. This presents an additional barrier to the reaction. It also means molecular oxygen is relatively unreactive at room temperature.*

http://en.wikipedia.org/wiki/Radical_(chemistry)

However, Fridovich, in a second paper entitled "Hypoxia and Oxygen Toxicity," which he delivered to an audience of neurologists in 1979, suggests that it is lack of oxygen, that is *hypoxia*, that is associated with free radical damage.[8] Unfortunately, this paper is rarely cited, although we now know that it is actually correct; insufficient oxygen is, paradoxically, associated with the release of free radicals. Hypoxia is actually difficult to define but refers to lack of an adequate level of oxygen, *hypo* indicating less and *oxia*, of course, referring to oxygen. Its association with free radicals obviously needs to be explained, but first it is necessary to outline the role of oxygen in normal metabolism.

The energy we need is derived from the glucose we obtain from food, and it is used to build the molecule at the centre of life, ATP, by a process known as *oxidative phosphorylation*. It is used for actions as diverse as powering muscle contractions to building proteins; even our thinking depends on this molecule. The process by which oxygen gains the energy contained in the glucose molecule involves removing its electrons; *loss* of electrons is known as *oxidation*. In the reaction, oxygen gains an electron; *gain* of an electron is known as *reduction*. Together, these effects are known as *redox* reactions. However, if glucose powder is dusted onto a surface it will not react with the oxygen present in the air, nor would it react if the air was replaced by pure oxygen. Equally, iron will not rust in 100% oxygen in the absence of water. However, if activation energy is provided by a flame, both glucose and iron will react in air and pure oxygen; in other words, they will burn. Burning glucose releases energy and produces carbon dioxide and water. The body cannot use fire to produce energy for obvious reasons, and instead uses an enzyme reaction and the enzyme is known as *cytochrome oxidase*. The reaction takes place in the mitochondria of our cells and the end result is the same as combustion; the glucose molecule is oxidised to carbon dioxide and water. A small amount of its energy is dissipated as heat, but most is used for the chemical reactions essential to life. What is so remarkable is that cytochrome oxidase is able to transfer electrons onto the oxygen molecule *safely*, avoiding the formation of free radicals. In other words, in providing energy it is acting as a powerful *antioxidant* producing water from oxygen without toxicity.

Although cytochrome oxidase is supremely effective in safely removing electrons from glucose, some free radicals escape from other proteins in mitochondria and it is usually stated that 1–2% of the oxygen we consume forms free radicals. To deal with this threat, cells have developed a sophisticated defence system of free radical *scavengers*. However, the scavenging molecules require energy for their production because they have to be synthesised by cells. This needs ATP and the production of ATP, of course, needs oxygen. The problem arises when oxygen levels fall because free radicals continue to be produced when there is less energy available to synthesise the complex scavenger molecules needed. And so, in the absence of effective scavenging, free radicals persist and cause cell damage. Conversely, if oxygen levels are increased above normal levels, for example when oxygen is given to a patient, ample energy is available for the production of matching levels of scavenger molecules. The dynamic balance between free radical production and free radical scavenging is central to life. To add yet another tier of complexity it appears that free radicals are involved in signaling within cells. Debunking the many myths and legends regularly cited about oxygen and free radicals is a key objective of this book, and is certainly needed to establish the use of higher levels of oxygen in treatment.

When a molecule of glucose is oxidised in mitochondria, it yields 18 times more ATP than is produced when it is converted to lactate in the absence of oxygen. This process later is termed anaerobic *glycolysis* and it has been assumed that glycolysis only occurs when lack of oxygen has reduced the mitochondrial production of ATP to zero. However, despite this being widely believed, it is not the case. The switch from oxidation to glycolysis is actually an active process, one of many controlled by a key protein hypoxia-inducible factor 1 alpha (HIF 1α),[9] which simply translates as low oxygen-induced factor 1 alpha. The hypoxia-inducible factor proteins are, paradoxically, increased when oxygen levels fall because their rate of destruction is reduced and, as will be seen later, this is the key to the existence of both multi-cellular plant[10] and animal life. Fibroblasts, genetically modified so that they cannot produce this protein, were cultured in a gas containing only 1% oxygen.[11] Although they continued to produce ATP, they died because of an increased release of electrons before their final transfer to complex IV and the production of carbon dioxide and water could take place. This release of electrons resulted in the production of the superoxide radical, which was responsible for the cell death—it appears that Fridovich was correct; paradoxically, hypoxia—lack of oxygen—is associated with free radical damage.

This information can actually explain the results of experiments reported in 1995,[12] which are of immediate relevance to the disease known as multiple sclerosis, because they confirm the vulnerability of *oligodendrocytes*. They are the cells which are responsible for producing the myelin sheaths in the nervous system which wrap around nerve fibres to increase the rate at which impulses are transmitted. Oligodendrocytes are the cells most commonly damaged in multiple sclerosis and the disease features in Chapter 13. When tissue cultures of the precursor cells that form oligodendrocytes were exposed to a gas not containing any oxygen at all, a state called *anoxia*, the cells astonishingly survived for 24 hours using anaerobic glycolysis. However, when the same cell cultures were incubated with a gas containing 1% oxygen, there was evidence of severe damage from lipid *peroxidation*. Lipids are forms of fat, and lipid peroxidation is the free radical chain reaction that makes butter rancid. In the body this process of peroxidation damages cells by attacking the lipids in their membranes. It became clear that the oligodendrocyte damage was due to the formation of the superoxide radical associated with lack of oxygen and indicates failure of the normal scavenging of free radicals. It seems reasonable to suggest that although at very low oxygen levels free radicals continue to be produced, there is insufficient energy to construct the complex scavenger molecules. The investigators found that when the oxygen content of the culture gas was *increased* to just 2%, there was no peroxidation of lipids, and metabolism was normal. And so doubling the oxygen level to 2%, far from increasing free radical production, actually abolished it! An oxygen level of 2% in culture gives a concentration of about 14 mm Hg, which represents a normal oxygen concentration for most cells in the body. It is clear that it is hypoxia, or too little oxygen, not too much oxygen, that is so dangerous. The retention of genes by mitochondria referred to earlier is needed to allow them to reproduce within the cell, retaining some of the characteristics of an independent life form. However, when oxygen levels are very low, the mitochondria of cells die and are absorbed into spaces called vacuoles within the cell. In the skin disease known as scleroderma, which is associated with an increase in connective tissue, the cells have been found by biopsy to contain very few mitochondria. A course of treatment with a high level of oxygen under hyperbaric conditions has been found to restore normal numbers of mitochondria in skin cells, confirming that they are capable of reproduction within the cytoplasm of cells.[13]

In recent years, astonishing proof that higher levels of oxygen are actually beneficial has come from the study of fossils. About 300–400 million years ago, the atmosphere of our planet was about 35% oxygen; much higher than the 21% value it is today. Dragonflies, like the fossil found in 1977 near Bolsover in Derbyshire, England, were able to achieve wingspans of more than 30 inches. Many other insects also grew to a much larger size, so it is clear that, far from being harmful to living things, a higher level of oxygen can be very advantageous. Unfortunately, many in medical practice today appear to regard such an increase to the concentration of oxygen as clinically insignificant. However, chemists employing air as the source of oxygen for an industrial process would certainly disagree; such an increase is *highly* significant and would dramatically alter the dynamics of a chemical reaction. This is all brought into sharp focus with the recognition that the genes that have shaped our existence on earth were able to develop when the earth's atmospheric oxygen concentration was much higher than it is today. Confirmation of the importance to the brain of breathing higher oxygen concentrations came from studies of brain damage associated with anaesthesia in the 1960s.[14] It was found that key areas of the brain were vulnerable to a slight reduction in the blood flow if only 21% oxygen was used in the gas supplied to patients in anaesthesia. A minimum level of 30% oxygen in the mixture used was introduced, which is now the required standard. It is notable that in the eighteenth century, such an increase in the concentration of oxygen was achieved by using compressed air and employed as a medical treatment.

The use of an increased air pressure in treatment has a long and controversial history, which dates back to the experiments of the English clergyman Henshaw in 1662.[15] He believed that acute diseases could be treated with an increase in pressure and chronic diseases with a reduction. As will be seen later, he was actually correct, although he had no idea why pressure has such effects. Changes in air pressure directly alter the pressure of oxygen it contains. A descent to the Dead Sea, which is below sea level, increases the concentration of oxygen breathed and an ascent to altitude reduces it. Interestingly, the reduction of the density of air by an ascent to a modest altitude—a few thousand feet, improves lung function because human lungs use a "push-pull" system, with the incoming air being mixed with the gases being exhaled.[16] Henshaw's research into the effects of air pressure predated the discovery of oxygen by more than a hundred years. The Polish alchemist Michael Sendivogius (1566–1636) should probably be credited with the discovery of oxygen. The English chemist Joseph Priestley also isolated it in 1774, although he called it dephlogisticated air. Priestley breathed the gas and anticipated some of the comments made by the customers of oxygen bars today (Figure 1.5). The term oxygen or, prophetically, *oxygene* was applied to the gas by the celebrated French chemist Antoine Lavoisier in 1778.

It is common knowledge that most of us feel better during a period of high pressure, and our aches and pains often increase if barometric pressure suddenly falls. The benefits from being in compressed air were rediscovered in France in the 1830s by Junod, Tabarie, and Pravaz, beginning the extraordinary era of the compressed air baths. They flourished in Europe and America until the outbreak of WW2, and persisted in Germany until the 1970s. The movement reached its zenith in the US with the construction of an enormous hyperbaric hotel by Dr. Orville J. Cunningham, a professor of anaesthesia at the University of Kansas. Apparently in 1918, Cunningham had successfully treated a young doctor in his hospital suffering from severe influenza in a hyperbaric chamber that had been used for animal experiments. He then built a large horizontal chamber and treated patients with a variety of conditions. His hyperbaric hotel was a 900-ton sphere 64 feet in diameter, with 38 rooms and 350 portholes. It was built in 1928 by the Melbourne Construction Co. at a cost of $1 million and financed by a patient Cunningham had treated, H.H. Timken, the owner of the Timken Roller Bearing Co. of Canton, Ohio. The sphere was attached to a series of large cylindrical chambers, and the entrance was via a three-story sanatorium hotel. A history of hyperbaric medicine was the subject of a remarkable book called *The Uncertain Miracle* by the Pulitzer Prize winner Vance Trimble, published by Doubleday Press in 1973. The grasp of the principles he displayed is exceptional and the author is delighted to have been given a signed copy.

Patients stayed in the sphere for days at increased pressure in luxurious rooms with a library and restaurant provided. They were even allowed to smoke! Cunningham treated patients with syphilis, diabetes, and cancer, arguing correctly that lack of oxygen was an important factor in these diseases. It is now known that they are all associated with lack of oxygen and with inflammation, a critical feature of the response of the body to a variety of challenges. Cunningham was making a good deal of money, and this attracted the attention of the American Medical Association. They undertook an investigation and their report claimed that there was no scientific evidence to support the treatment, obviously discounting the increase in the level of oxygen from compressed air. The facility closed in 1937, and Cunningham died a penniless and broken man.

EXPERIMENTS
AND
OBSERVATIONS
ON DIFFERENT KINDS OF
AIR
AND OTHER BRANCHES OF
NATURAL PHILOSOPHY
CONNECTED WITH THE SUBJECT.
IN THREE VOLUMES;

Being the former Six Volumes abridged and methodized, with many Additions.

By Joseph Priestley, L.L.D., F.R.S.

BIRMINGHAM,
PRINTED BY THOMAS PEARSON;

AND SOLD BY J. JOHNSON, ST. PAUL'S CHURCH-YARD, LONDON.
MDCCXC

"I have gratified that curiosity by breathing it, drawing it through a glass siphon, and, by this means, I reduced a large jar full of it to the standard of common air. The feeling of it to my lungs was not sensibly different from that of common air; but I fancied that my breast felt peculiarly light and easy for some time afterwards. Who can tell but that, in time, this pure air may become a fashionable article in luxury. Hitherto only two mice and myself have had the privilege of breathing it." [p. 162.]

"... From the greater strength and vivacity of the flame of a candle, in this pure air, it may be conjectured, that it might be peculiarly salutary to the lungs in certain morbid cases, when the common air would not be sufficient to carry off the putrid effluvium fast enough." [p. 168.]

"But, perhaps, we may also infer from these experiments, that though pure dephlogisticated air [oxygen] might be very useful as a *medicine*, it might not be so proper for us in the usual healthy state of the body; for, as a candle burns out much faster in dephlogisticated than in common air, so we might, as may be said, *live out too fast*, and the animal powers be too soon exhausted in this pure kind of air. A moralist, at least, may say, that the air which nature has provided for us is as good as we deserve." [p. 168–169.]

Figure 1.5:
Title page and quotations from Joseph Priestley's book.

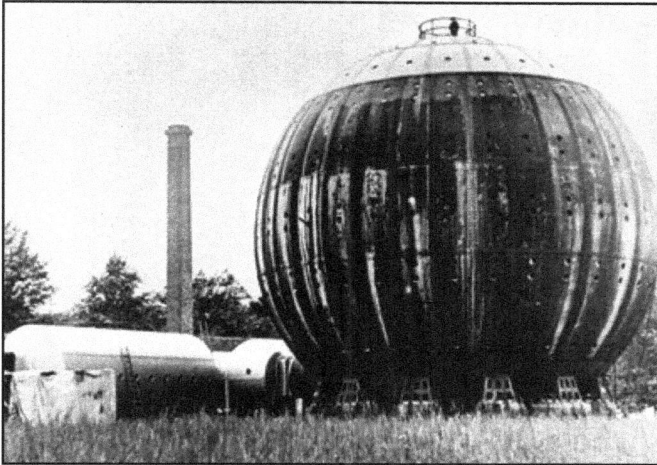

Figure 1.6:
Dr. Orval Cunningham's hyperbaric sphere.

The sphere was dismantled in 1942, and the steel used to build Liberty ships for the war effort. It would be 60 years before the key role of oxygen in the control of inflammation would be discovered, and it explains why compressed air can be an effective treatment.

A startling vindication of Cunningham's assertion that a modest increase in pressure improves health has come from a study in Israel of patients with advanced lung disease, published in the journal *Chest* in 1996.[17] The patients who were all receiving supplemental oxygen in Jerusalem were taken down to the Dead Sea to see if they would benefit from the higher level of oxygen in the denser air. Jerusalem is 2,600 feet (800 metres) above sea level, and the Dead Sea is 1,300 feet (402 metres) below sea level, giving a total reduction in altitude of about 3,900 feet (1,200 metres). On the satellite image in Figure 1.7, which shows the Red Sea's Gulf of Suez and Gulf of Aqaba, the Dead Sea is the stretch of water on the right below the Mediterranean.

The general health of the patients improved with better quality sleep, and they were able to walk significantly further, despite the fact that the use of supplementary oxygen in Jerusalem actually increased their blood oxygen values considerably above those achieved by being at the Dead Sea. Why, then, did the patients benefit so much more, despite the denser air at the lower altitude is harder to breathe? The answer may lie in the fact that at the Dead Sea, the patients were breathing a higher level of oxygen all the time whether they were awake or asleep. Patients rarely tolerate the constant use of oxygen masks or nasal spectacles, especially during the

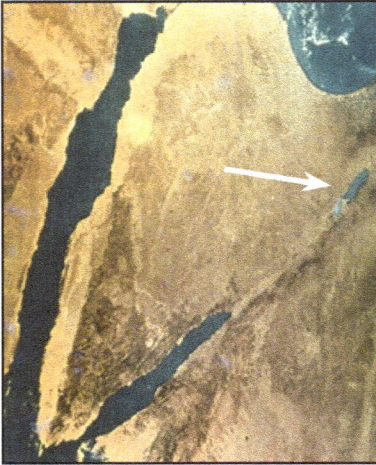

Figure 1.7:
The Dead Sea (arrowed) imaged from a satellite.

night. When we are asleep we all stop breathing, albeit for a short time. As a result the oxygen blood content falls, and the delivery of oxygen to the tissues decreases. As the normal leakage of water from capillaries and small veins increases when the oxygen level breathed falls, the tissues of the body become slightly swollen, although not enough to see with the naked eye. This "micro" tissue problem exacerbates chronic inflammation, and may not have been reversed by breathing supplementary oxygen just during the daytime in Jerusalem. In contrast, the additional oxygen associated with the increased air pressure at the Dead Sea was breathed 24 hours a day, avoiding intermittent reductions of oxygen level as when patients remove the nasal spectacles to eat and to sleep. The researchers found the evidence to support this suggestion; the patients maintained better oxygen values sleeping at the Dead Sea than when they were in Jerusalem. (The median haemoglobin oxygen saturation increased from 85% to 95%, and the percentage of sleep time with a saturation above 90% almost *doubled*, increasing from a median of 24% to 73%.) It is very important to note that the benefits of the very modest increase in the level of oxygen breathed at the Dead Sea unexpectedly lasted for *several weeks after* the patients returned to Jerusalem. Dr. Cunningham had been right and the naysayers, including many now involved in hyperbaric medicine, have been proved wrong.

Today, only saturation divers working in the oil industry experience the benefits of living in an atmosphere providing a similar level of oxygen to that used in the era of compressed air treatment. They live at constant high pressure in chambers usually built into ships, known as diving support vessels (DSVs), undertaking what is commonly known as saturation diving. A diving bell is attached to the chambers and lowered through an aperture known as a moon pool in the centre of the ship so that the divers can be transferred into the sea. Synthetic atmospheres of helium and oxygen are used, with a level of oxygen equivalent to breathing about 35–45% at normal atmospheric pressure. Many North Sea divers have now worked in the industry for decades and experience the usual aches and pains associated with getting older; they find that the pains disappear after a few days of breathing the higher oxygen level. Now, because the science is in place, we know why: Inflammation causes pain, and oxygen actually *controls* inflammation.

Our understanding of the fundamental role of oxygen in the development of life has come from intensive research in the last few decades. Far from just providing us with energy, oxygen controls much of our physiology and many of our most important genes. It is now well established that oxygen is the molecule that has underpinned the development of the biological world, and it has been equally important in making us. We all start life as a single cell, the fertilised egg, and it must embed in the lining of the womb to obtain the oxygen, glucose, and other nutrients essential for growth, from the blood of the mother. The oxygen, of course, comes from the mother's breathing, and is carried in her blood to the womb and thence to the developing embryo. The final transfer is into the mitochondria of the cells of the embryo to provide the energy needed for growth, that is, cell multiplication. Over 50 years ago it was shown that the first part of the process in which one cell divides into two can take place at very low oxygen concentrations.[18] However, a higher level of oxygen is needed to complete the division of the chromosomes, which contain the genes carried by our DNA. With the exception of the sex cells (eggs and spermatozoa), all our cells carry the full complement of 46 (23 pairs) of chromosomes in the nucleus. Every one of our cells, even the humble skin cells we discard into the air in their thousands every day, contain a complete set of the instructions needed to build another one of us; hence, the developing science of cloning.

The fertilised egg cell divides rapidly and soon becomes a ball containing many thousands of cells. Initially, the oxygen from the mother has to pass into this mass of cells by simple *diffusion* from the blood vessels in the lining of the womb. However, this process is not sufficient to sustain the embryo as it continues to grow; it needs its own circulation, and this means that blood vessels have to form, together with blood itself, and a pump, that is, a heart. The development of the components that form the circulation is actually triggered (signaled) in the rapidly growing embryo by the falling level of oxygen. This is, without question, the *central paradox of life*; a falling level of oxygen means that the energy that can be made available *reduces*, and there is the possibility that metabolism may stop altogether. To rescue the situation, something must *increase* to allow life to continue. The obvious problem in using oxygen itself as a signal is that if the level of oxygen falls too quickly, there may be insufficient energy available to power the actions necessary for survival. This critical balance determines whether an embryo lives or dies and, when we are older, if parts of us live or die.

What actually increases when the oxygen level in our cells falls is the protein hypoxia-inducible factor 1 alpha (HIF 1α). Every cell in the body produces HIF 1α, only for it to be continually destroyed when oxygen levels are normal, by another protein named after its discoverers, the von Hippel-Lindau protein (VHL). The following is a simplified explanation from a 2003 review in the journal *Nature*[19] of complex events which are still unfolding. A reduction of the oxygen available within a cell reduces the production of the von Hippel-Lindau protein, and so *less* HIF 1α is destroyed and, consequently, its level *rises*. HIF 1α is then able to bind with a second protein known as hypoxia-inducible factor 1 beta and this binding is also oxygen dependent. Two similar proteins have been discovered, also regulated by oxygen in a similar way—hypoxia-inducible factor 2α[20] and hypoxia-inducible factor 3α,[21] which is present in lung epithelial cells that form the gas side of the lung membrane. However, it appears that HIF 1α is present in all of our cells, HIF 2α in certain specialised cells, whereas HIF 3α is only present in cells in the lungs. This is for a very special reason: In contrast to every other location in the body, the blood vessels in the lungs contract, rather than dilate, in response to lack of oxygen; this reduces the transit time of red blood cells giving them more time to collect oxygen and improves the distribution of blood flow. In all, the HIF system proteins are now known to be responsible for regulating over 8,000 genes.

This is the answer to what must be the *central paradox of life*: Less oxygen equals, at least for a short time, *more* of the master proteins HIF 1α, HIF 2α, and HIF 3α. In the developing embryo, hypoxia begins the activation, or *upregulation*, of the necessary genes that control many growth factors via the HIF protein system. This includes the gene responsible for the production of blood vessels—vascular endothelial growth factor (VEGF), which translates as blood vessel lining cells growth factor. It is only one of several agents involved in the formation of new capillaries when we begin life as an embryo in the womb. But the system remains in control of the formation of new capillaries throughout our lives—for example, to form new capillaries to repair tissues after injury. The word *tissue* simply refers to a collection of cells, and it is important to note that, when a tissue is damaged, not only are its cells destroyed, the blood vessels the tissue contains are also damaged. The key message is that a *fall* in the oxygen level actually initiates the action needed to correct its own deficiency. Imagine a drug that can automatically ensure that it is delivered in the right concentration to the cells that need it! On the other hand, when we breathe a higher level of oxygen, the body is able to reduce the level of oxygen delivered to normal tissues by reducing blood flow, and the output of the heart is also reduced. This introduces another important principle yet to be recognised in medical practice or to influence treatment, which is also a central theme of this book: Giving oxygen is a unique treatment in not only being able to *reduce blood flow*, but actually *improve* its own transport into the tissues. A detailed explanation of why this happens and the scientific measurements that have confirmed it will be given later.

As the oxygen in the developing embryo falls, the level of HIF 1α rises, upregulating the key genes to initiate capillary formation—without creating a blood supply further growth would be impossible. Capillaries form as tiny tubes, pushing forward into the spaces between clusters of cells in tissues and branch out like a growing tree. Some invade the lining of the womb to form the placenta to gain much-needed oxygen from the mother. As more tubes form, they begin to come together, some will be arteries which carry blood away from the heart, whilst some remain as capillaries, and others become veins. Blood is forming and soon one capillary curls back on itself to begin forming the heart and the piping begins to join up to form a continuous loop. By the fifth week after conception, the tiny heart begins to beat and the pumping action forces blood round the newly formed circuit. The developing brain, heart, and spinal column are clearly visible.

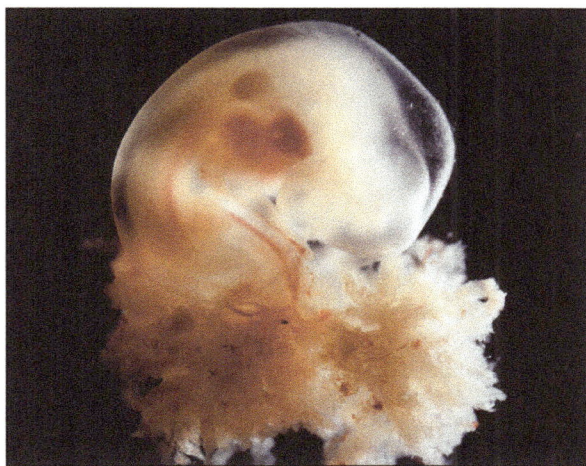

Figure 1.8:
Human embryo at five weeks.
(From *Behold Man,* courtesy of Dr. Lennart Nilsson.)

The development of this fine tubular transport system dramatically increases the surface area for the critical transfer of oxygen and nutrients to take place from mother to baby across the placenta and to the cells of the embryo itself. The embryo would, of course, soon die if a system to transport vital oxygen and nutrients was not organised in time to support its continued growth. The network of blood vessels in the body is truly enormous, especially within the brain. It is said that if all the blood vessels we possess were placed end to end they would easily surpass the circumference of the earth.

To illustrate the function of blood vessels, it may be useful to utilise an analogy from the organisation of human societies, the development of what we call civilization—of villages, towns, and cities. Villages formed when the value of collective agriculture made it easier for people to survive living together as a group. At first, the villagers grew crops and kept animals captive for food locally and they did not need roads; in fact, roads could bring the threat of invasion, allowing marauders to steal their belongings. However, as the number of people in villages became greater, outside resources became necessary and paths became roads and connected villages. Security was met by employing groups of strong men, who were the forerunners of our modern police forces. Now we can not only transport over land and sea, we can transport by air, which means that produce can be distributed quickly to anywhere in the world, sometimes with very unfortunate consequences. Blood vessels are our roads and not only transport oxygen, nutrients, and waste products, they are also responsible for transporting the white blood cells responsible for our defences against invading microbes. Ironically, microbes themselves may also be transported in blood and, as will be seen later, the effects of one, *Treponema pallidum*, the spiral bacterium responsible for syphilis, has profoundly altered the course of human history. The genetic control of new capillary formation, programmed by the lack of oxygen referred to as hypoxia, and the actions of the HIF transcription proteins are the key to recovery from disease and injury.

The term *anoxia*, which has already been introduced, should really be reserved for a situation where oxygen is completely absent, but it has been found that a level of less than 1% oxygen (at sea level), which is less than about 7.6 mm Hg, has the same adverse effects on cells in culture as true anoxia. This is because, for most cells, this concentration of oxygen is simply not sufficient to maintain their metabolism. Curiously, the term "hypoxia" cannot be related in this way to a specific level of oxygen—it does not represent an *absolute* concentration of oxygen. So the expression of the hypoxia-inducible factor proteins relates to a reduction in the oxygen concentration in cells and it is the *rate of change* that is important. In a clinical situation which will be discussed in Chapter 11, newborn children were often nursed in incubators breathing 80% oxygen, which was abruptly reduced to air with a normal oxygen level of 21% oxygen.[22] This caused a rise in the level of the HIF system proteins and, tragically, blindness due to an overgrowth of capillaries in the retina. In this case, the 21% oxygen in air is the normal concentration we breathe at sea level—and, therefore, not "hypoxia."

Of course, if we are *abruptly* starved of oxygen there is insufficient time for the growth of blood vessels to compensate and, unless the deficiency is rapidly corrected, vulnerable tissues, especially those in the brain, will eventually die from anoxia. The highest dosage of oxygen it is possible to give normally, that is, without a pressure chamber, is determined by the air pressure that surrounds us—barometric pressure. What does this mean for us as potential patients? It means that if we are rendered close to death, for example, by being strangled, and given pure, that is 100% oxygen in an intensive care unit, the concentration of oxygen we actually receive depends on the barometric pressure *at that moment*. This is determined by two factors, the *altitude* of the hospital and the *weather*. In the UK at sea level, barometric pressure varies by more than 10%; the lowest recorded pressure is 925 millibars and the highest 1,054 millibars. This means that 10% less oxygen enters the body on a very low pressure day than on a very high pressure day and the variation is even larger in other areas of the world.

Although the lowest pressure on our planet is at the top of Mount Everest, the brain cells of an asphyxiated patient may have oxygen levels far lower than those climbing to the summit who, of course, remain conscious. Most Himalayan climbers know that an increase in the level of oxygen they breathe of just a few percent when they are in the Death Zone above 28,000 feet may mean the difference between life and death. Unfortunately, asphyxiated patients are dying unnecessarily in our hospitals, simply because doctors in routine medical practice have no other choice than to give 100% oxygen at whatever the barometric pressure is on the day; the vast majority remain unaware that they may not be doing the best for their patients. So the take-home message for someone threatened by asphyxia from being grasped warmly by the throat—is make sure it is on a high-pressure day! But, as will be seen, a much bigger dose, equivalent to say 300%, may save a strangled patient from otherwise certain death, and this is *only* possible using an enclosure; a hyperbaric chamber.

If we are going to argue the case for hyperbaric oxygen treatment, then it is necessary to define *baric* oxygen treatment. This will be met by blank stares for two reasons: first, because the word "baric" is rarely used, and second, because giving more oxygen is rarely thought of as a treatment. Fortunately, in contrast to using drugs, giving more oxygen to restore viable levels in damaged or diseased tissue does not require detailed knowledge of the complexities of the body's repair mechanisms. But the baric oxygen in the air we breathe is treating our injuries and illnesses all the time and the use of more oxygen may extend the envelope of normal healing. For many people, their only experience of being given oxygen is by a flimsy mask or prongs pushed up their nose, and most assume they are getting 100% oxygen. The pipes in hospital wards deliver close to 100% oxygen, but the harsh reality is that a mask or prongs add only a few percent to the 21% oxygen in the air, when much more may be needed.

A hyperbaric chamber is simply an enclosure that allows the administration of oxygen to patients to be *independent* of these two factors. Many people, including doctors, allege they have never seen a hyperbaric chamber, but they have—aircraft are pressure chambers, and they must be equipped with oxygen breathing systems in case cabin pressure is lost at altitude. If aircraft were denied the use of pressurisation they would be limited to an altitude of just 10,000 feet and so the technology has to be accepted by every country in the world for aviation to continue. However, if today's aircraft were pressurised on the ground using their auxiliary power unit (APU) they could transform intensive care by allowing critically ill patients to benefit from the higher levels of oxygen possible. A new initiative is certainly needed in intensive care and this has been acknowledged by the team undertaking medical research on Everest. A leading critical care doctor in London interviewed for a magazine in 2010[23] has highlighted the failure of many recent "innovations" for patients in intensive care which, he claims, have been responsible for worsening outcomes. Put bluntly, they have not helped; they have hindered recovery.[24]

The remarkable information about the role of oxygen in gene control, largely the result of the work of biological scientists, has yet to alter medical acceptance of the use of oxygen as a treatment. In mainstream medicine, oxygen is used simply as a *supplement* given to ensure that blood is as red as it can be. The term used, which is not strictly correct, is haemoglobin *saturation* and 100% has assumed the status of a *clinical constant*. The redness is due to the combination of the pigment known as haemoglobin, which is carried in red blood cells. However, when oxygen is combined with haemoglobin it forms a compound and it is not available—just as the oxygen bound to hydrogen in water is not available. It is only the oxygen dissolved in the liquid component of blood, the plasma, that can be transported to tissues and cells. This means that for the oxygen bound to haemoglobin to become available it has to dissociate—leave the red blood cell and enter the plasma. The concentration of oxygen in plasma can only be significantly increased by breathing more oxygen and, curiously, when used as a treatment it does not need to be given continuously; sessions of a high level for just an hour a day are often very effective. It is important to emphasise at this juncture that the *principles* underpinning the use of oxygen are *not* a matter of opinion; they are derived from the basic physical laws that govern the universe.

Knowledge is advancing so rapidly that it is next to impossible for doctors to stay abreast of developments, even in their own specialised fields. The eye, for example, is a globe just a few centimetres in diameter, but years of training are needed to become a fully-fledged ophthalmic surgeon, and their knowledge and techniques must be constantly updated. Accumulating research data is hard work and often, unfortunately, those who produce it are jealous of its interpretation. This is usually because it has been collected to support a theory, which is often regarded as sacrosanct. The theory may dictate that a particular approach is correct, and so the test is then to see if the data collected fit the theoretical model. The best example of this is the still-fashionable theory of "auto" immunity in which, it is claimed, the immune system normally used to kill infecting microbes will attack healthy, normal tissue. This has led to the development of a raft of drugs to suppress the immune system, which all risk blunting resistance to infection. However, evidence accumulated over the last 60 years indicates that this approach is mistaken—the problem is due to inflammation. The word is derived from the Latin word *inflammatio*, meaning flame.[25] Oxygen is required for combustion and it is ironic that inflammation in the body is actually associated with *lack* of oxygen,[26] and, in contrast to anti-inflammatory drugs, giving more oxygen as a treatment can control inflammation safely.

The evidence that high levels of oxygen benefit healing has been published in many thousands of papers over the last hundred years and needs to be assessed by open minds aware of a simple principle: Lack of oxygen can only be corrected by giving more. Oxygen, like water and glucose, is unique; there are no substitutes. Many interventions in medical practice make more oxygen available by improving blood flow such as, for example, coronary bypass surgery, but there are many situations where improving blood flow is not possible. It is then necessary to breathe more, and the objective is absolutely clear: It is to bring the level of oxygen in the affected tissues *towards* normal, just as we give water to patients who are dehydrated. It is here that conflict arises with what is termed *evidence-based medicine* because, some allege, oxygen should be viewed as a *drug*[27] and subjected to the same rules in trials as drugs, especially if it is delivered at increased pressure as hyperbaric oxygen treatment. Rebutting this contention is so important that it merits separate coverage in Chapter 10; nevertheless, it needs to be stated here that it is *nonsense*. Molecular oxygen is not changed by a modest increase in pressure and is not an adjunct to recovery; it is essential. The principles involved appear simple and, in many ways, they are; we are all aware that the oxygen in air keeps us alive, but are much less likely to recognise that it also determines if we get better when we are sick or injured.

Until very recently, medical information was locked away in institutional libraries accessible only to professionals. Today medical publications are accessible on computers via the Internet and the words, if not their meaning, are accessible to all. To understand the words needs training and, for the most part, patients still have to rely on professionals for their interpretation. However, at least now they can ask relevant questions based on the information they have accessed. Patients who have discovered many of the publications that stress the importance of using oxygen under hyperbaric conditions are often perplexed and dismayed when there is a brusque dismissal of the basic facts from medical professionals. It is, of course, implicit in medical practice that no doctor will deny a patient a treatment that may be of benefit—it is a failure of the duty of care. The defensive response to oxygen treatment so commonly encountered is the result of the failure to teach the importance of oxygen and barometric pressure in our medical schools. The overriding problem facing society is obvious: Who can teach the teachers? It is to be hoped that after reading this book, the reader agrees with the suggestions made in the last chapter to find a way out of this terrifying impasse.

CHAPTER 2

The Brain: The Ultimate Oxygen Machine

The thorough aeration of the blood by free exposure to a large breathing surface in the lung is necessary to maintain that full vital power on which the vigorous working of the brain in so large a measure depends.

Self Help (Oxford World Classics). Samuel Smiles, 1859.

The oxygen the brain needs clearly comes from the air we breathe. It is the product of plant photosynthesis with the energy of photons from the sun acting on the green pigment chlorophyll. A molecule of oxygen breathed in the UK may well have been released from a plant in the Amazon rainforest and carried across the Atlantic by the trade winds. Entering the nose or mouth, pushed in by atmospheric pressure as we take a breath, it passes down the throat into the voice box—through the triangular space formed by the vocal cords in the larynx—on into the trachea. Descending a few inches, the oxygen molecule enters the right or the left bronchus continuing down to the smallest tubes known as the bronchioles. There are 23 generations of branching from the trachea to the final air sacs—the *alveoli*, where gas exchange takes place and oxygen transfers into the blood.[1]

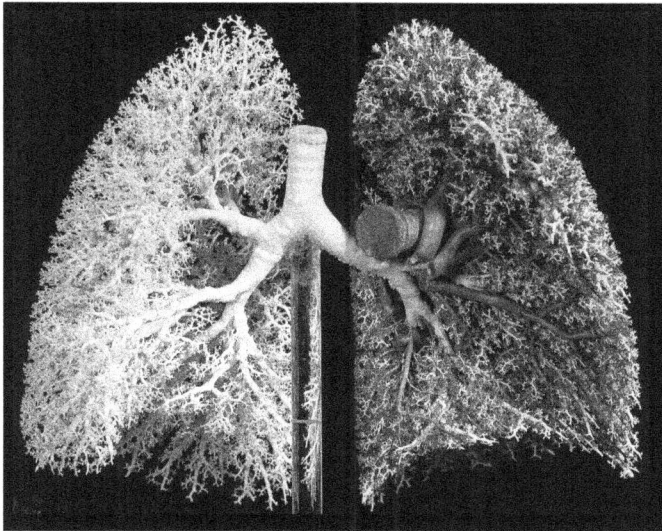

Figure 2.1:
A resin cast of the airways of human lungs. (Courtesy of Professor Brian Hills.)

During its journey down these air passages, the oxygen molecule will be buffeted against molecules of other gases, mainly those of nitrogen and water vapour, but also against molecules of carbon dioxide, which need to leave the lungs to be exhaled. Finally, the molecule reaches one of the clusters of alveoli, and here the oxygen *dissolves* in the membrane of the lung. This is formed by just two cells, one contributed by the lung itself and the other which abuts this cell is that of a capillary, as shown in Figure 2.2.

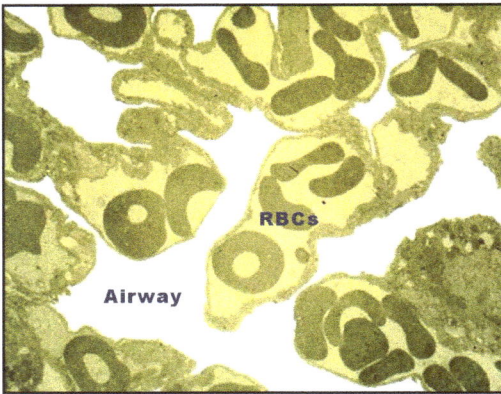

Figure 2.2:
Lung tissue showing red blood cells and plasma with the lung membrane separating blood from the air spaces.
(Courtesy of the late Dr. R. Alistair Bennet.)

Passing through the two cells of the lung membrane, which together are only 0.35 microns (0.000018 of an inch) thick, the oxygen molecule then dissolves in less than a second in the watery plasma of the blood flowing through the lungs. The surface area of the lung membrane is a truly astonishing 755 square feet (70 square metres), which is about the area of a tennis court. This lung membrane area has gas on one side, and on the other blood. It is, of course, essential for the alveolar membrane to be as thin as possible to allow gases to pass through easily. The blood pressure in the vessels of the lungs is very much lower than the blood pressure in the rest of the body—in fact, about eight times less. This is important because the membrane is so thin that a higher pressure would tend to force water through the lung membrane into the gas space and drown us. Some water from blood does pass into the lung tissues but it escapes via tiny lymphatic vessels to the lymph nodes in the centre of the chest. The low pressure in the blood vessels of the lung circulation is important for a second reason: Debris in the blood flowing into the capillaries can be easily trapped, and then removed by white blood cells. This secondary function of the lungs as "the guardian angels of the circulation" has been forgotten, and will feature in later chapters.[2] Rather surprisingly, trapping debris in the blood in the lungs is critical to protecting the brain and spinal cord from damage.

The constituents of air and Henry's law were discussed in Chapter 1 and it is necessary to introduce a second gas law, Dalton's law of partial pressures (John Dalton, 1766–1844). Because the actual molecules of gas are incredibly small, they occupy a very tiny part of the volume of any container and, in effect, each component gas molecule of a mixture like air has access to virtually the total volume. Possessing kinetic energy, gas molecules are in constant motion bombarding the walls of a container, thus creating pressure. The total pressure of air in a container is, therefore, made up of the sum of the pressures of each of the gases present; that is, the sum of the *part of the pressure* exerted by each gas, hence the use of the term *partial pressure* when describing a mixture of gases. As oxygen is 21% of air, it contributes a partial pressure of 21% of the total pressure. It is then possible to calculate the oxygen pressure at sea level on a day when the barometric pressure is at 760 mm Hg, which has been adopted as the standard reference value for atmospheric pressure, 1 ATA. The partial pressure of oxygen will be 20.9% of 760 mm Hg, which is close to 160 mm Hg. As we have seen in the previous chapter, the quantity of a gas that will dissolve in a liquid is directly proportional to the pressure of the gas. Oxygen is poorly soluble in water, and so the actual quantity of oxygen that dissolves in the plasma of the blood passing through the lungs is quite small. Nevertheless, it has been measured experimentally and assigned a value known as the *solubility coefficient.*

To sustain our level of activity, especially the demands of the brain, much more oxygen must be transported in blood than can be carried dissolved, that is, in solution in the plasma. This is achieved by storing oxygen attached to the molecules of haemoglobin in red blood cells and at this point, it is important to give some values. Imagine taking a very large syringe, withdrawing 100 millilitres (ml) of blood from an artery, and then measuring the volume of oxygen it contains. In a healthy person, it will be found that the volume of gaseous oxygen carried by 100 ml blood is about 19.3 ml, of which *19 ml* are carried attached to haemoglobin, and just *0.3 ml* dissolved in the plasma. The volume of dissolved oxygen stored in plasma is so small that it is even suggested that it should be ignored, as it is for example in the reference text *Scientific Tables*, published by Geigy.[3]

This fundamental error is a very significant factor in the academic rejection of the use of increasing pressure to give oxygen as a treatment and it needs to be understood at this point. To illustrate the importance of this factor an analogy is needed and the pressure of the dissolved oxygen in plasma can be compared to a *voltage.* The pressure of oxygen *dissolved* in a liquid, in this case blood plasma, is referred to in physiology as the *oxygen tension.* Tension is the term used by electrical engineers for voltage, as in the high-tension overhead cables used in a national electricity grid. Imagine possessing a small transistor radio that normally uses a tiny 9 volt battery but, not having one, connecting it to a very large 6 volt battery, for example, of a size that could be used to power a submarine. Despite the enormous amount of electricity in the 6 volt battery, the radio simply will not work. Substitute the tiny 9 volt battery and, despite storing only a fraction of the power that is in the submarine battery, the radio will spring to life. The reason is that the series of resistances in the circuits of the radio requires 9 *not* 6 *volts* for it to operate. In the body, a molecule of oxygen entering the airway, at a pressure of about 160 mm Hg, also meets a succession of resistances when passing through the lungs into the blood and then transferring into the tissues until it finally powers our cells. The oxygen pressure, or more correctly, the oxygen *tension* may fall down to as little as 5 mm Hg and yet be sufficient for some cells, like those in the skin.

Although some oxygen molecules are transported around the body dissolved in the watery plasma, we have seen that a much larger number are transported attached to the molecule haemoglobin. Oxygen combines four binding sites on the haemoglobin molecule to form the compound oxyhaemoglobin. Again, it is important to emphasise that the molecule oxyhaemoglobin is a *compound*, just as water is a compound of hydrogen and oxygen. The oxygen that oxyhaemoglobin carries is not free to be transported into our cells until it *dissociates* from haemoglobin and enters into solution in the plasma. Only this dissolved oxygen is then free to pass through the capillary wall into tissues and their cells.

The relationship of the level of oxygen in solution to the oxygen bound to haemoglobin as oxyhaemoglobin is illustrated graphically by the dissocia-

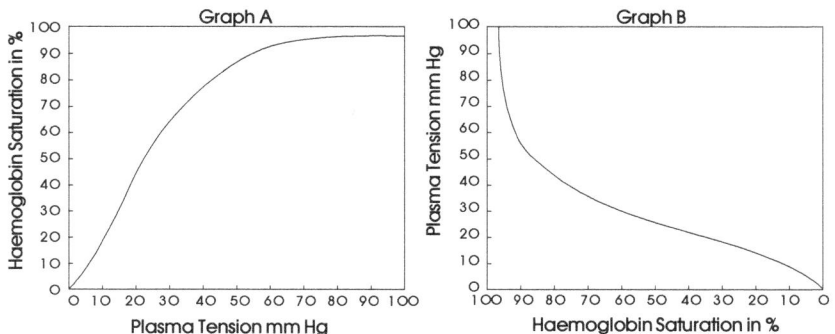

Figure 2.3:
The dissolved oxygen in plasma versus the oxyhaemoglobin level.

tion graph A, which is faithfully reproduced in every textbook of physiology. Saturation is plotted on the vertical axis and the oxygen tension on the horizontal axis in graph A, with the first point logged as zero. However, this state never exists in the body—there is never any time when the oxygen tension in the body is zero; it would mean that there was no oxygen present at all, and this is not the case even when we die. Also it is the dissolved plasma oxygen that leads, because oxygen first dissolves in the plasma in the lung capillaries, and then some transfers into the red blood cells. So graph B is a better representation of what actually happens and shows the plasma tension on the vertical axis and the oxyhaemoglobin level on the horizontal axis. The volume of oxygen carried in arterial blood is about 19.3 millilitres (ml) per 100 ml of blood, with 19 ml carried attached to haemoglobin and 0.3 ml being carried in solution. However, the blood that returns to the lungs under normal resting conditions is still carrying about 15 ml of oxygen and this is "topped up" with more oxygen when passing through the lungs, as shown in Figure 2.4.

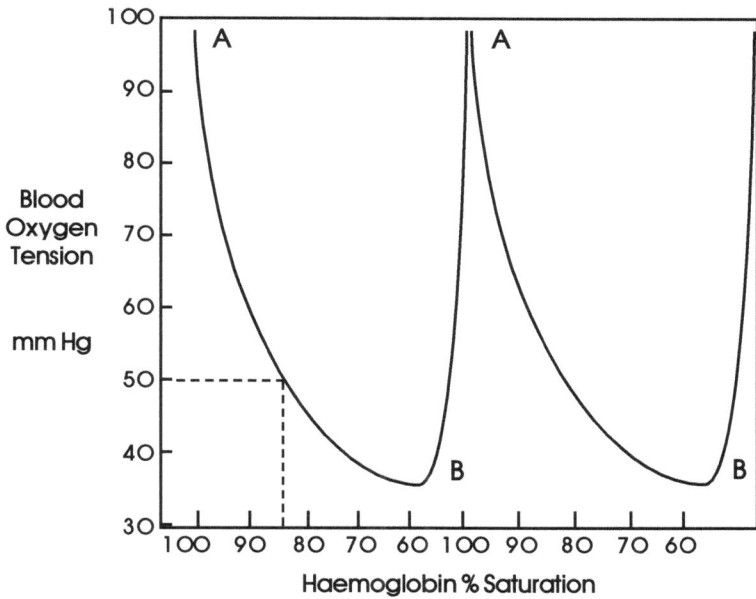

Figure 2.4:
Changes in blood oxygen tension on two passes round the circulation:
Blood leaves the lungs at maximum oxygenation (A) and is at its lowest oxygen level (B) in the veins entering the heart.
The increase in oxygenation—B to A—takes place in the lungs.

Note: When the oxygen tension falls to half its maximum value (50 mm Hg), haemoglobin saturation is still 85% (dotted line).

The misrepresentation of actual events in the body, implicit in the dissociation curve A, is reminiscent of the graph drawn by Edwin Hubble of measurements made of the expanding universe. He drew the regression line to zero, which has been claimed to indicate the Big Bang that started the universe. It seems that most astrophysicists now accept that this was not the beginning, as was discussed in the BBC programme "The Big Bang," broadcast in the *Horizon* TV series in October, 2010. In fact, oxyhaemoglobin is just one oxygen store; the molecule myoglobin, which is present in muscles, also stores oxygen and is responsible for the redness of red meat. It has been suggested that similar molecules store a limited amount of oxygen in the brain.

To continue tracing the route of an oxygen molecule from the lungs to the brain we will follow a molecule that simply remains dissolved in solution in plasma. Leaving the lung capillaries, blood flows into the chambers of the left side of the heart, entering the left atrium, or entrance chamber, before passing through the mitral valve, named after its resemblance to a bishop's hat, into the left ventricle. The left ventricle is the high pressure pump that circulates blood everywhere in the body except, of course, the lungs themselves, that are served by the right ventricle.

Blood leaves the left ventricle passing up the aorta, which is the largest artery in the body. After a short distance, the aorta begins to curve like a shepherd's crook. A large artery leaves it at this point known as the brachiocephalic artery, which is so named because it divides into the artery supplying the right arm, the subclavian artery, and the artery that passes up the right side of the neck, the right carotid artery. A little further around the curve of the aorta is the opening for the left carotid artery, and the next is the opening of the left subclavian artery, which supplies the left arm.

Let us assume that the oxygen molecule is pumped in the blood which passes up into the right carotid artery and then on into the skull to the point where the artery divides. It divides into three branches and for the sake of this account we will assume that the oxygen molecule then passes into the branch known as the middle cerebral (brain) artery. The oxygen molecule then passes down successively smaller branches until it reaches those with the smallest diameter, the capillaries, where it can finally transfer from the blood through the capillary wall into the liquid which surrounds brain cells. It finally passes through the wall of one of these cells to reach one of the hundreds of mitochondria it contains to oxidise a glucose molecule releasing energy for the nerve cell activity we need to think.

The route taken by an oxygen molecule from the lungs to the brain is, of course, exactly the same whether it is breathed in at sea level, in a hyperbaric chamber, or on the top of Mount Everest, where the air pressure is only a third of the barometric pressure at sea level. Everest, as the highest point on earth, is still a magnet for climbers and others who simply want to be able to say that they have been to the top of the world. It is a distressing place; there are more than 200 bodies frozen to the mountain at over 28,000 feet in what, not surprisingly, is known as the Death Zone. A group of doctors involved in intensive care are undertaking expeditions to the mountain to study the effects of lack of oxygen using the latest scientific techniques (see http://www.xtreme-everest.co.uk/). They were puzzled as to why some patients in their hospitals in London died, despite their blood oxygen values being higher than other patients who survived. However, the oxygen values in blood do not indicate the oxygen levels *in the tissues* of the body. The research objectives of the expedition were stated in a BBC *Horizon* television programme "Doctors in the Death Zone" in 2007 and in effect, by invoking genes, they imply that we should choose our parents wisely!

It might for the first time reveal how the body becomes more efficient when faced with a lack of oxygen allowing a treatment to be developed that can recreate this life saving effect in critically ill patients. In our wildest dreams what we would love to see is that some people have genes which allow them to use oxygen more efficiently than others and target treatment to poor oxygen users.

Unfortunately, being on Everest inevitably introduced many variables into the research that could not be controlled, not least the emotions generated by tending distressed and dying climbers. A gas-tight enclosure that could allow pressure to be reduced safely under controlled conditions, known as a *hypo*baric chamber, would have allowed their research to have been done in London under more scientific conditions but, of course, without the spectacular scenery. Ironically, a medical ethics committee would almost certainly not allow such extreme experiments to take place in a medical school because of health and safety legislation. The requirement for a minimal level of oxygen in the workplace would be flouted because low levels of oxygen may render an individual unconscious.

All mammalian brains share the same basic layout with symmetrical left and right hemispheres, and range in weight from less than 0.5 grams for a shrew to the massive 7,500 grams of a sperm whale. At about 1,350 grams, the human brain is actually considerably smaller than the brains of elephants, bottle-nosed dolphins, and whales. Although about 15% of the weight of the adult brain is contributed by blood, curiously no estimate has been made of the weight of the vast network of the blood vessels the brain contains. When the author was a medical student in the 1960s, blood vessels were viewed as simple tubes—they even look like soft plastic when they are opened. In fact, they are amazingly complicated, and their lining cells manufacture many important compounds, including a gas, nitric oxide (NO), involved in regulating their diameter.

The most complex blood vessels in the body are those that supply the brain, because they form a crucial barrier between blood and the delicate cells of the nervous system. Until recently, the blood-brain barrier has had little attention in neurology, although the first question asked in pharmaceutical companies about a new drug is whether it crosses the blood-brain barrier. We shall see later that understanding the blood-brain barrier is vital to finding effective treatment for several conditions that affect the nervous system and the barrier is, in fact, damaged in the commonest disease of the brain and spinal cord, multiple sclerosis.[4,5] When, after damage, the blood-brain barrier does not recover, the escape of toxic components from blood into sensitive nerve tissue may cause damage and, in patients with multiple sclerosis, the progression of disability.

The brain has a second circulation involving the colourless liquid known as cerebrospinal fluid. It is this fluid which is removed from the base of the spine in the procedure known as a lumbar puncture. The developing cells of the embryo in the womb form two humps which eventually bridge over to enclose a liquid-filled cavity. It is this cavity that is present in the centre of the developing spinal cord as the central canal and forms the ventricles present in the brainstem, mid-brain, and the two hemispheres of the forebrain. The cells of all tissues must be in a water-based environment known, logically, as extracellular fluid. In most tissues of the body, this liquid is produced by the minute leakage of water through the walls of capillaries and the small veins known as *venules*. The rate of leakage in the skin changes with temperature, which is one reason why swelling may accompany exposures to high ambient temperatures. This transport of water carries with it molecules that dissolve readily in water, like glucose.

In most tissues, extracellular fluid drains into the tiny tubes of the lymphatic system, but the nervous system does not have lymphatic vessels and, in fact, the blood vessels of the nervous system severely restrict such leakage. However, it has recently been reported that during sleep the space between the cells of the brain increases in volume. This facilitates the drainage of liquid and metabolites including ß amyloid, which is associated with Alzheimer's disease.[6,7] Figure 2.5 shows an artery in the brain of a mouse with the transport of fluid (green and yellow colouration)along the wall.

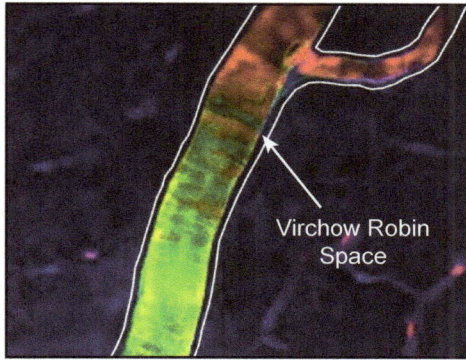

Figure 2.5:
An artery in the brain of a mouse:
The green and yellow represents the
flow of cerebro-spinal fluid along the
wall.
(Redrawn from J. Illif, University of
Rochester.)

Virchow Robin
Space

The lining cells of capillaries abut tightly together, and a cell called an *astrocyte* wraps around the capillary, inserting a process into the junction rather like the bung in a barrel. The blood vessels supplying the nervous system are said to have *tight junctions*, which allow very little leakage of water from blood. This means that an alternative supply of liquid is needed to bathe the cells of the nervous system. It is provided by the specialised tissue of the choroid plexus in the large ventricles of the two hemispheres and on the roof of the third ventricle in the mid-brain. This tissue provides a continuous flow of the necessary extracellular liquid inside and outside the nervous system and it drains away into small veins. If the drainage of cerebrospinal fluid is hampered, for example by brain inflammation, the pressure of the fluid rises. The condition that results is known as "hydrocephalus," which translates simply as "water on the brain." When, in the 1960s, tubes known as shunts were placed in children developing this problem, they limited the enlargement of the head but often did not prevent the ventricles from expanding. This was revealed when CT imaging became available and a series of children were followed in Sheffield by Professor John Lorber. His work featured in an article published in the journal *Science* in 1980 under the catching heading of "Is your Brain Really Necessary?" Lorber stated "There's a young student at this university, who has an I.Q. of 126, has gained a first class honours degree in mathematics, and is socially normal, and yet the boy has virtually no brain." There was, in fact, normal grey matter present but the bulky myelin sheaths of the white matter were absent.

The constituents of cerebrospinal fluid are very tightly controlled, ensuring a very constant chemical environment to allow the cells of the brain to function properly. The complexity of the blood-brain barrier defies belief and its relationship to disease has recently been reviewed. Take, for example, the simple molecule glucose. Glucose is the key fuel for the activity of the brain—if a diabetic patient injects too much insulin and causes the level of glucose in the blood to fall, he will rapidly lose consciousness and may even convulse. Glucose readily dissolves in water, and so is known as a water soluble molecule. Such molecules do not cross the blood-brain barrier and, in fact, glucose is *actively* transported by five proteins, dubbed the GLUT proteins.[8] This transport system itself uses energy. In contrast, fat soluble molecules such as ethanol, the alcohol present in our drinks, readily diffuse into the brain across the barrier—sometimes with unfortunate effects!

The development of the early neural cleft in the embryo, which forms the neural tube, defines the left and right sides of the developing nervous system. The lobes which develop at the front of the tube become the cerebral hemispheres, with the spinal cord forming at the rear. Viewed from above, an adult's hemispheres appear like a large, wrinkled walnut. The wrinkles, known as convolutions, are needed to allow the brain to be compressed into the limited space in the bony skull; otherwise, the head would be impossibly large. The rim of the outer part of the hemispheres, known as the cortex, can be up to six layers of the nerve cells known as neurons, which make up the grey matter. Underlying the grey matter is the white matter, which appears white because of the presence of the myelin forming sheaths around the nerve fibres that emanate from nerve cells. The myelin sheaths are formed by a parent cell called an *oligodendrocyte*, and one cell may be responsible for up to 30 sections of myelin sheath. Each sheath projecting from the parent cell is rather like the tentacle of an octopus and may wrap around a nerve fibre as many as 30 times. The impression is often given that the fibres of the nerve cells in the grey matter of the brain's cortex do not have myelin sheaths, but this is not true—there is just much less myelin present than in the white matter. Myelin sheaths are often said to insulate nerve fibres, but this is also not true—they actually increase the speed at which impulses are conducted, which is up to several hundred times greater than fibres that possess only thin sheaths. However, the trillions of fibres that are associated with the nerve cells occupying the tiny space available in the skull *must* be insulated in some way, otherwise interference from cross talk would render clear thought impossible! The most likely explanation is that the insulation is provided by the presence of double-charged insulating molecules called surfactants in the cerebrospinal fluid which bathes all the cells and fibres. An indication that mammalian brains possess large quantities of surfactant is that the surfactants used for laboratory experiments are usually extracts of bovine brain. Their general importance in the body[9] will be discussed later.

The two cerebral hemispheres are connected by a bridge of fibres known as the *corpus callosum*. If this communicating pathway is cut, as it is sometimes surgically in an attempt to control severe epilepsy, then the patient finds that their hands may obey independent instructions, even though they are only conscious of the action taken by their dominant hemisphere. Below the hemispheres are the mid-brain regions containing clusters of neurons called the *basal ganglia*. It is fortunate that we have two of many of the important structures in the brain as much, but not all, function can be preserved if one side is damaged. Passing through these areas are the large groups of nerve fibres known as tracts, which pass down to the brain stem and to the cerebellum, which lies under the rear of the two hemispheres. The cerebellum is connected by large tracts of nerve fibres that wrap around the brainstem, giving the appearance of a bridge and so is known as the *pons*. These structures and the spinal cord also have subdivided left and right pathways without the clear distinction obvious by the large cleft seen between the cerebral hemispheres.

The brain requires approximately 20% of the total blood flow from the heart, and needs a truly colossal network of arteries, capillaries, and veins. The complexity of the genetic programme controlling the growth of this immense pipe work beggars belief. As the embryo grows and organs develop, the growth of cells must be matched by the growth of blood vessels. The arteries penetrate from the outside of the brain and pass down through the complex folds and lobes into the depths of the cortex to supply a dense matrix of capillaries. A cubic millimetre of the grey matter of the brain cortex contains hundreds of capillaries. The illustration below of the blood vessels of the grey matter of the cortex of a mouse brain shows their extraordinary density. A blockage of just the one small penetrating artery may cause a stroke.[10]

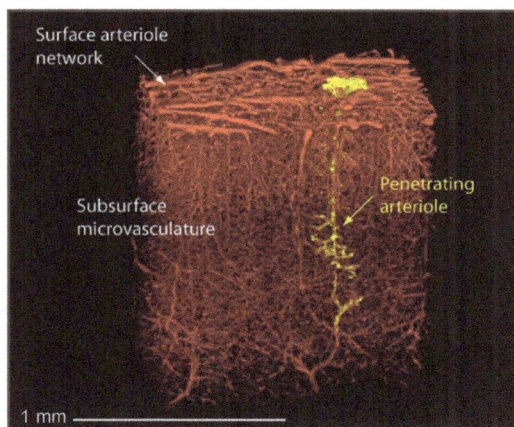

Figure 2.6:
Blood vessels of the cortex of a mouse brain.
(Courtesy Drs. Tsai and Blinder.)

The average distance of any cell in the cortex to a nearby capillary is 13 micrometres. In order to oxygenate nerve cells and fibres, they need to be within 80 micrometres of a capillary which indicates that individual capillaries can be blocked without a significant fall in the oxygen level risking damage. The significance of this safety factor will become clear later. Like the astronomical numbers of nerve cells and nerve fibre connections, the density of capillaries in the brain is difficult to comprehend. It is estimated that the total length of all the capillaries in just a *cubic millimetre* of the grey matter of the human brain may be an astonishing 50 centimetres—almost 20 inches.[10]

Inevitably, given the complexity of the architecture of the nervous system there are some compromises in the layout of blood vessels and their far-reaching consequences are not widely appreciated. The front and middle areas of the brain's two hemispheres are supplied from continuations of the left and right carotid arteries in the neck after they pass through their respective holes in the base of the skull. Each carotid artery divides to form the two arteries that supply the corresponding hemispheres and are known as the left and right anterior (front) and middle cerebral arteries; the word cerebral simply refers to the brain.

The supply to the rear of the hemispheres is by the posterior (rear) cerebral arteries, which are derived from a single vessel, the basilar artery. The basilar artery is derived from the union of two arteries, the vertebral arteries which pass up through holes in the vertebra in the upper neck and join together to form the basilar artery before passing into the cranium through the large hole in the base of the skull, the foramen magnum. The anastomoses ensure that if blood flow in one artery is crimped by neck movement, the reduction of flow can be compensated for by an increase in flow in the other artery. Even in situations where one of the vertebral arteries does not develop properly, the blood flow up to the basilar artery might remain constant but a serious reduction in blood flow to the vital centres in the brain stem can be fatal. The same principle is used in the electrical supply of our houses, where the power points derive from a ring circuit to maintain the voltage.

At the base of the brain, branches of the two internal carotid arteries connect to each other and also to branches from the basilar artery. The connections are known as anastomoses. This well-known arterial loop was first described by the anatomist Thomas Willis (1621–1673), and so is known as the Circle of Willis; however, the stylised textbook illustration of the anatomy is only found in about a third of brains examined at autopsy. Anastomoses are a feature of many sites in the body, occurring, for example, in the palms of the hands, soles of the feet, ends of fingers and toes, and in the tip of the nose. Not surprisingly, in view of the disaster that may follow blockage of an artery in the brain, it has many such connections.[11] Figure 2.7 shows the connections of most of the larger arteries in the brain.

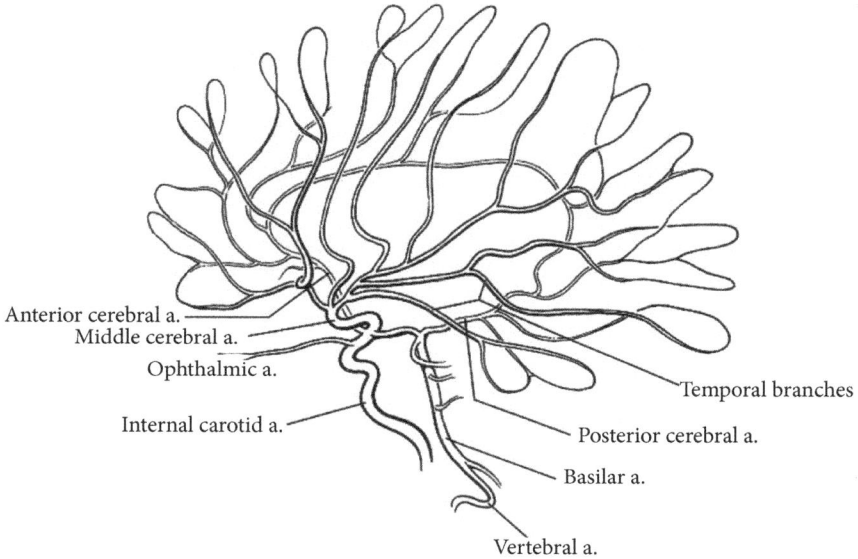

Figure 2.7:
The anastomoses of the arteries of the brain.
(From *Cerebrovascular Disease*, courtesy of Dr. James Toole.)

In fact, there is considerable variation in the arrangement of blood vessels in the body—just look at the differences in the pattern of the veins on the back of one person's hands. Arterial patterns vary less than veins, and the anatomical layout of arteries in the human arm and hand reproduced in textbooks are, like the Circle of Willis, only found in about a third of the population. Although most arteries in the brain connect to other arteries, it is little known that there are notable and rather unfortunate exceptions both in the brain and in the spinal cord. The *lenticulostriatal arteries* supply critical areas in each of the areas in the middle of the brain's hemispheres. They are branches of the middle cerebral arteries, and are "end" arteries because they do not connect to other arteries, as shown in Figure 2.8.

The lack of artery-to-artery connections for the lenticulostriatal arteries is central to explaining the vulnerability of these areas, which can be fairly termed the Achilles heels of the brain. The direction of flow is also important in the blood supply to tissues. Again, because of the complexity of the convolutions and lobes of the brain, sometimes a zone can have flow entering from opposing directions. This creates what have been termed "watershed territo-

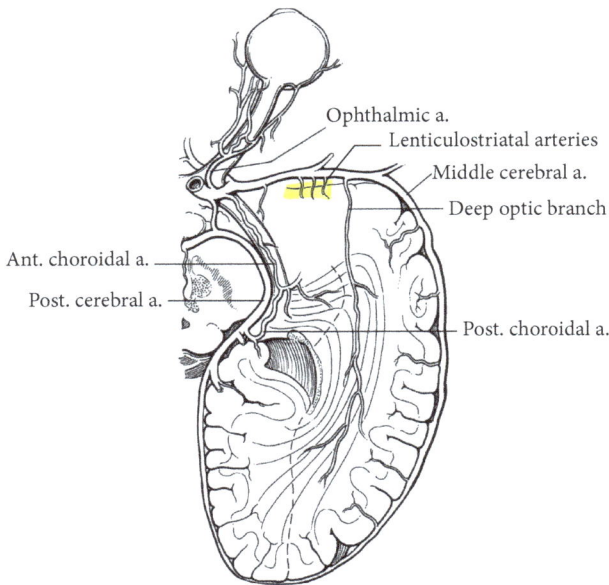

Figure 2.8:
The lenticulostriatal arteries (highlighted) of one hemisphere.
(From *Cerebrovascular Disease*, courtesy of Dr. James Toole.)

ries"[12] and in the spinal cord they may be associated with dire consequences. The region just above D8 in Figure 2.9 in a vertical section of human lower spinal cord[13] can truly be termed the Achilles heel of the nervous system—blockage of one small blood artery can cause paraplegia. A similar area is arrowed at D6. The diameter at this point is about the same as a little finger and D6 and D8 refer to the dorsal or *thoracic* segments and so today they would be labeled T6 and T8.

The arrows show where blood flows in opposing directions up and down the spinal cord and some of the watershed territories, where tissues are in

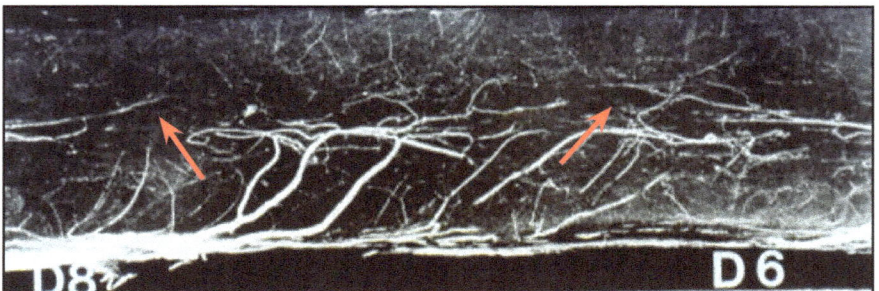

Figure 2.9:
Arteriogram of lower spinal cord. (Courtesy of Dr. O. Hassler.)

between the areas supplied by two arteries. The watershed territories of the brain are frequently involved in brain injuries such as the birth injury known as cerebral palsy, in patients with multiple sclerosis, and in the strokes that usually affect older people. These and other conditions will be discussed in later chapters.

Arteries form branches and their diameters reduce successively until, by the time they are about half a millimetre in diameter, they are renamed *arterioles*. Arterioles are the site of blood flow control; the muscle in their walls is able to contract, reducing their diameter. Blood flows from them into the multiple branches of the smaller vessels known as capillaries. Most of the exchange between tissues and blood takes place across the thin walls of capillaries and this, of course, includes the transport of oxygen. However, some exchange of nutrients takes place across the walls of veins. A paper by the German anatomist Pfeifer published in 1929[14] shows that the areas surrounding the small veins which pass through the white matter deep in the brain are actually devoid of capillaries. The tissue immediately surrounding these veins therefore depends on the blood flowing through them for oxygen and nutrients, and it will be seen that it is a critical factor in many diseases and injuries of the brain.

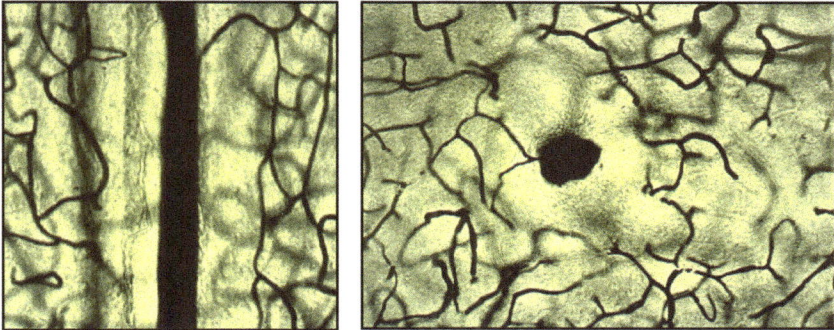

Figure 2.10:
Capillary-free zones around the veins in the deep white matter of human brain.
(From: Pfeifer RA. *Grundlegende Untersuchungen für die Angio-Architektonik des menschlichen Gehirns.* Springer: Berlin, 1930.)

Curiously, despite most of the tissues of the brain and spinal cord requiring a high level of blood flow, they actually need to be protected from blood itself. This raises the obvious question: Protection from what in blood? The answer may come as a surprise: It is from large molecules such as proteins, and especially from red blood cells. They are dangerous because if they are allowed to enter tissues and their capsule ruptures, iron is released from the breakdown of the haemoglobin molecules they contain. Haem, of course, stands for iron (haematite mines extract iron ore); and globin means a protein. Haemoglobin is an example of a group of compounds widely distributed in living organisms called *metalloproteins*. The chemists Max Perutz (1914–2002) and John Kendrew (1917–1997) were jointly awarded the Nobel Prize in 1959 for determining the structure of haemoglobin by crystallography. Iron is dangerous because when released it is involved in the formation of highly-toxic free radicals, and even a small amount of bleeding into the brain is often fatal.

The oxygen present in blood must finally be transported across the walls of blood vessels in order to reach cells and their mitochondria, but the wall of capillaries and the liquid that bathes our cells form resistances to this transfer. The current clinical fixation on measuring the "saturation" of haemoglobin with oxygen neglects the importance of the dissolved oxygen pressure to this critical process. When the walls of capillaries become thickened as they do, for example, in diabetic patients, less oxygen is transported. Less oxygen is also transported when the water content of the extracellular fluid surrounding cells increases, which happens in many injuries and diseases—the cells are effectively drowning. As already discussed, when less oxygen is transported, the fall in the concentration of oxygen leads to an increase in the level of hypoxia-inducible factor 1α and the associated genes are upregulated. This means that when we suffer a cut in the skin, new capillaries can be grown to allow repair to take place.

It is important here to again highlight an obvious and important principle that has yet to be properly recognised; simply, when tissues are injured, not only are the cells of the tissue damaged, the capillaries *within the tissue* are also damaged. This may reduce blood flow and, as a consequence, oxygen delivery to critical levels, thus slowing, or in some cases even preventing, recovery. The word *may* is needed here because, in lesser injuries, blood flow sometimes increases. Hence, the changes in blood flow and oxygen delivery that result from injury depend on its severity. In very severe injuries, of course, large arteries may be torn and surgery may be needed to repair them to re-establish blood flow. Generally in severe trauma, just when more oxygen and nutrients are needed to begin a repair, their supply is often seriously reduced. This introduces the concept of an *oxygen threshold* that needs to be overcome to initiate recovery.

Nowhere does this need to be emphasised more than in the treatment of the brain because, without sufficient oxygen, its cells cannot function and may die. Nevertheless, brain cells may survive for years in a state best described as "not dead, but sleeping." In other words, they have enough oxygen to continue to exist, but not enough to allow them to function. The term that has been adopted to describe this state is the "idling neuron." The record for the duration of a coma after head injury with the return of consciousness appears to be 19 years.[15] Such patients show that the potential for recovery after brain injury is much greater than is often thought possible, and oxygen is the key to the door. But without sufficient oxygen, many patients who may be capable of regaining consciousness will remain in a coma. This does not, however, mean that all coma patients can be saved, because in many cases the damage to the brain will have been too severe.

The neurological concept of idling brain cells has been confirmed by rather macabre research in the University of Amsterdam, which was reported in a letter published by the *Lancet* more than a decade ago.[16] Tissue from human brains was removed eight hours after death at a normal post-mortem examination. Slices of the brain tissue were incubated with oxygen and glucose, and, astonishingly, it was found that nerve cells were still functioning—in some cases, they were kept alive for many hours. This does not mean that resuscitation is possible over such an extended time, although it obviously raises critical issues that need to be discussed. The author wrote to the *Lancet* about the report, but publication of the carefully constructed and detailed letter was declined. Intrigued, the author made contact with a deputy editor at the journal who revealed that they had received no other correspondence about these astonishing observations. This research forms one piece of an astounding jigsaw that defines the importance of using oxygen at high concentrations—not only in the treatment of injuries and diseases of the brain, but in a wide range of other conditions where tissues fail to recover because of lack of oxygen. So, when was the importance of pressure and oxygen to brain function first recognised? The answer will undoubtedly come as a surprise: It was discovered by balloonists in the middle of the nineteenth century!

CHAPTER 3
The Importance of Pressure and Oxygen

We live submerged at the bottom of an ocean of elementary air, which is known by incontestable experiments to have weight.

Evangelista Torricelli, 1608–1647

It may come as a surprise to many that the importance of pressure and oxygen to the brain was actually discovered by balloonists in the nineteenth century. The Montgolfier brothers, Joseph and Étienne, had proved that balloon flight was possible in 1783 by using the lift provided by the hot air from a brazier. Their first unmanned balloon, made out of sackcloth and paper and held together with 1,800 buttons, managed to reach the impressive altitude of 6,000 feet before landing several miles away in a field. It was summarily destroyed by local villagers, who viewed it as an instrument of the devil. Human flight became a reality when the brothers persuaded a surgeon, Jean-François Pilâtre de Rozier, and an army officer, François Laurent, the Marquis d'Arlandes, to ascend in a much larger balloon. It measured 2,200 cubic metres, and was propelled by the hot air generated by a large iron furnace. The flight, from the outskirts of Paris on November 21, 1783, lasted just 25 minutes, reached a height of nearly 3,000 feet, and traveled over six miles. Just 10 days later, Alexander Charles and his assistant Monsieur Robert made the first ascent in a hydrogen balloon. They took off from the Jardin des Tuileries in the centre of Paris as a crowd of 400,000 people looked on. Hydrogen balloons proved capable of much higher altitudes than the early hot air balloons which were prone to catch fire, usually with tragic consequences.

In 1862, James Glaisher, a Fellow of the Royal Society and Superintendent of the Greenwich Observatory, and Henry Coxwell, a dentist and amateur balloon engineer, undertook a series of balloon ascents carrying scientific instruments. Their third and most sensational ascent was to just over 29,000 feet, which is about the height of Everest. It took place from Wolverhampton on September 5, 1862, and the pair left the ground from the gas works of the city at 1:03 p.m. The site is now used for gas pipe storage by British Gas PLC, and the arches carrying one of the main West Coast railway lines to Scotland can be seen in the background of Figure 3.1.

By 1:34 p.m. the pair had reached an altitude of about 17,900 feet, where the pressure was recorded at about half normal barometric pressure at sea

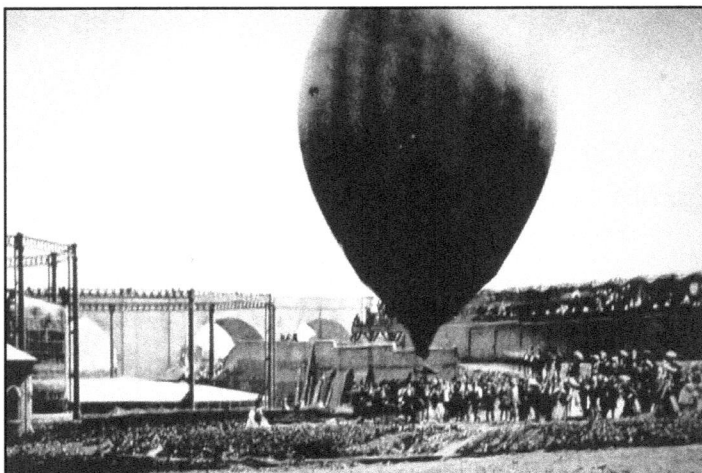

Figure 3.1:
The balloon *Mammoth* at Wolverhampton
gas works prior to the ascent.

level. They had become aware of the first physiological changes: Glaisher noticed that Coxwell, who was working hard managing the balloon, was "out of breath," although he was not panting. Glaisher did not actually record the breathing rate; he chose to log their pulse rates, which had risen from about 70 on the ground to over 100 beats per minute. Clearly, the decision to record the pulse rather than the breathing rate had been influenced by their experience of earlier ascents. They had noticed that, although they felt breathless at altitude, it was not accompanied by an increase in their rate of breathing.

At 1:39 p.m., they had reached a height of 21,000 feet and, having thrown out some of their sand bags, they continued their ascent. Up to this time, Glaisher records that he had taken his observations "without any difficulty," although he noted that Coxwell "seemed weary." Then, suddenly, Glaisher found he could not see the column of mercury in the wet bulb thermometer, or the hands of his watch, or the fixed divisions of any of the instruments. He calmly asked Coxwell to help him get the figures, but Coxwell was otherwise engaged—the balloon had rotated during the ascent, and the cord of the hydrogen valve had become entangled. He had left the safety of the basket to climb up onto the ring of the balloon to untangle it. Glaisher managed to see that the barometer registered 10 inches of mercury, and "was falling rapidly." The final pressure reached was about 9 and 3/4 inches of mercury (247.65 mm Hg), indicating that their height was over 29,000 feet.

Curiously, and perhaps appropriately, their paper was published in a med-

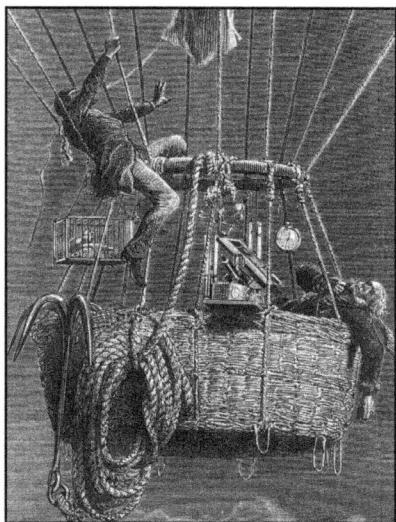

Figure 3.2:
A lithograph showing Coxwell releasing the hydrogen from the balloon.

ical journal—the *Lancet*[1] the following year. Glaisher graphically described for the first time the profound effects of lack of oxygen on the functioning of the brain.

> *Shortly afterwards I laid my arm, possessed of its full vigour, upon the table, and, on being desirous to use it, I found it powerless; it must have lost its power almost momentarily. I tried to move my other arm, and found it powerless also. I then tried to shake myself, and did shake my body but I did not seem to be aware of having any legs; I could only shake my body. I then looked at the barometer, and whilst doing so my head fell on my left shoulder. I struggled and shook my body again, but could not move my arms. I got my head upright, but for an instant only, when it fell on my right shoulder; and then I fell backwards, my back resting against the side of the car, and my head on its edge; in this position my eyes were directed towards Mr. Coxwell in the ring. When I shook my body I seemed to have full power over the muscles of the back, and considerable power over those of the neck, but none over either my arms or my legs; in fact, I seemed to have no limbs. As in the case of the arms, all muscular power was lost in an instant from my back and neck.*

Glaisher then records even more dramatic effects on his nervous system, and feared he was about to die as the balloon continued its perilous ascent:

> *I saw Mr. Coxwell in the ring, and endeavoured to speak, but could not; and then, in a moment, intense black darkness came: The optic nerve lost power suddenly. I was still conscious, with as active a brain as at the present*

moment whilst writing this. I thought I had been seized with asphyxia, and that I should experience no more, as death would come, unless we speedily descended. Other thoughts were actively entering my mind, when, like every other symptom, I suddenly became unconscious, as if going to sleep. I cannot tell anything about the sense of hearing; the perfect silence of the regions six miles from the earth (and at this time we were between six and seven miles high) is such that no sound (from the earth) reaches the ear.

Glaisher had heard the words "temperature" and "observation," and realised that Coxwell was trying to speak to him, but he could not actually see him. When Coxwell tried to descend from the ring, he found he could no longer use his hands—he was forced to let himself slide on his elbows to get back into the basket, where Glaisher was stretched out unconscious. This is the sequence in which the loss of function occurs with a reduction in the level of oxygen breathed and the same sequence occurs with the administration of a general anaesthetic. Surprisingly the mode of action of anaesthetics is still "controversial" and it is possible that the shared feature is that they may reduce oxygen transport by changing the characteristics of the lipid membranes of neurons.[2] The effects of alcohol, which is, of course, lipid soluble, are reduced by increasing the level of oxygen breathed.[3] In the same experiments it was found that breathing 100% oxygen reduces the effects of a hangover and this was widely used by Allied aircrew in WW2. Regardless, the balloon ascent over Wolverhampton had demonstrated the extreme sensitivity of the brain to lack of oxygen. The lack of oxygen resulted from the fall in pressure that occurs on an ascent to altitude. Exactly the same sequence follows a reduction of the oxygen available to the brain, regardless of the cause, as in the effects of black damp in coal miners. Glaisher's account of the events continued:

Mr. Coxwell told me that on coming from the ring, he for the moment thought I had laid back to rest myself; that he spoke to me without eliciting a reply; that he then noticed that my legs projected, and my arms hung down by my side; that my countenance was serene and placid, without the earnestness and anxiety he had noticed before going into the ring and then it struck him I was insensible. He wished then to approach me, but could not; as he felt insensibility coming over him; that he became anxious to open the valve, but was unable, in consequence of having lost the use of his hands; ultimately, however, he effected his object by seizing the cord between his teeth, and dipping his head two or three times.

Fortunately, Coxwell was able to bleed off the hydrogen by pulling on the release cord with his teeth, because he too had lost the use of his arms.

Coxwell recovered his strength quickly as the balloon descended, and Glaisher recovered consciousness. Coxwell told him that he had been seized by the extreme cold, and said later that "icicles hung around the orifice of the balloon, like a terrible candelabrum, worthy of the polar seas." They were not harmed by their close encounter with death and, landing some eight miles from Wolverhampton, they had to walk back to the gas works.

Climbers on Everest, of course, ascend to this altitude very slowly after weeks of acclimatisation although, despite this, many still become ill and some die. The onset of the effects of the lack of oxygen in Glaisher and Coxwell was very rapid, and their treatment and recovery from an *abrupt* increase in pressure and the level of oxygen they were breathing on their rapid descent was certainly dramatic. It has been found that a very modest increase in pressure can be equally effective in seriously ill climbers: A 37-year-old climber, who had reached the North Col of Mount Everest at an altitude of 22,945 feet, developed severe mountain sickness.[4] He was treated in a portable pressure chamber, known after its inventor, Professor Igor Gamow, as the Gamow bag. As in the case of Glaisher and Coxwell's rapid descent, it was successful simply because it was able to increase the air pressure; no supplementary oxygen was available. The casualty was placed inside the bag and a foot pump used to increase the pressure for just two hours. The increase in pressure was just 103 mm Hg, (130 millibars or two pounds per square inch), which is equivalent to a descent down the mountain from 19,662 feet to 14,300 feet. The treatment was dramatically effective; the mountain sickness associated with the fluid build-up in his lungs known as *pulmonary oedema* disappeared. He was then taken further down the mountain to 6,500 feet, by which time he had fully recovered. Not surprisingly, the authors recommend the use of the Gamow bag for the treatment of acute mountain sickness in their paper. The Gamow hyperbaric bag was not a new idea; the US Air Force had developed the same equipment during WW2 for a different problem, as will be seen in Chapter 6.[5]

In 2000, a group of medical students from the University of Edinburgh on an expedition to Mount Chacaltaya in Bolivia were featured in the "Mountain Madness" episode of the BBC TV programme, *Tomorrow's World*, aired on May 30, 2001. There is a laboratory at 17,900 feet (0.5 ATA) used for conducting altitude experiments. The BBC producer, a young lady who had stayed in La Paz, which is the highest city in the world, decided to visit the laboratory to see the students at their work. Shortly after reaching the high altitude she developed acute mountain sickness with nausea and a severe headache. She was eventually forced to descend and was driven at night down a precipitous mountain road lying prostrate in the back of a 4x4 vehicle. The vehicle had only descended a few thousand feet when she suddenly sat bolt upright and said she "felt fine." The lights of La Paz were still far below. The increase in pressure on the descent was about 100 millibars, and the increase in the oxygen pressure was, therefore, equivalent to an increase of about 2% at sea level. This was even less than the pressure found effective using the Gamow bag on the North Col of Everest in the case reported above. The relief of the serious symptoms of lung oedema and brain swelling from very modest descents from high altitude is now well known in mountaineering circles.

In another account of the epic ascent over Wolverhampton, Glaisher recalled making his last scientific measurement at about 29,000 feet and wrote:

> *That is within two metres of the height of the highest peak on the surface of the earth, the Gaourichnaka of Nepal, (now renamed Mt. Everest), at the foot of which the Brahmin pilgrims who are seeking Nirvana come to die; one may say that no human being ever could drag himself to this height following uneven terrestrial surface.*

Despite having been close to death, Glaisher had faithfully recorded the steady reduction of air pressure associated with an ascent to high altitude. He also noted that the effect on the body was not, as might be expected, an increase in the rate of breathing, but of the *pulse rate*. We now know that a reduction of air pressure exerts this effect because it inevitably reduces the concentration of oxygen in the air being breathed. The pulse rate as well as the output of the heart are controlled by the dissolved concentration of oxygen in the blood and, surprisingly, exactly how this occurs remains to be discovered. It should be noted that the percentage of oxygen in the air does not change at these altitudes; it remains at about 21%. It is the part of the air pressure due to oxygen that is important, that is, the *partial pressure*.

Ten years after the expedition by Glaisher and Coxwell, the renowned French physiologist Paul Bert discovered that breathing pure oxygen could prevent the effects on the brain of an ascent to high altitude, and had recommended that balloonists use oxygen equipment. In his book *La Pression Barométrique* (translated simply as barometric pressure), Bert[6] gives details of the first expedition in 1875 using a balloon equipped with "oxygen breathing apparatus." The gas contained in the reservoir bags of the equipment would have actually been a mixture of oxygen with air rather than pure oxygen. Two of the three balloonists, Sivel and Croce-Spinelli, died because as the balloon ascended they did not have the strength to reach for their oxygen apparatus. They lost consciousness and stopped breathing, having waited too long to conserve the precious oxygen. The third balloonist, Gaston Tissandier, managed to reach his apparatus and he survived. Paul Bert had an astonishing grasp of the physics and biology of oxygen and pressure. He anticipated the discovery of oxygen in gene regulation by hypoxia-inducible factor proteins, and the reduction of the oxygen content of the atmosphere that probably signaled the end of the dinosaurs.

> *The barometric pressure and the percentage of oxygen have not always been the same on our globe. The tension of this gas has probably been diminishing and no doubt will continue to diminish. This is a factor which has not been taken into account in biogenic speculation.*

Gases and liquids are known as *fluids*, and it is easy to forget that air has density, although a strong wind soon reminds us of it. There has to be a standard for atmospheric pressure at sea level and it has been equated to a 760 mm high column of mercury, which exerts a force of 14.7 pounds for every square inch of our body surface—1 kilogram per square centimetre. The average body surface area of an adult is about 18 square feet (1.73 square metres), and so our bodies are subject to a total force of about 17 Imperial tons (15.4 metric tonnes).

Getting to grips with units of pressure is a somewhat painful experience, as physicists have changed the units many times. Nevertheless, all are expressions of force per unit *area*—easily remembered when holding a door that is caught by the wind. The unit millimetres of mercury has already been introduced in this text, but the old Imperial units of pounds per square inch are the norm in the US, and often used in the UK. The metric equivalent is kilograms per square centimetre, although the more recently adopted *Systeme International* names units after the scientists who first described them which, in the case of pressure, is the Pascal, after the Frenchman, Blaise Pascal, and millibars equate to hectoPascals. Despite this, most weather charts on television still show the barometric pressure in millibars, one bar being normal atmospheric pressure at sea level also known as one atmosphere absolute or 1 ATA. A standard atmosphere is defined as the pressure which supports a column of mercury 760 mm (29.5 inches) high. The mercury barometer was invented by the Italian scientist Evangelista Torricelli, who was the first to measure barometric pressure and to demonstrate that it falls as altitude increases. In his honour, millimetres of mercury (mm Hg) are now known as Torr. However, to make life easier, it is customary to use the term atmospheres absolute (ATA) and the unit 1 ATA to represent normal sea level pressure in hyperbaric medicine. In this text, millibars are used for height and altitude measurements because they are still the units most commonly employed around the world.

Atmospheric pressure falls with increasing altitude, actually by one millibar for every 33 feet or 10 metres of an ascent. Equally, descending 33 feet down a mine, the air pressure increases by one millibar. As Torricelli pointed out in his famous quotation "air has weight," in fact, a cubic metre of air weighs 1.2 kilograms at normal barometric pressure; almost as much as the brain. Air is made up of about 21% oxygen, 78% nitrogen, and almost 1% of argon, with the rest being small amounts of carbon dioxide, water vapour, and other noble gases such as neon, krypton, and helium. The partial pressure exerted by oxygen is 0.21 bar or 210 millibars at normal sea level pressure. If we breathe 100% oxygen at sea level, then 100% of 1 is, of course, 1, and so the oxygen pressure is 1 ATA or 1,000 millibars. The fixed relationship between gas pressure and volume first described by Robert Boyle (1627–1691) means that, at constant temperature, the volume of a gas varies inversely with the absolute pressure. Doubling the pressure of a quantity of gas will, therefore, halve its volume.

The lungs and chest wall form a "breathing machine," and Robert Boyle would have understood the pressure changes involved in breathing, as he invented the vacuum pump. Breathing relies on atmospheric pressure; when we breathe in, we lower the pressure in the chest *below* that of the air that surrounds us, and so it is atmospheric pressure that moves air into the lungs. To breathe out, the pressure in the chest must go *above* atmospheric pressure to move gas out, and this is produced by elastic recoil and muscle action. Doctors ventilate patients with a machine that increases pressure to force gas into the chest and, logically, this is known as *positive-pressure* ventilation. The changes in atmospheric pressure that are responsible for the weather are due to the sun heating the air, which becomes less dense, reducing its pressure. Hot air, of course, rises and creates thermal winds. Water vapour due to evaporation from oceans and lakes is also a major factor in the weather. Unfortunately, such is the lack of awareness of atmospheric pressure that many people, including some doctors, talk about patients "going under pressure" in a hyperbaric, or pressure chamber, as if we actually live in a vacuum. Some even think that when patients are pressurised in a chamber, blood is squeezed from the surface of the body to the inside; a theory popular over a hundred years ago! Fortunately, the liquids of the body are incompressible and the body is not squashed like a prune. In Figure 3.3, the diver Theo Mavrostomos holds a board indicating he has reached a pressure of 71.1 ATA, 71.1 times

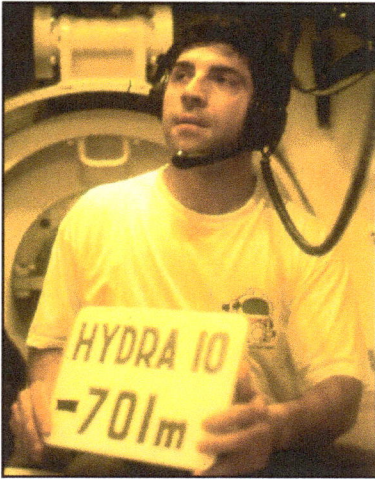

Figure 3.3:
Theo Mavrostomos at a pressure 71 times
normal atmospheric pressure.
(Courtesy of Comex SA Marseille.)

sea level atmospheric pressure, which is equivalent to the pressure at a sea water depth of about 2,300 feet (701 metres) He is the only man in the world to achieve this feat, and he sometimes features in watch advertisements in *National Geographic* magazine.

The pressure acting on his body exerted a force of over 1,208 Imperial tons (1,227 metric tonnes), yet he looks quite normal. It is just as well that liquids are incompressible! He was breathing a gas containing just 0.9% oxygen mixed with 50% hydrogen, the balance being helium. The hydrogen was added to make the gas thin enough to breathe, as a mixture of just helium and oxygen at this enormous pressure would be so dense that a diver would not have the strength to breathe it. Figure 3.4 shows part of the hyperbaric chamber complex used for the world record in the Comex SA facility in Marseille.

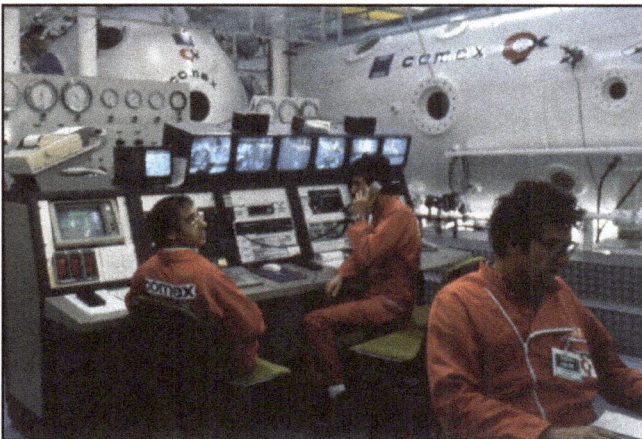

Figure 3.4:
The Comex
SA Hyperbaric
Research Facility
in Marseille.

Chapter 3: The Importance of Pressure and Oxygen ~ 49

The density of air as a gas is important in many ways and the resistance it creates can be easily felt at sea level by moving a hand quickly backwards and forwards. Repeat the movement in the cabin of a jet airliner at cruising altitude, and there is virtually no resistance because air becomes thinner the higher we go. The maximum altitude allowed for the operation of *non-pressurised* commercial aircraft is just 10,000 feet, whereas the cabins of *pressurised* aircraft are allowed to use an equivalent of 8,000 feet.

The problems created by the lack of training in our medical schools about barometric pressure were graphically illustrated on the BBC Radio 5 live programme "Up All Night" on May 16, 2013; a listener to the radio show, asked guest guru, Dr. Carl why his feet swell on long-haul flights. After discussing the role of immobility, Dr. Carl said that the second reason was actually the reduced pressure in the plane:

> *So normally the pressure (the air pressure acting on the body) is 10 tonnes per sq metre and you have 2 sq metres of surface area if you are a big person, so the air is pushing on you with 20 tonnes per square metre and the inside of your body is pushing out with 20 tonnes per square metre. Go into an aeroplane, suddenly the outside pressure is 8 tonnes per square metre, so your whole body is pushing outwards with a force of 4 tonnes per square metre; so you just swell slightly in all directions and I think that is the other reason. The pressure does equalise, so it is not a full 4 tonnes of course, nowhere near it, otherwise things would break, but you do swell slightly.*

The standard of an 8,000 feet equivalent cabin "altitude" introduced in the 1950s by civil aviation authorities is for the well-being of passengers; principally to ensure that they have sufficient oxygen. However, because today aircraft are now able to fly for much longer than the early jets, higher cabin pressures are being introduced as passengers would risk becoming ill flying as long as 16 hours with the reduced level of oxygen at a pressure equivalent to 8,000 feet. The new Boeing 787 Dreamliner uses a cabin pressure equivalent to an altitude of only 5,500 feet for this reason. The technology developed for use in the latest combat jet aircraft, which can exceed 60,000 feet, allows aircrew to be exposed to cockpit "altitudes" as high as 24,000 feet. Although the cockpit is pressurised it is not to the level used in commercial jets and the crew must wear pressure suits and breathe 100% oxygen. The oxygen is also supplied at a slightly increased ambient pressure to assist breathing, especially as the latest combat aircraft can reach 9-G in turns, risking a "blackout."

A tragedy, which unfolded over the Mediterranean in 2005, graphically illustrates the importance of maintaining air pressure and a safe oxygen level in an aircraft cabin; an aircraft on a flight from Cyprus to Greece actually failed to pressurise after taking off. Late on the morning of Sunday August 14, 2005, the author saw a moving ribbon on an Internet website page which spelled out "Oxygen and Pressure Believed to be Involved in Aircraft Crash." A Boeing 737 operated by the Cypriot airline, Helios, had crashed at Grammaticos, near Athens. The aircraft was not faulty and, as investigations have proceeded, it appears that it simply failed to maintain pressure as it climbed to its cruising altitude. It has been suggested that the pressurisation control in the cockpit was in the manual position, not the automatic. When an aircraft is on the ground and the doors are open, the air in the cabin is obviously at the same pressure as the surrounding air at the airport, and the air pressure is obviously retained when the doors are closed.

The Helios jet took off from Larnaca, which is close to sea level, and so the pressure in the cabin on the ground would have been about 1 ATA, that is, 1,013 millibars. However, this pressure cannot be maintained when an aircraft ascends to its cruising altitude; a fuselage constructed to be strong enough to sustain sea level pressure at altitude would be too heavy to fly. As aircrafts climb, some of the air in the cabin is allowed to vent from a "waste gate" in the tail, and the air pressure is allowed to fall by about a quarter of an atmosphere to about 750 millibars. This pressure is equivalent to being on a mountain at an altitude of about 8,000 feet. Although this ensures that the oxygen pressure is maintained at a safe level for normal healthy people, passengers with diseases of the heart or lungs may need supplemental oxygen, or they may become ill. As the aircraft flies, air from the engine compressors is used to refresh the cabin atmosphere and maintain the pressure at a safe level. At cruising altitude, the pressure inside a commercial jet aircraft is, therefore, considerably higher than the outside air pressure and so aircraft are, by definition, hyperbaric chambers. Being regularly pressurised and decompressed, in addition to being subjected to regular impacts with the ground on landing, aircraft become liable to metal fatigue and rigorous inspections must be made of vulnerable areas. They are also regularly pressure-tested for leaks, which are usually related to the door seals. Apparently, the Helios jet had needed servicing in Larnaca because of a problem with a door seal.

The jet took off just after 9:00 a.m., with the pilots handing over control to the aircraft's autopilot as it continued to ascend to 34,000 feet. Because the pressurisation control was in the manual position, the cabin air continued to vent from the aircraft and so the cabin pressure simply followed the air pressure outside. As an altitude of 12,000 feet was passed, the oxygen masks for the passengers automatically dropped from the cabin ceiling. Unfortunately, the masks for the pilots are not deployed automatically. They are more complex and use harnesses which fit over the head to ensure that they can be pulled firmly onto the face. The masks are stored in a small cupboard and the pilots would have had to reach forward, open the door, pull them out, and then fit them. They had been alerted to a problem by a klaxon sounding in the cockpit, but it was a general alarm and did not specifically indicate that the aircraft was not maintaining pressure. Their attention was also diverted by a warning light, which lit up to indicate that the cockpit instrumentation was not being cooled properly. It is very unlikely that the pilots recognised that the aircraft was not pressurising and, in any case, it would have been too late to act, as the balloonists Sivel and Croce-Spinelli had found in 1875; they would not have had the strength to be able to reach and fit their oxygen masks. The passengers, although getting very cold, would have used their masks until the oxygen supply ran out after about 20 minutes. This left the cabin staff using portable oxygen sets, to investigate the lack of response from the flight deck; they would have eventually realised that the aircraft was not descending to a safe altitude. Two flight attendants were seen in the cockpit by the Greek Air force F-16s who had scrambled to intercept the aircraft when it failed to respond to air traffic control communications. The aircraft crashed when it finally ran out of fuel, killing all 121 people on board. Mercifully, the passengers would have been unconscious from the combination of lack of oxygen and extreme cold. The disaster appears to have occurred simply because one control had been left in the wrong position.

More recently, a Boeing 747 of the Australian airline Quantas suffered a sudden decompression at an altitude of 28,000 feet apparently when one of the emergency oxygen bottles located in the hold exploded. It blew a large hole in the starboard side of the aircraft in front of the wing (Figure 3.5). The

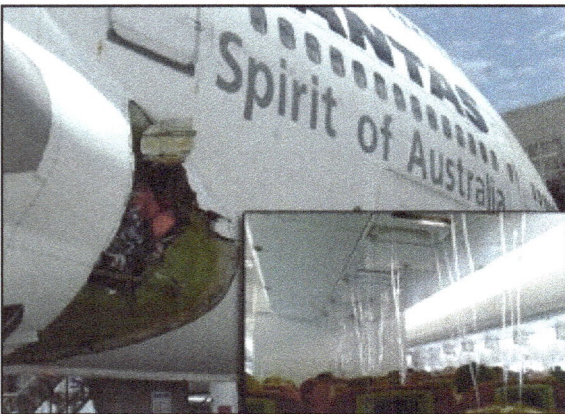

Figure 3.5:
The damaged Quantas Boeing 747 in the Philippines showing (inset) the cabin oxygen masks deployed.

loss of cabin pressure could not have been overlooked because of the noise generated, and the passenger masks dropping from the cabin ceiling as shown in the photograph. The pilots would have immediately donned their oxygen masks and initiated a rapid descent to a safe altitude of about 10,000 feet, where there is ample oxygen to maintain consciousness. They were able to land the aircraft in the Philippines. It is testimony to the superb design and strength of the Boeing 747 that, despite considerable damage, the aircraft remained airworthy. Quantas stated that the aircraft would be repaired and it has since been returned to service.

Barometric pressure falls consistently with altitude. At base camp on Mount Everest, the air pressure is about half the 1 ATA normal value at sea level, that is, 500 millibars. However, the oxygen percentage in the air remains the same (at about 21%) as the pressure falls, and so the part of atmospheric pressure exerted by oxygen at base camp is then 21% of 500 millibars, which is 105 millibars. Because of the low pressure of oxygen very few people live permanently at this altitude. Travellers to La Paz, which is at an altitude of about 13,500 feet, who have flown directly from sea level may develop mountain sickness; some have even died because they have not had time to acclimatise.[7] In fact, deaths from mountain sickness have occurred at altitudes as low as 9,000 feet, albeit associated with very hard exercise. Surprisingly, when acclimatised, it is possible to work at very high altitude; in the Andes, men work in silver mines at 19,000 feet. However, they live at 17,500 feet, the same altitude as base camp on Everest, preferring to make the 1,500 foot climb for their working day! Some birds can soar to extreme altitudes using favourable winds. Bar-headed geese have been seen as high as 33,383 feet above sea level. An aircraft flying over the Côte d'Ivoire collided with a Rüppell's vulture at the astonishing altitude of 37,073 feet; the highest recorded avian altitude. Birds have inherited the breathing system of dinosaurs, filling air sacs which discharge using a counter-current flow system through the lungs, which allows much greater uptake of the oxygen in air. However, the birds cannot fly up to these high altitudes because the air being too thin cannot provide enough oxygen—they will have been carried up by the high altitude winds known as jet streams.

The pioneering adventures of the balloonists had firmly established the importance of pressure and, specifically, the pressure of oxygen needed to maintain brain activity and consciousness, paving the way for today's global aviation industry. They had also recorded the steady rise of the pulse rate with increasing altitude, and the need to breathe additional oxygen to compensate for the thin air at very high altitudes. It remained for Edmund Hillary and Tenzing Norgay to follow the "uneven terrestrial surface" up Everest nearly a hundred years later in 1953 and disprove James Glaisher's prediction that "no human being ever could drag himself to this height following uneven terrestrial surface." They reached the summit using specially designed oxygen apparatus. The discovery of the body of George Mallory in 1999 led Graham Hoyland to assert that the mountain was first conquered by Mallory and Irvine in 1924 (*Sunday Telegraph*, September 30, 2007). However, as they did not complete the descent, it would not be regarded today as a valid climb.

In 1978, two Alpine climbers, Reinhold Messner and Peter Habeler, stunned the world by climbing Everest without supplemental oxygen. How was this possible? If, like Glaisher and Coxwell, we were now to ascend to this altitude and stay more than a few minutes, we would surely die. The reasons are now known and the science is in place. To understand it again requires an appreciation of the *principle of disease* already introduced—that, paradoxically, lack of oxygen causes the growth of new blood vessels due to the upregulation of hypoxia-inducible factor proteins. It is common knowledge that, although lack of oxygen affects the whole body to some extent, it is the brain that suffers the most. Injuries and many diseases of the brain affect its blood vessels, reducing the supply of vital oxygen. There is universal recognition that the blockage of arteries reduces the supply of oxygen. Indeed, damaged areas of the brain, for example in a patient with a stroke, may be struggling to recover with oxygen levels lower than those in the brain of a mountaineer on the top of Everest. What is still not generally recognised is that lack of oxygen in the brain can also be due to the dysfunction of *veins* because they leak, thus allowing the cells to become waterlogged; in effect, they are drowning. The pressure on the summit of Everest is very low; about a third of normal atmospheric pressure at sea level. As we have seen, despite the air still containing about 21% oxygen, its pressure and therefore its *concentration* is also a third of the value at sea level. Not surprisingly, many Himalayan climbers develop mountain sickness due to the lack of oxygen. However, on rapid ascents to high altitude without the necessary acclimatisation mountaineers, like pilots, may suffer from a second problem—bubble formation and decompression sickness, which will be discussed in Chapter 7.

A group of doctors who work in intensive care in London are currently studying the problems of lack of oxygen on climbing Everest on the Caudwell Xtreme Everest Expedition (www.xtreme-everest.co.uk). They wondered why some of their patients suffering from severe oxygen deficiency survived when others, with a more serious lack of oxygen, did not. At the moment, it would appear that they are looking for genes that increase oxygen efficiency. However, while genes are obviously important because, for example, they allow the construction of forms of haemoglobin with different affinities for oxygen, the outcome of high altitude ascents is not likely to be related to the oxygen levels in their *blood*, but to those actually in their *tissues*. It can probably be stated with some degree of certainty that those involved in this research will not have thought of looking at a barometer to see if more patients in intensive care die on low pressure days when the weather is poor. Nevertheless, an association has been shown between deep venous thrombosis (DVT) and a reduction of barometric pressure.[8] Small changes in barometric pressure are certainly relevant, and there is good evidence that the multiple deaths that occurred in the Death Zone on Everest in 1996 were due to a sudden fall in barometric pressure on the summit. It was estimated to have fallen *just 16 millibars*; contrast that with a fall of 129 millibars from the highest to the lowest pressure barometric pressure that has occurred at sea level in the UK. Is it relevant to patients close to death in intensive care units? It is; the 1996 tragedy was referred to in the 2007 BBC *Horizon* television programme "Doctors in the Death Zone" mentioned in Chapter 2, and it was stated, correctly, that "in patients, a minor improvement in oxygen utilization would have dramatic benefits!" As we have seen in Chapter 1, there can be no doubt whatsoever that this is true; there is a threshold in the level of oxygen at which cells will fail to function properly, yet can still be rescued. It is, however, very unlikely that we can alter how the body actually uses oxygen, but we can easily give patients more.

The oxygen apparatus used for mountaineering only adds a few percentage points to the level of oxygen in air, but it can make an enormous differ-

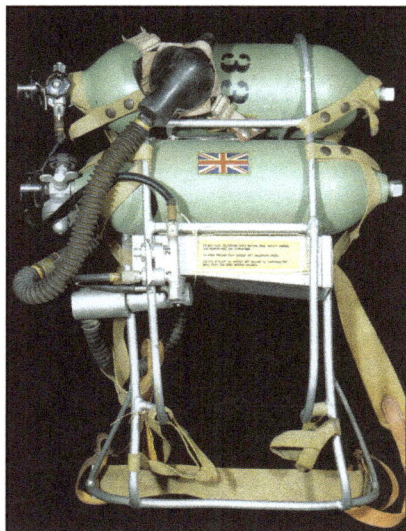

Figure 3.6:
The oxygen apparatus used on the first successful ascent of Everest in 1954, with the oronasal mask which can be seen strapped to the upper cylinder.

ence to man's ability to climb to very high altitudes. The greatest explorer of our times, Sir Ranulph Fiennes, who failed on two attempts to climb Everest tantalisingly close to the summit, was allowed to use oxygen equipment climbing from camp three to camp two. Normally, climbers do not use supplemental oxygen at this altitude, conserving the precious gas for the "attack" on the summit. The young climbers accompanying Sir Ranulph found it difficult to keep up with him over this stretch, and one actually said, "[Ranulph] was on rocket fuel today" which, in a sense, he was—oxygen is used in rocketry, except that it is not actually a fuel. Happily, he finally succeeded in climbing the mountain on his third attempt. If climbers develop mountain sickness, the small increase in the level of oxygen breathed may ultimately mean the difference between life and death. This clearly indicates that for some patients in intensive care a 10% increase in barometric pressure associated with a high pressure weather system will improve their chance of survival.

Most of our understanding of the physiological effects of pressure and oxygen is based on work begun in the nineteenth century by a handful of intrepid scientists, who were renowned for experimenting on themselves. Paul Bert, who worked in Paris, can, justifiably, be called the father of pressure physiology and students of the subject should certainly read his book, which was translated into English in the 1950s.[9] However, it was the Scottish physiologist John Scott Haldane who studied, first-hand, how lack of oxygen affects the body, and especially the brain. An excellent biography of Haldane by Martin Goodman, now professor of creative writing at the University of Hull, was published in 2007.[10] It is entitled *Suffer and Survive*, which is the motto on the family crest that adorns the front door of the house at Cloan, near Gleneagles, where Haldane spent his boyhood. The next chapter details some of the many contributions this astonishing man made to human physiology and the practice of medicine.

CHAPTER 4

John Scott Haldane: A Giant of Medicine

Lack of oxygen not only stops the machine, it wrecks what we take to be machinery.

John S. Haldane. *British Medical Journal,* 1919.

Although well known for his work on gas analysis and diving, few know of the contributions made by John Scott Haldane to our understanding of the effects of lack of oxygen or the value of oxygen used as a treatment. The family that Haldane was born into has been deeply involved in the history of both England and Scotland for over a thousand years, and influential in many walks of life. Haldane is a Viking name, and the Hal Danes may have been among those who sacked Lindisfarne Abbey on the coast of Northumberland in 793 A.D. Some of the Vikings settled in the Kelso area of Roxburghshire, but there was a migration north to Perthshire two centuries later when the youngest son of a descendant of the Haldanes, Robert, married the heiress of Gleneagles.[1] The Haldanes fought against Cromwell but, in 1526, they supported the distribution of the first copies of the New Testament in English, which had been translated and published abroad. They were in the forefront of the reformation in Scotland, joining the Calvinist movement. They were, nevertheless, strong advocates of religious freedom.

John Scott Haldane was born at 17 Charlotte Square Edinburgh in 1860, but his childhood was spent at Cloan, a large house in extensive grounds near Gleneagles and Auchterarder in Perthshire, Scotland (Figure 4.1).

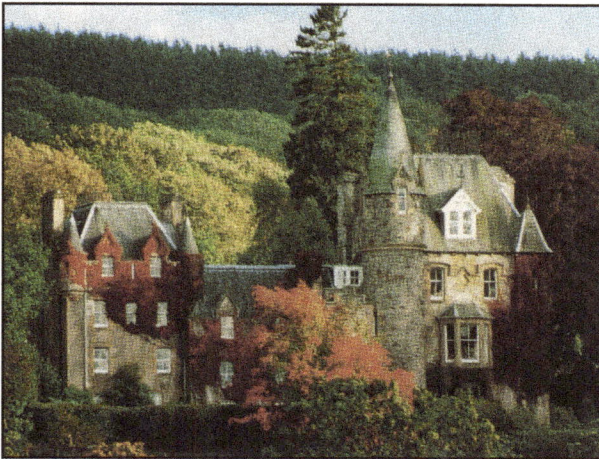

Figure 4.1:
The Haldane family house at Cloan. (Courtesy of Richard Haldane MBE.)

Haldane's father was a widower who already had five children when he married Mary Elizabeth Burdon Sanderson, who had six children by him, the first dying soon after birth. The next, Richard (b. 1856), became a barrister, and was granted the title Viscount Haldane in 1911. He served as Secretary of State for War and then as Lord Chancellor in the government of Prime Minister Herbert Asquith, and reorganised the Army before WW1, establishing the Territorial Army in 1907. The third son, George (b. 1858), known as Geordie, whose great love was music, tragically died of diphtheria at the age of seventeen. John Scott was the fourth, followed by a sister, Elizabeth (b. 1862), who subsequently gave him a great deal of practical help with his early experiments. She became the manager of the Royal Infirmary of Edinburgh, then the largest hospital in the United Kingdom, and was the first woman to be appointed a Justice of the Peace in Scotland. Later, she was elected as the Privy Council representative on the General Council of Nursing, and became a formidable social reformer. The last child, William (b. 1864), became a writer to the signet and carried on the family law practice at 4 Charlotte Square, Edinburgh. Their mother, Mary Haldane, was a truly remarkable woman who entertained many famous people at Cloan after the death of her husband, including the British Prime Ministers Asquith and Ramsay MacDonald. She was a strong supporter of women's rights, writing to the *Times* on February 16, 1909, at the age of 84, under the name "Octogenarian" to point out that, as a taxpayer, she should be entitled to the vote. She lived to be 100 years old, dying in 1925.

John Haldane entered the University of Edinburgh in 1876, when he was just 16, and was awarded an M.A. in 1879. After a period of study at the University of Jena in Germany, he enrolled in the medical school at Edinburgh, which may have been prompted by the untimely death of his brother George. He became friendly with fellow student Arthur Conan Doyle, who went on to write his famous novels featuring the detective Sherlock Holmes. Haldane failed his final examination in midwifery, and his sister recorded that he finally graduated "after a tumultuous time of controversy with his teachers in Edinburgh." He had apparently found the professorial lectures very boring, and even wrote anonymously to the *Scotsman* about the standard of teaching as if from a dying medical student, protesting about the facts taught that "Were to us students little else than rubbish formed from skeletons of dead theories." His pamphlet, "A Letter to Edinburgh Professors Signed by a Medical Student" was edited, with preface, by a "graduate of eminence," and published in London by David Stott, of 370 Oxford Street, in 1890. It drew attention to the lack of science behind many of the fashionable explanations of diseases, and the medical obsession with patented pills and potions. If he were alive today he would probably feel much the same way about treatments based on the popular theory of auto-immunity. Haldane registered with the General Medical Council in 1884. After six months as house physician in the Royal Infirmary of Edinburgh he decided not to enter medical practice, but to become involved in research.

Haldane was well known in Auchterarder for his talks on many topics allied to medicine, delivered at the local village hall under the auspices of the Order of St. John. It is recorded that on one occasion there was great excitement when he produced a skeleton to illustrate his subject. His enthusiasm for communicating to his fellow man was to influence his equally brilliant son J.B.S., "Jack" Haldane. J.B.S. became a card-carrying member of the Communist Party after witnessing the social injustice evident at the time of WW1, and he later fought with the partisans against Franco's forces in the Spanish Civil War. Jack became very well known in the 1930s for popularising science, writing articles for the *Daily Worker*, and giving many talks on BBC radio. The author first became aware of the Haldanes as a teenager from reading a 1941 wartime utility version of *Keeping Cool and Other Selected Essays*, a compilation of short articles written by Jack Haldane.[2] It had been borrowed, for a rather extended period, from the Army 13th Light Field Ambulance Station library in Palestine, by my late brother, Ivan, who was injured in 1948 during his time in national service.

Together with his son Jack, Haldane was to work on a wide range of projects until he died of pneumonia shortly after returning from Persia in May 1936. He developed the infection after sustaining a chest injury after falling out of bed at his home in Oxford. Jack erected an oxygen tent over his father's bed to ease his distress, and J.S. passed away peacefully at the age of 76. Jack continued his father's work on diving for the Admiralty during WW2, and became much better known than his father. Indeed, because they share the initials J. and S., they are often confused. In subsequent chapters, "Haldane" will always refer to the father. Haldane's extraordinary genius was fortunately recognised during his lifetime as he received many awards, including Fellowship of the Royal Society in 1897, at the age of 37. He was also a recipient of the Copley Medal, an honour bestowed on many eminent scientists including Albert Einstein. In 1925, he was made a Companion of Honour, a gift of the sovereign, George the IV. His astonishing curriculum vitae is reproduced in Appendix 1. His unfashionable interest in the health and welfare of workers ranged over 50 years, from the effects of explosions in coal mines, to his last investigation in 1936 of heat stroke in workers in the oilfields of the Anglo-Persian Oil Company, which later became BP. The company had its origins in the shale industry of West Lothian in Scotland, an area close to the village of Broxburn. This is not far from where Sir George Bruce had mined coal under the Firth of Forth in the seventeenth century, using the world's first offshore terminal. Haldane had flown out to Persia with his sister Elizabeth in Hengist, a four-engine Handley Page aeroplane. It was the extraction of shale in West Lothian by James "Paraffin" Young that started the world's petroleum industry. Young invented the refining process and became wealthy, not so much from his shale mines, but from the royalties he received from companies such as Standard Oil, owned by the Rockefellers. It is ironic that shale and oil both involve hydrocarbon extraction, and their use has made a substantial contribution to the rising carbon dioxide levels that so concern us today.

Although best known for his contributions to the physiology of breathing, especially the role of carbon dioxide[3] and, of course, the decompression tables used to allow divers to safely ascend back to the surface,[4] Haldane was truly an intellectual giant, with interests ranging from philosophy to physics. In fact, he even wrote a textbook of physics,[5] *Gases and Liquids: A Contribution to Molecular Physics*. Not surprisingly, being written by a physician, it caused considerable controversy among contemporary scientists. The textbook was inspired by the work of the little-known Scottish physicist, John James Waterston (1811–1883). Haldane was fulsome in his praise of Waterston's work on the kinetics of gases; the paper Waterston had submitted to the Royal Society had originally been retained in the archives after being rejected. It would appear that Haldane was the first to suggest that gases could be responsible for osmotic pressure, a subject that will be discussed later. Haldane wrote many papers on the philosophy of science, including one with his brother Richard whilst he was still a medical student in 1883. He continued this interest into the last decade of his life.[6] The controversy generated by the theory of evolution had engaged Haldane but, unlike his son Jack, he felt that while evolution could account for human development, there was much more to the story of the force of life itself. Charles Darwin's book was, of course, entitled *The Origin of Species*, not *The Origin of Life*. Although, as a boy, he had been a Baptist, Haldane formally resigned from the congregation, and later in life did not follow any religious persuasion. He felt that the totality of the universe was his God.

Haldane's first appointment after qualifying and his "house" job, as an intern in Edinburgh, was as demonstrator in physiology at University College Dundee. The town has strong connections with the Haldanes; Admiral Duncan, famed for his victory at the battle of Camperdown, was the son of the Provost of Dundee, Alexander Duncan, and Helen Haldane of Gleneagles. The Admiral is buried with several other Haldane family members at Lundie, a hamlet a few miles north of Dundee. There was a high infant mortality in the city, especially among the jute workers and it was suspected that the infants were dying from lack of oxygen during the night, as many families shared a bed in the rooms of the meager tenements. Working in the chemistry laboratory with the new head of department, Professor Thomas Carnelley, Haldane analysed samples of the room air taken from the tenement rooms during the night. They were accompanied, understandably, by a policeman. The samples showed that the lowering of the oxygen content was so small that it was barely recordable, and they realised that most infant deaths were probably due to "overlaying" and suffocation, which is hardly surprising when as many as eight people often shared a bed. By the 1880s, the government had become aware of the problems of contaminated air, and a House of Commons Select Committee commissioned studies of the air in the sewers of London and later of Dundee. The city engineers of Dundee were proud of their innovative large bore, intercept sewer, which ran under the Murraygate in the centre of the city.

Haldane took samples of air from the sewer system and his son J.B.S. recalled that when the pair went to the city for J.S. to give a British Association lecture in 1921, his father remembered his way around the city from the layout of the sewers!

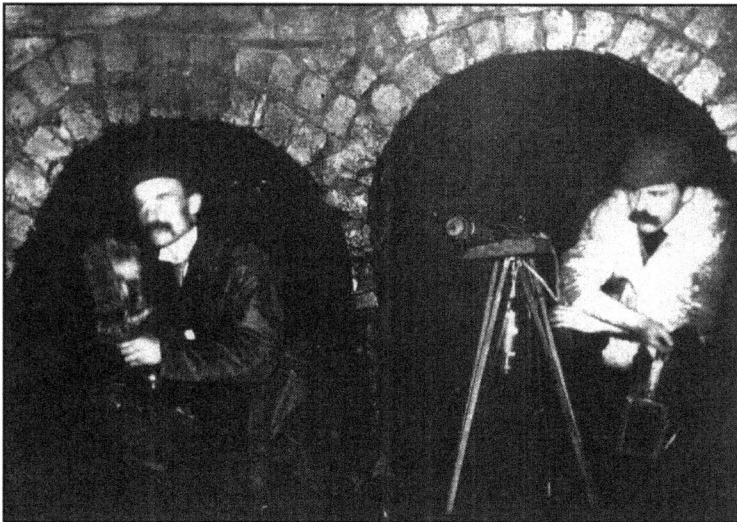

Figure 4.2:
Carnelley and Haldane (right) in the Intercept Sewer in Dundee.
(Courtesy of Richard Haldane MBE.)

Chapter 4: John Scott Haldane: A Giant of Medicine ~ 61

Following the report of their work in Dundee, Carnelley and Haldane were asked to investigate the smells originating from the main London sewer, which discharged into the river Thames alongside the Houses of Parliament, to the great annoyance of its members. Later, they tackled a similar problem affecting the centre of Bristol. At the time, it was thought that foul air caused disease, including cholera, as the seminal work of John Snow, who showed it was a water-borne disease, had yet to be accepted. However, the pair found that there were fewer bacteria in sewer air than there were in the outside air, and Haldane was quick to use the data to dismiss the popular notion that cholera was an air-borne disease. Leaving Dundee in 1887, he sailed to the continent from Leith, Edinburgh, and worked for a few months in Berlin. His next appointment later in 1887 was as demonstrator in physiology at the University of Oxford, where his uncle, John Burdon Sanderson, was professor of physiology. Haldane was recorded in the 1901 census as "M.D. (not practicing) living in Oxford, in the parish of St. Giles."

In 1894, Haldane, already well known for his work on gases, was asked to investigate the events which take place during a mining explosion, following a disaster at the Albion Colliery in South Wales that claimed many lives. He went on to work on mining safety with the Inspector of Mines for North Staffordshire, W.N. Atkinson. The atmosphere encountered in mines could produce suffocation in the absence of an explosion and "black damp," as it was termed, was found on analysis to be a mixture of 87% nitrogen and 13% carbon dioxide. It was the residue left when the oxygen in the air, which had penetrated the coal, had been removed by the oxidation of the carbon. It causes death by asphyxiation; in fact, a few breaths of black damp are rapidly fatal, as is the breathing of any gas not containing oxygen. Many divers involved in oilfield diving have died from being delivered pure helium. It is now mandatory, at least in European waters, for helium to be supplied containing at least 2% oxygen.[7] Despite medical scaremongering, the *only* pure gas that is safe to breathe is oxygen itself!

Analysis of the gas left after an explosion, known as "after damp," showed that it contained the lethal gas carbon monoxide. Haldane was able to show that carbon monoxide combines with the haemoglobin in red blood cells to form carboxyhaemoglobin, and this prevents the haemoglobin taking up oxygen. He investigated the effects of the gas on himself, carefully noting the symptoms, and devised a method to analyse the amount of carboxyhaemoglobin present in blood. In 1896, Haldane submitted a report on colliery explosions and underground fires to the Home Secretary, based largely on his investigation of an explosion in the same year at Tylorstown Colliery in

South Wales. Of the 57 bodies recovered, only four had died from traumatic injury; the remainder had died from burns and carbon monoxide poisoning. This was the start of Haldane's long association with the mining industry that culminated in his appointment as President of the Mining Association in 1925 and an honorary chair at the University of Birmingham, which finally gave him the title of professor. He was apparently disappointed not to be awarded the chair in physiology his uncle had occupied at Oxford, but his close links to workers in industry would certainly have been frowned on in the academic quadrangles of power. His involvement in the controversy about vitalism and evolution may have counted against him. Haldane had also built a laboratory at Cherwell, his home close to the river Cherwell, to conduct his experiments free of "official" interference; a course of action also taken by Nobel Prize winner Sir Peter Mitchell, honored for his discovery of cellular proton pumping.

In 1895, Haldane published one of several of his remarkable papers on carbon monoxide in the *Journal of Physiology*,[8] detailing the mechanisms of poisoning. Haldane was the first to employ the benefits of oxygen in the treatment of carbon monoxide poisoning, not for men, but for birds. He had introduced the use of canaries to detect carbon monoxide in coal mines. The canary was housed in a small transparent box, which he fitted with a small oxygen cylinder.

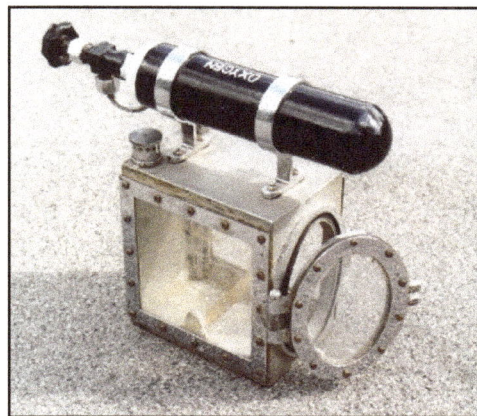

Figure 4.3:
Haldane's humane apparatus for the detection of carbon monoxide. (Courtesy of Robert Gardiner.)

When a bird was taken down a mine and breathed air containing a dangerous level of carbon monoxide, it fell off the perch. It was immediately revived by oxygen from the cylinder, and so constituted a reusable biological monitor. This illustrates an obvious, important, but much-neglected principle: The faster that lack of oxygen is corrected, the better the result. As will be seen in Chapter 22, carbon monoxide poisoning is still rarely treated with oxygen using hyperbaric conditions, despite official directives. Robert Davis, later Sir Robert Davis, worked with Haldane to develop a breathing apparatus for use in mines at the Siebe Gorman premises close to Westminster Bridge. They also developed apparatus to allow escape from a sunken submarine. Haldane employed his son Jack as an experimental subject in his tests of the method at the tender age of 13. It had become a family tradition to be one's own rabbit and Haldane constantly experimented on himself. Figure 4.4 shows him in a boiler suit, wearing a hard hat and testing breathing equipment down a mine.

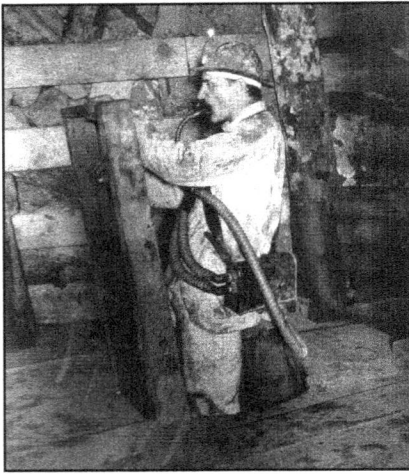

Figure 4.4:
Haldane testing his breathing apparatus down a coal mine.
(Courtesy of Richard Haldane MBE.)

When as a medical student in Edinburgh, Haldane had criticised the standard of teaching in letters to the *Scotsman,* he named two scientists as great teachers who not only made great discoveries, but also made their pupils think. They were Joseph Black (1728–1799) of the University of Glasgow, the discoverer of carbon dioxide, and Joseph Priestley (1733–1804), one of those credited with the discovery of oxygen. Much of Haldane's life was to revolve around these two gases. He was to highlight the consequences of lack of oxygen and also discover that carbon dioxide controls breathing.

In the 1890s, Haldane devised an apparatus to sample the gases from deep within the lungs close to the final air sacs, the alveoli, at the end of the tubular airways. He constructed an airtight wooden chamber in the private laboratory at his home, Cherwell, in Oxford for his experiments. It was lined with lead and had rubber seals on the door to prevent leaks, and measured three feet by four feet and six feet high. The occupants could be observed through a small window, and the atmosphere sampled through a pipe led through the wall. In the first experiments to study lack of oxygen, Haldane and his colleague, James Lorrain Smith, sat in the chamber at rest and closed the door. The oxygen in the air was steadily depleted as they breathed, and the carbon dioxide level began to rise. After about three hours, they had developed a violent headache with shortness of breath and severe panting. The longest time the pair endured in their experiments was seven and a half hours, by which time the oxygen level had fallen from 21% to about 13%, and the carbon dioxide level had risen to 6.5%. Obviously, the oxygen had been used up by their metabolism which, in turn, produced the carbon dioxide they exhaled.

The question they needed to answer was: What was responsible for the headache and the panting? Was it the lack of oxygen, or the high level of carbon dioxide? To eliminate the latter, a tray containing a mixture of slaked lime and caustic soda, which absorbs carbon dioxide, was placed in the chamber. Further experiments were performed. After three hours, the oxygen level had fallen so low that a struck match simply fizzled and would not light. There was no panting, even after more than seven hours, so the lack of oxygen did not increase the rate of breathing. It appears that Haldane did the final experiment on his own, eventually becoming blue and falling down unconsciousness inside the box.[9] Thankfully, his collapse was observed, and help was on-hand to open the door and pull him out. He was soon revived by the fresh air.

Contrary to popular belief, the first response of the body to lack of oxygen is not to increase the rate of breathing, it is the *pulse rate* that increases together with the output of blood by the heart, as the balloonist Glaisher had found.[10] This means that organs can receive more blood flow to compensate for a lower level of oxygen in the blood. Dramatic increases in the size of arteries have been found using ultrasonic equipment in climbers in the Death Zone on Everest. The same increase in pulse rate can be detected ultrasonically in a distressed baby short of oxygen in the womb. So, if lack of such a vital substance does not drive breathing, what does? Again, we can turn for an explanation to Haldane's brilliant research into gases and breathing, which developed from his first studies with Professor Carnelley in University College, Dundee. Haldane, working with his colleagues in Oxford, devised the first apparatus to measure the levels of the metabolic gases dissolved in blood.[11] In 1911, he travelled on his second visit to the US to collaborate with the celebrated American physiologist Yandell Henderson. Haldane met Professor Henderson at a meeting in Vienna and had explained the difficulty of taking his equipment to altitude, having braved the weather on the summit of

Ben Nevis in Scotland. Henderson pointed out that Pike's Peak on the eastern edge of the Rockies in Colorado, which reaches an altitude of 14,115 feet, would be an excellent location for such a study because an entrepreneur had actually constructed a hotel near the summit serviced by a funicular railway. An expedition was duly organised, and the finance obtained. Haldane's brother, Lord Haldane, provided diplomatic assistance for the importation of the considerable equipment and supplies needed into the US. The railway proved invaluable in carrying the teams and their equipment up the mountain. During their stay at Summit House, Haldane and his colleagues watched one of the new flying machines attempting to fly over the mountain. It lacked sufficient power, but it would not be long before aircraft were able to exceed this altitude and become formidable weapons of war. The original hotel on Pike's Peak has all but disappeared but, in 1969, the US Army established a second laboratory on the mountain, the Pike's Peak Research Laboratory. Ironically, in view of the continuing war in Afghanistan, its stated aim is still to study the impact of high altitude on warfare. It may have had some influence, as the US Army has apparently purchased portable hyperbaric chambers for treating soldiers who develop altitude sickness.

Because oxygen is so central to life, and especially to the function of the brain, it seems logical for it to control the rate at which we breathe but it does not, indeed it *cannot*, because it would be both *ineffective* and *dangerous*. It would be ineffective because breathing faster without an increase in the flow of blood through the lungs would actually be pointless; the amount transferred to the blood would barely change. It would be dangerous because it would wash out carbon dioxide from the body. Breathing faster when we exercise is due to stimulation of the centre in the stem of the brain, which controls respiration. However, the primary stimulus is not lack of oxygen, it is an increase in the acidity of blood associated with a rise in the level of carbon dioxide, largely produced by our muscles. The reason it is actually dangerous to breathe faster, or hyperventilate, without an increase in the carbon dioxide level produced by exercise, is because the carbon dioxide already present in the body is rapidly exhaled, the acidity of the blood falls, and it becomes alkaline. This, in turn, causes a change in calcium levels, eventually triggering dangerous muscle spasms, known as *tetany*, to develop. Voluntary over-breathing, as it is often called, may even precipitate a full-blown grande mal convulsion; that is, a fit identical to those seen in severe epilepsy. Haldane commented that if an animal were forcibly ventilated to remove carbon dioxide from its blood, "It would die from 'want' of oxygen without drawing a single breath." Hyperventilation *can* relieve hypoxia *safely*, but *only* if the exhaled gas is rebreathed using a mixing chamber; the carbon dioxide maintains normal blood acidity.[12] This is clear evidence that a hypoxic respiratory drive does not exist.

The increase in the rate of breathing from exercise increases the intake of oxygen, because the flow of blood through the lungs is increased as the output of the heart rises. The increase in breathing not only allows us to generate more energy from the oxygen we breathe in, but also it allows the carbon dioxide produced to be exhaled. This keeps the acidity of blood normal, which is critical to the health of our cells. The mechanism is astonishingly accurate in controlling the hydrogen ion concentration responsible for its acidity. However, a fall in the level of oxygen breathed does have one immediate action: It causes the arteries supplying the lungs to narrow. This slows down the transit of red blood cells through the capillaries of the lungs, giving them more time to take up oxygen. The passage of red cells through the brain is also slowed down for just the opposite reason: To give oxygen time to escape from red blood cells into the brain.

If a gas not containing any oxygen is breathed, consciousness is rapidly lost with no increase whatever in the rate of breathing. Haldane had witnessed the effects first-hand down in the coal mines of South Wales: "Thus it is a common experience with miners going into an atmosphere of nearly pure fire damp [methane, CH_4], or climbing up so that their heads are in the gas; they drop suddenly as if they were shot." The response to rapidly halving the oxygen level breathed is actually an increase in *pulse rate* and *blood flow*, not an increase in the rate of breathing. The increase in pulse rate had first been recorded by Glaisher and Coxwell in their epic ascent from Wolverhampton gas works; it had risen from 70 on the ground to 100 at altitude. Unfortunately, by the time Haldane had begun his investigation of the control of breathing, it was already a commonly accepted opinion that the "want of oxygen," which is now referred to as hypoxia, was the stimulus to the respiratory centre, and acted quite independently from carbon dioxide. Haldane certainly did not subscribe to this view; he had experienced loss of consciousness after just 50 seconds breathing the "air," which was afterwards found to contain 1.8% oxygen. He noted that he had no increase *whatsoever* in his urge to breathe.

The lack of stimulus from an abrupt and severe deficiency of oxygen in the gas subjects breathe was shown in a remarkable series of experiments published in 1923 by Drs. Edward E. Schneider and Dorothy Truesdell,[13] working at the School of Aviation Medicine and the Wesleyan University in Connecticut. Schneider had collaborated with Haldane and Henderson on the Pike's Peak expedition, when he had been professor of biology at Colorado College. These unique and dangerous experiments would certainly not be allowed today. They gave seventeen volunteers pure nitrogen to breathe until they reached the point of unconsciousness. Surprisingly, the time varied from 47 seconds to as long as 112 seconds, and the subjects often exhibited some bizarre symptoms:

> *In the experiments the subject was permitted to breathe the nitrogen until unconsciousness was impending, at which time the eyes tended to converge and sometimes the pupils to dilate . . . In our experience none of the subjects fainted; although a number of persons twitched in the early stages of the asphyxial decrease of muscle tone.*

But there was no increase in the rate of breathing, indeed Schneider and Truesdell reported that;

> *In some instances the breathing began to slow and in some subjects even stopped, but by slapping the back of the subject a deep inspiration was immediately obtained. It was our custom to prompt the subject, on restoring him to air to take deep breaths until he had taken five or six.*

There can be no doubting the courage of the subjects; some even did several experiments! The effect of the lack of oxygen associated with fire damp in coal mines was much more rapid than in these experiments simply because the miners were exercising; whereas, in Schneider and Truesdell's experiments, the subjects were seated and completely at rest. Exercise *dramatically* increases the need for oxygen.

The highest altitude where people live constantly is the Tibetan plateau, which averages 14,763 feet (nearly three miles) above sea level. Tibetans avoid disabling altitude sickness because they correct the lack of oxygen in the tissues by greatly increasing blood flow and the output of the heart. With broader arteries and more capillaries carrying higher levels of blood flow, they are able to deliver *normal* levels of oxygen to their muscles and organs. Astonishingly, the heart output and blood flow of Tibetans is generally twice that of people who reside at sea level. The increase in blood flow in the tissues of the body is because of the action of another gas, nitric oxide, which relaxes blood vessels. It has been found that these Tibetans, acclimatised over generations by genetic changes, actually have much higher levels of nitric oxide in the circulation.[14] Similar adaptations have been found in other populations living at high altitude,[15] although curiously the genes involved may be different.[16] It is produced by the cells that line blood vessels, and it is inactivated when it binds to oxygenated haemoglobin. However, when the level of oxygen breathed falls, haemoglobin takes up less oxygen and so binds less nitric oxide, which is then free to react.[17] It relaxes the muscle in the wall of blood vessels in the body by increasing their diameter and increasing blood flow through the tissues to compensate for the lower level of oxygen carried in the blood. When lower oxygen levels are breathed, the heart needs to pump harder to increase blood flow and this, of course, includes through the lungs, otherwise blood would pool in the blood vessels they contain. As the heart rate increases as the level of oxygen breathed falls, it seems likely that the response is due to the oxygen sensors called *chemoreceptors*, which are located in the large blood vessels above the heart and act by increasing the heartbeat, rather than the rate of breathing. Curiously, this possibility does not seem to have been investigated, perhaps because the response to changing oxygen levels has been the preserve of *respiratory* physiologists, scientists involved in the research of breathing, rather than those who study the heart and the circulation.

If the response of the heart rate to the level of oxygen breathed is plotted on a graph, it is a straight line. Lower the level and the rate increases; breathe a higher level and it will slow down. The heart is, of course, a muscle, and so its activity produces some carbon dioxide. As the workload of the heart increases, the carbon dioxide it produces will increase and this will stimulate breathing. Of course, breathing itself involves muscle activity, which again produces carbon dioxide and, as the oxygen availability falls, lactic acid is produced. A fall in the oxygen content of the gas being breathed to almost half the level in air at sea level certainly has little effect, although, in some people there is an increase in the respiratory rate as the level of oxygen breathed falls further, probably in response to the extra carbon dioxide produced by the increased heart action. Nevertheless, in others the increase in breathing rate is negligible. If the hypoxic stimulus was significant, then it would surely be present in all of us. As we have seen from the experience of the balloonists, as the level of oxygen in blood falls further, the activity of the nervous system fails and, eventually, becomes too low to allow the respiratory centre in the brainstem itself to function.

The controversy over the hypoxic drive is far from being academic to a very large number of patients with lung disease, especially when it is associated with chronic obstruction of their airways and, therefore, known as chronic obstructive pulmonary disease (COPD). This illness is a major health problem, affecting millions of patients. They struggle to stay alive because of lack of oxygen. For many years it has been believed that when such patients are having an acute attack with severe breathing problems, giving oxygen may be harmful, although no one seriously doubts that they are dangerously short of oxygen. Generations of medical students have been indoctrinated that giving oxygen to such patients reduces their drive to breathe and may worsen their condition, even when they are in a stable condition. The allegation, which dates back to the 1950s, was greatly reinforced in 1960 by what would, today, be regarded as a totally inadequate study by Dr. E.J.M. Campbell. It was published in the *Lancet*[18] and involved just four patients, only two actually suffering from COPD. No actual measurements were made; he simply drew extrapolations that were based on his theory. In a second article in the same issue of the journal, he describes the apparatus needed to deliver more oxygen, but limiting the percentage of oxygen.[19] It is still in use today around the world. Such was the impact of these articles, detailing the hypoxic drive and Campbell's subsequent crusade to restrict the use of oxygen, that the allegation is still featured in textbooks of medicine and is taught to every medical student. It was the only concern expressed in online correspondence prior to the publication of the British Thoracic Society's (BTS) guideline for emergency oxygen use in adult patients, released in 2008.[20]

Surprisingly, the controversy has raged for over 50 years, and there are demands for still more research. In 2007, Australian doctors[21] referred to it as "a major issue at our university teaching hospital." They had studied the difference between acutely ill COPD patients admitted to their hospital receiving more than 4 litres of oxygen a minute and those receiving less than 4 litres a minute, and claimed that those given the higher level of oxygen fared less well. However, the patients in the group given more oxygen were more seriously ill, and more of them needed assistance with their breathing. The difference in the amount of oxygen carried in plasma between the two groups would actually be very small, simply because oxygen is so poorly soluble in the water of the plasma. There can be no doubt that the level of carbon dioxide in the blood of such COPD patients *will* increase when they are given oxygen therapy, because they have accumulated an oxygen *debt*. Lack of oxygen leads to *anaerobic* metabolism, that is, metabolism without the use of oxygen, resulting in the build-up of lactic acid in the body. Patients with acute respiratory problems on top of already existing chronic obstructive pulmonary disease will have high levels of lactic acid, and given more oxygen, they will for a short time produce a large amount of carbon dioxide. This will have to be exhaled which will dilute the oxygen in the incoming air, a phenomenon known as *diffusion hypoxia*.[22]

There can be little doubt that Haldane would have argued, based on his experience as an experimental subject, that these patients *desperately* need oxygen because, even though it may temporarily increase the level of carbon dioxide in the blood, without sufficient oxygen everything undoubtedly fails. Obviously, lack of oxygen will cause breathing to stop, as it does in all of us eventually. However, carbon dioxide in high concentrations is also a poison. In 1905, Haldane was asked by the Admiralty to investigate unexplained loss of consciousness in deep sea divers. The traditional helmet used required a constant supply of compressed air piped from the surface provided by hand-driven pumps. When divers worked harder there was ample oxygen in the air they were supplied, but the exhaled carbon dioxide accumulated in the helmet. The divers often experienced hallucinations and some lost consciousness, although they almost always recovered. Haldane, again experimenting on himself, was able to determine the flow rate through the helmet necessary to prevent the build-up of carbon dioxide and it is in the Admiralty report.[4] In the 1970s a North Sea diver, who was using equipment designed to reclaim and recycle the expensive helium and oxygen mixtures used for deep diving, attempted to breathe on open circuit. Unfortunately, he failed to open both of the necessary valves, and was forced to re-breathe the very small volume of gas contained in his helmet. This meant that the carbon dioxide quickly accumulated, causing a dramatic acceleration in his breathing rate. As with the hard hat divers Haldane had investigated, despite having plenty of oxygen in his breathing mixture, he stopped breathing. Fortunately, at this point he was expertly rescued back into the clean atmosphere of the diving bell by the bellman who was the standby diver. Once in the safety of the bell, the bellman removed the diver's helmet and he rapidly recovered. Within minutes, he was talking normally to the supervisor via the communications system. Carbon dioxide is certainly poisonous and *very* high levels will actually stop breathing. So this is yet another paradox: Both lack of carbon dioxide and too much carbon dioxide in the blood may stop breathing. Life is not simple!

As long as doctors continue to rely on poor quality clinical studies of the use of oxygen in patients with COPD, the controversy about oxygen supplementation will never be resolved. It is a perfect example of the need for science, that is, measurement, not double-blind controlled trials, and they have already been made in a group of COPD patients by French doctors in the 1980s.[23,24] It is notable that this work is referenced, but not discussed, in the 2008 BTS guideline. The measurements were made in COPD patients with severe breathing problems given supplementary oxygen, and they showed that the oft-quoted reduction of breathing was only present for a few breaths and in only in half of the group. It is, of course, easy to provide assistance with breathing. The studies were reviewed in an article in *Intensive Care World* as long ago as 1987 by

Drs. Schmidt and Hall,[25] two American physicians working in New Jersey, who concluded:

The purportedly devastating hypoventilation (reduction of breathing) after oxygen is, in fact, trivial and of no demonstrated relevance.

Nevertheless, what is highly relevant and certainly not trivial is failing to give sufficient oxygen to patients who desperately need it to survive. Schmidt and Hall recognised this, pointing out that the most severely affected patients given oxygen may get worse anyway. They continued with this dramatic statement of the obvious:

Oxygen is good and necessary, particularly in incipient ventilatory failure, (i.e. when patients are not breathing properly), not a treacherous commodity to be sparingly meted out.

A decade later, in an editorial in *Critical Care Medicine* entitled "Debunking Myths of Chronic Obstructive Lung Disease," Dr. John Hoyt drew attention to the matter again in no uncertain terms.[26]

There are examples of mythology that float about in the atmosphere of medical information that desperately need to be debunked because they influence the care of patients. One sample of medical mythology is the commonly told story that the administration of oxygen to a patient with chronic obstructive lung disease will shut down the patient's hypoxic respiratory drive and lead to apnea, cardio respiratory arrest, and the subsequent death of the patient.

Curiously, Dr. Hoyt does not appear to be aware of the historical background to the COPD controversy.

It is not clear where this fallacious information comes from, but it seems to enter the medical information database at an early age, at the medical student or resident level, almost like a computer virus corrupting the appropriate function of the equipment. In addition, this myth becomes very difficult to extinguish during the career of the physician, even with clear factual information of long standing. The danger here is that this medical mythology will inappropriately influence treatment decisions in patients.

The editorial was about an article in the same journal which had shown that giving oxygen to some COPD patients during an acute attack changed the matching between gas movement and blood flow in the lungs, which is known as a *ventilation/perfusion* mismatch. Uniquely, the blood vessels of the lungs actually constrict in response to lack of oxygen. If this constriction is released by giving more oxygen, it may cause the diversion of blood through the lung to areas which are not being ventilated with air. There is another problem: These patients adjust to a higher level of carbon dioxide, and the kidney retains the bicarbonate ion to buffer the acidity of blood caused by the dissociation of carbon dioxide into carbonic acid. When these patients have an acute respiratory problem, such as infection, and are given oxygen, the metabolism of the high level of accumulated lactic acid is likely to liberate a large volume of carbon dioxide and this has to be exhaled impeding the incoming oxygen in the airways. This phenomenon is better known when nitrous oxide is used for anaesthesia. On completing an operation anaesthesia needs to be reversed and the body burden of nitrous oxide has to be exhaled. If patients are left to breathe air they will suffer from lack of oxygen again due to diffusion hypoxia.[22] It is one of the reasons patients are given 100% oxygen to breathe after being given a general anaesthetic. Unfortunately, oxygen is still being withheld from patients with acute exacerbations associated with COPD: Campbell's long standing crusade and the unthinking acceptance by the rest of the profession has meant that thousands of patients have suffered needlessly.

The physicist Edward Teller, who was a patient of Dr. Richard Neubauer, had a Vickers clamshell chamber installed in his home to continue his rehabilitation after a stroke. He enquired if hyperbaric oxygen treatment could possibly be of value to his wife, Mici, who had emphysema and COPD after smoking for many years. In a letter, published in the *Journal of American Physicians* in 2003,[27] he wrote:

> *A totally unexplored area with which I have personal experience requires extensive investigation. This is the application of hyperbaric oxygenation in chronic obstructive pulmonary disease. My wife of many years suffered from this, and when the chamber was installed in my home, she was bedridden and severely emaciated. Her pulmonologist expected her to die within two months. Drs. Richard Neubauer and William Maxfield suggested hyperbaric oxygenation at very low pressures of 1.1–1.25 ATA for 20 minutes twice a day. This was indeed helpful, Mici became more alert, began to gain weight, and no longer needed constant supplemental oxygen, although she did use oxygen at night. The pressure was gradually increased to 1.35 ATA for 40 minutes twice a day. Mici gained 35 pounds and became bright, alert, and ambulatory. If the technician missed a single treatment, she would deteriorate. She had five wonderful unexpected years. One hopes that home chambers may become readily available.*
>
> *I also wish to comment on the overwhelming evidence of the effectiveness of hyperbaric oxygenation in cerebral palsy and the brain-injured child.*

Reproducibility of results from around the world is compelling. Although double-blind cross-over controlled studies are the standard of the scientific community, effectiveness has been demonstrated by Dr. Neubauer and a number of others, using each patient as his own control, and documented by sequential functional brain imaging. Experience is such that a double-blind study may be immoral.

In the long-term history of hyperbaric oxygenation, many of the problems have resulted from inappropriate pressures and treatment protocols. The proper dose in many conditions has not been fully ascertained and may vary as does insulin dose in a diabetic. I feel that the lower-pressure protocol and use of functional brain imaging will eventually make hyperbaric oxygenation a standard treatment.

A commentary in the *Lancet* in 1995[28] asked, "Why Do Patients with Emphysema Lose Weight?" It is simple; they are hypoxic and will also suffer from chronic low grade inflammation. Those who live at very high altitude suffer the same problems and it is known as Monge's disease.[29] Not surprisingly, a controlled study of patients with breathing problems from advanced cancer has shown that giving oxygen administration relieves breathlessness.[30]

Surprisingly, despite their bold attempt to educate colleagues and debunk the dangerous myth that often prevents sufficient oxygen being given to COPD patients, Schmidt and Hall actually stated that they were not advocating any great change in practice! The reason is abundantly clear in their paper and centres on the critical failure to understand the importance of the concentration of *dissolved* oxygen in the plasma. They stated that "All physicians make *haemoglobin saturation* a treatment goal." Indeed, the argument is regularly used by doctors to deter patients from accessing more oxygen. One patient in the UK who attended her family doctor to discuss hyperbaric oxygen treatment had her haemoglobin saturation measured—it was 99%. The doctor reassured her that her oxygen level was normal and, being so close to 100%, could not be improved. Of course, her blood levels were normal, but this does not mean that the level of oxygen in her tissues was normal. This starkly illustrates why those who advocate using high levels of oxygen in treatment face such enormous difficulties.

Haemoglobin oxygen saturation, which determines the redness of blood again, in effect, it has become a *clinical constant*, not least because it is easy to measure using a simple light device called an oximeter. However, many doctors remain blissfully unaware that the redness of blood can be produced by the combination of haemoglobin to *methyl* groups derived from a wide number of drugs to form *methaemoglobin*. Most will remember that carbon monoxide also binds readily with haemoglobin, producing carboxyhaemoglobin. So, although the measurement of the redness of blood may not reflect the saturation of oxygen with haemoglobin, the problem does not even rate a mention in the 2008 BTS guideline on using oxygen.[20] Chemists would also point out the use of the term "saturation" applied to the combination of oxygen with haemoglobin is actually incorrect, and it certainly adds to an already confused situation. The guideline fails to acknowledge the importance of the oxygen transported dissolved in the plasma, simply stating that "Oxygen is transported in blood bound to haemoglobin." Although acknowledging that, "For critically ill patients, high concentration oxygen should be administered immediately," the requirement is only that it should only be prescribed "to achieve a target saturation of 94–98%."

Physicians can only be as effective as the information they are given, and this highlights the failure of proper scientific teaching in our medical schools. The author suspects that he would have failed his second professional examination in the 1960s for not stressing the importance of the transport of oxygen dissolved in the blood plasma. The BTS guideline admits the woeful ignorance about oxygen still present in medical practice:

> *Audits of oxygen use and oxygen prescription have shown consistently poor performance in many countries. One major problem is that health care professionals receive conflicting advice about oxygen use from different "experts" during their training and during their clinical careers, and many are confused about the entire area of oxygen prescription and use.*

We are not discussing something of questionable importance here—oxygen is central to our health. It is an incredible indictment of medical education in the twenty-first century that there such confusion reigns and the reader will surely understand the need for this book.

Haldane had demonstrated that lack of oxygen did not control the desire to breathe, and his experiments, both in his laboratory at Cherwell and on Pike's Peak, had shown the importance of the gas, especially to the function of the brain. He returned to England with speculation about the possibility of war with Germany rife. In February 1912, he accompanied his brother Richard, Lord Haldane, who represented the UK Cabinet, on a secret peace mission to Berlin to see the German Chancellor and the Kaiser—Wilhelm II, and the German hierarchy.[31] Hostilities were soon to follow and the lungs would become the target of a new and terrible weapon in what, regrettably, did not live up to the promise of being "the war to end all wars." The details in the next chapter illustrate the immense difference that giving a high level of oxygen can make to patients, especially with acute, severe lung disease.

CHAPTER 5
Oxygen Treatment: When Air is Not Enough

The living body is no machine, but an organism constantly tending to maintain or revert to the normal, and the respite afforded by such measures as the temporary administration of oxygen is not wasted, but utilised for recuperation.

John S. Haldane. *British Medical Journal*, 1917.

At 5:00 p.m. on April 22, 1915, the Germans changed the face of warfare by discharging the highly toxic gas chlorine from 6,000 high-pressure cylinders brought to the front at Ypres in Belgium. The greenish yellow cloud rolled into the trenches, disabling hundreds of unsuspecting soldiers; the gas caused extreme irritation of the eyes and convulsive coughing. The War Cabinet was immediately informed of the attack, and Lord Kitchener telephoned Haldane at his home in Oxford. Haldane packed his trusty Gladstone bag and boarded a train to London, heading for an emergency meeting at the War Office. The following day, he sailed across the channel to France accompanied by Professor Baker, a chemist from Imperial College, London. They attended post-mortem examinations of the soldiers and saw first hand, the dreadful effects that the chlorine had on the lungs. They found that the lungs were severely inflamed, and the air spaces full of fluid. The fluid came from the leakage of water and proteins from blood across the lung membrane. Thousands of men were to die from this dreadful form of chemical warfare, and many of the survivors were disabled, suffering permanent damage to their lungs. Haldane had a very personal interest in events at the front—his son Jack had volunteered for active service upon the outbreak of the war. Enlisting in the Black Watch, he was rapidly promoted to the rank of captain and served in the explosives unit. It was not long before a second gas was used at Ypres, mustard gas, which became known by the troops as "Yperite." British scientists soon produced it, but the politicians apparently rejected its use on ethical grounds, although they were prepared to allow the use of chlorine. Ironically, many years later Jack Haldane[1] claimed that Yperite was "the most humane weapon ever invented" because only 2.5% of the casualties died and 0.25% remained incapacitated. He contrasted these effects with those of high explosives and shrapnel, which kill or maim about half their casualties.

The first priority for Haldane, having seen for himself the devastating effects of inhaling chlorine, was to make protective masks. He returned to England and set about testing various devices by breathing different concentrations of chlorine himself in his laboratory at Cherwell. His second priority was to design equipment to give oxygen to treat victims of the gas attacks, as he realised that protection was of only limited use. Although the logic of this approach may seem inescapable, Haldane was certainly aware that breathing a high level of oxygen may itself be associated with inflammation of the lungs i.e. an objection to the use of oxygen treatment which is constantly raised today. After Joseph Priestley and his mouse, it was probably the balloonist Gaston Tissandier who was next to breathe pure, or nearly pure oxygen, and by the late 1800s oxygen was routinely used in balloon ascents to high altitude. At the outbreak of the WW1 in 1914, oxygen equipment had been introduced in some aircraft and, like the balloonists, the pilots also had to breathe oxygen from a tube. With the introduction of chemical warfare, oxygen breathing apparatus was needed on the ground. Haldane had already designed oxygen breathing equipment for workers employed in making munitions who were exposed to toxic gases in the factories, and he set about adapting the equipment for use on the battlefield. It is still not an easy matter to deliver pure, that is, 100% oxygen to patients and Haldane was to admit later; "Like many others I did not at first realise the practical difficulties of oxygen treatment." He designed the first tight-fitting oronasal mask to cover both the mouth and nose, and fitted it with a reservoir bag to allow the storage of sufficient oxygen for each breath.[2] Leonard Hill had constructed an improved oxygen delivery system in 1912 but it lacked the tight-fitting oronasal mask employed by Haldane. Nevertheless his report in the *British Medical Journal*[3] gives some remarkable case histories and confirms that we have made little progress in the last 100 years. In Haldane's apparatus, the oxygen was supplied by two small cylinders and a box provided convenient portability.

Haldane taught medical orderlies at the battlefront how to use the equipment, and a colleague later commented that nurses could be trained to use the equipment in just three minutes. This was the first time that pure oxygen was systematically used as a *treatment*, rather than simply as a supplement.

Haldane was actually convinced that the body had a way of actively transporting oxygen across the membrane of the lung. The theory, known as oxygen secretion, generated much controversy. Active transport has since been demonstrated in other processes in the body, for example, cells use energy to maintain different concentrations of sodium, potassium, and calcium ions across their boundary membranes and without these ion pumps, life would be impossible.

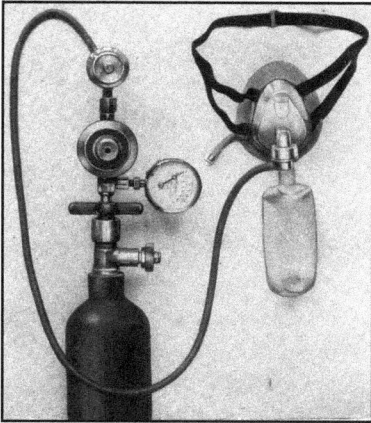

Figure 5.1:
Haldane's oxygen apparatus with its
tight-fitting oronasal mask.

Haldane knew that fish have developed oxygen secretion in the swim bladder; they are able to mysteriously concentrate the small amount of oxygen in the water—equilibrated with an oxygen pressure of a tenth of an atmosphere, to pressures of over a hundred atmospheres! They use the gas in the bladder to adjust their buoyancy. The mechanisms involved in concentrating oxygen in this way would, in the author's opinion justify a major research programme. However, human lungs do not secrete oxygen from the air into the blood; the gas is transferred by simple diffusion and not only can be transported from the lungs into blood, but also in the opposite direction when any pure gas other than oxygen is breathed. Many deaths occurred in deep diving when, by mistake, pure helium was supplied to divers instead of the appropriate mixture of helium with oxygen. A discovery made in the 1970s has added another twist to the story, which would have delighted Haldane; the lungs actually *do* produce substances which facilitate oxygen transport—they are known as surfactants. They work by keeping the gas side of the lung membrane dry, because water would be a significant barrier to the transport of oxygen. Credit for this discovery is due to the late Professor Brian Hills, who saw that their structure as zwitterions—double-charged molecules, is similar to the surfactants synthesised by the chemical industry to induce water repellency in fabrics.[4] Hills used the analogy of the fabrics used for camping tents to illustrate water repellency in his ground-breaking book, *The Biology of Surfactants*, published by Cambridge University Press in 1988.

A tent can, of course, be constructed out of totally waterproof material such as plastic, but would be very uncomfortable to use because, not being gas permeable, it would not exchange gases—it cannot "breathe." Tents are made of porous fabric and treated with surfactants to repel water, using just the same technology that keeps the gas surface of the lungs dry, allowing the ready transfer of oxygen and carbon dioxide across the membrane of the lungs. Unfortunately, many scientists cling to the old theory still published in every textbook of physiology—that the gas surface of the lung membrane is actually wet. It was postulated in the 1950s that the surfactants produced by cells in the lungs were dissolved in a liquid film on the gas surface of the alveoli to reduce surface tension, just like the detergents used in washing-up liquid. The claim was that lowering surface tension would reduce the work of breathing. However, the theory does not take into account the fact that *any* water on the gas side of the lung membrane would form a formidable barrier to the transport of oxygen. It would, therefore, limit the rate at which oxygen can be transferred by breathing into the blood flowing through the lungs and, as a consequence, severely restrict our ability to exercise.

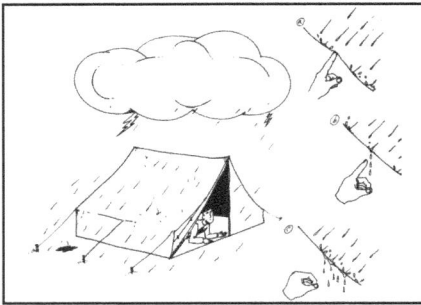

Figure 5.2:
The tent analogy—surfactants induce water repellency.
(Courtesy of the late Professor Brian Hills.)

Unlike the gills of fish, in which water flows continually past the blood vessels, and the through-flow system used by birds, our lungs use an inefficient push-pull system in which the air breathed in mixes with the gas being breathed out. The astonishing tubular network was shown in Chapter 2, Figure 2.1, where it was explained that the membrane of the air sacs, known as alveoli, have gas on one side and blood on the other. It is vital that the water in the blood flowing through the lungs does not escape through the lung membrane into the air spaces. When chlorine contaminates the air breathed, it forms hydrochloric acid in the lung passages which not only causes severe irritation to the air passages, it also destroys the surfactant protection of the lung membrane. The alveoli then flood with water from the blood passing through the lungs, a condition known as *pulmonary oedema*. As oxygen is poorly soluble in water, the transport of the gas from the airspaces into the blood flowing through the lungs would have been greatly reduced. And so, the soldiers at Ypres actually died from lack of oxygen. This cascade of events also occurs from the inhalation of a surprisingly small amount of water in drowning, which, even after a delay, may trigger fatal oedema of the lungs.

The administration of oxygen is the cornerstone of treatment for water-logged lungs, but it does more than simply increase the transport of oxygen, it actually assists in restoring the critical "barrier" function of the lung membrane, and so improves its own transport. The ability of the administration of a high level of oxygen to *initiate* healing was implicit in Haldane's article on the use of oxygen as a treatment in 1917. It was written after the success of his oxygen apparatus in treating victims of the German gas attacks, and answers criticisms that are still made of oxygen treatment today, indeed, it clearly indicates a duty of care.

> *From the foregoing remarks it seems clear that a physician ought to make every effort to avert the effects of want of oxygen or cut them short. It may be argued that such measures as the administration of oxygen are at the best only palliative and are of no real use, since they do not remove the cause of the pathological condition. As a physiologist I cannot for a moment agree with this reasoning.*

A colleague of Haldane's, Dr. C.G. Douglas, joined him at the front treating the casualties with the new oxygen apparatus. In 1932, at a meeting attended by Haldane, he spoke about his success in giving oxygen continuously for three days to a soldier[5] who "was already far gone." He found that the soldiers most severely affected by the gassing often "fought against the mask," clearly because covering the mouth and nose evokes a primitive, and powerful, reaction aimed at preventing suffocation. However, Douglas found that with persuasion and patience he was able to "secure its tolerance." He was dismayed to discover that some of the junior army doctors were limiting the use of oxygen to just five minutes in each hour, because the masks were prone to fill up with secretions brought up by coughing. He went to great lengths to ensure that they understood the need for a continuous supply of oxygen. The problem caused by secretions entering the masks led Captain Adrian Stokes of the Royal Army Medical Corps to develop the nasal prongs that are so popular today. Unfortunately, this was a backward step because air mixes with the oxygen and they only allow the oxygen level breathed to be increased from the 21% present in air to about 28% at a tolerable flow rate of about 4 litres a minute. Haldane had stressed the importance of using the tight-fitting mask he devised to deliver close to 100% oxygen to ensure the maximum concentration entered the airway and he would have been dismayed to find his concepts are still not understood today.

Modern perceptions of Haldane's contribution to the use of 100% oxygen in treatment are often very far off the mark. For example, in 1987, the group of Australian anaesthetists writing about oxygen therapy in the *Lancet*,[6] after raising the usual fears about oxygen's "toxicity," alleged that Haldane had "described a loose-fitting mask for oxygen delivery and emphasised the importance of keeping the inhaled oxygen concentration as low as possible." In fact, this is just the opposite of Haldane's advice—he was fully aware of the need to give as high a concentration to correct a sudden lack of oxygen— acute hypoxia, and he had also gone to great lengths to design the first tight-fitting oronasal mask. It is not a surprise to find that the authors of the article actually give the wrong reference in their paper. Haldane was aware that high levels of oxygen may eventually cause problems, but only advised loosening the mask when oxygen is administered over many days. One paragraph in his seminal paper in 1917[2] should feature in the training of *every* doctor, because it explains, simply and clearly, the reason why using oxygen as a treatment is so important. Haldane emphasised that lack of oxygen, the hypoxia that he refers to as "want of oxygen," may not only kill, it may *maim,* causing problems which sometimes develop after a delay.

> *The mistake is often made of not grasping the serious, widespread, and lasting effects caused by want of oxygen. Even when the want of oxygen is completely removed these effects remain.*

Haldane's development of the equipment needed to deliver 100% oxygen, as well as the clear reasoning for its use given in his paper, establishes him as the father of oxygen treatment. And, being involved in both diving and aviation, he was well aware of the importance of barometric pressure to the use of oxygen in medicine.

It is truly ironic that Haldane developed the first apparatus to deliver 100% oxygen *specifically* for the treatment of the lung inflammation caused by gas attacks, because the almost universal fear today is of oxygen being poisonous to the lungs. Indeed, most physicians have been thoroughly indoctrinated about pulmonary oxygen toxicity. What little research is undertaken today is usually done to support this assertion. For example, in 2005, a paper from prestigious institutions in the US and Germany,[7] after stating that giving oxygen is "life-saving," then alleges that it has dangerous side-effects in patients with lung inflammation. They tested their theory in a genetically modified mouse model in which severe inflammation had been induced, and used continuous exposures to 100% oxygen for 48-60 hours, which is far in excess of what is ever used clinically. Curiously, they observed that; "It remains to be determined, however, whether the much longer time course of the direct toxicity of 100% oxygen in healthy, non-inflamed lungs could be explained by the recruitment of immune cells." As will be seen, the recruitment of neutrophils, which of course are immune cells, is the key factor which has been overlooked. Their results fly in the face of vast clinical experience: The *British National Formulary* has for decades stated that "High concentration oxygen therapy is safe in pneumonia, pulmonary thrombo-embolism, pulmonary fibrosis, shock, severe trauma, sepsis, or anaphylaxis." In fact, it is *not safe to withhold it*, but the reader will be dismayed to find that in 2012 it was actually stated that there is little rational foundation for using oxygen in medical disease and anaesthesia.[8]

The first recorded use of pure oxygen in a pressure chamber was as a treatment for pneumonia which, of course, is associated with severe inflammation due to infection. The successful treatment was described in an editorial in the *Lancet* in 1887;[9] Don Francisco Valenzuela, a physician in Madrid, saved the life of a young man dying of pneumonia. Oxygen is probably the most widely prescribed agent in medical practice, but, as we have seen, the constant emphasis is to use as little as possible and only to ensure that the haemoglobin in red blood cells is carrying the maximum amount of oxygen. In other words, it is simply to ensure that blood is as red as possible.

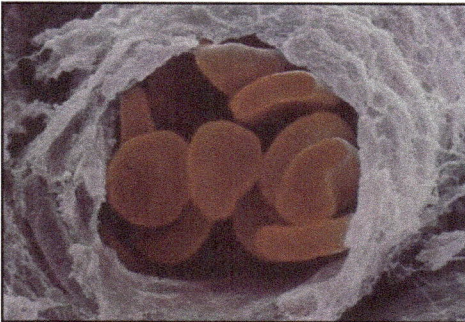

Figure 5.3:
Normal biconcave red blood cells in a small vein. The space around the cells would be occupied by plasma.

As a consequence of today's oxygen phobia, a continuous dribble of oxygen is now used for prolonged periods, often with a maximum level rarely above 35%, when what is needed is a much higher level of oxygen, but for just a short time. Ironically, this may mean using *less* oxygen in total, especially because when using nasal prongs or a loose-fitting mask, most of the gas cascades onto the patient's bed and the floor!

It is clear that the fears raised about oxygen must have some basis and it has been known for more than 100 years that if oxygen is breathed *continuously*, patients will eventually develop a dry cough and some discomfort in the centre of the chest, under the breast bone. Animal experiments have also shown that days of oxygen breathing may eventually cause fatal lung damage. Nevertheless, it is also well known that if nitrogen is introduced by using short breaks breathing air, the lung damage does not occur. This clearly indicates that oxygen is not a simple poison. In the 1930s, when oxygen began to be used more widely as a treatment and pure oxygen breathing was introduced for aircraft pilots and divers, proper data was urgently needed. Comprehensive experiments were undertaken during WW2 by Dr. Julius Comroe and his colleagues in the US using human volunteers.[10] Although their landmark paper was published in the *Journal of the American Medical Association* as long ago as 1945, it is rarely referenced and was not even mentioned in the 2008 BTS guideline.[11] A total of 90 healthy men between the ages of 19 and 31 participated in the experiments. Full face masks were used with the test group breathing 100% oxygen, and the controls breathing compressed air, although both groups were actually told that they were breathing pure oxygen. The protocol was rigorous; removal of the mask was not permitted; liquids and liquefied food were provided by tube. It came as a surprise that after a few hours *breathing either air or oxygen* the volunteers developed sore throats, dry eyes, and nasal congestion. Clearly, as both groups were affected, these effects cannot be due to so-called oxygen toxicity. It is most likely that these symptoms were due to the dryness of the gases, and humidifiers are now used when oxygen is given for long periods. However, and this is a critical observation, only the oxygen group complained of discomfort under the breast bone and, moreover, it developed in *all* the subjects by the end of a 24-hour period. It rapidly disappeared when oxygen breathing was stopped and normal air breathing was resumed, which is entirely consistent with the observation that intermittently breathing air can greatly prolong the time that oxygen could be breathed.

These experiments had clearly shown that 100% oxygen can be breathed continuously for 24 hours with only very minor symptoms, and it is likely that these would not occur if the oxygen was humidified. There is more recent evidence that is also rarely cited: In a study published in the *New England Journal of Medicine* in 1970, 20 of 40 patients after cardiac surgery received up to 42% oxygen, and 20 100% for at least 20 hours.[12] No differences were found in tests of lung function or in the clinical recovery. In a second study in the same issue of the journal, five patients with irreversible brain damage were given air to breathe and five 100% oxygen for a mean of 52 hours.[13] The oxygen group demonstrated the expected lung collapse known as "atelectasis," but at postmortem examination there were no differences in pathology between the two groups. Sadly, the conclusion of the authors has gone unheeded.

Fear of pulmonary oxygen toxicity should not prevent use of elevated inspired oxygen concentrations in critically ill patients requiring artificial ventilation.

It is perfectly obvious that if breathing high levels of oxygen posed a serious problem, these were just the patients that should have been affected. It is truly reprehensible that, despite an enormous amount of research spanning more than 150 years into the alleged toxicity of oxygen to the lungs, the sequence of events that begins with chest discomfort has not been properly explained. Oxygen is certainly *not* a poison in the conventional sense; a North Sea diver breathed oxygen for a short time at a depth of 80 metres of sea water (260 feet), when he was supplied with pure oxygen rather than a helium and oxygen mixture. This represents a total pressure of 9 ATA, a level *45 times* greater than breathing air at sea level, but it had no effect whatsoever on his lungs. In contrast, patients during anaesthesia and in hospital intensive care units may develop lung problems breathing little more than the normal percentage of oxygen in air.

Despite the lack of evidence, it is still assumed by many that the effects of oxygen on the lungs are due to the formation of the ever-fashionable free radicals and that they are produced directly from breathing a higher level of oxygen. This is despite good evidence having been available for many years showing that this is simply not true. Divers breathing compressed air may breathe levels of oxygen on deep dives well in excess of the concentration produced by 100% oxygen at normal sea level, but they do not develop lung absorption collapse, confirming that, when nitrogen is present, it splints the air sacs of the lungs. It is only possible to breathe a very high level of oxygen in the presence of nitrogen under *hyperbaric* conditions; that is, at a pressure greater than normal barometric pressure. In contrast, collapsed lung tissue is present in almost all anaesthetised patients given 100% oxygen, either when breathing spontaneously or being ventilated. Absorption collapse resolves if the level of oxygen breathed is lowered but if it is then increased again to 100%, atelectasis rapidly reappears.[14] There is also a clear correlation between the extent of atelectasis and the shunting of blood through the lungs in anaesthetised patients. Divers are, of course, healthy, and breathe more deeply than seriously ill patients.

However, a truly dramatic discovery published in 1998[15] has unravelled the mystery and it can finally end years of controversy. Ironically, in view of the 2005 paper[7] cited above, it was made in a mouse model. Injecting a monoclonal antibody known as CD40-CD40 can allow a high level of oxygen to be breathed *indefinitely*, and the antibody can even reverse early damage. Given the *immense* importance of this finding, the authors probably expected some publicity for their discovery, especially as the work was undertaken in the prestigious University of Rochester School of Medicine and Dentistry in New York. It certainly deserved coverage in a widely read journal like the *Lancet* or the *New England Journal of Medicine*, but there appears to have been no comment in *any* other journal. The finding could well be of commercial importance, although a massive marketing campaign would be needed to change the prevailing medical mind set about oxygen. Given this problem, it would probably not make commercial sense to risk the investment needed.

But why would oxygen, which is able to quell inflammation, as Haldane demonstrated in treating the soldiers gassed in WW1, appear to cause it in the lungs? The answer can be provided from already well-known data and it involves neutrophils, the white blood cells also referred to as granulocytes, and the oxygen free radicals they produce. What follows is an example of Occam's razor; that is, finding a single explanation to link what appears to be a jumbled assortment of facts. The starting point is a property unique to oxygen; it can disappear from the gas spaces of the lungs simply because it is used up in metabolism. It appears that the absorption collapse associated with oxygen breathing leads to the white blood cells (neutrophils) being attracted to the area. They cause damage to the capillaries by releasing free radicals, as they are programmed to do in fighting infection.

No mechanism has actually been identified to explain the "toxic" factor in so-called oxygen "poisoning" and evidence has been overlooked that atelectasis may trigger the events that lead to lung damage from breathing high levels of oxygen. The most important fact in support of this concept is that the first changes after prolonged oxygen breathing do not involve the cells on the gas side of the lungs, they begin in the cells of the capillaries in the lungs, and so involve the cells of the capillary lining—the *endothelium*. The epithelial cells on the gas side of the lung membrane are obviously exposed to a higher oxygen level than any other tissue in the body simply because they meet the gas being breathed. Remarkably, epithelial cells in the swim bladders of fish living at extreme depths can tolerate contact with oxygen at pressures of hundreds of atmospheres. In order to follow the argument that *molecular* oxygen is not directly poisonous to the lungs, it is first necessary to understand the basic physiology of breathing.

Our total lung capacity, that is the maximum quantity of air we can breathe in, is about 4.5 litres for the average male, with women averaging about 3.5 litres. Breathing at rest, we do not use this full capacity, and only move about half a litre of gas with each breath. This expands the areas of the lungs closest to the main bronchi so other areas are less well ventilated. The gas spaces of our lungs contain some nitrogen derived, of course, from the nitrogen in the air we breathe. On changing to breathing pure oxygen, the nitrogen is slowly replaced by oxygen. Although it does not react chemically in the body, nitrogen has a very important role. As discussed, anaesthetists often refer to it as a "splint" propping the airways open. If oxygen breathing is continued over a period of a few hours, almost all the nitrogen in the lungs and much of that dissolved in the body tissues is eventually breathed out. The dissolved nitrogen is transported in blood from the tissues to the lungs where it comes out of solution, becoming a gas in the alveoli, and is then exhaled. The oxygen that accumulates in poorly ventilated areas of the lungs disappears, most being transferred into the blood flowing through the lung capillaries, although some will be metabolised by the cells of the lung itself to produce carbon dioxide.

Because of these effects, the volume of oxygen contained in the static areas of the lungs is reduced, which leads to the collapse of groups of alveoli, that is, atelectasis. Chest X-rays actually taken in human experiments have shown that this usually happens in the lower lobes of the lung, just above the diaphragm. Despite the lower lobes being affected, it is associated with the well-recognised first symptom of so-called lung oxygen toxicity—discomfort under the breastbone, usually known medically as substernal pain. The longer oxygen is breathed, the greater the effect, and eventually damage occurs. Many experiments have shown the resulting inflammation in animal models. The following blocked section discusses the evidence implicating absorption collapse and the inflammation derived from free radical release by neutrophils in the lung damage associated with continuous oxygen breathing. The irony is that it is not the molecular oxygen we breathe that is toxic; the effects of prolonged oxygen breathing are actually due to inflammation caused by *neutrophils* attracted to the collapsed areas of lung which then release free radicals.

Human experiments into absorption collapse of the lung, which were conducted as part of an anaesthetic research programme in 1965,[16] can provide a logical explanation of the effects of pure oxygen on the lungs. It was found that if a subject forcibly exhaled as much of the air in the lungs as possible and then breathed from this starting point, rather than allowing the chest to normally re-inflate, collapse of the alveoli would occur in several minutes and the subjects developed pain under the sternum. The lung collapse was clearly seen on a chest X-ray. The experiment was repeated in one subject breathing 100% oxygen rather than air for just two five-minute periods. After the expected initial rise in the blood oxygen level to 676 mm Hg, by the end of the second period it had fallen dramatically to 433 mm Hg. A chest X-ray showed severe collapse at the lung bases with elevation of the diaphragm. Astonishingly, it was found that the total lung capacity had actually fallen by 30%.

Despite his chest discomfort, the subject walked over a mile in the four hours following the experiment, although his inability to take a deep breath actually lasted for 12 hours. Because of these worrisome findings, the oxygen experiments were discontinued.

In 1978 the experiments were resumed by the same investigators, and the six subjects who volunteered were all doctors.[17] As in the case of one of the subjects in the 1965 experiments, oxygen instead of air was breathed, again with the lungs at residual volume and, because it was known that it would be uncomfortable, the experiments were limited to a duration of only five minutes. There were no changes at five minutes in two subjects, but the remaining four developed substernal pain which, as in the subject in the previous experiment, *prevented them taking a deep breath*. They also had decreased lung capacity on exhalation, a reduction in the level of oxygen in the blood, and there was the same evidence of lung collapse on their chest X-rays. This is highly relevant to the tests developed at the University of Pennsylvania used to determine the effects of oxygen on the lungs in diving.[18]

The explanation is that breathing 100% oxygen prior to reaching residual volume and small airways obstruction, alveoli will contain only oxygen, carbon dioxide, and water vapour. The combined tension of the carbon dioxide and water will be less than 100 mm Hg, and so at a normal atmospheric pressure of 760 mm Hg, the alveolar pO_2 will be about 660 mm Hg when the pO_2 of the mixed venous blood passing through the lungs is less than 50 mm Hg. The alveolar/mixed venous pO_2 gradient will therefore be over 600 mm Hg, or about 80% of an atmosphere. This results in a rapid transfer of oxygen and atelectasis: The absorption collapse, occurring in the absence of nitrogen which acts as a "splint" to maintain inflation. It is, therefore, clear that when areas of the lungs collapse because the blood flow through the affected area has transported the oxygen away, paradoxically, the local tissue becomes hypoxic. This, as we have already seen, attracts white blood cells, which stick to the lining cells of the capillaries. They then migrate into the tissues causing inflammation by releasing free radicals, as they are programmed to do normally in fighting infection. The role of neutrophils in producing the effects seen with oxygen breathing has been demonstrated in an animal model.[19] These experiments have confirmed that neutrophils are recruited to the lungs after hours of oxygen breathing. Further studies were then undertaken in which animals' neutrophils were depleted using a toxic agent, and it was found that oxygen breathing could be tolerated for 72 hours.[20] The ventilator breathing "pattern" used also influences the degree of lung collapse.[21]

Neutrophils, attracted to an area of atelectasis, cause damage to the air/blood barrier formed by the lung membrane at alveolar level, and this allows plasma to leak from the blood flowing through the lungs into the air spaces. If oxygen breathing is continued, death eventually occurs from lack of oxygen associated with pulmonary oedema—in effect from internal drowning. This phenomenon does not actually pose a problem in clinical hyperbaric oxygen treatment, because the time breathing oxygen is well below the time for these problems to occur. For example, breathing pure oxygen at 2 ATA, the time to the development of pulmonary problems can be extended if oxygen breathing is interrupted for short periods. The problems seen in current practice are being caused by using a low dose of oxygen over an extended period. The key message of this text is that high levels of oxygen can be effective when given for short periods.

Further supporting evidence that can assist in explaining the sequence of events in the lungs can be found in studies undertaken of the effects of oxygen on the ear. Comroe and his colleagues[10] called it "aural" atelectasis in their paper describing the effects of continuous oxygen breathing. The effect is regularly experienced by military divers using closed circuit oxygen breathing equipment, and it is mentioned in the diving manuals of the US Navy. When oxygen replaces the air in the middle ear cavity, it is absorbed just as it is in causing absorption collapse in the lungs. This reduces the volume of gas held in the ear cavity, causing the ear drum to be drawn inwards; the bone of the skull, of course, holds the cavity open. Sometimes this causes mild deafness, which can be simply relieved by opening the eustachian tube to equalise the pressure, for example, by swallowing. This allows air back into the middle ear and is just the same action that is needed to equalise middle ear pressure in an aircraft descending to land. However, with oxygen breathing, inflammation may complicate matters just as it does in the lungs because it attracts neutrophils and they release free radicals. Sometimes the middle ear appears as a bright area on MRI of the head in patients undergoing regular sessions of hyperbaric oxygen treatment. This indicates that some local inflammation is present, but it is very rare for it to cause any symptoms. There is also growing recognition of atelectasis because it can be readily seen on CT imaging of the chest.

It appears, therefore, likely that what is loosely termed pulmonary oxygen toxicity is *not* due to a direct action of oxygen on the lining cells of the airways and the cells on the gas side of the lung membrane, it is produced by neutrophils attaching to the lining of the capillaries in the lungs and causing damage by releasing free radicals. Oxygen free radicals are involved, but *not* as the result of a direct attack from breathing a high level of oxygen. Again, as

Fridovich had emphasised,[22] molecular oxygen itself is not toxic, indeed he emphasises that it is surprisingly unreactive. The involvement of neutrophils in causing the pathology is strongly supported by the protection given by the injection of CD40-CD40 monoclonal antibody, which, as discussed, can allow pure oxygen to be breathed indefinitely, and even lead to a reversal of the early pathology.

There may be a way to determine if atelectasis is at the root of the problem associated with prolonged oxygen breathing and an alternative treatment to using a monoclonal antibody. In infants born prematurely, the lungs often do not expand properly because they are not fully developed. It is now standard practice to blow an aerosol of lung *surfactant* into the airway. The results are usually dramatic: The infant turns from blue to pink within minutes as oxygen transport into the body greatly improves. Could blowing surfactant into lungs affected by prolonged oxygen breathing reverse atelectasis and the associated capillary changes? If this is the case, then the technique may prove invaluable by allowing greater use of oxygen in intensive care patients. As the treatment has proved to be safe in the newborn, it can certainly be used with confidence in adults; in fact, it has been investigated as a treatment for asthma, based on the ideas of the late Professor Brian Hills.

Despite massive funding, the research undertaken into the effects of oxygen in aerospace and diving medicine has only served to muddy the waters. By the 1950s, the demand for diving in the exploration for oil and gas in the Gulf of Mexico began to increase dramatically and the laboratory in the University of Pennsylvania undertook studies of oxygen breathing under hyperbaric conditions using volunteers.[18] The lung function tests used before and after the periods of oxygen breathing required the subjects to take a full breath, and then exhale forcefully into a machine. This recorded both the volume of gas exhaled in one second and the total volume exhaled. It was found that both figures were reduced when oxygen was breathed. However, this is perfectly understandable. It is explained by the experiments discussed above: The discomfort under the sternum limits the depth of a breath taken, and also the rate at which gas is exhaled in the tests, but the reduction is *not* due to the direct action of oxygen poisoning the lungs; it is due to atelectasis. By the 1970s, the US Navy wanted a guide to oxygen exposures for diving. An arbitrary unit pulmonary toxicity dose (UPTD) was devised in which breathing 100% oxygen at a pressure of 1 atmosphere for one minute was assigned a value of 1 unit. A limit was suggested for a single oxygen exposure of 615 units, but without any indication of the time to recovery; that is, when the count subsequently returned to zero. In fact, the clinical studies already discussed have shown that the UPTD is not a valid measurement. In actual practice and certainly in the personal experience of the author from measurements in experimental diving trials, the method simply does not work. Unfortunately, in 1972, the US Navy Experimental Diving Unit, then located in the Washington Navy Yard, issued an internal report[23] that was soon appropriated by the commercial diving industry and led to the incorporation of the procedure into diving manuals and protocols. It is of note that no research group has ever been able to repeat the University of Pennsylvania results, and the UPTD has never been mentioned in *any* of the diving manuals subsequently published by the US Navy or the Royal Navy.

It is vital to stress at this point that, regardless of these details, the problem referred to as lung or pulmonary oxygen toxicity is easily avoided by using well-established protocols developed over many years for hyperbaric oxygen treatment, because they use intermittent exposures to high levels of the gas. Although the final event in the poisoning of the lung from the prolonged use of oxygen is leakage of fluid into the air spaces, or lung oedema, Haldane demonstrated that this does not prevent oxygen being used as a treatment when lung oedema is present due to other causes. He showed conclusively that exposure to chlorine or mustard gas can be treated by breathing high levels of oxygen. Conversely, lung oedema is *always* associated with hypoxia, especially in fire victims with smoke inhalation. Smoke is a powerful irritant because it contains particulates and also carbon monoxide, which itself causes hypoxia in cells by blocking the enzymes that use oxygen. The combustion of plastics may release other toxic gases, like isocyanates and hydrogen cyanide. In such patients, the high levels of oxygen possible under hyperbaric conditions can mean the difference between life and death. The treatment was adopted as the standard of care in the city of Milwaukee where the late Dr. Eric Kindwall, a former US Navy submarine medical officer, championed the use of hyperbaric treatment for the fire fighters of the city. Unfortunately, many physicians involved in intensive care units still oppose the use of hyperbaric oxygen treatment in patients with smoke inhalation, alleging that it will exacerbate free radical damage in the inflamed lungs although this has been comprehensively rebutted.[24] Nevertheless, Haldane had shown by treating the victims of gas attacks in WW1 that this is not the case; paradoxically, correcting lack of oxygen is essential to reducing inflammation and this includes the lungs.

There is a growing recognition that many modern innovations in intensive care are not beneficial—they are causing harm. It is a very difficult area to study, and the public needs to be made aware of the emotional cost to medical and nursing staff caring for acutely ill patients. The problems raised by current strategies were discussed in a remarkably frank interview with Dr. Mervyn Singer, a consultant in University College London by the journalist Dan Jones. It was published in *New Scientist* in 2010[25] and included the appropriate title "Heal Thyself." It featured a paper co-authored by Dr. Singer entitled "Treating Critical Illness: The Importance of First Doing No Harm," which was published in 2005.[26] It argued that the mortality of soldiers with battlefield trauma in the nineteenth century was actually lower than for patients with similar injuries today. He also points out the astonishing lack of evidence to support many accepted acute interventions. In the *New Scientist* article, Singer is quoted as saying that "Virtually all the advances in intensive care in the past 10 years have involved *doing less* to the patient," and "Patients often survive in spite of medical interventions rather than because of them." He is not alone; others feel that little progress has been made in the last 40 years. Singer's logical argument is that the body is adapted to deal with critical illness and modern medicine might be interfering with natural protective mechanisms. It is stressed that a local immune response can lead to the systemic inflammatory response syndrome (SIRS) mentioned in Chapter 1 and, if this is not controlled, to multi-organ failure—the *leading* cause of death in critically ill patients. Dr. Singer and his colleagues submitted two papers on a rat model demonstrating the critical importance of oxygen levels to survival to a meeting of the International Society on Oxygen Transport to Tissue (www.isott.org), held in Scotland in 1996. Founded by scientists interested in measuring tissue oxygen levels in 1973, sadly, this organisation has had little impact on clinical practice.

Prolonged inflammation and the associated hypoxia may lead to mitochondrial damage and programmed cell death; hence, the need to establish normal metabolism which, of course, requires sufficient oxygen to be available. However, there is no mention in the article of the critical role of oxygen in the control of inflammation, the importance of the hypoxia-inducible factor proteins or that oxygen is the ultimate anti-inflammatory agent. But there is more; oxygen is the antibiotic of the body and so lack of oxygen also impairs the ability of white blood cells to deal with infection. This information is not taught in our medical schools but now, faced with antibiotic resistance, it will soon be critical. It was the subject of two seminal articles by Bernard M. Babior, published by the *New England Journal of Medicine* in 1978.[27,28]

One almost universal aspect of current practice was singled out for criticism by Singer: "We haven't evolved to cope with being sedated, put on a ventilator and pumped full of drugs." He is correct. Patients are sedated to allow a tube to be placed in the windpipe and the use of a ventilator. The tube secures the airway, but the sedative drugs used do not just reduce the level of consciousness—they also suppress the patient's metabolism. The lung is certainly not adapted to cope with positive-pressure ventilation, and there is growing awareness that ventilation itself causes lung damage and inflammation. As described in Chapter 2, in normal breathing the ingress of air into the lungs follows the creation of a negative pressure within the chest. This can actually be replicated by the external device known as an iron lung and a patient can be safely ventilated using an iron lung without a tube in their throat for many years. However, the method is cumbersome and no longer in fashion.

The three recognised complications of positive-pressure ventilation relate to traumatic injury to the delicate fabric of the lungs. They are the lung collapse known as pneumothorax, the entry of gas into the middle of the chest known as mediastinal emphysema, and air embolism where gas bubbles are forced into the bloodstream through tears in the blood vessels in the lungs. All of these are well-recognised complications of abrupt pressure changes in divers, where they are macroscopic injuries from large changes in pressure. However, recent research has shown that positive-pressure ventilation causes micro trauma and inflammation in the lungs, and there is growing recognition of the problem clinically. In fact, it has been argued that many of the lung problems commonly attributed to oxygen are more likely to be due to damage from mechanical ventilation.[29] It is disturbing that such a universally-used technique may contribute to a poor outcome in some intensive care patients and this featured in an eight-page article entitled "Ventilator Assisted Lung Injury" in the *Lancet* in 2005.[30] Is it possible that it is better to leave patients breathing on their own? There is good evidence that in many cases, it would with the patient given a higher level of oxygen and this will be discussed later. The benefits from a small increase in dissolved oxygen to a biological system are demonstrated convincingly by increasing the oxygen content of polluted lakes. The British Oxygen Company developed this technology many years ago. Their advertisement taken from a British Airways in-flight magazine is reproduced in Figure 5.4 and flying features in the next chapter.

The intrepid pioneers Glaisher and Coxwell had experienced the dramatic effects of lack of oxygen on the brain first-hand when they ascended to the height of Everest over Wolverhampton in 1862. Little did they realise what the future held for flying machines and how they would change the course of history. There are many relevant lessons to be learned from the extensive use of oxygen in aviation and in diving and, as we shall see, Haldane made pivotal contributions to both fields.

SINCE WE'VE BEEN DUMPIN
INTO THIS LAKE, IT'S (

First, the lake was black. Then it turned a murky brown.

Then green. Then almost overnight, a vivid shade of pink.

Yes, at The BOC Group we have a product which we dump

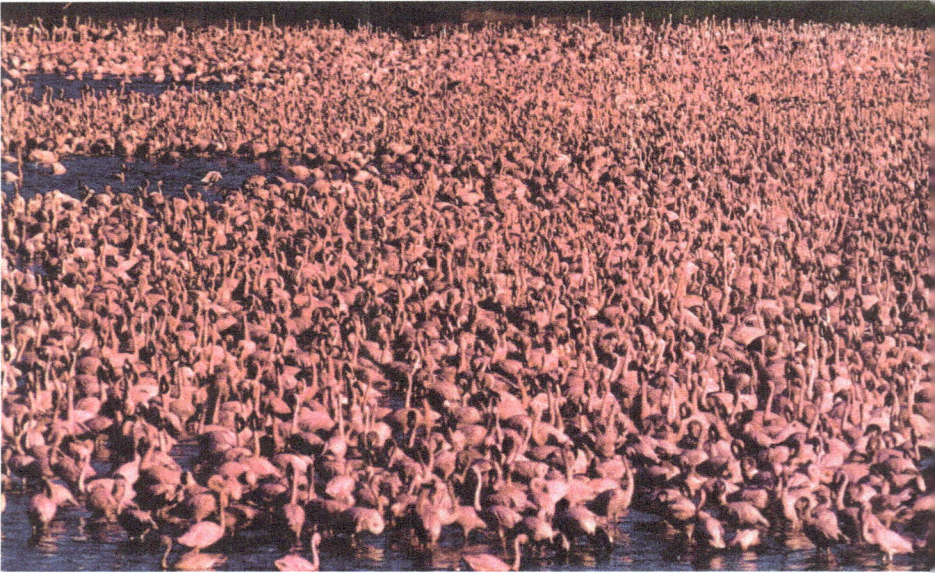

into rivers, lakes and seas all over the world. And just look

at the effect it can have on the environment.

A lake in Africa, polluted and devoid of life for 30 years, is

now a haven for flamingoes. Fish can now live in Hong Kong's

Kowloon Harbour. And we've even helped to revive the Thames.

Figure 5.4:
Oxygen Treatment: When Air is Not Enough. The importance of oxygen to life is vividly
illustrated in this advertisement by the BOC Group of the dramatic benefit of increasing the
dissolved oxygen in a lake devoid of life in Africa.

...G ONE OF OUR PRODUCTS ...NE A FUNNY COLOUR.

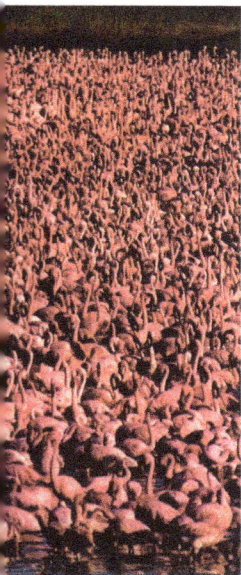

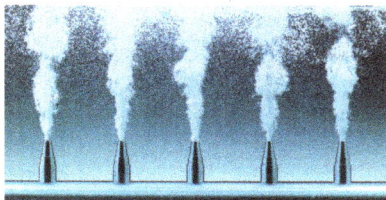

(Reproduced with permission from BOC Ltd.)

CHAPTER 6
Taking to the Air

Heavier-than-air flying machines are impossible.

William Thomson, Lord Kelvin, 1824–1907

Aircraft have arguably had a greater impact on our lives than any other invention and there are few places in the world that the vapour trail of a jet cannot be seen making its contribution to global warming but few would connect the technology involved with the care of patients. The scale of airline operations is staggering; it is said that the number of passengers flights over a three year period is equivalent to the population of the earth, which is now over seven billion. As we have seen, the hot air and hydrogen balloons invented in the eighteenth century began the conquest of the air. They were the forerunners of airships and appeared to be set for a bright future until the Zeppelin *Hindenburg* disaster in 1937. The airship caught fire coming into dock at Lakehurst, New Jersey on its tenth Atlantic crossing. The escaping hydrogen burned vigorously and 36 of the 92 people on board were killed. The tragedy signalled the end of the use of hydrogen for airships, but they are actually slow and cumbersome and it was the development of fixed wing aircraft that paved the way for today's aviation industry. The Wright brothers were the first to succeed in controlled powered flight, taking to the air near Kitty Hawk, North Carolina on December 17, 1903. Their longest flight on the day was just 852 feet. The military soon recognised the potential for aircraft to be used in warfare and by 1908, Orville Wright had begun trials with the US Army at Fort Myers. It appears to have been the Turks who were the first to use aircraft offensively. They created terror in their war with Greece by dropping hand grenades on their troops, and when they ran out of grenades they apparently used melons to similar effect. The outbreak of the WW1 in 1914 saw aircraft in use as spotter planes for artillery fire, but they were soon fitted with guns and equipped to carry bombs.

The engines of early aircraft were not sufficiently powerful to allow them to fly much above 10,000 feet, but with improvements in engine performance during the Great War, they soon became capable of exceeding 15,000 feet. As already discussed, with increasing altitude the barometric pressure falls and so, although the percentage of oxygen remains the same at about 21%, the *concentration* of the gas falls as the air becomes thinner. At an altitude of 17,900 feet the air pressure is half the value at sea level and, as a consequence, engine power is greatly reduced as is the efficiency of a propeller. In 1917, the British ace Major James McCudden, VC, who had been an engineer before he trained as a pilot, fitted the engine of his Sopwith SE5a fighter with a supercharger. This allowed him to achieve altitudes as high as 21,000 feet and so gain a considerable advantage in aerial combat; he achieved 57 kills. Superchargers are simply pumps which compress the air and so increase the concentration of oxygen to be delivered to an engine. This, of course, means that fuel can be burnt more efficiently to increase the power output.

However, it was obviously not possible to supercharge the air to the pilots, because breathing air at a higher pressure than the surroundings would tear the lungs, causing the same problems encountered in diving and positive-pressure ventilation in anaesthesia. The only alternative possible at the time was to give pilots more oxygen to breathe, and it was the Germans who were the first to introduce oxygen breathing equipment in aircraft. Paul Bert's suggestion[1] that it is the part of the pressure exerted by oxygen that is important, the gas partial pressure, had apparently created a storm of controversy among physiologists in the 1870s, despite being based on Dalton's law. However, the Austrian von Schrötter and Berson in Germany understood the concept well and collaborated to make serviceable oxygen equipment that was first used for high altitude balloon ascents between 1894 and 1901. The equipment, using flasks of liquid oxygen, was installed in a few German military aircraft during WW1. By this time, Haldane, working with Robert Davis of the Siebe Gorman Company at their Westminster Bridge works, had also designed oxygen equipment for British warplanes. They used either flasks of liquid oxygen, or high pressure oxygen cylinders. In the event, very few aircraft of either side were equipped with oxygen breathing apparatus but the principle had been proven; to achieve high altitudes in aircraft more oxygen was needed for the engines and for the pilots.

During WW1 a curious phenomenon had been found to affect pilots undertaking regular flights which rendered them temporarily or, sometimes, permanently unable to continue flying duties. It was recognised that their problems in some way related to altitude, but lack of oxygen was not thought to be responsible. Perhaps in view of the stresses involved in aerial warfare, this is understandable and it must also be remembered that high altitude mountaineering was in its infancy. Few people had Haldane's appreciation of the ill effects and symptoms associated with lack of oxygen. The pilots who were flying on a daily basis found that the altitude they were able to reach and function properly was successively reduced week by week. They experienced headaches with excessive fatigue and the symptoms often persisted for hours, or even days. Contrast this with the instant recovery made by Glaisher and Coxwell in 1862 as they descended from 29,000 feet over Wolverhampton in their balloon.[2] However, the symptoms are now well known to Himalayan mountaineers, especially those who do not take sufficient time to acclimatise to altitude. Eventually, a study of repeated daily flights up to 16,000 feet was undertaken by US military pilots at Randolf airfield in Texas[3] which established that it is unwise for pilots to make daily flights to more than 10,000 feet. This, of course, is just the opposite of what would be expected if acclimatisation to altitude were taking place. Nevertheless, it established an altitude limitation for unpressurised commercial aircraft which is still imposed by aviation regulatory authorities. It was being recognised, at least in the US, that pilots were not being looked after properly; a US War Department publication in 1919 actually stated:

Wonderful has been the development of the airplane; inconceivable has been the neglect of man in the airplane.

Although the reason for the altitude limitation was not understood at the time, it was soon found that it did not apply when pilots breathed oxygen. MRI studies of climbers have since shown, just as early experiments in aviation physiology had found, that the brain becomes swollen at high altitude; because of lack of oxygen the blood vessels leak.[4,5] Recent studies have shown that the reduced level of oxygen at altitude is associated with increased free radical production and dysfunction of the blood-brain barrier.[6,7] Although the swelling of the brain may be very rapid, it is most important to appreciate that it takes *much longer* for the accumulated water to resolve.

By the end of WW1, the importance of both supercharging engines and providing oxygen breathing for pilots had been established beyond any doubt. The urge to fly ever higher continued in the 1920s and in 1933; two biplanes equipped with the oxygen breathing apparatus designed by Haldane and Robert Davis succeeded in flying over Everest at 32,000 feet.[8] The Houston Everest expedition had been sponsored by Lady Houston and the Royal Air Force team received medals at a celebratory luncheon given by the *Times* at Grosvenor House on the 1st of June, 1932. One of the pilots, Squadron Leader Lord Clydesdale, said: "They had a duty to do and did it. They had demonstrated that a British machine with a British engine could fly over the highest mountain in the world." The race for the world altitude record had begun in earnest and Haldane had already designed a pressure suit (Figure 6.1) for use in aircraft at high altitude and it was also built by the Siebe Gorman Company.

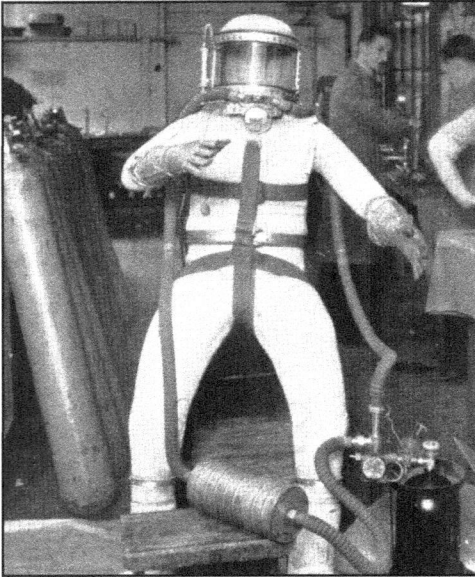

Figure 6.1:
Haldane's stratospheric suit used in high altitude aircraft.

Known as the "stratospheric suit" it was the forerunner of the modern space suit and was used by Wing Commander John Swire to capture the world altitude record at over 53,000 feet in 1937. Haldane also produced the first design for a pressurised airliner. The passengers would have had the benefit of the increased pressure in the cabin, but the pilots would have had to wear his stratospheric pressure suits. It is hardly surprising that the aircraft was not built. The drawing was commissioned by the Siebe Gorman Company.

The first scheduled commercial airline flight was by the St. Petersburg-Tampa Airboat Line and took place on January 1, 1914. The service flew between St. Petersburg and Tampa in Florida, the journey taking just 23 minutes. In 1917, Chalk's Airlines, now Chalk International Airlines, began a service between Miami and Bimini in the Bahamas. The Dutch airline KLM made their first flights out of Amsterdam in 1919 and the commercial market began to increase rapidly in the 1920s, especially in the US. The altitude achieved by aircraft was limited by the lack of engine power and the airlines did not provide the pilots with oxygen equipment. This, of course, saved weight, which is always a serious consideration for flying machines. However, by the 1930s there was a growing sense of unease in commercial aviation because aircraft were being lost in unusual circumstances. As it was usually associated with bad weather, mechanical failure was usually blamed. But there were also complaints from pilots of excessive fatigue and attacks of nausea and vertigo reminiscent of the experience in WW1. It became increasingly obvious that there was a clear association between the symptoms and repeated high altitude flights and it began to be suspected that lack of oxygen was involved. The importance of the earlier research in WW1, which had shown the marked effects of hypoxia on the performance of skilled tasks by pilots at altitudes over 10,000 feet, was beginning to be recognised; mild degrees of hypoxia actually induce a sense of euphoria clearly adding to the dangers. Oxygen breathing equipment was introduced although pilots initially opposed the development, arguing that it would make them bald, loosen their fillings, and render them impotent; allegations reminiscent of arguments used by some today when it is suggested that patients can benefit from hyperbaric oxygen treatment! There was actually some truth in the claims by the pilots as in early military aircraft the pilots had to breathe the oxygen by tube and the cold, dry, gas caused pain in their teeth and chapping of the lips.

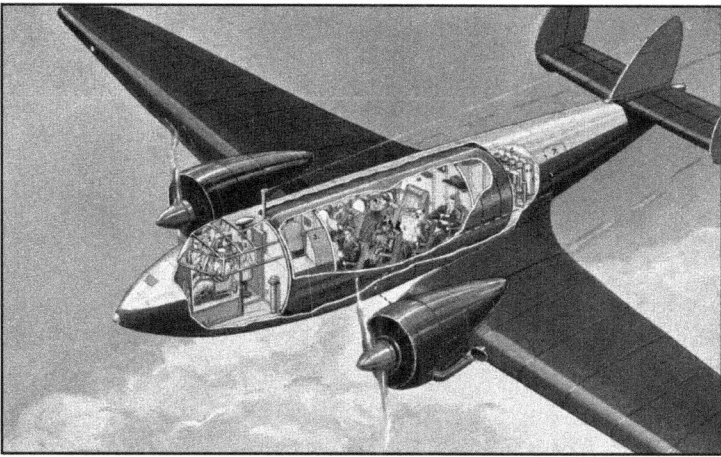

Figure 6.2:
Haldane's design for a pressurised aircraft drawn in the 1920s.

By the 1930s, it became a requirement for commercial pilots to use oxygen breathing when aircraft exceeded an altitude of 15,000 feet and oronasal masks were introduced to cover the mouth and nose based on Haldane's design. There was a growing appreciation of the need for cabin pressurisation and Haldane designed an aircraft with a pressurised cabin in the 1920s which required the pilots to wear pressure suits! The basic equipment requirements were detailed by Dr. Harry G. Armstrong in 1935.[9] His design criteria were used for the Lockheed XC-35 experimental "sub-stratospheric" aircraft commissioned by the US Army Air Corps and flown in 1937, the same year Boeing flew the world's first pressurised airliner, the B307.

At the outbreak of war, only 19 had been built and, although none were used by airlines, the technology allowed Boeing to build the B29, the first pressurised military aircraft to enter service. The bomber was set to change the course of history as it was able to fly high enough and fast enough to drop the first nuclear bomb and escape the blast. The Germans had also recognised the importance of pressurising aircraft to enable flights to very high altitudes and introduced the Junkers 86 for reconnaissance missions. It was not armed because it was able to fly too high to be intercepted by the fighters used by the Royal Air Force. However, improvements to the Spitfire allowed one to be intercepted and shot down. Hitler ordered the flights to be cancelled immediately. In Britain, Barnes Wallis, famous for his bouncing bomb, also experimented with pressurisation using the Wellington bomber he had designed for the Vickers company. Using the "geodesic" method of construction he had pioneered in the R100 airship, which enabled the aircraft to fly at 40,000 feet.

Today, with just a few exceptions, all commercial aircraft are pressurised but, unseen by passengers, pilots are required by law to don masks and breathe oxygen when flying at altitudes in excess of 40,000 feet. This is in case there is a sudden loss of cabin pressure, because the time to loss of consciousness at this altitude is measured in seconds. The technology reached its zenith with the development of the Anglo-French Concorde, which had to maintain a safe cabin pressure at altitudes as high as 64,000 feet. Kept on the ground with the cabin pressurised it would make a superb intensive care unit, large enough to provide all the required facilities for many patients.[10]

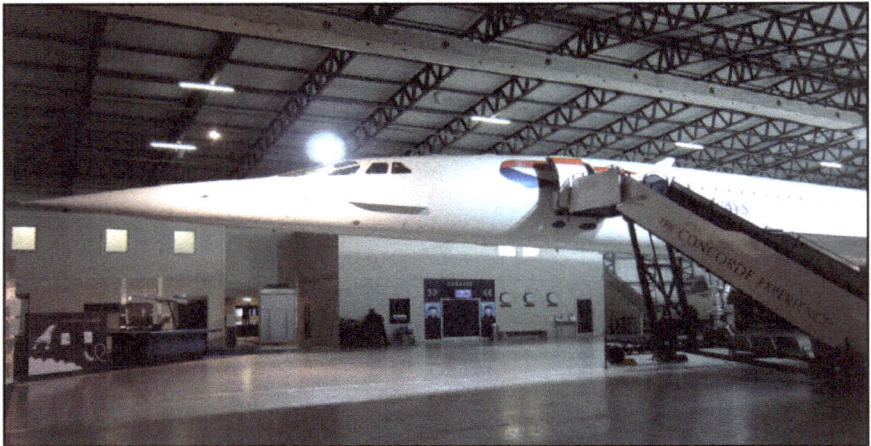

Figure 6.3:
A retired British Airways Concorde at the East Fortune Aircraft Museum near Edinburgh, Scotland.

Concorde pilots were exempted from the 40,000 foot rule for wearing masks because it would have meant that they would have had to wear them for almost all of the flight over the Atlantic! The aircraft used a higher cabin pressure at altitude than other jet aircraft, equivalent to 5,000 feet, despite being able to fly as high as 64,000 feet. It was a truly astonishing machine. Because of the extreme high altitude capability of Concorde, the various scenarios that would have resulted from it losing pressure had to be carefully examined by the design teams. The windows in Concorde were made smaller than those in normal aircraft to limit the rate of depressurisation in the event of a failure. It is a tribute to the engineering excellence that, in fact, in more than 30 years of operation, not a single window failed. The window apertures in the fuselage were actually machined into a single metal casting to prevent the metal fatigue failure and explosive decompression which caused the loss of three de Havilland Comets in the 1950s.[11] The engineers had calculated that the rate of decompression due to loss of a window at Concorde's highest cruising altitude would have given the pilots just four minutes to don their oxygen masks and descend to a safe altitude without losing consciousness. The Comet had been the first jet airliner to enter service but its initial success was blunted by the tragedies, leaving the Boeing 707 to dominate the early years of jet travel. The pressure in the cabin of a passenger jet at cruising altitude is required to be no lower than is equivalent to an altitude of 8,000 feet. This means that at cruising altitude, passengers are at the same pressure as they would be at 8,000 feet up a mountain; about a quarter less pressure than at sea level, and the level of oxygen entering the body is reduced in the same proportion. The Comet and early Boeing 707s were only able to fly for about six hours, which was just enough to allow them to cross the Atlantic, and so even elderly passengers were able to tolerate the lowered oxygen pressure. Now, some of the latest commercial aircraft can fly for up to 18 hours and may, perhaps, be able to cross both the Atlantic and Pacific oceans on one flight. At a cabin "altitude" of 8,000 feet, passengers on long duration flights risk being made ill from the lack of oxygen. Not surprisingly, aircraft like the Boeing 787 are now engineered to use a higher cabin pressure, equivalent to an altitude of 5,500 feet, which equates to a lower cabin "altitude," to improve passenger safety and comfort. So, not only the degree of oxygen deprivation, but also the *time* spent breathing low oxygen levels is important, especially for older passengers and those suffering from illness.

By the 1930s, the pioneers of aviation medicine had established if an unpressurised aircraft climbs at a rate of 1,000 feet a minute to an altitude of 25,000 feet the pilot becomes rapidly disabled. Unless a descent is made, or oxygen is breathed, death can occur in as little as 20 minutes. We have little tolerance of an abrupt lack of oxygen and the early aviation research showed the variation between pilots in the time to unconsciousness at 25,000 feet is negligible. The conquest of Everest in 1953 by the late Edmund Hillary and Tenzing Norgay was achieved with a period of acclimatisation at altitude but also using oxygen apparatus. They overturned James Glaisher's prediction in 1862 that "no human being ever could drag himself to this height following uneven terrestrial surface." As discussed in Chapter 3, Reinhold Messner and Peter Habeler succeeded in climbing Everest without supplemental oxygen in 1978, a feat that Haldane actually thought possible. Their success was initially disbelieved, especially by Tenzing Norgay, and it was even suggested that Messner and Habeler had hidden small oxygen cylinders under their clothing! Many climbers have now succeeded in this prodigious feat and the record for the ascent from base camp was set on May 23, 2003 by Pemba Dorje at the age of 39. He climbed from base camp at 17,500 feet to the 29,040 feet summit in 12 hours and 46 minutes. The total time for his climb was just 21 hours and it was his tenth ascent of Everest—all completed without supplemental oxygen! So, if pilots die after about 20 minutes at 25,000 feet, how is it possible for climbers to reach the summit of Everest without breathing more oxygen?

Given that pilots had found that their ability to reach high altitude *reduced* with daily flights it would seem that acclimatisation is not possible, but it clearly does occur and it is the *rate of change* of the level of oxygen that is critical. Climbers take many weeks to acclimatise for an ascent of Everest; they climb slowly and stay at altitude and make regular upward excursions. This has profound effects both on both their blood and their blood vessels. In contrast, pilots spend at most just hours a day at altitude and usually return to sea level, or close to it. Studies of the effects of sudden ascents to a modest altitude have shown, as Glaisher and Coxwell had found, that the first changes manifest as a very significant increase in the pulse rate with only a slight increase in the rate of breathing. In some people, a mild degree of anxiety may occur as low as 12,000 feet. As these changes are rapidly relieved by breathing oxygen, it is clear that they are due to the reduction in the oxygen concentration breathed. It is important to understand why, if the problems are not reversed quickly, they can persist. When the brain of an anaesthetized animal was observed through a hole in the skull in the experiments undertaken by Armstrong and colleagues at the School of Aviation Medicine in Texas in 1916, it was seen that on reaching about 17,000 feet the blood vessels of the brain became large and congested. Brain tissue then expanded through the hole. The effects are due simply to lack of oxygen and exactly the same effects can be seen on the ground, by the addition of a few hundred parts per million of the gas carbon monoxide to air. Carbon monoxide simply prevents oxygen being used by the cells of the brain, and the lack of oxygen causes the same brain swelling due from leakage of water from the circulating blood.[12]

The effects of a sudden reduction of air pressure are very complex and reveal a paradox; an abrupt reduction of the level of oxygen is stressful because of the formation of oxygen free radicals! In other words, a sudden lowering of the oxygen level paradoxically *increases* oxidant stress. An increase in free radical production from suddenly lowering the level of oxygen was demonstrated in an elegantly simple experiment in the University of Porto in Portugal.[13] Six young men sat in a chamber that was engineered to allow air to be removed from it—a "hypobaric" chamber. The removal of air from the chamber allows the simulation of the low pressures associated with high altitudes. The subjects were decompressed to a pressure equivalent to an altitude of 18,000 feet, that is, about half sea level atmospheric pressure. Blood samples were taken before, during, and after the period at low pressure. There was an *increase* in the markers of oxidative stress at the low pressure showing, paradoxically, that on lowering the oxygen level, more free radicals formed. Again, Fridovich's hunch expressed in his paper "Hypoxia and Oxygen Toxicity" had been confirmed.[14] At the end of four hours at low pressure, the chamber was then compressed back to sea level. This, of course, doubled the level of oxygen the subjects were breathing, but no increase in free radical formation was found. The researchers thought that perhaps the levels would actually increase because of the increased level of oxygen. At very high oxygen levels there is energy available to increase the production of the free radical scavengers which are able to maintain the status quo. In contrast, the level of scavengers cannot match free radical production if oxygen levels fall, because there is less energy available to construct the complex scavenger molecules. This will certainly be true in rapidly developing severe hypoxia. However, there is an issue which adds another dimension to an already complex situation; it is now known that changes in the level of free radicals are used for signaling corrective actions—for example, to increase capillary formation and blood flow, the key factors essential in acclimatisation to the lack of oxygen at high altitude.

The biology of oxygen has been studied intensively over the last three decades and it has been shown that the diameter of blood vessels, blood flow and the output of the heart are all governed by oxygen. Astonishingly, it has recently been found that another gas is involved in these changes—nitric oxide (NO), which is actually manufactured by the lining cells of blood vessels and causes blood vessels to enlarge.[15] Before it was recognised that nitric oxide was involved, the agent had originally been called endothelial-derived relaxing factor (EDRF). So the response to a reduction in the level of oxygen in blood is for the blood vessels in the brain to enlarge their diameter. This increases the volume of blood within the skull and takes up the space normally occupied by the fluid, known as cerebrospinal fluid, which surrounds the brain and spinal cord. The enlarged blood vessels tend to leak and the brain tissues swell due to the increase exceeding the rate at which the fluid can drain away. Swelling of the brain is responsible for the typical headache that may develop at altitude and it is due to irritation of the coverings of the brain, known as the meninges. So the headache is due to a mild, but obviously not infectious, form of inflammation; an aseptic meningitis. However, although the brain swells very quickly, it may take some days for the increased tissue fluid to drain away and this is the reason for the reduction found in the capability of pilots to achieve high altitudes on successive flights already discussed. Since the days of the early Alpine climbing undertaken by the British in the 1800s, climbers, especially those climbing in the Himalayas, have recognised the importance of acclimatising to altitude, which was a critical factor in the conquest of Everest in 1953. So what changes occur in the body in acclimatisation?

It has been known for many years that the number of red cells in the circulation increases with increasing altitude in climbers who normally live close to sea level. Research has now shown that this and other changes are due to the fall in oxygen levels and it appears that oxygen free radicals actually signal the need for change. The key proteins we have already met in Chapter 1, the hypoxia-inducible factor proteins, are in control. Normally only 45% of the volume of blood is made up of cells—the remainder is the liquid known as plasma. After acclimatising at base camp on Everest, the volume of red cells in the blood of climbers may increase to become more than 60% of the total volume of their blood, as Haldane and Douglas had observed on the Pike's Peak expedition in 1911.[16] However, if someone living at sea level actually had a transfusion of packed red blood cells on the ground to achieve the same volume of red blood cells (60%), and then ascended to the height of Everest in a balloon, they would not be able to stay conscious for much longer than Glaisher and Coxwell, despite their blood containing much more oxygen. The reason is simple; the extra haemoglobin would not increase the *oxygen pressure*, that is, the concentration, of oxygen available in the plasma to transport oxygen from blood into the cells of the brain. Another adaptation to altitude is actually more important than the formation of extra red blood cells, a very remarkable adaptation also controlled, not surprisingly, by oxygen via the hypoxia-inducible factor proteins. During the time climbers stay at base camp on Everest and undertake excursions to higher altitudes in preparation for an ascent to the summit, the same genes that are responsible for the growth of blood vessels in the developing embryo are upregulated. They ensure that, over the weeks spent at base camp, climbers actually grow *50% more capillaries* in the brain to counter the lack of oxygen.[17] The increase in the number of capillaries greatly increases the surface area available for oxygen to diffuse from the blood into tissues and reduces the distance that oxygen has to travel from the blood to cells.

By the 1940s, it began to be suspected that the effects of a rapid reduction of atmospheric pressure on the brain extended beyond lack of oxygen—it was being recognised that gas bubbles may form in the body at altitude. In other words, that pilots may actually get the "bends," that is, decompression sickness. Proof of this came from investigations begun in the turbulent years of WW2 following the experience of bomber crews on missions over Germany. The crews would complain of knee pain after long duration flights and there were reports of pilots collapsing over the controls. Experiments in hypobaric chambers in the UK at the Institute of Aviation Medicine at Farnborough and also in the US had shown that the pain was due to gas present in the ligaments and tendons around the knee joint. X- rays of the aviators' knees were taken on the ground and compared to those taken in the chamber when the pain was present at the low pressures equivalent to being at altitude. The X-rays showed gas formed in sheets within the capsules of the joint. Both the pain and the gas disappeared when the aviator descended because it was compressed to sea level conditions. Sometimes the gas formed into a pocket behind the knee, as shown in Figure 6.4 from Wing Commander David Fryer's superb NATO monograph.[18]

The loss of aircraft over Germany prompted a series of experiments using a converted B24 Liberator bomber in California. Having had its guns and armour removed, the aircraft was able to reach an altitude of 35,000 feet.[19] An increase in pressure had been validated in the treatment of the bends in divers and so the USAF scientists developed a pressure bag—a portable hyperbaric chamber. It was carried in the aircraft for the treatment of decompression sickness during flights.

Altitude decompression sickness became of critical importance with the introduction of the jet engine. If aircraft have changed our world, it is largely because of the gas turbine engine, their combination of power and

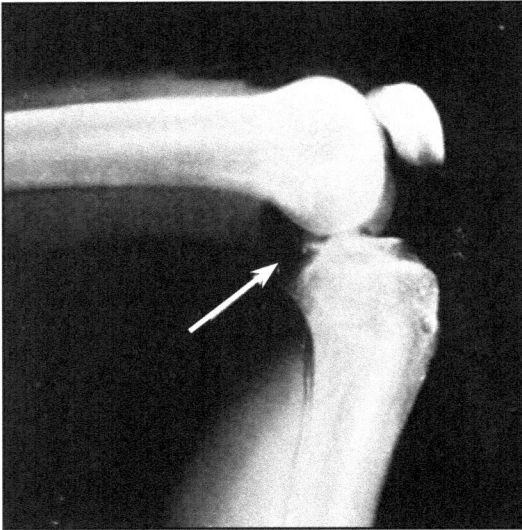

Figure 6.4:
X radiograph of a gas pocket in the joint fluid behind the knee. (From Fryer DI. "Subatmospheric Decompression Sickness in Man.")

reliability has been truly astonishing. Sir Frank Whittle's patent, published in 1930, covered the first practical design. Following the customary lack of interest from the British government, Whittle formed a company in 1936, Power Jets Ltd., to develop the technology. Valuable time had been lost as the storm clouds were gathering over Europe. The importance of Whittle's invention was quickly understood in Germany. Hans Joachim Pabst von Ohain also published a patent for a gas turbine engine and in 1936, he was recruited by the aircraft company, Heinkel. Von Ohain's experiments, carried out in secret at Heinkel's factory, resulted in the bench test of an engine by 1937, and a fully operational jet aircraft, the He 178, which made the world's first jet-powered aircraft flight on August 27, 1939. Although the landing gear of the plane failed to retract, preventing the test pilot from accelerating to the planned speed, the centrifugal-flow engine performed perfectly. The centrifugal compressor was less efficient than the axial-flow compressor developed by Whittle and, in Germany, Anselm Franz had also developed an axial flow engine. It seems most likely that the Whittle invention was the basis of the design. The engine powered the Messerschmitt 262, the world's first operational jet fighter aircraft, which saw action in the last throes of the war against the American Boeing B29. The early jet aircraft were not pressurised, although a few Me 262s were fitted with prototype equipment. However, they were only capable of reaching very high altitudes for minutes rather than hours and oxygen breathing proved to be sufficient for the pilots to avoid serious problems. The last Luftwaffe pilot trained during WW2 was the Austrian Franz Gerstenbrand, who became a professor of neurology in Vienna. He flew the Me 262 in the final stages of the War and the author discussed his experience with him at one of the meetings held by the Aviation, Space, and Underwater Medicine section of the World Federation of Neurology in Florida. A revolutionary air to air missile had been introduced and saw action against the Boeing B29 bombers flown over southern Germany by the USAF.

With more efficient engines, longer flight times became possible and, not surprisingly, cases of decompression sickness began to occur. They were often misdiagnosed and details of British experience are covered in Fryer's monograph. It was generally believed by the military doctors involved that, even if gas bubbles did form at altitude, they would disappear as the aircraft returned to the ground, the descent obviously being a re-pressurisation. In the 1950s and 60s, many jet pilots and crew developed symptoms from what is now known to be altitude decompression sickness and some died after suffering bizarre and inappropriate treatment. However, no attempts were made to use recompression treatment, despite the fact that in 1941, the brilliant US Navy physician, Albert Behnke, had successfully treated a seriously ill aviator in a pressure chamber after deciding that he had decompression sickness.[20] It was not until 1967 that recompression treatment was formally recognised and became standard practice in US and European Air Forces following a review by Col. Jefferson Davis at Brooks Air Force Base in San Antonio, Texas.[21] There was a reason for the reluctance to accept that bubbles were involved in the syndrome; it was because the pilots did not develop the paraplegia, the typical paralysis of the legs, which is the hallmark of decompression sickness in divers. It was, therefore, argued that the problems could not be due to the "bends." They were wrong, and the possibility that aviators could develop the bends had been raised by Haldane as long ago as 1908.[22] Reports of pain in joints at altitude actually date back to the ascents made by balloonists in the late 1800s. A remarkable paper from the USAF, published in 2013, has confirmed the risk of brain damage using MRI in 102 pilots flying the U-2 high altitude reconnaissance aircraft. The pilots had three times the number of UBOs (unidentified bright objects) in the brain when compared to 91 matched controls.

In 1905, Haldane was commissioned by the British Admiralty to investigate decompression sickness and he recruited Dr. A.E. Boycott and the Superintendent of Diving in the Royal Navy, Lt. G.C.C. Damant, to help in his investigations. They were to highlight a key principle of disease that can solve many of the unsolved mysteries that remain in medicine.

CHAPTER 7
Bubbles, the "Bends," and the Lungs

If small bubbles pass through the lung capillaries and lodge in a slowly desaturating part of the spinal cord they will there increase in size and cause blockage of the circulation or serious mechanical damage.

Boycott AE, Damant GE, Haldane JS. *Journal of Hygiene*, 1908.

Diving using breath-holding has been undertaken for thousands of years, but the risk of such divers forming bubbles and developing "the bends" is very low because they do not breathe compressed gases. When pressurised gases are breathed underwater, the reduction of pressure on returning to the surface risks bubbles forming, just as bubbles form in a bottle of fizzy drink when the cap is removed. The space in the bottle above the liquid contains the gas carbon dioxide at increased pressure, and the noise produced when the cap is removed is due to its escape. Bubbles that form in the body on decompression may enter the circulation and may damage the nervous system which, as the quotation above indicates, includes the spinal cord.

It was the invention of the diving helmet by two brothers in London, Charles and John Deane, that allowed men to accomplish work underwater for the first time.[1] The brothers successfully adapted their design of a smoke hood for use in diving, after showing that it was possible to pump sufficient air to sustain a man wearing their device at depth. They had helmets constructed by Augustus Siebe in Soho and became known for salvaging wrecks. They were soon commissioned to work on the wreck of the H.M.S. *Royal George*, which had foundered at Spithead, Portsmouth in 1782, with great loss of life. Theirs was not the first attempt to salvage the vessel: Shortly after it sank, William Tracey made an attempt using a copper atmospheric diving suit, which simply enclosed a man leaving his arms out in the water. The arms were pushed through sleeves and subjected to the pressure of the water, whilst the body remained at normal atmospheric pressure. The depths achieved were very modest, being limited by the pain that could be endured. Little was achieved. As the wreck of the *Royal George* was partially obstructing the entrance of Portsmouth harbour, it had to be removed, but the Deane brothers were more interested in retrieving the many fine cannons still on the site. In 1835, they actually held an exhibition of the many artifacts they had recovered, in premises in Regent's Street, London. The following year the salvage was taken over by Colonel Charles W. Pasley, director of the Royal Engineers Establishment at Chatham, and his team of sappers. They adopted the full diving dress, which Augustus Siebe had developed by 1837. The bolted corselet with the traditional copper hard hat has become the symbol of diving around the world. As is often the case, it was a contemporary development that had made this further advance possible—the rubberised canvas invented by Charles Macintosh allowed the construction of a waterproof enclosed suit.

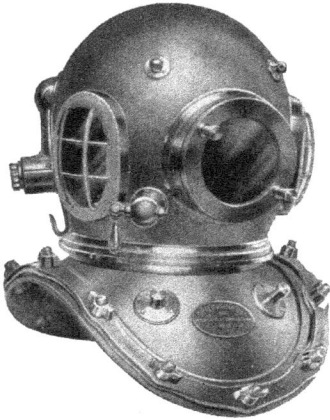

Figure 7.1:
The traditional hard hat helmet made by Siebe Gorman Ltd.

Two experienced civilian divers from Whitstable, George Hall and Hiram London, were recruited by Colonel Pasley and began training the sappers who were to form the first team of military divers. The team lifted the last of the bronze cannons from the wreck, and several were melted down to form the plinth, or capital, of the monument to Lord Nelson, which stands in London's famous Trafalgar Square. The divers destroyed the wreck using explosives triggered electrically, which was the first time that the method had been used underwater. The salvage was not without problems. Pasley reported that his men often suffered from "severe rheumatism," especially in the knees, after long periods working underwater and often required "therapeutic Cognac on surfacing." This was probably the first description of the joint pain typical of "the bends." Some of the Army divers also suffered mysterious paralyses, as had Charles Deane, who spent some time in a lunatic asylum in Peckham.

Another development essential to the industrial revolution had been the use of compressed air to exclude water from mines and tunnels under rivers. It also allowed the construction of bridge foundations using caissons, which had been invented in England by Cochrane in 1830. The caisson was first used by the French mining engineer Alain Triger in the late 1830s, and many of the men employed developed strange symptoms. In 1848, Triger hired two French doctors, Pol and Watelle, to examine them on one of his projects. In their paper[2] they described the illness as *la maladie de caisson* and used the oft-quoted phrase "*en payes de sortie,*" translated as "one pays on leaving." They noted that the men would only become ill after they had decompressed and left the site. The doctors observed that some of the workers developed problems affecting the nervous system, and wondered "what the great Professor Charcot would have made of the disease." Jean-Martin Charcot was the renowned neurologist working in la Hôpital Pitié-Salpêtrière in Paris, who was the first to properly describe both the clinical and pathological features of *la sclerose en plaques*, the French term for multiple sclerosis—the disease that features later in this book.[3] The men found that their symptoms would resolve when they returned to pressure in the workings and so discovered recompression therapy.

Many divers and compressed-air workers died from decompression sickness in the eighteenth century, and the great French physiologist, Paul Bert, chronicled their tribulations in his epic book *La Pression Barométrique* [Barometric Pressure], which was published in 1878. It was translated into English in 1941.[4] Physicians, traditionally shy of physics, had little idea of the cause of the affliction. In fact, Drs. Pol and Watelle thought that the increased pressure alone was responsible for the problem, in some way redistributing the blood in the body by squeezing it away from the skin. In 1881, a well know physician boldly stated in the *British Medical Journal*:

> *It hardly needs an experiment to show that the pressure drives blood away from the surface of the body.*

Incredibly, this misinformed explanation, which was confidently asserted by many physicians involved with diving and compressed air work at the time, is still encountered today. But Paul Bert, however, had realised that bubbles were involved in decompression sickness, and demonstrated them in his experiments. He simply watched them appearing in the blood that flowed out of a cut in the external jugular vein in the neck of a dog that had been exposed to compressed air. The term "the bends" was coined during the construction of the foundations of the Brooklyn Bridge under the Hudson river.[5] There was a ladies' dress in fashion in the 1870s known as the Grecian bend, which used a bustle that caused women to stoop forward when walking.

Compressed-air workers with painful decompression sickness were forced to adopt the same posture, hence the description of "the bends."

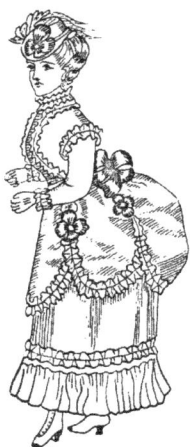

Figure 7.2:
The nineteenth century dress known as the Grecian bend.

However, some men developed serious respiratory symptoms, which became known as "the chokes," some weakness of the legs, or "the staggers," but a few convulsed and died.

To return to diving; it is now well known that most dives to significant depths breathing compressed gases risk gas forming in the body. It may form as sheets between tissues, for example, in the tendons and ligaments of a joint like the knee, or as small bubbles in the blood. By the turn of the nineteenth century, the number of divers in the Royal Navy rendered paralysed by decompression sickness had become a matter of serious concern to the Admiralty. The paralysis of the legs was termed diver's palsy, and is due to an injury to the *spinal cord*, a critical, but neglected, part of the nervous system. An afflicted diver would often be confined to a wheelchair, which today has become the symbol of the disease multiple sclerosis which, in Haldane's day, was a rarity.

The spinal cord runs in a canal in the bony spine from the base of the skull to the level of the first of the lumbar vertebra. Most people will remember the late Christopher Reeve as Superman. He was paralysed from the neck down after damaging his spinal cord falling from a horse, and was to fully exemplify his character's persona by the courage he showed in his fight to recover and to help fellow sufferers. The injury, which affected the spinal cord in his neck, made him lose the function of both arms and legs. An injury further down the cord would have restricted the loss of function to the legs. Unfortunately, in both cases, other functions, such as control of the bladder, are usually affected. The spinal cord weighs only 50 grams, which contrasts starkly with the 1,350 gram weight of a typical human brain. The spinal cord is rather like a telephone cable, relaying signals to and from the brain. With the dense concentration of nerve fibres in the spinal cord, which is little larger in diameter than a little finger, a small amount of damage almost invariably gives rise to symptoms such as weakness of an arm or a leg or loss of sensation.

It was in 1905 that Haldane, by now well known for his work on the physiology of breathing and industrial disease, was commissioned by the British Admiralty to investigate a number of problems affecting Royal Navy divers.[6] His remit ranged from the investigation of loss of consciousness underwater to the cause of decompression sickness. He found that the loss of consciousness was due to a build-up of carbon dioxide in the helmet, and it was easily solved by increasing the flow of air. Solving the problem of "the bends" proved to be much more difficult: Haldane first devised a classification with joint pain termed Type 1, the respiratory and neurological problems as Type 2, and convulsions and death classified as Type 3. He recognised that when a diver breathes air pressurised to match the surrounding pressure underwater, additional nitrogen dissolves in the body, and it has the potential to form bubbles on returning to the surface. Haldane decided that the best way to reduce or prevent them from forming was for a diver to stop at predetermined depths on the ascent in the water, which is equivalent to letting the gas out of a bottle by unscrewing the cap at intervals so that it escapes very slowly. He arbitrarily divided the body into five tissues, or as he called them, "compartments," and drew exponential curves for them to indicate a rate at which different tissues took up and gave off nitrogen; some, like the brain, being very fast and others, like bone, being very slow. He then allocated stoppages of increasing duration for the ascent to the surface based on what he considered to be a tolerable level of excess gas dissolved, known as supersaturation, in the body. In the 1907 Admiralty report he stated that bubbles *would* actually form, but that they would not cause any symptoms. The decompression tables he devised for the Admiralty have formed the basis for almost all procedures used in diving today.

The five compartments that Haldane divided the body into were not specified, nor attributed to actual organs or tissues. He argued that with an increase in pressure the body would take up the additional nitrogen exponentially—rapidly at first, becoming progressively slower as the nitrogen reached equilibrium. He drew five upward curves on his graph paper, one for each of his compartments, with five downward curves to represent the elimination of gas on decompression as a diver returned to the surface. Here the methods used become hazy. In fact, a distinguished contemporary, Dr. Leonard Hill,[7] complained that he could not find the basis for the tabulated stoppage times. It has even been suggested that they were calculated by his young son Jack, who by the age of 16 was a competent mathematician!

The decompression tables were based on determining the maximum depth at which a diver could remain indefinitely underwater and then return to the surface "without symptoms due to bubbles," as it is stated in the Admiralty report. This, known as the no-stoppage or no-stop depth, was found by experiments, first using goats and then Royal Navy divers, to be about 5 fathoms or 42 feet of sea water (fsw). The figure was soon reduced by experience to just 33 fsw, or 10 meters of sea water (msw), which is just 1 atmosphere of extra pressure—it became known as the 2 to 1 rule. In other words, a diver could remain indefinitely at 33 fsw, which is 2 atmospheres absolute, and decompress back to 1 atmosphere absolute at the surface. Two things must be considered here: First, Haldane admitted that bubbles *would* form on decompression after an indefinite stay at 33 fsw (10 msw). Second, that he thought they would not be likely to cause symptoms. "Indefinite" was a relative term when applied to a stay underwater; divers wearing traditional standard gear—a hard hat and the rubberised canvas suit—despite wearing woolly underwear would be overcome by cold after a few hours in the water. As for bubbles being present in the body that did not cause symptoms, Haldane found this to be true by observing the goats used in his experiments, just as Paul Bert had done in dogs 30 years earlier.

After a time at depth, a diver must ascend in the water, decompressing to reach the surface. During the ascent, the excess dissolved gas taken up during the dive, which is nitrogen in air diving, is transported in the blood from the tissues to the lungs. There, it diffuses into the gas spaces of the alveoli and simply escapes by being breathed out. Therefore, most of the excess gas remains in solution in the blood until it finally escapes across the membrane of the lung to be exhaled. However, the elimination of the nitrogen from body tissues takes time, and may continue for some hours after a diver leaves the water. During this time there is the potential for some of the excess gas to come out of solution in the capillaries of tissues as bubbles. This is what happens when the top of a bottle of fizzy drink is removed. If the cap is removed slowly, most of the extra gas dissolved in the liquid remains in solution, and it will leave from the surface of the liquid over many hours, with very few bubbles forming. However, if the bottle is gently tapped, bubbles form, and they rise to the surface. If it is shaken, there is an explosive release of bubbles as froth. In the body, gas that forms in the tissues on decompression may remain where it forms, or it may enter a blood vessel and be carried as bubbles

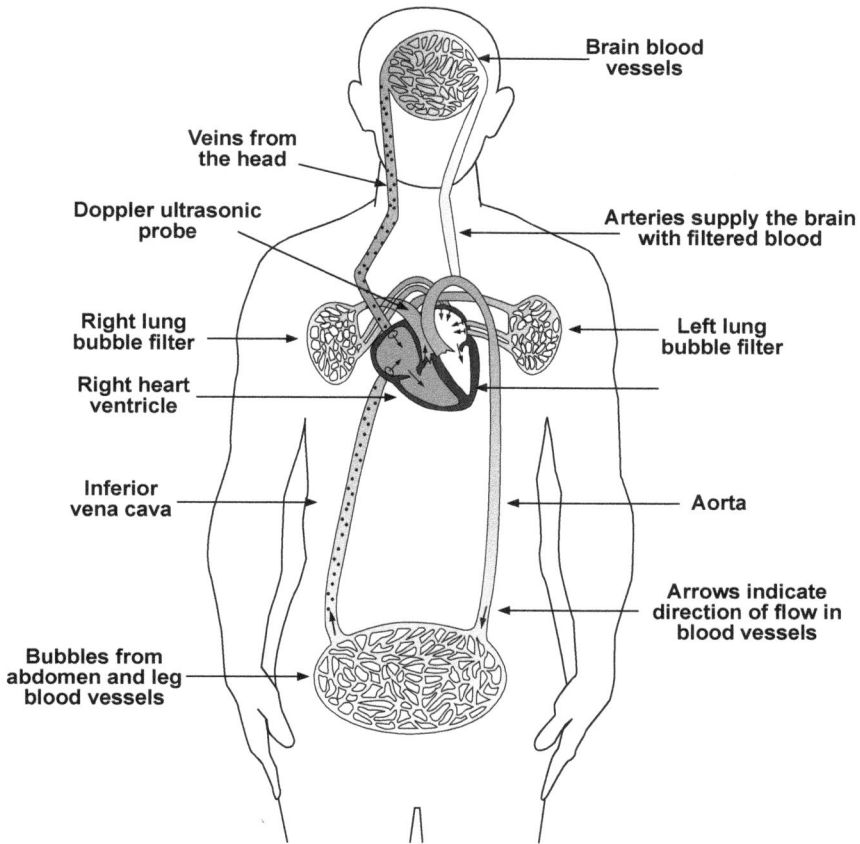

Figure 7.3:
The circulation showing the two pumps and the position of the lungs.

in the veins, which return blood to the heart. The route taken from the tissues by bubbles in blood is shown by the arrows in Figure 7.3.

After passing through the right side of the heart, the right atrium and the right ventricle, the blood containing bubbles is pumped up the pulmonary artery flowing into the capillaries of the lungs where the bubbles are normally trapped. The gas molecules then transfer across the membrane in the lungs and are breathed out. This is just the opposite of what happens during a descent when nitrogen dissolves in the body from the compressed air breathed through the lungs. The dose of the extra nitrogen taken up depends on the depth of a dive, which determines the pressure and its duration. There are many physiological variables that cannot be controlled, which determine whether or not bubbles are produced on decompression, their quantity, and the number that may enter the circulation on a given dive. The most significant variation is in blood flow through certain tissues, which can alter both the amount of gas taken up during a dive such as when a diver exercises, and also the rate at which the gas is released during the decompression on the ascent to the surface. Unfortunately, variations in blood flow for a given tissue cannot be predicted or controlled, especially those tissues which do not need a constant supply of blood, like ligaments and tendons. As discussed in Chapter 6, X-rays of the knee joints of aviators during WW2 showed that gas forming in these tissues is responsible for the characteristic pain of the bends. It may affect the knee or shoulder or, much less commonly, other joints such as the finger, wrist, elbow, or ankle.

An outline of Haldane's method and his decompression tables was included in the 1907 Admiralty report on deep water diving.[6] The tables were adopted by the Royal Navy in 1908 and made available to the public as a Blue Book. In 1912, they entered use in the US Navy. Haldane's methods have been the basis for decompression table development since, with the sole exception of the tables developed by the pearl divers in Australia which were studied in the 1960s by the late Professor Brian Hills.[7] The success of Haldane's tables led him to make an uncharacteristic error after a successful visit to the US. WW1 had begun in 1914 and, surprisingly, he crossed the Atlantic in 1916 to give a series of lectures at Yale University, which had been endowed in memory of Mrs. Hepsa Ely Silliman. Haldane had been invited to give the lectures in 1915, the year that the *Lusitania* had been sunk by a German U-boat off the southern coast of Ireland. Not surprisingly, he postponed the trip, feeling that the danger was too great. He was far from idle that year, however. As we have seen in Chapter 5, he was fully occupied with developments at the battlefront at Ypres.

When Haldane returned home to Oxford from the US, he assembled the notes from his four lectures, added other material, and published his well-known book, *Respiration*. The war delayed its release, but it was finally published by Yale University Press in 1922.[8] In chapter 12, he again pointed out that decompression from the no-stoppage depth on his 2 to 1 rule gave immunity from *symptoms* due to bubbles, but then without any explanation, he claimed that bubbles of nitrogen are actually *not liberated* within the body under these circumstances. This was almost certainly based on the resounding success of his decompression tables during WW1, but the use of ultrasonic techniques has now shown that it is certainly not true. Unfortunately, Haldane's mistake led to a plethora of mathematical models of decompression and, in recent years, an almost unquestioned reliance on his concept for the software programs used in the decompression computers by amateur divers.

They undoubtedly reduce the risk of decompression sickness by reducing the bubble count, but the risk can never be completely removed. It does not take many bubbles in the blood stream to cause havoc, and, perhaps, just one if it reaches the spinal cord.

The formation of the blood vessels and the heart constituting the circulation in the developing embryo is discussed in Chapter 1. Bubbles or other particles, for example clots, which may circulate in the blood are known as *emboli*. The word bolus means a lump of material passing along a tube and is used, for example, to describe the passage of food down the gullet. Emboli in blood can range in size from just a few microns to several centimetres in diameter and many centimetres in length, as in the clots that can form in the legs. Most people have heard of deep vein thrombosis, and know that it is associated with sitting in cramped conditions for too long as, for example, on long-haul aircraft journeys. Clots may form in the veins deep inside the legs because the muscles are not exercised, and the blood flow becomes sluggish. However, a second factor is that the reduction of pressure in the cabin typically reduces the plasma oxygen concentration by about 25%. Curiously, a recent Scottish study has shown that a fall in barometric pressure is associated with an increased risk of deep venous thrombosis.[9] The risk apparently increases by 2% with just a 10 millibar fall in atmospheric pressure. Such reductions are common in Scotland, where atmospheric pressure ranges from 925 to 1,054 millibars.

Fortunately, most clots in the deep veins of the legs do not give rise to any symptoms, because blood from the legs can easily return to the heart by other routes and over time they are usually resolved. However, a clot may break free and travel in the blood via the large veins, passing through the abdomen to the heart and on into the lungs. This is known as pulmonary embolism. If such a clot is large enough, it may block the pulmonary artery, which is the main blood vessel leading to the lungs. This abruptly stops the heart from pumping blood and causes sudden death. The trapping of smaller clots by the lungs actually protects the nervous system, because if a clot were to pass through the lung and reach the left side of the heart it could travel to the brain or spinal cord and cause a catastrophic stroke. The role of the lungs as "the guardian angels of the circulation" is a critical concept that has been forgotten in modern times[10] and it will be discussed in detail later. Another phenomenon that has been linked to barometric pressure is subarachnoid haemorrhage with, again, reductions of as little as 10 millibar increasing the risk.[11]

Decompression problems not only occur in divers, but also in military pilots and astronauts. Although their symptoms are usually less severe than in divers, decompression sickness may, nevertheless, be fatal. As of yet, no studies have looked for bubble formation in climbers who ascend rapidly to high altitude, but it is the author's conviction that in some circumstances they contribute to mountain sickness. Gas also enters the circulation in many medical procedures. For example, air always enters the circulation when the heart and major blood vessels are opened during surgery. Blood has to be removed from them to create a bloodless field, so that a surgeon can see to operate. The illnesses caused by bubbles in blood provide a unique opportunity to study the diseases caused by other material that may enter the circulation. The blood may also carry infection. Although it is not usual to regard bacteria in the circulation as emboli, they can impact in capillaries either singly, as in the case of syphilis or, in staphylococcal infections, as clumps, and may then spread into the surrounding tissues. Today it is easy to forget the horrors of infection, as we are better able to resist them than our forebears, and epidemics are now counted in tens rather than thousands of victims. We also have powerful antibiotics, although their indiscriminate use has allowed the development of super bugs such as methicillin-resistant Staphylococcus aureus (MRSA). When they are carried in blood, bacteria, like cancer cells, can spread causing distant problems; that is, they can *metastasise* to other remote sites.

One of the most dramatic stories in the history of medicine, which has important lessons for us today, was the discovery of the cause of childbed fever by Ignaz Philipp Semmelweis[12] (1818–1865). During his time as assistant physician to Professor Klein in the General Hospital in Vienna, he was tasked with finding the cause of the illness. Women were admitted to hospitals in the final stages of labour in the late eighteenth century, so that midwives and doctors did not have to attend a woman at home to deliver the child. This seemingly forward-thinking step was eventually responsible for the deaths of hundreds of thousands of mothers and often their babies. It was the first example of the dreadful hospital-acquired infections that so trouble us today. The infection was introduced by vaginal examinations of the mother made after the baby was delivered, and hence was known as childbed fever. However, only the medical wing of the hospital had the hallmark of "death in rows"—the nursing wing had many fewer deaths. Many improbable explanations were given for the difference in mortality between the two wards, which was well known to the women of Vienna, including cosmic radiation. Semmelweis was alerted to the fact that medical staff was responsible for spreading the infection, by the death of his friend Jakob Kolletschka, the professor of forensic pathology. The professor was infected by material from a corpse of a mother after his finger had been cut by a medical student during the postmortem examination. Kolletschka died after developing all the features of disseminated childbed fever; the bacteria would spread in the blood to many sites, sometimes even to the eye. Semmelweis realised that, despite washing with soap, the material from the corpse still clung to the hands, because they retained the characteristic odour. He had bowls of chlorinated lime placed at the entrance of the ward for all the staff to rinse their hands before entering the ward. The disease was soon controlled but, despite his monumental discovery, it was not long before Semmelweis was derided as the "Fool from Pest," although he was actually from Buda. Professor Klein had introduced the rigorous policy of dissection and, despite the success of Semmelweis in solving the problem of childbed fever, he was demoted and returned to Hungary to practise in Budapest. He went to Vienna some years later, and died of metastatic infection in a mental asylum. The world of medicine is not kind to whistleblowers.

It is said that at the turn of the last century one in ten people had syphilis caused by the bacterium *Treponema pallidum*, which is also blood-borne. There can be no question that the reason the infection has had a major impact on the course of history is because it affects the brain. Vladimir Lenin apparently died from the disease he contracted from a prostitute in 1902, a fact known to a famous contemporary, Professor Ivan Pavlov. The evidence has been assembled by Helen Rappaport in her book, *Conspirator: Lenin in Exile*, which was published in 2009.[13] Lenin died in 1924, and examination of the brain is said to have confirmed the diagnosis although, not surprisingly, the Soviet regime did not release the information. It has also been claimed that Joseph Stalin had the disease, and that the body of Benito Mussolini tested positive for it. The megalomania and neurological symptoms exhibited by Adolf Hitler are typical of the tertiary stage of the disease. Judged by his ravings in *Mein Kampf*, which was published in 1925, with volume two in 1926, Hitler was obsessed with syphilis. In the film made of the 1936 Olympics by Leni Riefenstahl, both his left hand and left leg can be seen to be trembling, and later he often held his left hand to minimise its shaking. It has been claimed, as it has been with Mao Tse-tung, that Hitler had Parkinson's disease, but this label simply describes a collection of symptoms and is not strictly a diagnosis. Syphilis is known as "the great mimic," and may certainly cause the symptoms typical of Parkinson's disease.

The organism responsible for syphilis is a *spirochaete*, a spiral, rod-shaped bacterium. The reason for it invading the brain and spinal cord is because the capillaries in the nervous system are smaller in diameter than those elsewhere in the body. The spirochaete may arrest in the capillaries in a form of embolism, and then slowly invade the surrounding tissues. It is a very slow growing organism that proved extremely difficult to culture outside the body, until it was recognised that its growth is inhibited by oxygen.[14] Once this had been identified and a low oxygen gas substituted for the air previously used, studies were soon made. The early symptoms in stages one and two are usually concealed by the patient. The insidious development of tertiary syphilis may be delayed for decades, causing knowledgeable victims to agonise for years over their fate. The reappearance of the disease in the brain may well be due to the spirochaete growing again when chronic inflammation reduces the tissue oxygen level.[15]

Another important form of embolism occurs in malaria associated with infection of red blood cells by a parasite of the genus *Plasmodium*, which is carried by mosquitoes. The parasite does not invade the brain like syphilis—its neurological effects are due to the increased size and reduced deformability of red blood cells when they are invaded by the parasite. The red cells actually cause damage to the lining of the capillaries *in transit*, in a similar way to the tiny bubbles responsible for decompression sickness. In the severest form of the disease, cerebral malaria, there is damage to the blood-brain barrier and its opening allows water, plasma proteins, and even red blood cells to transfer into the brain causing hypoxia, inflammation, and swelling.[16,17] This suggests that, as with the damage to the barrier caused by bubbles, the brain swelling in malaria will respond to hyperbaric oxygen treatment. Oxygen is also involved in the destruction of the malarial parasite by the herbal drug Artemisinin. Within the structure of the molecule, two oxygen atoms form an endoperoxide bond. This bond is split in contact with iron released in the red cell causing a free radical reaction which kills the parasite. The discovery was made by the Chinese scientist, Professor Tu Yuyu, who received the Lasker-DeBakey Clinical Medical Research Award in 2011 for her excellent work.

Embolism associated with clots that form in the deep veins of the legs are on the low pressure side of the circulation in which blood flows to the right side of the heart, and the lungs. There are other forms of embolism that arise on the arterial side of the circulation, for example, from clots forming on the walls of the left atrium or left ventricle after their lining has been damaged in heart attacks. Emboli may also arise from fatty material deposited in the lining of the aorta and other major arteries, especially in the neck. Being already on the arterial side of the circulation, these emboli cannot be trapped by the lungs, and so travel along arteries until they may impact in the smallest branches, often causing a stroke. Some may even flow back to the arteries of the heart and cause a heart attack. Larger emboli are most likely to travel to the organs of the body that have a large blood supply, such as the brain, which is determined by hydraulic principles. Again, emboli that are too small to cause a blockage may still inflict damage to the blood-brain barrier in transit, just as bubbles do in divers.

The involvement of the spinal cord in decompression sickness has caused some to doubt Haldane's idea that bubbles circulating in the blood are involved because, it is claimed, it is rare for circulating emboli to affect the spinal cord. However, it certainly does occur in syphilis, where the lodging of the bacterium gives rise to a condition known as *tabes dorsalis*. Nevertheless, it is true that the brain is the usual target when air emboli enter the circulation, such as when a diver's lungs are torn by the expansion of gas in too rapid an ascent, or if air enters the circulation in an operation, such as during cardiac surgery. The bubbles responsible for decompression sickness are very much smaller, and are certainly able to reach the spinal cord. How do we know? We know for sure because red and white blood cells, which are effectively emboli suspended in plasma and also very small, certainly travel to the spinal cord in the blood supply. A number of alternative theories have been proposed to explain the involvement of the spinal cord in decompression sickness, including the suggestion that the veins draining the spinal cord may become blocked by bubbles. Another suggestion is that there may be a spontaneous eruption of gas within the substance of the cord itself. By far the most credible explanation is the one at the head of this chapter from the 1908 publication by Boycott, Damant, and Haldane in the *Journal of Hygiene of London*[18] that Haldane had founded. Although the three authors are listed alphabetically, there can be little doubt that the ideas were those of Haldane, as many appear in the 1907 Admiralty report. They are so important in defining *a principle of disease* that they deserve detailed discussion.

Haldane and his co-workers had devised an extensive testing program using goats in the chamber at the Lister Institute in London. They undertook post-mortem examinations of the animals and, after piecing together the information, finally made the remarkable statement reproduced below the heading of this chapter, beginning, "If small bubbles pass through the lung capillaries…" What is being suggested for the first time in the history of medicine is that the lungs are a trap, in this case for bubbles, and for other particles in the circulation. However, they are a trap that can fail and it is a contention of this book that this principle has been overlooked and that material that escapes being trapped in the lungs contributes to a number of diseases where the cause is said to be unknown, which are labeled auto-immune. Haldane would have been very aware of embolism, as he was a scientist with an interest in gases and liquids. He would also have recognised the critical importance of the *size* of emboli because of the presence of very small blood vessels in the body, and that blood is in reality a suspension of small emboli: red and white blood cells. In fact, it would really be better not to have any particles in the circulation because they increase the pumping force required, and some clump together to form clots obstructing blood flow. Despite its name, the red cell is not truly a cell because after being formed in the bone marrow, the nucleus is pushed out and the cell assumes the configuration of a biconcave disc. This is the optimal shape to allow the uptake of oxygen and the ability to deform. Red blood cells are slowed down in deforming to squeeze through the capillaries in the brain, which gives time for them to give up the oxygen attached to haemoglobin. The constant deformation eventually damages the membrane covering the red cell, as does colliding with the leaflets of heart valves. When red cells are damaged, the surface roughness ensures that they are removed from the circulation by the spleen. The average life expectancy of a red cell is said to be just 120 days.

Haldane's analysis of the journey of bubbles was simple but brilliant: Small ones may pass through the lung capillaries and once they have done so, they may be transported to the nervous system. Larger bubbles, however, would be trapped in the lung, allowing their gas to be exhaled. The primary function of the lungs in exchanging the gases oxygen and carbon dioxide has been studied exhaustively. The features needed to fulfill their function as gas exchangers, such as a large number of capillaries and a low blood pressure, are also important characteristics that facilitate filtering of the blood. Being located between the right and left chambers of the heart, the lung capillaries are ideally placed to entrap circulating debris, so cleaning blood going to the main arteries supplying the rest of the body. This is especially important for the health of the blood vessels of the nervous system, which being small are peculiarly vulnerable to damage from small emboli. In contrast to the research of gas exchange, this function of the lungs as traps, cleaning blood of dangerous particles, has only been investigated in relation to the effects of bubbles in diving and aerospace research. These are, of course, highly specialised fields outside mainstream medicine, which have only given employment to a very small number of scientists and physicians in the world.

The lungs are actually very efficient and, surprisingly, even blockage of 90% of the capillaries of the lungs has been found to be compatible with survival. Some 80 years after Haldane's perceptive observation of this property of the lungs, trapping has been found to be of special *physi-*

ological importance in the body. Cells in blood called megakaryocytes, which translated means large carrying cells, are produced in the bone marrow and released into the draining veins. Like bubbles occurring in divers, they are transported in blood to the right side of the heart and then pumped into the capillaries of the lungs. Being rather large, they are trapped and broken down to release platelets, ensuring that they are well-mixed in the arterial blood and thoroughly distributed around the body.[19] Platelets are essential to clotting and if they were released into the slow-moving, deoxygenated blood leaving the bone marrow, it is likely that clots would form in the deep veins returning blood to the heart.

Haldane continued his explanation of the effects of bubbles in divers stating that they may "lodge in a slowly desaturating part of the spinal cord, where they may cause blockage of the circulation or direct mechanical damage." Here, he introduces two important concepts: first, the arrest of blood flow and second, damage to the lining of blood vessels. From the additional knowledge gained from experiments over the last few decades, it appears that direct mechanical damage to the lining of blood vessels is the most significant factor. If emboli are small enough not to arrest in the low-pressure capillaries of the lungs, then it is likely that the much higher pressures in the capillaries of the rest of the body will force them through other organs. Animal studies in Canada in the 1950s by the distinguished neurologist Dr. Roy L. Swank and his colleagues[20] showed that emboli much larger than blood cells can actually squeeze through the microcirculation of the brain, although they often damaged the lining of the blood vessels. They also found that the emboli could be retained in the capillaries of the animal's brain indefinitely without causing damage. Since a cubic millimetre of brain tissue can contain many hundreds of capillaries, their presence would be unlikely to cause lack of oxygen to nerve cells. However, the smaller size of the capillaries in the brain is a significant factor in the damage that small emboli cause to their lining cells. As already discussed, the blood vessels in the nervous system are different to those in most organs of the body; the lining cells fit together tightly, forming the blood-brain barrier. It has been shown experimentally that the *passage* of small bubbles causes damage to the lining cells of blood vessels in the brain and opens the barrier. This attracts white blood cells, which invade the tissues releasing free radicals, just as they do to combat infection and the end result is, of course, inflammation.[21]

Experiments undertaken in the University of Texas in the 1980s have confirmed the accuracy of Haldane's prediction.[22] Carefully graded small bubbles in the size range known to be released into the circulation in decompression sickness were introduced into the carotid artery of a guinea pig. One hour following their injection, an injection of a special blue dye, which binds to the proteins present in plasma, stained the tissues of the brain hemisphere supplied by that artery. Controls injected with plasma alone, without bubbles, did not show this effect. This provides unequivocal evidence that bubble micro-emboli open the blood-brain barrier, as did adipose tissue and mineral oil micro-emboli. Experiments undertaken at the Cleveland Clinic have extended these observations to peripheral nerves.[23] Carefully sized emboli were injected into the femoral (leg) artery of a rat. The largest dose of emboli injected caused death of the sciatic nerve whereas the smallest dose had no effect. However, the middle dose of emboli injected caused demyelination—damage to the myelin sheaths of the nerves. The emboli opened the blood-nerve barrier, which is the equivalent of the blood-brain barrier. These barriers protect the internal environment of the nervous system and are present in other sensitive tissues.

When the blood-brain barrier is breached, the proteins in plasma leak into the tissues of the brain and cause inflammation by triggering the complement pathway.[24] A technology from chemistry and the invention of X-ray computed tomography came together in magnetic resonance imaging (MRI), to allow the detection of the small areas of inflammation and swelling due to an increased water content, and known in neurology as unidentified bright objects (UBOs). They can be found in the brains of divers who suffer from what is known in Haldane's classification as Type 2 decompression sickness.[25] Figure 7.4 shows a typical "bright object" in a key position in the brain of a diver who had developed decompression sickness. It is likely that this MRI from 1984 is the first time the technology has been used in a case of decompression sickness.

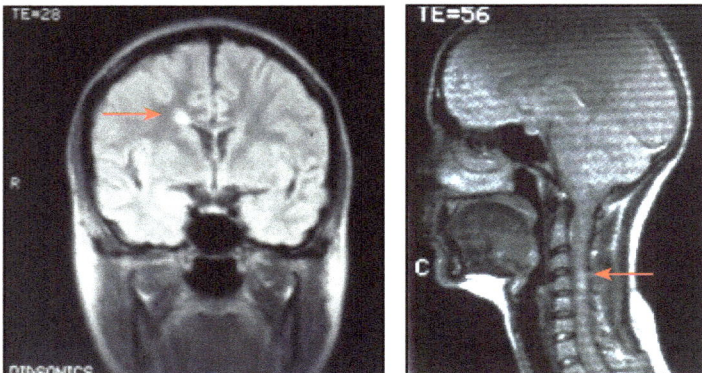

Figure 7.4:
Damage in the brain and spinal cord of a diver (arrowed).

What is remarkable is that the diver concerned now does not have any symptoms. UBOs are actually common in the general population but much commoner in patients who have been told they have multiple sclerosis. By repeating MRIs in multiple sclerosis patients every two weeks over many months, it has been found that UBOs come and go on a regular basis.[26]

The next question is obvious: What does the tissue damage look like under the microscope? Figure 7.5 shows the appearance of the spinal cord in experimental decompression sickness with haemorrhages surrounding the draining veins.[27] These haemorrhages are also found in patients with acute multiple sclerosis in the same locations and resolve leaving tissue damage.

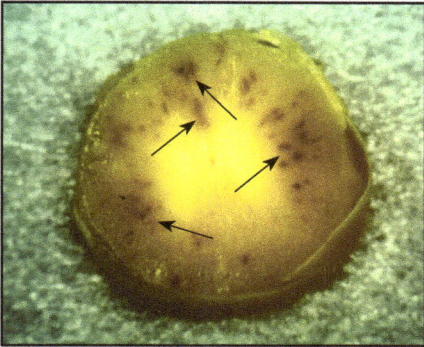

Figure 7.5:
The spinal cord in acute decompression sickness. (Courtesy of Professor D.H. Elliott.)

The spinal cord of a diver who actually recovered after an episode of Type 2 decompression sickness[28] is shown in Figure 7.6. The areas arrowed are where the stain for myelin sheaths has not been taken up. They are in the same locations often involved in patients with multiple sclerosis.

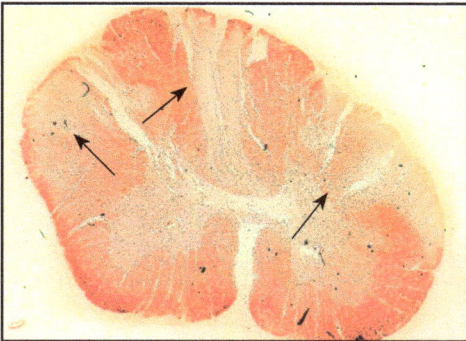

Figure 7.6:
Section of the spinal cord at C5 from a diver post-decompression sickness.
(Courtesy of Dr. I.M. Calder.)

Many thousands more men have been employed in civil engineering projects using compressed air than have been employed in diving and they also risk decompression sickness. Because of the proximity of Lake Michigan to Milwaukee, civil engineering excavations in the city are undertaken using compressed air to prevent the ingress of water. Although the monitoring of the health of compressed-air workers has not been as rigorous as it has been for divers, an MRI study in the US has revealed that they have a much higher prevalence of UBOs than the normal population.[29]

The study was of 19 workers who had been involved in tunnelling projects in the Milwaukee area. Eleven men who were also employed in the tunnel contracts were used as matched controls because they had not worked in compressed air. The 19 compressed-air workers had a total of 152 UBOs on MRI, compared to only 22 in the control group. However, the 22 UBOs were in only two men, whereas the 152 were in 10 of the 19 compressed-air workers. Seven men had more than 20 lesions each. This data is very important, because it shows that the bubbles produced by decompression do indeed produce UBOs, and also that as in multiple sclerosis patients they usually do not give rise to symptoms or correlate with disability. The key part of the nervous system that gives rise to disability is the spinal cord. UBOs found in the brain on MRI have been given an undeserved status in trials of drugs introduced for patients with multiple sclerosis. Professor George Ebers[30] recently pointed out that for many doctors undertaking these studies of multiple sclerosis, the MRI findings have "been regarded as the disease."

The unique link between diving flying and multiple sclerosis patients has recently been reinforced by a study of pilots flying the very high altitude reconnaissance aircraft, the Lockheed Martin U-2. First flown in 1955, the U-2 came to international attention when, on May 1, 1960 an aircraft flown by Francis Gary Powers was shot down over the Soviet Union. The pilots undertake flights lasting many hours at a cabin altitude equivalent to 28,000 feet. They prebreathe oxygen for several hours on the ground and continue oxygen breathing during the flight, but, nevertheless, they can suffer from bubble-induced decompression sickness. As mentioned at the end of the previous chapter, a remarkable paper released in August 2013 compared the brain MRI findings in 102 pilots with 91 carefully matched controls. The pilot group had a 394% greater volume of white matter tissue affected with 295% more areas of damage than the controls.[31] The authors draw attention to the fact that micro-particles have been detected in blood on decompression[32] but fail to mention the key information: Micro-embolism opens the blood-brain barrier.[33]

The Admiralty had tasked Haldane to solve the problem of diver's palsy, and he succeeded with the introduction of his decompression tables—cases of paralysis then became rare. Haldane had, for the first time in medicine, drawn attention to the ability of the lungs to trap material that could endanger the brain. As will be seen, the trapping of debris in the capillaries of the lungs is of critical importance to the health of the nervous system. The first event in the development of symptoms in both decompression sickness[22] and multiple sclerosis is damage to the lining of blood vessels, which opens the blood-brain barrier, and leads to a fall in the oxygen level in the area. This is the signal for the white blood cells, known as neutrophils, to stick to the lining of the blood vessels and then invade the tissues releasing free radicals, as they are programmed to do against infection. This causes inflammation, which is the hallmark feature of both diseases. Haldane prophetically called the damage to the spinal cord caused by bubbles in divers "an unusual form of embolism," and he was certainly right. It raises a key question: If bubbles in the blood reaching the brain can cause this damage, is it possible that something else carried in the circulation is responsible for multiple sclerosis? It will be seen that it is certainly possible and has been confirmed by a number of pathologists over the last hundred years. The evidence will be covered in detail later.

In 1936, Haldane undertook his last project—an investigation of heat stroke in men working in the oilfields of Persia travelling with Imperial Airways in the Hengist, a four-engine aircraft, accompanied by his sister Elizabeth. Shortly after returning home, Haldane fell out of bed and, after a short illness, died of pneumonia aged 76. Thirty years later his decompression tables for divers were to play a critical part in the exploitation of oil and gas resources offshore, especially those of his native country, Scotland. In 1969, drilling for oil began in the UK in the Firth of Forth just a few miles east of Broxburn where James "Paraffin" Young had mined shale. Little oil was found, but soon much further north off the Scottish east coast, dramatic finds were made. The hostile waters and extreme depths of the North Sea were to claim many lives of many divers. However, thanks to Haldane's pioneering research, many were treated using oxygen at levels unheard of in mainstream medicine.

CHAPTER 8
Oxygen: Diving, Flying, and Medicine

Oxygen should be regarded as a drug . . . an inappropriate concentration can have serious or even fatal consequences.

The British National Formulary, 1996–2010

In a letter addressed to the committee responsible for the above quotation in the formulary in 1998, the author and a colleague, the late Dr. David Perrins, posed a question which could not have been simpler: By referencing "an inappropriate concentration," did they mean too much or too little? The letter was acknowledged by the secretary, but to-date no answer has been received from the committee. It would be difficult to imagine a better illustration of the nonsense that oxygen has generated in medical practice. Too little oxygen is obviously fatal; indeed, we all die from it, but it would be extremely difficult to find an instance of a patient dying from receiving too much. In fact, the *only* pure gas it is safe to breathe is oxygen—breathing *any* other pure gas is fatal within minutes, because it does not add oxygen and it removes the oxygen already present in the body.[1] Oxygen is certainly *not* a drug, although, like a drug, it can be given in differing dosages and has a variety of actions. However; very high levels have been used safely for decades in aviation, space exploration, and diving. Although the knowledge gained from these fields impacts on all of our lives, the facts in this chapter are known to only a handful of the world's physicians.

Pure oxygen was first used as a diving gas by a resourceful civilian diver in the 1870s when standard hard hat equipment was found to be too bulky for a difficult underwater task in a civil engineering project. By the 1930s, pure oxygen had been introduced in military diving using self-contained breathing apparatus, and this use continues today. Because oxygen can be recirculated through a scrubber to remove the exhaled carbon dioxide, cylinders of oxygen can provide much longer times underwater than an equivalent volume of compressed air. Known as closed circuit breathing apparatus, it has a second advantage for covert military operations—the release of tell-tale bubbles can be avoided. Millions of man hours have been accumulated by divers in the armed forces of many countries, breathing pure oxygen at levels regarded as dangerous, or even lethal, by most doctors. Military pilots also routinely breathe pure oxygen, as do commercial jet pilots when they fly at altitudes above 40,000 feet. Astronauts wear suits with helmets pressurised with oxygen for their extra-vehicular activities in space. Their equipment uses the same method of recirculation used by military divers to conserve the limited supply of breathing gas in the cylinders contained in the backpack.

During WW2, oxygen breathing equipment was used by the courageous X-craft submariners who managed to cripple the German pocket battleship *Tirpitz* near Tromso—its remains can be seen on Google Earth resting on the bottom of a fjord. The X-craft volunteers had been forced to dive to extreme depths to avoid anti-submarine nets and escape enemy action. As the pressure of the oxygen breathed by a diver has to match the surrounding water pressure, the deeper they went, the higher the concentration of oxygen they had to breathe. Some of the men convulsed, and, losing the mouthpiece of the apparatus, drowned. However, this extreme military situation is far removed from the clinical use of hyperbaric oxygen treatment, not only because of the absence of water, but also because the pressures needed for effective treatment are normally well below those that risk convulsions. As Paracelsus (1493–1541) wrote, "All things are poison and nothing is without poison, only the dose permits something not to be poisonous." However, to avoid any allegation that the risk is being downplayed, this chapter gives the necessary background and the most likely explanation for the effects that are loosely termed "toxicity." The way is then clear to introduce the vital lessons learned from the treatment of the bubble-related illnesses with oxygen at high pressures.

Paul Bert's animal experiments[2] had already shown in the 1870s that high levels of oxygen could cause convulsions. During WW2, as part of the development of oxygen diving, an extensive research programme was undertaken by the late Dr. Kenneth Donald.[3] He was later to be appointed professor of medicine at Haldane's old university in Edinburgh. Donald founded the Admiralty Experimental Diving Unit (AEDU) at Gosport, when he was working in the Royal Navy, simply by printing new headed notepaper. He showed that the risk of a convulsion was greatly increased both by hard exercise and also by being underwater rather than in a dry pressure chamber. Military diving usually involves hard work, and so combines these two factors. Testing for oxygen sensitivity was introduced for naval divers during WW2 both in the UK and in the US in an attempt to exclude those men most likely to suffer a convulsion underwater. The tests proved very unreliable; divers who showed no symptoms whatsoever on one test, would convulse on their next under exactly the same conditions. One diver descended to the bottom of Horsea lake near Portsmouth at 70 feet (21 msw) three times a week and stood breathing pure oxygen until he noted the onset of the symptoms that are usually attributed to oxygen toxicity. Measures were taken to standardise every possible factor, from the time he went to bed the night before, to the food he had for breakfast. The time to the onset of the early symptoms, usually lip switching—after the first few days when it was thought that apprehension played a part—ranged from 23 to 128 minutes! Clearly, oxygen is simply *not* toxic and there must be some major physiological variable involved to make such an enormous difference in the timing of the symptoms.

Despite this, oxygen tolerance testing continued to be used for many years, before it was finally abandoned because of its failure to predict the likelihood of convulsions. However, the experience gained confirmed that oxygen cannot be a poison in the conventional sense. Despite oxygen research continuing in military laboratories, the cause of the convulsions has remained elusive. It has been alleged that they are the result of a massive release of free radicals,[4] but this is certainly *not* true as it would cause severe brain damage, or even death. But no long-term effects on the brain have ever been reported following an oxygen convulsion. The author witnessed oxygen convulsions first hand in two divers in the former Admiralty Experimental Diving Unit at Alverstoke, near Portsmouth, when a mistake was made in a diving trial—oxygen was supplied instead of air at a depth of 132 feet (40 msw). Both recovered consciousness rapidly after the gas they were breathing was changed from oxygen to air.

The lack of serious consequences from a convulsion induced by high-pressure oxygen was graphically illustrated in the 1980s when a diver working in the now defunct Argyll field in the North Sea was supplied pure oxygen working on the bottom at a depth of 260 feet (80 msw). A mistake had been made on the diving support ship in coupling his umbilical gas supply to cylinders of oxygen, rather than the correct mixture of 7% oxygen and 93% helium. Again, the pressure of the gas breathed has to match the combined water pressure and sea level air pressure, and this combination gave a total oxygen pressure on the bottom of 9 ATA. The diver had been supplied the correct helium and oxygen mixture for the first few hours of his dive, and the change to pure oxygen can be heard on the tape of the incident from the noise made by his demand valve. Despite an enormous increase in the effort needed for him to breathe, as pure oxygen is much denser than a helium and oxygen mixture, the diver continued working for almost five minutes before reporting that he felt unwell. The diving supervisor at dive control in the ship found him difficult to understand because the pitch of his voice had become much lower. After about five minutes, the diver returned to the diving bell and after being helped inside by the bellman, the diver convulsed for about 20 seconds after his helmet was removed. Far from sustaining brain damage, he recovered consciousness within a few minutes and was soon conversing normally with the supervisor via the communication system. The dose of oxygen he received was *45 times* greater than the level of oxygen in the air we breathe at sea level—so much for allegations that oxygen is a deadly poison. Another clear indication of the lack of serious consequences from an oxygen-induced convulsion is evident from the advice given in the *US Navy Diving Manual*. The instruction given for managing divers who convulse during treatment for decompression sickness is simply to continue breathing oxygen after a lapse of just 15 minutes. Other relevant experience was gained in psychiatric practice in the US during the 1950s. High levels of oxygen were actually used to induce convulsions as an alternative to electrically-induced convulsions— again, important evidence of the safety of oxygen.

Are there any clues as to why very high oxygen levels cause convulsions? The evidence indicates that it is related to a *known property* of the gas, and the most obvious is its role in controlling blood flow by *constricting* blood vessels. Three gases are actually involved in the control of blood vessel diameter and, hence, blood flow: oxygen (O_2), carbon dioxide (CO_2), and nitric oxide (NO). Oxygen reduces the diameter of blood vessels reducing blood flow, whilst carbon dioxide and nitric oxide both cause them to enlarge by relaxing the muscle in the wall. Curiously, although the gas nitric oxide is produced by the lining endothelial cells of blood vessels, if it contaminates the air we breathe, it is a deadly poison. It forms nitric acid on entering the lungs and induces internal "drowning" from the leakage of blood plasma into the airspaces. The same process occurred in the troops gassed at Ypres in WW1, when hydrochloric acid was formed in the lungs from the chlorine gas inhaled. The control of blood flow by nitric oxide over the *normal physiological* range of oxygen levels involves a complex interaction between oxygen and haemoglobin.[5] However, at higher than normal oxygen levels and haemoglobin saturated, blood vessels continue being constricted because oxygen inactivates nitric oxide *directly*.[6]

The constriction of blood vessels by oxygen is likely to be the key factor in the production of a convulsion because when blood flow is severely restricted, the delivery of glucose, the other substance critical to metabolism, will be reduced. It is well known that a sudden fall in the level of glucose in the blood can itself precipitate a convulsion. It was in the 1970s that neurosurgeons in the University of Bonn found that as the level of oxygen increased, *glucose uptake by the brain was reduced*.[7] The dramatic reduction of blood flow seen in some patients breathing a high level of oxygen will inevitably reduce the delivery of glucose because it is transported in blood. This may well explain why oxygen divers are most likely to convulse when they are exercising hard and using up glucose and it only needs a small amount of dysfunction in the brain to trigger a fit.

The author had a unique opportunity to examine the retina in a patient who was breathing oxygen at 2.8 times atmospheric pressure and developed the early warning signs of apprehension and facial twitching which, if the oxygen breathing had been continued, would have been followed by a convulsion. The blood vessels in the eye were like pencil lines, and the normal redness of the retina had turned to a pinkish grey. This can be fairly described by a new term, *hyperoxic ischaemia,* translated simply as a reduction of blood flow associated with a high level of oxygen. This clearly contrasts with *lack of oxygen* caused by a reduction of blood flow, that is, hypoxia, as happens, for example, in a heart attack or a stroke. This very common disease process is known either as *hypoxic-ischaemia,* or, more usually, as *ischaemic-hypoxia.* Based on the available evidence, it is likely that oxygen convulsions are, indeed, due to lack of *glucose* associated with an extreme reduction of blood flow, and it would certainly account for the great unpredictability of the effect. It is likely that adding carbon dioxide to oxygen which dilates blood vessels would reduce the likelihood of convulsions.[8] Regardless of the mechanism, if very high levels of oxygen are breathed continuously for long periods, they may eventually threaten tissue damage. It may also exacerbate pre-existing disease, as in the Case Report that follows.

A Case Report

Experiments were conducted by a group at the University of Pennsylvania in the 1960s to determine the effect of four hours of continuous oxygen breathing at double atmospheric pressure (2 ATA) on the lung function of volunteers (see Chapter 5). One subject had a history of optic neuritis, and he was examined carefully by an ophthalmologist before being included in the experiment.[9] Only slight paleness of the optic disc was found and so he was allowed to continue. After 90 minutes of continuous oxygen breathing in the chamber, he complained that his field of vision in the affected eye was reduced. Surprisingly, the experiment was continued. After three hours he had severe tunnel vision, and by four hours he had completely lost vision in the eye. As the experiment had been completed, the volunteer was allowed to remove the oxygen mask and breathe the air in the chamber as he was decompressed to normal atmospheric pressure. As soon as he stopped breathing oxygen and breathed air, his vision began to recover. After 12 hours, it had returned to normal, although he was also given a steroid stimulating drug (ACTH) for eye discomfort.

The blood vessels are damaged in optic neuritis, as they are in areas affected in the brain and spinal cord in patients with multiple sclerosis. This often, as in this patient, causes pallor of the optic disc, which can be seen by looking in the eye using an ophthalmoscope. The loss of vision could not have been due to lack of oxygen, given the very high level he was breathing, but there is no question that the dramatic reduction of blood flow induced would have reduced the delivery of glucose. The change to breathing air at the end of the four hours would have rapidly relieved the constriction of the blood vessels, and returned glucose delivery to a normal level.

The convulsions induced by very high levels of oxygen are indistinguishable from the grande mal convulsions seen in epilepsy, where they may be associated with cumulative brain damage, and it is understandable that they should raise concerns. However, patients who suffer a convulsion associated with epilepsy actually lack oxygen after convulsing. Magnetic resonance spectroscopy (MRS) has shown that there is a build-up of lactic acid in the brain after an epileptic fit.[10] The presence of lactic acid conclusively indicates a failure of aerobic metabolism and it is due to a deficiency of oxygen. It is almost certainly due to tissue swelling when water enters brain tissue due to failure of the blood-brain barrier, and it is reversible.[11] It would, therefore, make sense to give epileptic patients oxygen to breathe after a fit, because it is likely that the cumulative brain damage is due to the inflammation and hypoxia that follows opening of the blood-brain barrier.

It is also important to note that hypoxia may itself cause a seizure, as it sometimes does with loss of consciousness when blood pressure falls in a simple faint. The abrupt lack of oxygen in the body that results from breathing a gas not containing oxygen may also cause a fit. On December 20, 1992, the *International Herald Tribune* reported the case of a 12-year-old boy who convulsed after breathing pure helium used for inflating balloons at a party. Again, this risk is present if *any* pure gas other than oxygen is breathed. In contrast, there is certainly no risk of patients having an oxygen-induced convulsion when they are receiving treatment for a severe deficiency of oxygen, as in acute carbon monoxide poisoning, and very high oxygen levels have been successfully used for such patients. In another case, a hypoxic patient, deeply unconscious and unresponsive after air had been introduced into the blood vessels of the brain, was compressed to six times atmospheric pressure breathing air. The object was simply to "squash the bubbles," but he did not regain consciousness. Pure oxygen was then administered at this pressure, as a last resort, and he immediately regained consciousness (personal communication, Dr. Robert Goodman, St. Luke's Hospital, Milwaukee).

At this point, the reader may well be questioning the need for a detailed discussion about diving. It is needed because the only use of pressure chambers and hyperbaric oxygenation accepted around the world is for divers. Admittedly, it is for the treatment of air embolism and decompression sickness where it is claimed that the rationale is simply the elimination of bubbles. Nevertheless, 100% oxygen is used routinely at high pressures, which may have much to do with the fact that divers are robust, self-reliant, no-nonsense individuals who demand the treatment. Commercial diving operations are required by law in many countries to provide hyperbaric chambers on site, and they are always equipped with oxygen breathing systems. The procedures developed for the treatment of divers are also those which use the highest pressures used in hyperbaric oxygen treatment. The objective is to compress the large bubbles that enter the circulation when the lung tears, a condition known as pulmonary barotraumas—such a tear may allow the gas being breathed direct access to the blood circulating through the lungs. It was originally thought that high pressures were simply essential to compress and re-dissolve the gas present. "Bubble squashing" provides a simple and biologically plausible mechanism to explain the benefit of hyperbaric treatment but, as will be seen, the effects of gas bubbles in the circulation are very complex. The concept of bubble squashing is widely accepted, especially among divers, and amateur divers are now using advanced techniques to achieve ever-greater depths. Nevertheless, studies undertaken of gas embolism both in the UK[12] and Australia[13] have actually shown that immediate compression to just 2 ATA breathing pure oxygen is more effective than the currently recommended high pressure military procedures, which use compressed air.

The recompression treatment of decompression sickness has evolved from the experience of the early caisson workers more than a hundred years ago and, in the absence of controlled studies, the evidence must be deemed anecdotal. Regardless, anyone foolish enough to question its value faces the wrath of many thousands of well-informed divers. In the UK and many European countries, commercial divers are empowered to treat acute decompression illness in their colleagues under government diving regulations. It is the only civilian profession in which life-saving treatment, well in excess of simple first aid, is under the control of non-medical personnel. In 1985, this was strongly reinforced by the government diving inspectorate in the UK, after mistakes in treatment made by inexperienced doctors caused the deaths of several divers. Under a Diving Safety Memorandum issued by the Chief Inspector of Diving,[14] the on-site diving supervisor was authorised to be "in control at all times," and could not be overruled by a doctor. This includes the management of divers paraplegic, or even unconscious, from bubbles. So divers are responsible for using oxygen at far greater levels than are used in our hospitals, both as a diving gas and in the treatment of the gas bubble-related illnesses.

It may come as a surprise to many that despite Haldane's brilliant research, the mechanism causing brain or spinal cord damage in divers is still said to be controversial. It would appear to be a simple matter to determine what happens, for example, when a diver loses the movement of his legs suffering from the "diver's palsy" of Haldane's day. After all, the circumstances are known—the depth of the dive and its duration, together with rate of the decompression, and so on. In fact, they are always carefully recorded in commercial diving. The dose of nitrogen, the offending agent, is determined solely by the depth and duration of the dive. Because events are often witnessed first hand and recorded, it would seem a simple matter to solve the mystery. It is at times difficult to escape the feeling that some do not want answers to be found. Equally, no one can seriously doubt the effectiveness of the recompression treatment used for divers using a hyperbaric chamber. The increase in pressure will certainly reduce the volume of any gas present, both by the direct effect of pressure (Boyle's law) and, because when gas is pressurised, it re-dissolves (Henry's law). These effects may seem to be enough, but sometimes the procedures available simply do not work. The value of returning to a high pressure was actually discovered by compressed-air workers in France. Triger, an engineer, designed the first practical caisson for use in bridge construction in 1839.[15] His workers soon discovered that they only became ill after leaving the caisson, and also that a return to pressure in the caisson usually created a cure. It was even recorded that when the workers became ill they returned to sleep in the caisson, and then continued working in the caisson the next day.

In the 1950s there was a boom in amateur diving, and people began to present for treatment in increasing numbers at military decompression chambers, especially in the US. The treatment offered was simply recompressed breathing air based on schedules developed in the 1930s. It became obvious by the early 1960s, however, that all was not well. In 1964, a study published by the US Navy[16] showed that compressed air treatment was failing to resolve almost one out of every two cases of serious decompression sickness affecting the nervous system. Recompression tables using compressed air add more nitrogen to the body during the treatment, and so it becomes a race to resolve a diver's problems before the additional nitrogen makes matters worse on decompression. Two US Navy doctors, Maurice W. Goodman and Robert D. Workman, decided to develop treatment tables using pure oxygen breathing at much lower pressures.[17] This avoids the addition of more nitrogen, and allows considerable shortening of the treatment time needed. The longest compressed air table took almost two days, whereas the equivalent oxygen procedure takes about six hours.

Two new US Navy procedures, tables 5 and 6, which became known as the Minimal Recompression Oxygen Breathing Tables, were incorporated in the *US Navy Diving Manual* published in 1970. Even by this time, two problems had been found to complicate their use: convulsions, which were fortunately very rare, and also a worsening of symptoms. Surprisingly, no one has suggested that there may be a connection between the two; in other words, that the events which can lead to a convulsion may in a lesser form be responsible for a diver becoming worse during the treatment. Another significant factor, which is constantly overlooked, introduces a large variable that affects the level of oxygen in these procedures. At the same pressure and using the same type of oronasal mask, a very wide variation exists in the level of oxygen actually present in the arterial blood of patients. Measurements have been made by sampling the blood from arteries of patients breathing 100% oxygen through a tight-fitting mask in a chamber at twice atmospheric pressure (2 ATA). The oxygen levels in the arterial blood samples ranged from 850 mm Hg (equivalent to 1.11 ATA) to 1,140 mm Hg (equivalent to 1.59 ATA), despite strict precautions being taken to ensure that the masks were properly fitted.[18] This means that under the strictest conditions there can be nearly a 44% difference in the plasma concentration of patients, or divers, all sitting in a chamber at the same pressure, and all using a properly fitting oronasal mask. Whilst this is a large difference, it will be seen later that there can be a 700% difference in the blood concentration of drugs in patients taking a drug by mouth!

The US Navy developed table 6 for the treatment of serious decompression sickness using oxygen breathing at 2.8 times atmospheric pressure (2.8 ATA), equivalent to a pressure of 18 metres (60 feet) of sea water. The principle was to use the maximum pressure possible to compress any gas bubbles present, while minimising risk of a convulsion. A pressure of 2.8 atmospheres was arrived at by analysing the experience of convulsions in US Navy divers training to use an oxygen breathing apparatus. The end point used when oxygen breathing was a warning symptom, usually twitching of the muscles of the face. However, sometimes a full-blown oxygen convulsion, which is identical to a grande mal epileptic seizure, occurred. A search of US Navy records was made, and it was found that the risk of a convulsion became significant after 30 minutes of oxygen breathing at 3 ATA. In the oxygen treatment tables, it was decided to reduce the pressure used to 2.8 ATA, and also interrupt the oxygen breathing after 20 minutes by removing the mask and allowing the patient to breathe air for five minutes. Oxygen breathing was then resumed again for 20 minutes, and the cycle repeated three, or sometimes four, times.

The final US Navy Research Report of the oxygen procedures developed by Drs. Goodman and Workman was released in 1965.[17] After a review of their use, which indicated they were more successful than compressed air, they were published in 1967 and incorporated in the next revision of the *US Navy Diving Manual* released in 1970 as tables 5 and 6. But a warning was included in the instructions for using the new tables—there was reference to a diver's symptoms worsening during the time breathing oxygen at 2.8 atmospheres. No explanation was given for the worsening, and the advice given was simply to stop the patient from breathing oxygen and revert to using the original approach using further pressurisation on compressed air. This, of course, means using a method of treatment proven to be less successful. The reference to worsening of symptoms breathing oxygen has been included in every subsequent revision of the diving manual, and still without any explanation. The author experienced this phenomenon treating a diver in 1976, and has raised it with several generations of US Navy medical officers, who have steadfastly refused to discuss the matter. It seems logical that if just a small increase in the pressure and the time spent breathing oxygen, that is, from just 2.8 to 3.0 ATA and from 20 to 30 minutes, means that a convulsion becomes likely, it is reasonable to suspect that the mechanism responsible for a convulsion is also responsible for the worsening of symptoms. There is a simple and now well-proven solution to the problem: Use less oxygen. Lower the level used to just 2 atmospheres, and use helium rather than nitrogen to give a total pressure of 4 ATA. This procedure introduced by the French diving company Comex in 1986[19] has been very successful commercially, and has completely avoided the problem of the worsening symptoms sometimes seen when very high oxygen pressures are used.

In the *US Navy Diving Manual* edition published in 1959, helium and oxygen mixtures had actually been recommended for serious cases, recurrence of symptoms, and when a diver had difficulty breathing. Helium and oxygen treatment has been well proven in the commercial oil field diving over the last 40 years, and the scientific basis confirmed by animal experiments.[20] When using oxygen, the message is simple: The dosage is important, especially in the treatment of the brain. Unfortunately, protocols now 40 years old used for the treatment of diving illnesses may cause convulsions and worsening of symptoms because of the very high oxygen levels designated. However, they are still current and even regarded as the gold standard, despite the fact that improved procedures using lower levels of oxygen have been proven in commercial diving. While this may again only seem relevant to diving, unfortunately the US Navy oxygen tables using 2.8 atmospheres of oxygen have influenced clinical treatment. For example, oxygen at 2.4 ATA is often used in wound healing, when just 2 ATA would be sufficient in a pure oxygen chamber or if a properly-fitting mask or hood is used.

Our understanding of the events that follow the formation of bubbles in divers has progressed dramatically in the last decade. Since bubbles were first seen on decompression in the blood of a dog by Paul Bert[2] in the 1870s, it has been assumed that they block blood vessels, and that the symptoms produced were simply due to lack of blood flow. This simple explanation is certainly wrong; even with the large bubbles that block large blood vessels, the story is much more complicated than simple lack of blood flow. However, although the bubbles formed on decompression are often small enough to pass through capillaries, this does not mean that they are harmless. In fact, Haldane's prediction in 1908 that they may cause "direct mechanical damage" has proved to be correct. Bubbles have been shown to damage the lining of blood vessels and cause them to leak. In the brain, this means that they open *the blood-brain barrier*,[21] and the tissue swelling is associated with inflammation. The illustration of the spinal cord already seen in Chapter 7, which looks rather like a kiwi fruit, is reproduced again in Figure 8.1.[22] It shows that the opening of the barrier may be so severe that red blood cells are able to escape; in other words, it causes tiny bleeds from veins and some are arrowed in the figure.

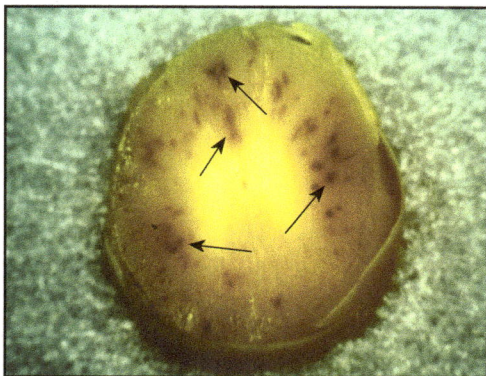

Figure 8.1:
The effect of bubbles on the veins in the spinal cord.
(Courtesy of Professor David Elliott.)

The breakdown of red blood cells in tissues is very harmful because free iron is released, which leads to the formation of the most dangerous of free radicals—the hydroxyl radical.

When an increase in pressure is used to treat decompression sickness, it will assist any gas still present in the body to re-dissolve and a high concentration of oxygen will also arrest inflammation by preventing white blood cells, the neutrophils, sticking and moving into the tissues. The oxygen will also constrict the blood vessels, reducing swelling, and allow capillaries that have been compressed by the swelling to reopen. Swelling and white blood cell injury occur as the result of most tissue injuries, and so the experience of hyperbaric oxygen treatment in decompression sickness is very relevant to other injuries. It is impossible to measure the concentration of any drug in the tissues of a patient, but in contrast the concentration of oxygen in the tissues can actually be measured. Drug concentrations can only be measured in blood, and this cannot possibly indicate how much of the drug is reaching the tissues targeted for treatment.

Astonishingly, it would appear that the changes in the oxygen level in the tissues of the nervous system under hyperbaric conditions have been measured only once. The experiments discussed below studied the use of hyperbaric oxygen treatment for injuries to the spinal cord. Spinal cord injuries are the worst nightmare, especially when all four limbs become paralysed, as they were with Christopher Reeve. As the spinal cord typically weighs just 50 grams, even a small amount of tissue injury can have devastating effects. Spinal cord injuries are fortunately not common, but because patients often have other injuries such as a head injury or fractures, they are easily missed and, consequently, difficult to study clinically. This frustration led neurosurgeons at the beginning of the twentieth century to develop a technique for use in an animal model, in which a known weight is dropped onto the spinal cord from a measured height to give a reproducible injury. This allows the resulting damage to be controlled and studied. The events that follow injury to the spinal cord are essentially the same as those that affect the brain but, because the cord is so much smaller, injuries are very much more difficult to treat. The following experiments are unique because actual measurements were used. They show that the level of oxygen in the spinal cord is reduced by injury, and that it can be raised by giving more oxygen at greater than atmospheric pressure. They also show that the additional oxygen improves the degree of recovery. In the author's view, it is impossible to overestimate the importance of this ground breaking study.

In the 1970s, a group of neurosurgeons in Bowman Gray Medical Centre in North Carolina adopted the dropped weight method in an experimental study designed to test the value of hyperbaric oxygen treatment in spinal cord injury. Their paper was published in the eminent journal *Neurosurgery* in 1972.[23] An animal was anaesthetised and the spinal cord exposed to allow electrodes to be placed in the area to be damaged in order to measure the tissue oxygen levels. Figure 8.2 shows the level of oxygen in the tissues of the cord when the dog was breathing air at normal atmospheric pressure as 25 units. The level can be seen to rise to about 80 units with the animal given 100% oxygen. However, over the next 20 minutes the oxygen level in the tissues falls back to the normal value, despite the animal continuing to breathe 100% oxygen. This is because the body reduces the flow of blood by constricting the blood vessels, a reaction known as autoregulation. The addition of 5% carbon dioxide to oxygen caused an even greater increase in the tissue oxygen value, but again the body responded by reducing blood flow, so that a normal level was restored in the tissues. The graph shows how the level of oxygen in the tissue falls following the bruising injury—a 20-gram weight was dropped from a height of 20 centimetres. Note that the oxygen level in the damaged tissue does not rise with the administration of 100% oxygen, or 95% oxygen with 5% added carbon dioxide at normal atmospheric pressure.

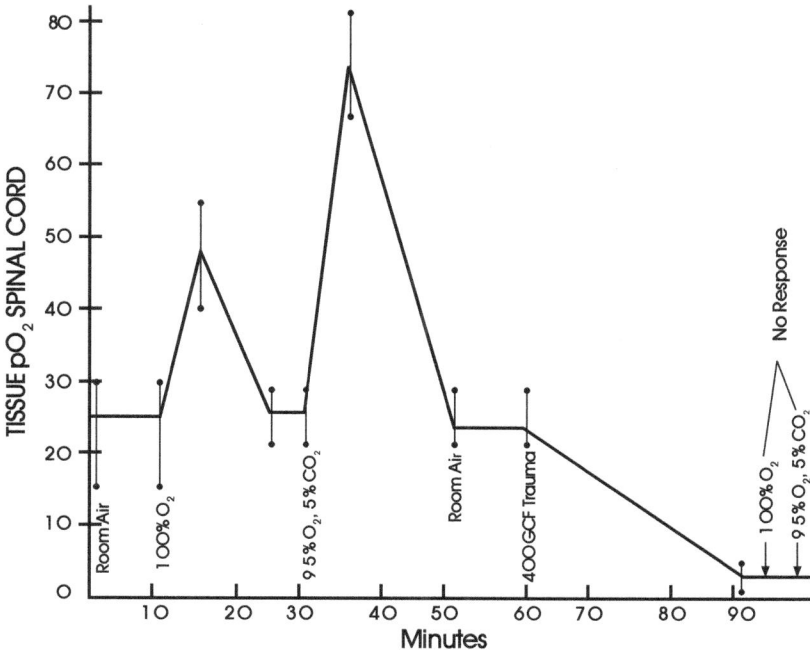

Figure 8.2:
Effect of giving 100% at normal atmospheric pressure on tissue oxygen levels in the spinal cord of a dog.

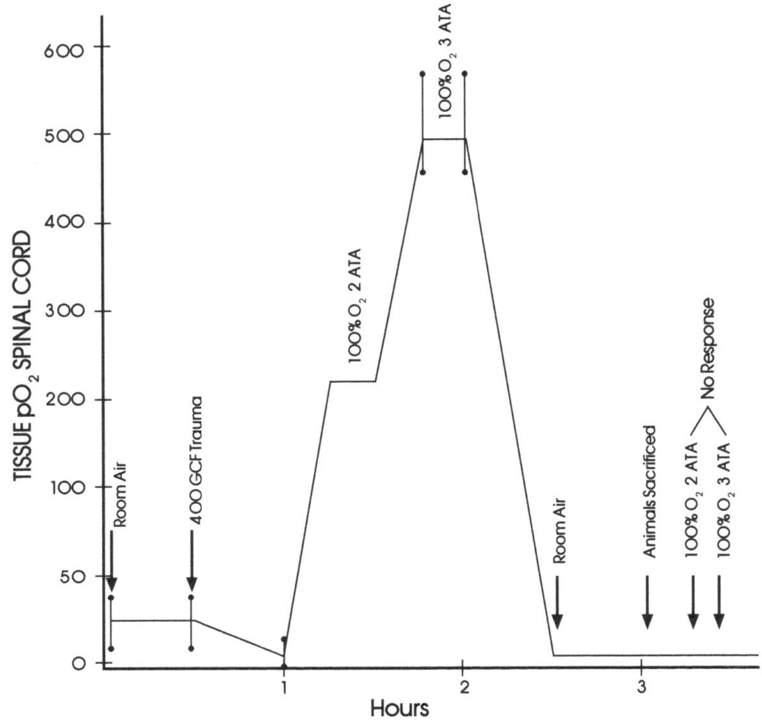

Figure 8.3:
Effect of giving oxygen at 2 and 3 atmospheres on oxygen levels in the exposed spinal cord after injury caused by a 20-gram weight.

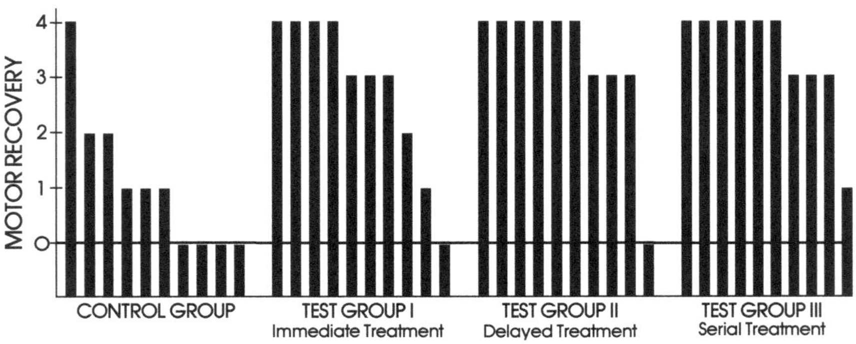

Figure 8.4:
Recovery of motor function three months post-injury (each vertical bar represents one animal). The treatment delay in group II was four hours: the better outcome compared to group I probably reflects random variations in the severity of the spinal cord damage, not benefit from delaying treatment.

However, if a pressure chamber is used, the oxygen level can easily be increased, as shown in Figure 8.3. This is simple physics; more oxygen is dissolved in the plasma at the increased pressure.

Did the extra oxygen help? Figure 8.4 shows that after a period of three months of nursing care, of the ten control animals that did not receive hyperbaric oxygen treatment, only one regained the ability to walk and did not have any residual disability, which is motor recovery grade four.

In contrast, nine out of the ten of the dogs given just three sessions of hyperbaric oxygen treatment (test group III) regained the ability to walk (grades three and four). This study shows that physics is reliable; the gas laws are correct. The results have been successfully repeated, in sheep[24] and dogs,[25] but without measurements of tissue oxygen levels. In the 1980s, a group in Texas have taken the work one stage further by studying spinal cord regeneration in a rat model.[26] They severed the spinal cord completely placing the ends together, closed the wound, and treated the animal with a course of hyperbaric oxygen sessions with the addition of dimethyl sulphoxide (DMSO). They demonstrated that nerve fibres in the central nervous system do regenerate. Figure 8.5 shows how the supporting scar tissue tends to trap the nerve fibres. In the treated group, nine of 37 animals regained the ability to walk but no animal in the control group recovered.

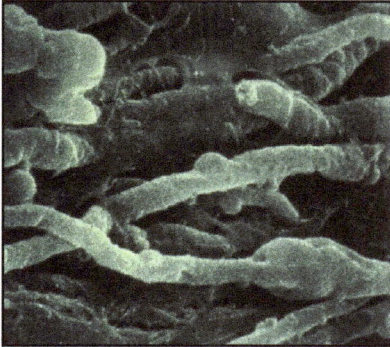

Figure 8.5:
Nerve fibre regeneration in a severed rat spinal cord after hyperbaric oxygen treatment with DMSO.
(Courtesy Dr. J.B. Gelderd et al.)

As already stated, the use of pressure to deliver a high dosage of oxygen for the treatment of both gas embolism and decompression sickness has been accepted around the world for many years on the basis of both biological plausibility, and truly massive anecdotal evidence. It will be recalled that Haldane suggested that bubbles may cause "direct mechanical damage" to blood vessels and the research discussed earlier in this chapter has confirmed that small bubbles may actually damage the lining of small blood vessels as they pass through. They open the blood-brain barrier, and agents normally retained in blood escape triggering inflammation. The story has finally been completed by some remarkable research from a former deep-diving research unit in the University of Pennsylvania, which was published in 2002.[27] It has shown that the local swelling produced by bubbles reduces the oxygen level, and the hypoxia attracts white blood cells—neutrophils. The researchers photographed the neutrophils sticking to the lining, and they can be seen in the image reproduced in Figure 8.6.

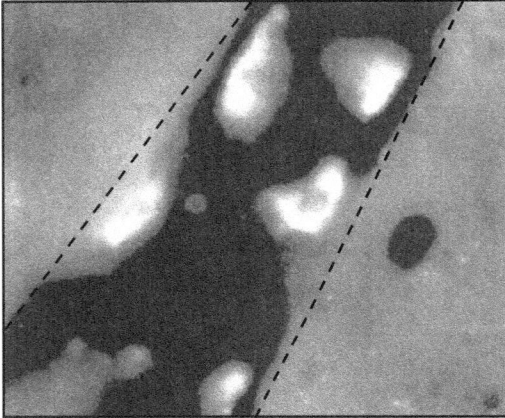

Figure 8.6:
Neutrophils sticking to the wall of small vein after the passage of bubbles on decompression. (Redrawn from Martin and Thom, 2002.)

An apparently simple event, the passage of a small, seemingly inconsequential bubble down a blood vessel triggers events of immense complexity with a fall in the available oxygen increasing the level of the hypoxia-inducible factor proteins. The benefit of using high levels of oxygen for decompression sickness is, therefore, two-fold: the restoration of normal metabolism, and the arrest of the inflammation caused by neutrophils.[28] However, the involvement of neutrophils in the bends is part of a much bigger picture and we need to go back to an event in 1987 that shook the world: A little girl called Jessica fell down a well in Midland, Texas.

CHAPTER 9
Jessica in the Well

Day by day those who are obliged to consume their best energies in the frequently so toilsome and exhausting routine of practice find it becoming less and less possible for them not only to closely study, but even to understand the more recent medical research.

Robert Virchow, 1858. *General Pathology as Based on Physiological and Pathological Histology.* 2nd Edition. Translated by J. Chance. London: Churchill, 1877.

In October 1987, a little girl shocked the world by falling down a disused well in Midland, Texas, a small town known for its association with the former US Presidents George H. W. Bush Sr. and his son George W. Bush Jr. Her name was Jessica McClure, and her rescue became the focus of the world's media. Only the death of Princess Diana in a Paris subway claimed a larger television audience in the last century. Jessica was only eighteen months old when she was playing with other children in the back garden of her aunt's house at 3309 Tanner Drive on the morning of Wednesday, October 14th. When her mother went to answer the telephone, Jessica pushed aside the cover of the well, climbed in the shaft, which was just eight inches in diameter, and promptly fell into it. Her cries were heard by her mother who frantically tried to reach her, but she slipped further down the shaft. The emergency services were called, and two policemen were first on the scene—they were not to leave until she was safely back above ground 58 hours later. The rescue brought more than 400 workers to the site, and the neighbourhood opened their homes to them in a moving demonstration of community spirit.

As the story spread, television and radio crews arrived at Tanner Drive from every corner of the globe. The fledgling news outlet CNN cut its teeth providing constant coverage of the rescue. The rescuers had to bore a second shaft close to the well because any attempt to widen the well risked collapsing the walls and burying Jessica alive. Having reached the required depth, a horizontal tunnel had to be dug, but a layer of hard rock was encountered, and hopes of an early breakthrough faded. The following day a bulletin from the authorities read, "Jessica might not be freed until 6:00 p.m. today," but Thursday passed with the rescuers still working around the clock. All through Friday they struggled, painfully boring the final tunnel needed to reach Jessica. Finally they broke through, and the rescuers could see her. A paramedic,

Robert O'Donnell, was able to reach her and extricate her from the confines of the well. Jessica was finally brought to the surface at 8:00 p.m. in the glare of television lights, and to an explosion of cheering from the hundreds gathered at the site. Car horns honked and church bells were rung with the huge relief at news of her rescue.

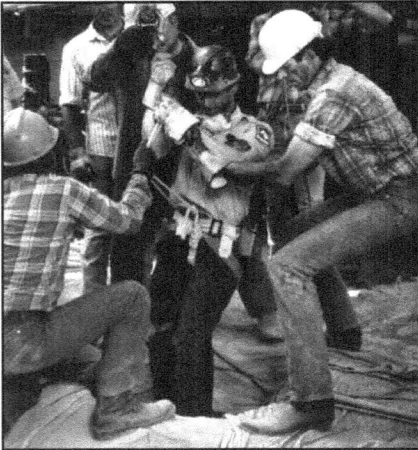

Figure 9.1:
A scene during the rescue of Jessica from the well on Tanner Drive in Texas.

All was not well, however; Jessica's right foot was black, and she was rushed to Midland Memorial Hospital. The surgeons feared there was no alternative to amputation, but a doctor in Dallas, the late John R. Maxfield, knew the hospital had a rare piece of equipment: A pressure chamber similar to the decompression chambers used by divers. It had been installed in the hospital by a Texan oil billionaire for the treatment of his daughter who has multiple sclerosis. Dr. Maxfield called pleading for hyperbaric oxygen treatment to be tried, in the hope that it would avoid amputation. That evening, Jessica found herself in the chamber breathing a much higher level of oxygen than is normally used in our hospitals. Although surgery was needed to help with the swelling of the foot, after a few days, it became obvious that Jessica's leg had been saved. Although she needed further surgery over some time, she only lost her little toe. A simple pressure chamber and oxygen treatment had made the difference, and an amputation had been avoided. The media events continued. Jessica was visited in hospital by George Bush Sr., then Vice President, with his wife Barbara. A week after the rescue, Oprah Winfrey broadcast her television show from the Midland Center, saying that the town had every reason to be proud of the support the community gave to the rescuers. At noon on November 20, Jessica left the hospital in a wheelchair surrounded by cheering crowds, with the president of the hospital close to tears.

It might have been expected that doctors would have been quick to endorse the success of the hyperbaric treatment this little girl received, and even keen to provide it for their own patients facing the trauma of leg amputation. What followed, however, is very difficult to comprehend. A letter appeared in the *Journal of the American Medical Association (JAMA)* from a doctor at the University of Miami,[1] alleging that it had been wrong to use hyperbaric oxygen treatment. Astonishingly, it was argued that the additional oxygen would have created free radicals, making Jessica's leg worse, despite the fact that the author must have known that her leg had actually been saved. This needs us to step back for a moment to analyse this extraordinary situation. Despite the evidence that hyperbaric treatment had been successful, the doctor's absolute conviction made him take the time to write a critical letter to the journal based on *his* understanding of the science involved. A brief search of the literature would have revealed that regular reports of the success of hyperbaric oxygen treatment in skin grafting have been published since the 1960s,[2] and none indicated that the additional oxygen used had been in any way harmful. Also, the editorial staff of *JAMA* would surely have known that Jessica's leg had been saved, so why did they accept the letter? It was because it struck a chord by invoking the latest fashion, the spectre of free radicals.

The allegation that giving oxygen may be harmful actually followed studies undertaken in the early days of heart transplant surgery. When the heart is removed from the body of a donor, its blood flow obviously stops and the clock is then ticking. If more than a few hours elapse before the organ is placed in the recipient, it will fail. Researchers were desperate to find out why, and undertook many experiments transplanting organs in animals. The reason for the failure associated with a delay came as a surprise: The damage, which was detected by enzyme markers, occurred when blood flow was re-established in the recipient animal. Return of blood flow is known as *reperfusion* and the damage was found to be due to oxygen free radicals.[3] This was confirmed by further experiments in which blood not containing oxygen was passed through the blood vessels of an isolated heart. The initial increase in the markers of free radical damage did not occur and so withholding oxygen prevented the damage to the heart, but only for a time. It is painfully obvious that without oxygen, a heart soon stops beating, and then, of course, its tissues die. Paradoxically, the very oxygen that a transplanted heart desperately needs to survive appeared to be responsible for its demise. The first theory attempting to explain the formation of free radicals implicated the energy molecule we have already encountered, adenosine triphosphate (ATP). It was suggested that the cascade of biochemical events resulting from lack of oxygen degraded ATP via adenosine diphosphate (ADP), and adenosine monophosphate (AMP), finally to hypoxanthine. It was suggested that hypoxanthine was responsible for the release of free radicals when blood flow was restored and oxygen became available.[4,5] This has turned out not to be the case, and it was events that followed the publicity surrounding Jessica's ordeal that led to the mystery being finally unravelled.

Returning to the story of Jessica and the letter published in *JAMA*, it must be pointed out, to be fair, that the editors did publish two letters answering the criticism. One was from the surgeon who was responsible for Jessica's care,[6] and the second was from an authority on hyperbaric medicine, who at the time worked in the US Air Force Hyperbaric Facility in San Antonio, Texas.[7] Neither letter addressed the science involved and the debate might have ended there without the intervention of a young plastic surgeon in Springfield, Illinois, Dr. William A. Zamboni. He had followed the controversy and seized the opportunity to apply for funding not, as he readily admits, to establish the importance of hyperbaric treatment, but to shore up the argument that giving oxygen to patients like Jessica, facing amputation, may be wrong. He was duly awarded a grant, and assembled a team to set up the necessary animal experiments.

Their first experiments looked at the effect of hyperbaric treatment used after skin grafting in rats. The blood flow to the graft was stopped for eight hours, and then restarted. Some animals then breathed air, and some oxygen under hyperbaric conditions. The length of time blood flow was arrested in these experiments, eight hours, would normally have led to the death of the skin grafts. To the investigators' surprise, hyperbaric oxygen treatment in a chamber ensured their survival, in marked contrast to the failure of the grafts in the animals that breathed only air. The results did not confirm the allegations of harm from hyperbaric oxygenation and free radicals. The paper written by Zamboni and his colleagues[8] stated,

Instead we found that hyperbaric oxygen therapy significantly improved skin flap survival.

Fortunately, the research in Springfield did not stop there. A crucial series of experiments extended the work to studying the effect of stopping the blood supply not just to skin, but also to muscle. It is impossible to overstate the importance of the results to both medicine and surgery. Imagine having a tourniquet pulled tightly around your leg, stopping all blood flow for four hours. It is undoubtedly a dangerous thing to do because there is a very good chance that the tissues may begin to die, and the leg would then need to be amputated. In effect, this is what Zamboni and his group studied; their paper[9] was published in the specialist journal *Plastic and Reconstructive Surgery*, which is probably the reason why these pivotal experiments have escaped discussion by others involved in free radical research. The details certainly need to be made available to as wide an audience as possible. Many will find discussion of the experiments uncomfortable, but the findings are unique and it would be impossible to obtain the information using patients.

All the experiments were conducted under anaesthesia using drugs given intravenously rather than anaesthetic gases, so that the oxygen content of the gas the animals breathed could be changed from air to 100% oxygen. The blood supply to the thigh muscle was stopped for four hours using a ligature, and the arrest of the circulation was verified by direct observation using a microscope. When the ligature was released, the return of blood flow was filmed using the video camera mounted on the microscope. This procedure was used for every experiment in the study. When the ligature was released at the end of the four hours, allowing blood to flow back through the blood vessels in the muscle, it was seen that white blood cells (actually neutrophils) began to stick to the lining of the small veins that drain the capillaries. The white cells are shown attaching to the vein wall in Figure 9.2.

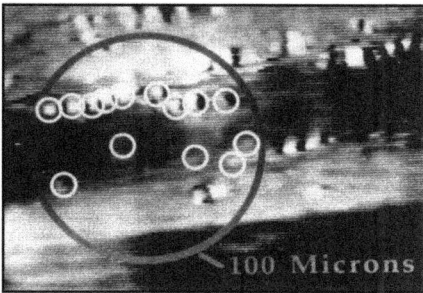

Figure 9.2:
Neutrophils, circled sticking to the wall of venules in one of the reperfusion experiments.
(Courtesy of Dr. W.A. Zamboni.)

The circle drawn in the photograph, which is taken from one of the video recordings, indicates 100 microns. White blood cells continued to accumulate, and some actually started to migrate through the wall of the vein into the tissues. Another event was also seen—the small arteries nearby started to constrict. After about two hours, the blood flow became completely obstructed by clumps of white blood cells. This happened in every experiment where air was the breathing gas. Deprived of a blood supply, the muscle tissue was, of course, certain to die.

Two groups of animals were given hyperbaric oxygen treatment using pure oxygen at 2 atmospheres. In one group this was done in the first hour *after* the ligature was released, but animals in the second group received the hour of hyperbaric oxygen treatment in the last of the four hours *whilst the ligature was in place*. The results in both groups were the same: The adhesion of white blood cells to the veins was prevented, and normal blood flow resumed. This means that the muscle would have survived. However, as we shall see, the benefit found when oxygen was used while the circulation to the muscle flap was stopped is profoundly important.

The accumulation of white blood cells that was observed is actually an amplified version of the normal response to infection. Neutrophil granulocytes, which are generally referred to simply as neutrophils, are the most abundant type of white blood cells in mammals and provide the critical first response of the immune system to infection but also to tissue injury. They have an average diameter of 12–15 micrometres, which is about double the diameter of a red blood cell. They account for approximately 70% of the white blood cell population, and we produce millions every day. They only survive in the blood for about 12 hours, although once in the tissues they may survive for days. They circulate constantly in blood, migrating within minutes to sites of injury or infection.

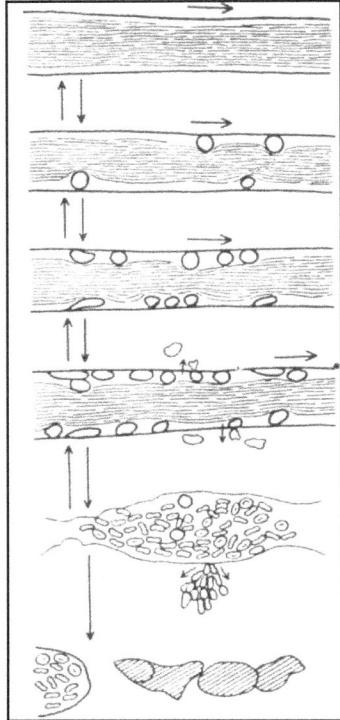

Figure 9.3:
Neutrophils adhering to a post-capillary vein wall in the tadpole tail and causing haemorrhage due to their release of free radicals.

The name neutrophil derives from the neutral result of staining with the dye hematoxylin and eosin (H&E). The white blood cells that stain dark blue are known as basophils, eosinophils stain bright red, but neutrophils remain very slightly pink. Confusingly, they may also be referred to as polymorphonuclear leucocytes because of the characteristic multi-lobed shape of their nucleus.

It is normal for neutrophils to enter the tissues from blood by first sticking to the lining of the small veins when signaled to do so by local hypoxia. They may then pass through the wall in just the same way observed by Zamboni and his colleagues. This sequence was observed in experiments conducted in 1935 in the small veins of tadpole tail, and it is shown in Figure 9.3.[10]

Neutrophils are truly remarkable cells. They actively migrate into tissues to kill microbes using oxygen derived free radicals, either after engulfing them (known as phagocytosis), or by excreting free radicals and enzymes into the surrounding tissue space. The release of these agents by neutrophils exposes the normal cells of a tissue to damage. Seemingly to minimise this problem, neutrophils are also capable of producing an astonishingly complex web of fibres, or neutrophil extra-cellular traps (NETs).[11] They allow microbes to be caught and killed in the tissues outside the neutrophil itself, allowing it to survive.

The experiments undertaken by Zamboni's group showed that providing hyperbaric oxygen treatment is used promptly, it can allow the muscle of a limb to survive even when its blood flow has been completely stopped for four hours. But the researchers had made an even more dramatic discovery: They showed that the reperfusion damage can actually be prevented by giving a large dose of oxygen *before* the circulation is released. This is now known as preconditioning. Just as in Jessica's treatment, to achieve the high dosage of oxygen necessary, a pressure chamber is needed. It is truly ironic that oxygen, the substance blamed by researchers in the 1970s for causing damage when blood flow returns to a transplanted heart, can actually *prevent* it. The results are indisputable: There can be no conceivable doubt about the benefit of giving oxygen under hyperbaric conditions—the events were watched using a microscope and recorded on video as they actually happened. Far from discrediting the use of hyperbaric oxygen treatment for Jessica, the experiments funded to show that the treatment was wrong, had finally shown that it was the right course of action and explained why her leg had been saved.

It is most important to note that the *timing* of oxygen treatment is critical to its success. Hyperbaric oxygen treatment was successful in saving the muscle in the first hour following the release of the ligature, but the effectiveness was reduced when treatment was delayed until the second hour, and by three hours there was no benefit at all. This critical timing must be kept in mind when considering hyperbaric oxygen treatment if the blood supply to any organ is interrupted, for example, when patients suffer a stroke or a cardiac arrest.

To his great credit, Zamboni soon incorporated the results into his surgical practice. He found that using hyperbaric oxygen treatment, it is possible to reconnect a severed arm or leg as late as 12 hours after amputation, when four hours is normally the limit using standard procedures. Since these studies were done, the sequence of biochemical events that follow stopping blood flow and the rescue of tissues by hyperbaric treatment have been researched in great detail.[12-14] The key question is: What causes the white cells to stick? They stick because of the expression of adhesion molecules. The research discussed here has shown that hypoxia—just a simple lack of oxygen—can trigger the genes regulating these events, and it can occur without preceding tissue injury or an infection. The lack of oxygen occurs when there is a reduction or stoppage of the supply of blood to a tissue that is called ischaemia, but also, and this is not yet appreciated, when tissues become waterlogged with oedema. The discovery of hypoxia-inducible factor 1α has finally allowed the sequence of events to be understood.[15] As we saw in Chapter 1, it begins with an increase in the levels of the hypoxia-inducible factor proteins when oxygen levels fall; circulating neutrophils stick to the endothelial cells lining the post-capillary veins because *adhesion molecules* are expressed on their surface. In the presence of sufficient oxygen, the master protein hypoxia-inducible factor 1α which is constantly produced by every cell is continually destroyed by the von Hippel-Lindau protein and what remains is rendered ineffective. The attachment of neutrophils to the vein wall in the sequence filmed by Dr. Zamboni and his colleagues is the basis of the *immune response* to infection and injury. Inflammation is therefore initiated by the release of free radicals by neutrophils. As was discussed in Chapter 8, the damage to the nervous system in decompression sickness is caused by bubbles damaging the lining of blood vessels, and this attracts neutrophils. Infection also produces a fall in the level of oxygen and triggers inflammation in the same way. However, the immune response occurs for a second reason, which is just as vital to us as the control of infection; it is the removal of debris, to begin healing damaged tissues after trauma.

Despite the drama of Jessica's story her case is, of course, just an anecdote. It is now almost 20 years since it was found that it is possible to extend the time for a severed limb to be successfully re-implanted from four to 12 hours—a truly staggering increase. Despite the detailed research that followed and similar dramatic results, hyperbaric oxygen treatment has still not been adopted for reattaching severed limbs and is probably due to the perceived constraints of evidence-based medicine.

Dr. Zamboni and his team have continued work into the molecular biology in reperfusion injury and the benefit of using hyperbaric oxygenation, but feel that before using the treatment is adopted controlled studies are needed:

Although this treatment has been used clinically with major limb re-implantation, resulting in improved limb survival with prolonged ischemia (low blood flow) times, this information is anecdotal and a controlled randomised prospective protocol will be necessary to delineate the HBO benefits.

Despite this assertion, it is actually *impossible* for a controlled trial to delineate the benefit to an *individual*; trials only give an indication of the overall value of a treatment to a group of patients. It is possible that Zamboni and his colleagues realised that this cautionary statement had to be included, because without it the paper may well have been rejected by the journal's referees. Nevertheless, the insistence on randomised controlled trials for oxygen, a biological agent, is not scientific, it is absurd. Fortunately, there are signs that the use of controlled trials is finally being questioned. The tenets of evidence-based medicine are an example of a belief system that has many features in common with religious dogma. It is, of course, impossible to show using scientific experimentation whether or not the cherished beliefs held by the religions of the world are true; they are the objects of faith. This is an admission that they cannot be understood and, if we admit that we do not understand something, then we have given up the right to say whether or not it is correct. Unfortunately, if the demand for controlled trials continues in re-implantation surgery, it is unlikely that hyperbaric oxygenation will ever be used. This may seem like an extreme statement, but it is based on the response to the use of hyperbaric oxygen treatment in other conditions when controlled studies have actually been undertaken, and will be discussed in later chapters.

The controlled trial is regarded as the gold standard in evidence-based medicine drug trials, but it has serious flaws and limitations that are rarely debated. In a controlled trial, two groups of patients with a defined condition are allocated to either a treatment group given the agent under test, for example a drug, or to a control group given an inactive placebo. In a double-blind controlled trial, neither the patient nor the physician are allowed to know to which group an individual has been assigned, and the allocations are usually randomised. The fundamental problem is that we are all different, and differences are often amplified when we are ill, or suffer an injury. It is, therefore, very difficult to match patients, and reliance must be placed on using large numbers so that the groups will include enough similar patients. Inevitably they are very expensive; running drug trials is very big business for academic institutions, and massive profits can be made by companies if a drug proves successful.

In the next chapter it is argued that controlled trials of using oxygen in treatment are not only unnecessary, they are unscientific, and that reliance must be placed on measurements which, of course, relate to individual patients. Today, case histories are often treated with derision and dismissed as anecdotes. The next chapter discusses the limitations of controlled trials and why anecdotes provide the necessary evidence for using oxygen in treatment. These statements are clearly controversial, and need to be justified.

CHAPTER 10

Anecdotes, Evidence, and Uncontrolled Double-Blindness

Thus the profession has been led to overlook or ignore oxygen as a medicine, even though chemical science tells us decidedly that it ought to be a most valuable remedial agent. A single trial, or several trials on several patients, are no evidence, if they fail, against its value; they are only proof either that it was not suited to the case, or that it was not properly exhibited.

SB Birch, MD. *Lancet,* August 1, 1857.

The information in this chapter is needed for the reader to be able not only to assess the evidence for using hyperbaric oxygen treatment, but also to understand the reaction of medical professionals to the treatment, especially in disorders of the brain. Most physicians are not familiar with the use of oxygen in treatment or the equipment needed and if the subject is raised, they usually respond by asking if there are any controlled trials. Attempts have been made to collate the published studies for the UK Cochrane Collaboration, a repository of evidence from controlled trials named after Archie Cochrane (1909–1988), a public health physician. Such reviews of the use of hyperbaric oxygen treatment are said to be needed to gain respectability for the modality and for those operating chambers to attract patient referrals from sceptical colleagues. The reports present the meagre evidence for each indication where hyperbaric oxygen treatment has been used; meagre because most indications predate the insistence on controlled studies. The principle involved is, of course, the same: lack of oxygen can only be treated by giving more. Absurdly, oxygen is referred to as an "adjunct" to recovery, when only a moment's reflection is needed to recognise that no treatment can be effective in the absence of oxygen. It is also most important to acknowledge that the placebo effect cannot occur in its absence. Although high-quality controlled trials of hyperbaric oxygen treatment have been performed, for example in patients with multiple sclerosis,[1] they are usually dismissed as unconvincing, or said to be too few, when just *one* properly undertaken study provides class 1 evidence.

But demands made for controlled trials of oxygen must be challenged because they are actually inappropriate and a very significant factor in preventing millions of patients from accessing this effective and safe treatment.

To question the effectiveness of giving oxygen to a patient with a known deficiency of oxygen is much the same as questioning the need for water in dehydration, or food when a patient is starving. Oxygen is indispensable to us, to all our cells, and, moreover, there is no substitute. Withholding water or food would obviously be a failure of the duty of care, but withholding oxygen escapes this censure. Blood oxygen concentrations are measured regularly in hospitals, but lack of oxygen in just a few grams of *tissue*, for example in the brain stem, or the muscle of the heart, may be fatal. Using today's jargon, giving oxygen is the most *biologically plausible* intervention possible, especially in the treatment of disorders of the brain.

When lack of oxygen has been proven by measurement, controlled trials are both unscientific and unethical: Evidence from the treatment of a *single patient* is sufficient, because we all use oxygen in the same way. Scientifically, this is represented simply as n=1, where n stands for number and 1 is obviously just one and remember, it may be you! A leading figure in the production of the Cochrane reviews of hyperbaric oxygen treatment, Dr. Michael Bennett, apparently, now agrees with this reasoning; he wrote that doctors in the Prince of Wales Hospital in Sydney, Australia, "went from a position of complete skepticism to enthusiastic support (for hyperbaric oxygen treatment) over a six-month period following the chance referral of a single patient who did well." Again, because the actions of oxygen are reliable and *universal*, another patient treated for the same condition *at the same stage* of the disease process will also benefit.

It is possible, even likely, that many will disagree with this logic and continue to insist that controlled trials must be done. This may seem to be taking the academic high ground, but it is not: The tactic is commonly used when treatments are controversial, and is often an excuse for denigration and inaction. Those who agree with the argument that controlled trials of oxygen used in treatment are inappropriate may want to have the necessary facts to be able to counter the arguments. Other readers may prefer to move on, although the two case reports in this chapter are essential reading.

To broaden the debate, it will be helpful at this juncture to outline the approach used for the acceptance of new drugs and why evidence-based rules can only be a guide to any form of treatment, because, in fact, they cannot possibly predict the result for a single patient. Put another way, a report from treating one patient even with a drug which has proven successful in several controlled studies will *always* be anecdotal.[2]

Regulatory authorities now require that all new drugs must demonstrate that they are safe, beneficial, and superior to placebo "under controlled conditions" before they are licensed. Testing drugs against a placebo is necessary to determine effectiveness and avoid bias in favour of a treatment on the part of both drug companies and prescribing physicians. It will be seen later that when using oxygen, the bias has often been *against* the treatment, which betrays trusting patients. Although it has been estimated that fewer than 15% of the medications currently in use have qualified by data from controlled trials, no one should dispute the need for proper evidence to establish the safety and efficacy of new drugs. Given the modern obsession with taking pills, the use of oral medication is a good starting point to illustrate the principles involved in controlled trials and show why they are *not* appropriate to using oxygen in treatment.

The first necessity for a drug given by mouth is to gain entry into the bloodstream, the second is for it to be transported to the target tissue, and the third is that the drug must move to the cells of a tissue to interact at the molecular level with cell receptors. Non-steroidal anti-inflammatory drugs (NSAIDs) are one of the most widely used classes of drugs and oral preparations are often prescribed for patients with arthritic joint pain. Figure 10.1 shows the blood concentrations in two patients given the *same* dose of a NSAID by mouth.

The concentration of the drug in the blood of the patients is shown on the vertical axis of the graph, and the time intervals after it has been swal-

PLASMA CONCENTRATIONS OF A NON-STEROIDAL ANTI-INFLAMMATORY DRUG

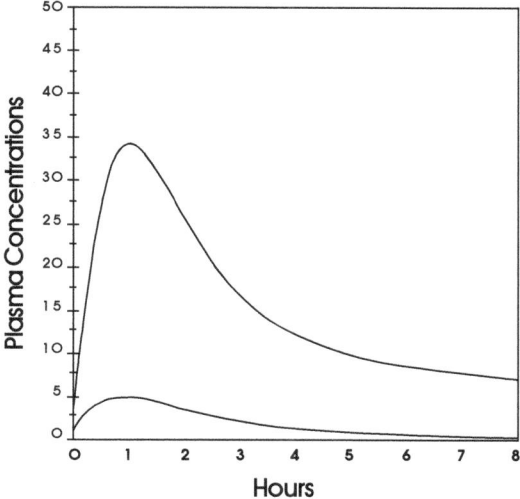

Figure 10.1:
Plasma NSAID concentrations for two patients given the same oral dose. Upper graph is one who absorbs well and the lower is one who absorbs poorly.

lowed are shown in hours on the horizontal axis. It can be seen that the concentration in the blood rises rapidly, until it slows to peak about one hour before it begins a slow decline over several hours. The two curves illustrate the huge difference in the blood levels of two patients given the same dose of the drug. Note also that the difference is not just in the peak value attained, it is actually in the total area under the two curves. A patient who absorbs the drug well maintains a much higher blood concentration for many hours longer than a patient who absorbs the drug poorly and so will benefit more.

To understand the reasons for the differences in blood levels, it may be helpful to chart the route taken by a drug taken by mouth. After passing down the oesophagus, the drug has to pass through the stomach so that it can be absorbed into the blood in the gut. There may be some degradation in the stomach, and in the gut some of the drug will be retained in any food present. Some will also be retained in the tissues of the wall of the bowel itself before the drug is finally absorbed into the blood. It is then carried in veins which pass into the liver, the organ entrusted with the task of dealing with any undesirable substances in the food we eat. The liver will remove some more of the drug from the circulation. All of these actions reduce the amount of a drug that finally enters the circulation of the rest of the body and, because they vary from patient to patient, are responsible for the huge differences seen in the graph. What remains of the drug after passing through the liver enters the large vein in the centre of the body known as the inferior vena cava. This vein drains blood into the right atrium of the heart, and from there passes through the tricuspid valve to be pumped by the right ventricle into the circulation of the lungs. A little of the drug will also be retained in the tissues of the lungs, but most will simply pass in the blood flowing through the lung capillaries into the left atrium and on into the left ventricle. This chamber of the heart is responsible for pumping blood to every organ and tissue of the body except, of course, the lungs. By now the concentration of the drug will have reduced substantially, as it becomes progressively diluted in the six litres or so of blood held in the circulation. As the drug circulates, the concentration in blood further reduces as it is lost to tissues, metabolised by the liver, and excreted by the kidneys. It should be noted that NSAIDs, like many other drugs, are prevented from accessing the nervous system by the blood-brain barrier.

Samples of blood taken to follow the changes in drug concentration are taken from veins and in the graph it can be seen that one hour after the drug has been taken there is more than a 700% difference in the maximum blood concentration between patients. The *peak* concentration defines the maximum rate of the transfer of the drug into the tissues, which is usually the key factor in determining any benefit. However, the concentration of a drug where it is needed, that is, in the target tissue, *cannot* be measured, and the variation in *tissue* levels of drugs is certain to dwarf those seen in blood. To understand why requires a principle of disease to be stated that is little recognised: It is that when a tissue is injured or diseased, the capillaries within the tissue are also almost invariably damaged. This reduces the flow of blood and of the substances it carries and this, of course, will include a drug. Ironically, a drug can often access most of the other tissues of the body where it is actually not wanted, but has great difficulty reaching the site where it is needed. A NSAID taken, for example, for joint pain will have great difficulty accessing the site where it is needed, simply because the capillaries are closed by the swelling associated with the inflammation.[3]

The contrast between the delivery of drugs and the delivery of oxygen could not be greater. Oxygen is rapidly absorbed through the enormous surface area of the lungs at a consistent level and directly into the blood in the lung capillaries. It is readily transported from blood into the tissues without being removed by the liver and, being a very small molecule, it can rapidly diffuse into an affected tissue. Also, unlike any drug, the oxygen level in tissue can actually be measured and measurements are, of course, the basis of the scientific method. Because of the enormous variation introduced by absorption and the transport of drugs to the tissues, patients given a drug in a controlled trial *cannot* receive the same treatment and to make matters worse, patients are usually given the same dose regardless of their weight. They may also be in different stages of a disease process, often with a broad range of pathology. These factors obviously reduce the scientific validity of drug trials, particularly of oral medications. To increase the possibility of a statistically valid result, large numbers are studied in the hope that sufficient numbers of similar patients are included. Statistics are then used to derive a numerical value for the *probability* that a drug is effective, which gives clinicians the comfort of a number— a probability, or p value, that can be quoted. A value less than 5% is required as an indication of a beneficial effect, which means that there is a less than 5% probability that the benefit is not due to chance.

If a coin is tossed a thousand times, then chance will determine that number of heads will be much the same as the number of tails, and so dividing the number of heads by the number of tails will give a value close to 1. The probability value, p, is then said to be 1, indicating there is no significant difference. However, if the number of heads greatly exceeds the number of tails, this number reduces, clearly indicating that some factor is disturbing the randomness of the effect. Tossing a coin a thousand times is more likely to result in an equal number of heads and tails than just ten. The larger number increases the "confidence" that a result is correct. If the value drops to 5% (e.g. five tails in 100 throws of the coin), then the p value drops to 0.05. This is regarded as the threshold at which the possibility that the observed effect is due to chance can be reasonably excluded. In other words, something is happening that is *not* due to chance. Clearly, the greater the number of throws used, the greater the likelihood of identifying an effect which is disturbing an equal distribution of heads and tails. Probability values less than 0.05 are required in controlled trials for regulatory authorities to accept that a drug is beneficial when it is compared to a placebo.

Needless to say, clinical trials are extremely expensive. A single trial may cost $100 million, and it has been estimated that the total cost of bringing a new drug into use, including several studies and final marketing, has now reached about $2 billion. The requirement for trials has created a very profitable research industry. In the UK, drug companies are required to pay overheads to medical schools and NHS teaching hospitals, which range from 50% to 95% of the actual trial cost. Less well known are patient recruitment fees, which range from $750 to as high as $5,000 per patient. This applies to patients receiving the drug under test, and patients who are given a placebo. It is not difficult to see that it is an extremely lucrative business for all concerned (except, of course, the patients), and few want the status quo disturbed. In fact, medical schools in the UK would collapse without this income, as successive governments have steadily reduced their funding in real terms over the last decades, and more is to come. Nevertheless, the reliance on trials has been attacked by Sir Michael Rawlins, chairman of the UK gate-keeping body, the National Institute of Health and Clinical Excellence (NICE), who has argued strongly for due recognition of observational studies.[4]

At this stage, it is worth outlining the stages needed to acquire an acceptable evidence base for a new drug. Drug formulations are based on a concept, that is, a disease *model*, where assumptions are made about how the disease arises and the way pathological changes are produced. Studies are first undertaken in animals, and then safety trials in human volunteers. Assuming that the results are satisfactory, regulatory authorities then require clinical trials involving patients, which are undertaken in several phases. After pilot studies, several large controlled trials are needed. In controlled trials, patients are allocated, usually randomly, into two groups: one group is given an inactive placebo, and the other a fixed dose of the drug being tested.

Only three outcomes are possible from a controlled trial, and it is important to recognise that this applies to both those patients given the drug being tested, *and* the patients given an inactive placebo.[5] Patients may benefit, they may remain the same, or they may get worse; the outcomes are qualitatively the same for both groups of patients. Assuming the drug being tested is actually beneficial, what is the difference between the two groups? Generally, for a drug to be regarded as effective, about 70% of the patients need to show improvement compared to about 50% of the patients given the placebo, and this evidence is usually sufficient to allow a drug to be approved and marketed.

It has also been found in controlled trials that side effects occur both in patients given an active drug and in those given the placebo. However, usually more patients given a drug actually get worse than those receiving a placebo and so, in reality, the biggest difference overall between the treated and control groups is that more patients in the placebo group stay *the same*, not getting either benefit or side effects. How is this dealt with in practice? To avoid unhelpful complications slewing the results against a drug under test, an *outcome measure* is chosen. This allows a more favourable statistical result—more patients will improve taking the drug, but only for the specific outcome being measured. This problem has been recognised, as this quote from a *Lancet* commentary in 2005[6] indicates;

> *. . . the authors are right to point out the need for trialists and journals to embrace clinically significant outcomes that are meaningful to patients, their attendants, and care organisations. Disingenuous surrogate markers and misleading composite outcomes may create good advertising material, but can obscure data and hinder genuine patient-centred care.*

A drug, for example, that improves walking distance in patients who have diseased arteries in their legs that proves to have statistically significant benefit under trial conditions may produce side effects that render its use unacceptable to many patients. As Einstein famously said, "Not everything that can be counted counts, and not everything that counts can be counted." Drugs marketed following controlled trials may be of little real benefit to patients in terms of improved quality of life, despite the fact that patients taking drugs should also gain from the placebo effect. This is because they are prescribed by a doctor who is biased to expect them to benefit and patients, of course, will feel that something is being done for them.

It is important to recognise that for a placebo effect to occur something *must* be done: An action must be taken and it is usually assumed that it must be known to the patient—the conscious brain must be involved. In the UK, the deliberate use of placebo is frowned on; the Parliamentary Select Committee on Science and Technology has stated that:

> *Prescribing placebos . . . usually relies on some degree of patient deception.*

It has also stated that:

> *Prescribing pure placebos is bad medicine. Their effect is unreliable and unpredictable and cannot form the sole basis of any treatment on the NHS.*

In fact, the benefits from a placebo are often comparable to those of many prescribed drugs. Recently, an extraordinary study undertaken at Harvard Medical School compared the benefit from a placebo to no treatment in patients with irritable bowel syndrome.[7] No deception was involved; the trial details were fully explained to the patients, including the fact that the pills used contained no active ingredient—they were even dispensed in a box clearly labelled "placebo." The patients in the treatment group given the inactive pills were told to take them twice a day. Both groups improved but, inexplicably, the group of patients taking the placebo pills showed greater improvement. The Nobel laureate Dr. Albert Schweitzer (1875–1965) understood the reason:

> *Each patient carries his own doctor inside him. They come to us not knowing that cure. We are at our best when we give the doctor who resides within each patient a chance to go to work.*

What must, however, be recognised is that, even if a drug has provided the necessary statistical significant evidence from controlled trials and is approved by regulatory agencies, it *cannot* ensure that an individual patient will gain benefit from it. A successful trial of a drug simply demonstrates that more patients in the treated group derive benefit when compared to a placebo. A group is, of course, a collection of individuals; they are not fused together to allow one large pill to be administered; treatment is *always* of an individual. This patently obvious fact seems to elude academics and in 2005, the *Lancet* actually carried a series of five articles on "Treating Individuals"; the first raised the question: To whom do the results of this trial apply?[8] The result of a treatment constitutes an *anecdote*, and the only way to find out if a drug is effective in an individual is to monitor the response in *each* patient. Each prescription is, therefore, an experiment, and the patient is their own rabbit, or guinea pig. This is where the practice of medicine actually resides; it is in the contract between the patient and their physician to gain the most benefit, in other words to get the best possible outcome. This contract is rather more obvious in surgery where there is eye-to-eye contact before cutting commences! However, anecdotes are not always positive and adverse results also introduce bias.[9]

After drugs have survived the long process to be regulated, it is essential for monitoring to continue as short-term benefits may be very deceptive. In the 1980s, cardiologists suggested that heart failure was not simple pump failure: changes in blood vessels were involved in producing a complex disease. This is an obvious fallacy when it is recognised that all the complex changes rapidly resolve if patients receive a heart transplant. Nevertheless, eight pharmaceutical companies developed drugs to dilate peripheral blood vessels to relieve the burden on the failing heart. From post-marketing surveillance it eventually became obvious that more patients were dying than would be expected without any treatment, and by 1993, all eight drugs were withdrawn. For the Boots Company, which marketed the drug Manoplax, it was a catastrophe, and they eventually sold their pharmaceutical division. A 1997 commentary in the *Lancet*[10] included a table with the heading "Drugs Associated with an Increased Mortality in Cardiac Failure." (It could have been phrased differently.)

Why is all this detail so important in a book about the benefits of using oxygen in treatment? It is because we take the oxygen in air for granted, failing to recognise that it is impossible for *any* treatment, whether it is drug-based, surgical, or even a placebo, to be beneficial without this gas; it underpins *all* recovery. While everyone recognises that we need to breathe to stay alive, few recognise the importance of breathing to getting better when we are sick or injured. If the quality of breathing reduces, as it does in patients with the lung scarring known as emphysema, they often lose weight[11] and need to be given supplementary oxygen. If the correct dose is given to a sick patient with an oxygen deficiency, they will certainly benefit, although sometimes it may prove difficult to measure. This logic applies to many other actions. For example, if a car journey is undertaken with a coin in the driver's pocket, the car will use more fuel, and if the complete details of the ride are known the energy used can be accurately calculated. It would, nevertheless, be impossible to measure the extra fuel used by matching the journey in an identical car driven in the same way, simply because uncontrolled variables will dwarf the increase in fuel used due to transporting the coin.

In the early days of evidence-based medicine, when academics were formulating the basis for the discipline, it was accepted that some interventions did *not* require formal trials. The examples quoted by one paper[12] were, blood transfusion in haemorrhage, insulin in diabetic coma, and, rather curiously, the reduction of a dislocated elbow in a toddler—adults obviously do not qualify! A longer list compiled in a more recent article[13] cited a drug, *streptomycin*, used for the meningitis associated with tuberculosis, but even included the use of a defibrillator for ventricular fibrillation. However, the use of oxygen treatment does not feature. The lists published are truly a hodgepodge with little apparent logic, and so it is worth compiling a list of criteria to assist in establishing *anecdotes as evidence* in acute conditions. It is similar to the list relating to causality drawn up by Bradford Hill.[14]

- A mechanism that can explain the changes, i.e. biological plausibility
- A clear relationship of the timing of the intervention to the benefit and of delay to poor outcome
- Objectively measurable changes
- Reproducibility
- Supporting experimental studies using (other) animals
- Evidence of a dose-response relationship

How does giving oxygen as a treatment fare when tested against this list? Mechanism and effectiveness cannot be questioned, especially when it is remembered that the object of giving more oxygen is to achieve *normal* values in an affected tissue, and the mechanisms that are brought into play are those involved in normal healing. Timing is the real issue because it determines the degree of irreversible tissue damage sustained and hyperbaric oxygen treatment is often given too late. Measurements can be made to give objectivity and reproducibility. The evidence of animal experiments is very much more relevant than for drugs, simply because they use oxygen in the same way that we do.

However, there is an additional reason for accepting oxygen in the group of interventions not requiring controlled trials that does not apply to drugs: It is simply that we know precisely what happens when oxygen is *withdrawn*—we, of course, cease to exist. However, what does not feature in this list is what is termed the "cost-benefit ratio" which is simply measuring whether it is worth the effort involved. This depends on your point of view, and differs widely from being a purchaser as a patient to being a provider as a hospital administrator or government health minister. It is critically dependent on the costs involved, which will be discussed later.

This leaves the question of a dose-response relationship, and it is obvious that giving more oxygen is an increase of the dose we receive from air. It will be helpful here to compare oxygen with another biologically essential molecule, insulin. Imagine that insulin has just been discovered, and under evidence-based rules the usual validation from controlled trials is demanded. Patients who will obviously be diabetic need to be divided into two groups, one to receive an insulin injection and the other an injection of an inert placebo. The patients who have received insulin injections will have one of three outcomes: benefit, no change, or they may lose consciousness and die. Those injected with the placebo will show a little benefit or worsening—most will not change. Clearly the reason for this variation is that the insulin dosage has to be adjusted to match the level of the patient's blood glucose. In other words, we must be guided by measurements made in *each patient*. The argument that n=1 is clearly correct and, as will be seen, this logic applies to using oxygen as a treatment. The neurologist V.S. Ramachandran, in writing the book *Phantoms in the Brain* with science writer Sandra Blakeslee,[15] highlights the gulf in diagnosis between the reality of observations in a single patient and the absurd academic statistical approach in this delightful paragraph:

> *A tension exists in neurology between those who believe that the most valuable lessons about the brain can be learned from statistical analyses involving large numbers of patients and those who believe that doing the right kind of experiments on the right patients—even a single patient—can yield much more useful information.*

> *This is really a silly debate since its resolution is obvious: It's a good idea to begin with experiments on single cases and then to confirm the findings through studies of additional patients.*

> *By way of analogy, imagine that I cart a pig into your living room and tell you that it can talk. You might say, "Oh, Really? Show me." I then wave my wand and the pig starts talking. You might respond, "My God! That's amazing!" You are not likely to say, "Ah, but that's just one pig. Show me a few more and then I might believe you." Yet this is precisely the attitude of many people in my field.*

It is not scientific, indeed, it is ridiculous to suggest that oxygen should be tested in the same way as a drug and n=1 is certainly valid for oxygen; the physics involved in using the gas and varying its pressure to control its dosage is not a matter of medical opinion, it is dictated by the gas laws first described by luminaries such as Robert Boyle and John Dalton hundreds of years ago. For most of the time, the atmospheric pressure of our planet gives a blood concentration of oxygen that is sufficient for us to recover from the huge variety of illnesses and injuries we may suffer. Sometimes, however, it is simply not enough because the dose reaching the affected tissue is too low. Unfortunately, as already discussed, the stated objective of oxygen administration in the 2008 BTS guideline on the emergency use of oxygen in adult patients[16] is simply to ensure that haemoglobin is saturated—that it is carrying as much oxygen as possible. Although haemoglobin saturation ensures that the dissolved oxygen concentration in the blood will be normal, as we have seen, this *cannot* guarantee that the level of oxygen in *any* body tissue, other than the lungs, is normal. Ironically, red blood cells do not, of course, suffer when haemoglobin "saturation" is low.

At this point, readers may well question why so many in medicine are sceptical of the benefits of increasing the blood concentration of oxygen when so many of the conditions that afflict us are associated with its lack in our tissues. There is a straightforward answer to this question. The current generation of doctors have not been taught at medical school the importance of pressure to the delivery of oxygen, or even about the critical role of oxygen in healing. Once qualified and the title of doctor conferred, there is great resistance to admitting the lack of such elementary knowledge. Rather like the dark side of the moon, the benefits of using oxygen treatment continue to remain unseen, rotating out of view to most in the world of medicine.

Given the clarity of thought, perhaps only possible with the uncluttered mind of a lay person, it must seem blindingly obvious that the most important use of a high level of oxygen is in the treatment of emergencies. Establishing this is far from simple; there are serious difficulties in attempting to apply the principles of evidence-based medicine to assess the treatment of acute illness and injury. Also, powerful emotions are aroused by emergencies, and the public remains largely unaware of the personal cost to medical and nursing staff of being involved in life and death situations. Another significant problem is that patients sometimes get better against the odds without any treatment. Major advances often meet a hostile reaction, because they challenge the status: study the history of medicine, from hand washing introduced by Semmelweis, to the discovery and use of penicillin by Fleming, Florey, and Chain. But there is another problem which is rather less obvious: Those who use oxygen as a treatment are, in effect, criticising the knowledge and competence of colleagues.

The distrust of the case reports that discuss individual patients has particularly restricted progress in emergency medicine: They are out of fashion, although, thankfully the tradition is continued by the superb series, Case Records of the Massachusetts General Hospital, published by the *New England Journal of Medicine*. The story of Jessica in the well and the controversy that followed occupied a good deal of the last chapter. The story of her treatment is by definition an *anecdote*, and, despite 20 years of research, hyperbaric oxygen treatment has still not been adopted in the reattachment of severed limbs. As we have seen in the last chapter, even those involved in the original work do not think it should be, and are insisting that controlled trials are needed. To illustrate the importance of oxygen treatment in emergencies, we need to return to the halcyon era of hyperbaric medicine that followed WW2.

In the 1950s, heart surgeons and brain surgeons, two of the most powerful professional groups in medicine, became interested in the use of hyperbaric oxygenation. In those days, eminent professors had the status immortalised by the character Sir Lancelot Spratt, brilliantly portrayed by the actor, James Robertson Justice, in the film *Doctor in the House*. The opinions of junior doctors were formed by their teachers in a well-hidden, but nonetheless real, form of educational coercion—they would need a good reference for their next post. Although many would argue that eminence-based medicine has had an undue influence on practice, leading thinkers like John Scott Haldane and his friend William Osler often challenged accepted medical myths and they have shaped much of modern medicine. Research, as the name suggests, implies a rehash, or a continued development of already established concepts. We are in desperate need of "searchers," but thinking today is generally confined within the comfort zone of accepted wisdom, which is hardly surprising given the immense complexity that exists in every field of medicine. Change requires open minds hungry to explore new ideas, but those who challenge accepted wisdom pose a threat to the established funding streams of the research industry.[17] As Caesar said of Cassius, " . . . he has a lean and hungry look; he thinks too much, such men are dangerous."

Cardiac surgeons became interested in hyperbaric oxygenation after WW2 because it raised the possibility that the time that the heart could be stopped without risking brain damage could be extended. The time had already been modestly increased by cooling patients, which reduces the oxygen demand of the brain, and it is still used in most cardiac surgical centres. The hope was that combining cooling with a high level of oxygen would allow enough time for a surgeon with a good pair of hands to open the heart and replace a diseased valve. There were many patients who had sustained valve damage from episodes of rheumatic fever. Large chambers were constructed in Amsterdam and then Glasgow, and many more followed in other countries. Few have survived because heart-lung machines soon became available, and surgeons were only too pleased to operate without being confined in a hyperbaric chamber. Ironically, the new machines that bypass the heart and the lungs and both pump and oxygenate blood were soon found to be associated with brain damage. Research over the last 30 years has shown that it is due to a variety of small emboli, including bubbles. Eventually blood filters were introduced, although they are by no means as efficient in filtering blood as the lungs. Brain damage is still a problem in cardiac surgery, and has been demonstrated by imaging patients by MRI before and after operations. A preliminary report of the study published in the *Lancet* in 1993[18] showed the areas of white matter damage on the images—unidentified bright objects (UBOs). Most, but not all of the UBOs resolved over a period of weeks; it is clear that surgeons discarded the use of hyperbaric chambers too soon as hyperbaric oxygenation is the only treatment for the localised areas of hypoxia caused by small emboli.

Two astonishing case reports from the 1960s illustrate the importance of accepting the evidence of anecdotes. The first predates the introduction of the heart-lung machine when operations were still being undertaken on the beating heart. In 1964, a 50-year-old man was admitted to the London Chest Hospital desperately ill, having coughed up half a pint of blood the day before. He had become progressively breathless because of damage to the mitral valve of the heart, which lies between the left atrium and ventricle. Although not stated in the paper, this was almost certainly caused by an episode of rheumatic fever in childhood that caused inflammation of the flaps of the mitral valve. They had fused together, restricting the flow of blood through the heart. If the valve does not close properly, back pressure is created in the blood vessels of the lungs, and they may rupture, causing the patient to cough up blood. The paper describing this remarkable case was published as a two page report in the *Lancet* in 1965[19] under the title, "Hyperbaric Oxygen in the Treatment of the Postoperative Low-Cardiac-Output Syndrome." The patient failed to recover consciousness after the operation, and his blood pressure was low. He was given 100% oxygen and placed on a ventilator, but his blood pressure continued to fall. When his death seemed inevitable, he was taken off the ventilator and loaded into the acrylic cylinder of a Vickers single person chamber. Astonishingly, when pressurised in the pure oxygen atmosphere of the chamber, he actually began to breathe spontaneously, and despite a turbulent 24 hours, eventually made a full recovery. The abstract in the following Case Report gives the details.

A Case Report

A 50-year-old man was admitted to the London Chest Hospital on October 23, 1964. He had a history of productive cough, recurrent haemoptysis (blood in his sputum), and dyspnoea (breathlessness) on exertion for 21 years. He had been discharged from the Army 20 years before with mitral valve disease. The operation was performed by Mr. J.R. Belcher on November 3, 1964. After the operation the patient displayed all the signs of a low cardiac output—failure to recover consciousness with no localising cerebral signs, severe peripheral cyanosis, and a very slow capillary refill in the limbs. In an attempt to lower the pulmonary vascular resistance and raise the cardiac output, he was artificially ventilated with 100% oxygen. This was ineffective, and the patient's death seemed certain.

Since the patient's condition was now desperate, it was decided to use hyperbaric oxygen therapy. He was placed in the Vickers mobile chamber at a pressure of 2 ATA. Since there were no facilities in the chamber for artificial respiration, transfusion, or drainage these had to be discontinued. The patient's condition began to improve after an hour inside the chamber; he was taken out of it every two hours to aspirate from his bronchial tree the considerable amount of heavily bloodstained sputum. After 12 hours of treatment, he began to move and gradually recovered consciousness for the first time since the operation.

Yacoub MH, Zeitlin GL. *Lancet.* 1965; i:581-3.

It was a truly miraculous recovery—little wonder, that it merited two pages in the *Lancet*! The surgery had been undertaken as a last resort and, because the patient could not sustain his breathing after the operation, he was ventilated with 100% oxygen. However, it failed to reverse the decline of his blood pressure, which at one stage it fell to just *50 mm Hg*, risking his kidneys shutting down. To take him off the breathing machine, disconnect the drains which were draining blood from his chest, together with the intravenous lines, and push him into the Vickers chamber required considerable resolve. The doctors involved could not possibly have known that he would start breathing when pressurised in the chamber, but the patient was dying in front of them and every other treatment option had been used. There is no indication in the paper of the time that had elapsed from completion of the operation to the use of the chamber, but it would have been hours, not minutes. The chamber was described in the paper as being "mobile," and it certainly was—it was in the back of an ambulance. It had been driven to the hospital from the Vickers Headquarters near Ascot, with a police escort and

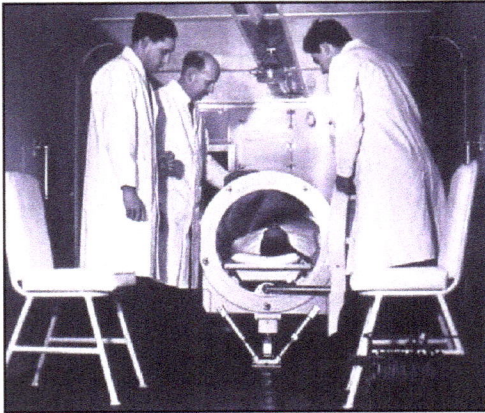

Figure 10.2:
The ambulance and the Vickers "mobile'" chamber.

the Chief Engineer of the Vickers Medical Division, the late John Hounsell, was in hot pursuit on what he described to the author as a "hair-raising" journey. He remained at the hospital through the night to run the chamber. However, what is not stated in the account in the *Lancet*, is that the patient was actually treated in the ambulance in the hospital car park (Figure 10.2). Perhaps the authors were simply too embarrassed to include this detail!

Despite the publication of this astonishing story, later in the same year a leading article about hyperbaric oxygenation appeared in the same journal.[20] It opened with the sentence:

Within a few years oxygen under pressure may prove to be one of the most useful, versatile, and dangerous forms of treatment.

No letters of protest were published by the *Lancet*, yet there could not be a more convincing demonstration of both the safety of hyperbaric oxygen treatment and its efficacy than the experience of this one dying patient. He actually received a total of 18 hours in the chamber over just two days with no suggestion of lung, or other problems. Many of the hyperbaric doctors practising today would, for sure, not have accepted him for treatment and would certainly regard the duration of this patient's exposure to oxygen as dangerous. In fact, after looking at the X-ray of his chest, most, especially in the US, would have excluded him as being unfit to go under pressure! In the US, a chest X-ray is often regarded as mandatory, a precaution in the pre-dive work-up for hyperbaric treatment, as if the patient is actually going underwater! If this is challenged, it is claimed that it is done to exclude lung cysts that may predispose a patient to problems from gas expanding on decompression. Experience from submarine escape training has shown this to be spurious; sadly, it has more to do with making money than a genuine fear of injury or a malpractice claim.

We now have the scientific knowledge to explain why the benefits to this cardiac patient in heart failure were so profound. The most important fact is that breathing oxygen at twice normal atmospheric pressure reduces the workload of the heart. The oxygen requirements of the body can be satisfied by pumping 20% less blood than when a patient breathes air.[21] There are other reasons why it is beneficial, and they were discussed in the *Lancet* paper. By correcting a lack of oxygen, the raised blood pressure in the pulmonary artery supplying the lungs is reduced. As discussed in Chapter 2, in contrast to every other blood vessel in the body, paradoxically, these arteries constrict when the oxygen levels falls. This is in order to slow blood flow through the lungs to allow time for red blood cells to collect as much oxygen as possible and ensure better blood distribution. If ever there was proof of principle needed to underpin hyperbaric oxygen treatment, this patient provided it— he was rescued from certain death. The primary function of the heart and circulation is to deliver oxygen and the principle involved in using oxygen as a treatment is that its delivery to tissues can be improved, and this may occur despite blood flow actually being *reduced*.

The authors of the 1965 paper concluded that the experience of using hyperbaric oxygen treatment in this dying patient "justified further trial of the technique in similar cases"—a very conservative statement in view of the miraculous recovery they had witnessed. This appears to be the only occasion when the Vickers mobile hyperbaric chamber was used for a patient following cardiac surgery, although it was also used for patients with gas gangrene. The service was continued by a team of anaesthetists at the Princess Alexander Hospital at RAF Wroughton, until it was finally withdrawn when the hospital closed in the late 1980s.

The surgeon involved in this first story was in the media spotlight recently as a co-author of another dramatic case report which the *Lancet* again published.[22] This time the anecdote merited six pages, demonstrating that the exception proves the rule, and featured in TV and newspaper reports around the world. In 1995 he had operated with colleagues on an 11-month-old girl who, like the patient in 1964, was in low-output cardiac failure. A heart was transplanted which was "piggy-backed" onto the patient's own heart to give it a rest, which clearly invokes the principle of natural recovery. This is now known to include the rebuilding of heart muscle by the patient's own stem cells. Irrefutable evidence of this has come from postmortem studies of patients who have died after receiving a heart from a donor of the opposite sex. Muscle cells with the recipient's chromosomes have been found in the

---

transplanted heart. They could only have come from the bone marrow of the recipient, and so must have migrated into the heart as part of a normal maintenance programme. In other words, the muscle cells of the heart are, like other organs, being continually replaced. However, this depends on improving the oxygenation of the heart, which is reduced when the muscle tissue contracts to pump blood.

After years on immune-suppressing drugs and many life-threatening crises, the young lady developed a persistent viral infection, which was associated with the development of blood cancer. Her drugs had to be stopped, and as a consequence the second heart had to be removed when she had reached the age of 16, because of rejection. Fortunately, despite the toxicity of the drugs she had received for over a decade, her own heart had recovered to be able to pump efficiently. Happily, she has been able to lead a normal life and has completed her school's GCSE examinations. She told reporters that it was strange to lose her second heart, "I could feel a bit more space inside me." (The *Sunday Times*, July 19, 2009.)

The second remarkable hyperbaric anecdote is the story of a mother and her unborn child from a report published in the *British Medical Journal* in 1968[23] under the title "Fatal Brain Damage Associated with Cardiomyopathy of Pregnancy, with Notes on Caesarian Section in a Hyperbaric Chamber." The patient was in the last weeks of her pregnancy when, because of bleeding, she was admitted for bed rest in a Glasgow hospital. The subsequent events were so dramatic that the journal allowed a very detailed report to be published, with an hour by hour account.

The patient was resting in bed at 6:50 p.m. on January 16, 1967 when she suddenly developed a severe headache with pins and needles and weakness down her left side. This clearly indicated a problem in the brain, which was confirmed when minutes later she abruptly lost consciousness. The most likely cause of her illness was not the heart problem suggested, but the escape of fluid and debris from the womb into the circulation, a condition known as *amniotic fluid embolism*.[24] This diagnosis was not discussed in the paper, but the bleeding had indicated that there was a problem with the placenta. After many investigations and the lapse of 24 hours, the mother was in a desperate state, having started to convulse. The baby had become distressed in the womb, and it was decided to operate to save the baby oxygenating the mother under hyperbaric conditions in the chamber that had been installed for cardiac surgery on the roof of the Western Infirmary by Sir Charles Illingworth (Figure 10.3).

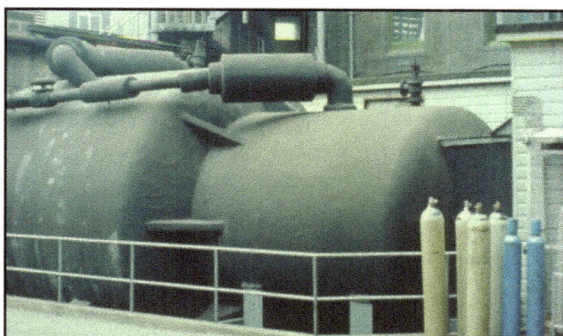

Figure 10.3:
The hyperbaric chamber on the roof of the Western Infirmary, Glasgow.

As the mother was pressurised to twice atmospheric pressure breathing 100% oxygen, she became pink, and the heart rate of her baby fell from an irregular 220 beats per minute to 165 and regular. A healthy baby girl was delivered by caesarian section which, it is stated, went remarkably smoothly. The remarkable details from the journal report are reproduced in the following Case Report.

A Case Report

On December 26 1966, a 22-year-old primipara in the 37th week was admitted to a maternity hospital for observation because of a minor antepartum haemorrhage. While in bed at 6.50 p.m. on January 16 1967, she complained of pins and needles in her left limbs, abruptly developed hemiplegia, and became unconscious and cyanosed with stertorous respiration. Because of the marginal nature of the improvement which had taken place in the patient's condition with 100% oxygen at normal pressure, and because of the onset now of fetal distress (the fetal heart rate had risen to approximately 200 per minute and was irregular), it was decided to assess the effect of oxygen administration at 2 ATA. Before compression started however, the patient began to have generalised convulsions, which became continuous in minutes, and her general condition deteriorated until death was thought to be imminent.

Following compression to 2 ATA breathing oxygen, there was a marked improvement in the patient's condition: The blood pressure rose to 100/70 mm Hg and the periphery became warm and pink. The fetal heart rate, which had been 220 and irregular immediately before compression, fell to 165 and became regular. Caesarian section was now performed (Professor Ian Donald, University Department of Obstetrics and Gynaecology), and proceeded remarkably smoothly, though it was noted that the uterus remained slightly cyanosed in spite of the high maternal arterial oxygen tension. A normal live female child was born with an Apgar score of 9.

Yet another truly astounding story—unfortunately, although the mother had improved from being in the chamber, it was her only treatment, and she died three months later. In contrast to the patient in the first Case Report, recordings had been made of the oxygen levels in the blood in her arteries before, during, and after the chamber session. An increase was, of course, to be expected with the patient breathing oxygen at twice normal atmospheric pressure, but it only rose to half the expected value. This shows that the mother had sustained damage to her lungs, and this is consistent with amniotic fluid embolism. Nevertheless, the heart rate of the baby fell in the chamber and the operation was successful; a normal, healthy girl had been delivered. Again, the principles involved are simple. A baby is at the end of the line for the delivery of oxygen, and any reduction in the concentration of oxygen from the lungs of the mother to the placenta places the baby at risk. How many infants with fetal distress have since died or sustained brain damage when the additional oxygen made possible by using a simple pressure chamber would have made a difference? There is no record of any other mothers being treated in the Glasgow chamber, and it was dismantled in 1995. Sceptics, of course, would claim this is just another anecdote, but readers who feel that this is an exaggeration to make a point need to know that, after reading the paper, one midwife asked if any controlled studies have been done in such cases!

We need to examine just what this implies—it would mean recruiting a series of such patients, and they would need to be divided into two groups, one receiving standard treatment, in other words 100% oxygen at normal atmospheric pressure, the other hyperbaric oxygen treatment. Time would be needed to stabilise the patients and randomise them to the two arms of the study. Ideally, some would argue for blinding—that to be scientific, neither the patients nor their doctors should know who received which protocol, but this would clearly be impracticable, as the clock is ticking in such emergencies. Apart from being impossible in practice to recruit a series of such rare cases, it would, in the author's view, be both unscientific and unethical. Again, the contention is that the evidence needed to treat patients in heart failure and distressed babies in the womb with a high level of oxygen has already been provided by each of these case reports. Some will argue that after 40 years the reports are out-of-date, but the timing is totally irrelevant—the benefits from giving more oxygen do not change.

Twenty years after the publication of this dramatic case in the Western Infirmary in Glasgow, a paper in the *Lancet*[25] described the results from giving more oxygen to mothers whose babies had stopped growing in the womb, a condition known as fetal growth retardation. What made this study especially important was that measurements were made of the oxygen concentration in the umbilical cord blood being delivered from the placenta to the baby. Five mothers were examined with one mother carrying twins. The measurements showed that the babies were suffering from lack of oxygen and, in two, this was so extreme that lactic acid was present. The transport of nutrients across the placenta to the developing baby is *active*, which means that it requires energy and, of course, this requires sufficient oxygen. If there is lack of oxygen, nutrients are not transferred and the growth of the fetus is retarded. By the time the mothers were given supplementary oxygen, one of the babies with acidosis had died in the womb. However, the lack of oxygen was corrected in the others and uncomplicated deliveries were undertaken by caesarian section with all five babies surviving with minimal requirement for intensive care. The authors observed that deaths in the womb in similar babies with growth retardation has been reported to be as high as 85% and in survivors, severe neonatal complications occurred, also in 85%. Yet, again, the report ended by stating that a prospective double-blind trial was planned. However, there is *no other treatment*; indeed, the authors stated that "the present management of such cases is simply to wait." The oxygen treatment used is inexpensive, safe and immediately available in every hospital. A controlled study would have to obtain consent from pregnant mothers that the baby they were carrying had stopped growing because of lack of oxygen, but that they would be given air or oxygen to determine if more oxygen would be beneficial. It truly beggars belief that any mother would give informed consent to be given air rather than oxygen when their baby is suffering from lack of oxygen and the results of the *Lancet* study are explained to them. As with so many oxygen initiatives it seems to have disappeared without trace. But the science is in place, many measurements were made, and the conclusion incontestable: Lack of oxygen requires more to be given, because air is not enough.

It is logical to argue that when a patient has been suffering from a chronic, long-standing, condition they can be their own control, but even this may be misleading. A patient with a fungal infection of the toenails was given a high dose of anti-fungal drug after suffering the problem for more than 20 years. It is usual for a low dose of the drug to be used in a prolonged course of treatment, but a dermatologist had suggested in a letter to the *Lancet* that a high dose could be successful.[26] All 10 toes were affected but, after the single dose of the drug, the nail of the patient's right big toe began to grow normally. However, the nail of the left big toe was unchanged, as were the other toes of both feet.

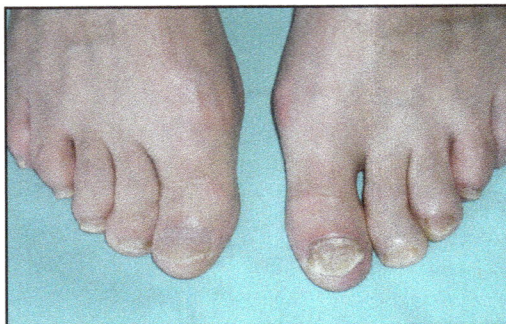

Figure 10.4:
Normal nail of the right big toe; effect of a single drug dose after 20 years of infection.

Perhaps, it could be argued, taking the drug was irrelevant, that the change in the nail would have occurred without treatment. This is most unlikely, because the infection had been present in both feet for over 20 years. Why did both toes of the patient not recover? An uncontrolled variable was obviously present. In fact, 30 years previously, the patient suffered damage to the left sciatic nerve, and since then the left foot has been consistently colder than the right. This means a lesser supply of blood to the foot, and so less of the anti-fungal drug delivered to the nail bed. This shows that even one leg of a patient cannot be used as a control for the other.

Oxygen is, of course, widely used in emergencies, but the dosage is limited by barometric pressure, and it is difficult to avoid the conclusion that hyperbaric equipment can improve outcome for many patients. In contrast, however, there is a perfectly understandable reason for some having difficulty accepting the value of oxygen treatment in chronic conditions. The question posed is simply this: Why can giving a high level of oxygen for just one hour a day possibly be effective when the lack of oxygen is present for the remaining 23 hours? The answer lies in the discovery of the role of oxygen in gene control, via the hypoxia-inducible factor proteins already discussed, especially in controlling inflammation. This, and other evidence, is woven into subsequent chapters.

CHAPTER 11

Suffer the Little Children

Hypoxia is the greatest danger to which the fetus in utero is exposed; it is the most common cause of intrauterine death.

Harry Prystowsky, 1959

Being born is a dangerous event. After months of growing in the protected environment of the womb, with oxygen provided via the life support system of the placenta, our entry into the world forces a change to breathing air to gain much-needed oxygen. We are at a disadvantage when compared to other primates, as the human birth canal is narrower; the downside of walking on two legs is the necessity for strong pelvic bones. The human brain and hence the head is also much larger than other primates at term, and so birth must take place when the brain is much less developed at birth than, for example, the brain of a chimpanzee. Baby chimpanzees are able to hold on to their mothers within days of being born, whereas human infants require many months to reach the same degree of independence. It is clear that everything should be done to ensure that birth is as safe as possible so that children are healthy and able to achieve their full potential. When it became possible in the 1980s to monitor the progress of a baby during pregnancy, it was soon recognised that if a child was not growing at the normal rate (a condition called fetal growth retardation), it was due to lack of oxygen[1] and usually associated with a problem in the placenta.

To give birth requires considerable physical fitness because the muscular contractions of the womb needed to expel the baby require a great deal of effort. Contractions reduce the blood supply to the placenta, simply because the pressure exerted by the muscles compresses the vessels that supply the womb with blood. This is the same effect as when a fist is clenched tightly; the tissues of the hand, being compressed, become white as the blood is removed. The contractions of the womb have to become most forceful in the final stage of labour, as the infant's head stretches the birth canal. It has not proved possible to obtain meaningful physiological data from a baby during this critical period, which is reminiscent of the radio silence of an Apollo spacecraft passing around the dark side of the moon. However, even if it were possible to accurately monitor the heart of a baby throughout a delivery, it would not provide the information needed to predict birth injury. Both extremely fast and very slow heart rates give an indication of risk, but large variations in heart rate are often recorded in babies in the womb who are found to be perfectly normal after delivery. Equally, babies who are very blue (cyanosed) at birth usually develop normally. Dr. Harry Prystowsky's comment in 1959[2] about using oxygen during labour, which is supported by animal data showing a clear reduction in mortality,[3] still holds true:

> *Hence, it would seem desirable to follow this procedure of routine oxygen administration in order to protect the welfare of the one baby in twenty who needs it and who may suffer some degree of hypoxia . . . there is no way of predicting which fetus might become embarrassed at this late stage of labor; an unfortunate event with which obstetricians are not unfamiliar.*

The provision of 100% oxygen during labour is an almost zero cost option, in stark contrast to the millions required to care for a brain-injured child over a lifetime and the emotional costs, which are incalculable. The astonishing story of the delivery of a baby in a pressure chamber in Glasgow[4] detailed in Chapter 10 shows beyond doubt the importance of increasing the dosage of oxygen breathed by the mother to counter fetal distress. Given that it only involves doubling atmospheric pressure, the equipment should be made available in every delivery room. Nevertheless, incredible though it may seem, obstetric opinion has moved away from regarding lack of oxygen in a baby during delivery as important.

In fact, in recent years it has been fashionable to assert that conditions such as cerebral palsy are actually not due to a problem during birth, reflecting the emotions generated, the culture of blame, and the enormous sums demanded in compensation. It is now common to claim that to be able to attribute a brain injury like cerebral palsy to a birth event, there must be evidence that the baby suffered from a severe lack of oxygen or a severely irregular heart rhythm during delivery.[5] Blood samples are often taken from the umbilical cord after birth to be analysed for possible *acidosis*, that is, a buildup of lactic acid.[6] This is to defend against allegations that an adverse event has occurred; evidence of acidosis may render staff open to a claim of negligence. If the samples are normal, it is claimed that this shows that there has not been a serious lack of oxygen in the brain.[7] However, the absence of acidosis in such a sample cannot rule out the possibility that lack of oxygen in a small area of the brain has resulted in damage that may lead to cerebral palsy. It is as absurd as claiming that an adult cannot suffer from a stroke unless the whole body lacks oxygen and there is a generalised acidosis. Acidosis in the blood is a sign of a general lack of oxygen in the body, not of an acute deficiency in a small volume of tissue. It is obvious that a reduction of blood flow to a small area of the brain may cause a stroke due to a local lack of oxygen when the level of oxygen in the blood is normal, and exactly the same reasoning applies if a patient has a heart attack.

Many myths have grown up around events at birth attempting to account for cerebral palsy, one being that the baby had the cord wrapped round the neck, evoking an image of airway obstruction associated with strangulation in an adult. However, during birth the baby is not yet breathing, and the mouth and nose are, of course, blocked by the mother's tissues. Breathing can only start after a baby has been delivered. In passing down the birth canal, the head of a baby is compressed or molded to reduce its size; the soft plates of cartilage that form the skull of the baby are pushed together to reduce the diameter of the head. This pressure inevitably reduces blood flow to the brain. If the compression is prolonged and very low oxygen levels are present when blood flow abruptly returns as the baby is delivered, this sequence of events may lead to *reperfusion injury*. This is, of course, the phenomenon covered in Chapter 9 researched by Dr. Zamboni and his team after the controversy over the use of hyperbaric oxygen treatment for Jessica McClure.[8] The abrupt return of normal blood flow after a period of restriction is paradoxically accompanied by tissue damage from neutrophils, and it is likely that exactly the same sequence occurs in the brain after cardiac arrest in an adult resulting in damage to the areas of the brain where blood supply is poorest. They are known as watershed territories, and include the areas in the middle of the brain where the nerve fibres responsible for movement pass.[9] Damage to the motor nerve cells in the cortex and the fibres in these pathways both give rise to the loss of muscle control known as cerebral palsy.

If a baby is born after the normal duration of a pregnancy, that is, at term, the blood vessels of the brain will have matured sufficiently to cope with the stresses of a routine delivery. However, premature infants have many fewer blood vessels in their brains,[10] and so there is less oxygen available to cope with the stress of coming into the world. There is a second problem: the lungs of preterm infants are also immature, and so are less able to oxygenate the blood after birth. Of course, most babies do fine, but sadly not all, and sometimes it is many months, or even years, before brain damage is formally recognised by medical staff. Mothers, however, often sense a problem in the first few days or weeks after delivery, although their fears are frequently dismissed. Unfortunately, the longer the interval before a problem is discovered, the less likely a link will be made to an event during birth. Despite this problem, there is one brain disorder that paediatric neurologists accept *is* due to birth injury and which may develop many years later. It is associated with muscle contractions and called dystonia.[11,12] This raises an obvious question: Why cannot other forms of brain dysfunction, such as cerebral palsy, also present years later? The answer is simple: They can.

What may go wrong? Labour may start early for unknown reasons before the blood vessels of the brain of the baby are fully mature. The separation of the placenta, which normally occurs after delivery, may also begin too soon, reducing the supply of oxygen during the final stage of labour, just when compression of the head is also reducing the blood supply to the brain. The disruption of the mother's breathing with the pain of labour reduces oxygen levels and, so, particularly in the last stage of labour, the oxygen supply to the baby falls. The longer birth is delayed, the greater the risk of brain damage in the infant, but it is not predictable. Labour may be prolonged because of a lack of physical fitness to sustain the effort required; unfortunately, general standards of fitness of both men and women have declined in the Western world. It is ironic that "labour saving" is a major selling point for our domestic appliances. Although the reduction of blood flow limits the supply of all the essential substances carried in blood, it is only the deficiency of oxygen that is critical and it is obvious that, with very rare exceptions, it is only the brain that suffers from this deprivation.

Another recently recognised problem is the timing of clamping the umbilical cord.[13] In a natural delivery, the baby is delivered, followed by delivery of the placenta, but other animals then chew through the cord in slow time. This natural delay allows time for the full transfer of what is quite a large volume of blood in the placenta to be "milked" into the circulation of the newly born baby. Clamping the cord too early deprives the baby of this blood and may actually precipitate hypovolaemic shock—low blood volume shock. The reduction of blood volume at this time may also cause brain damage and, in some children, contribute to events that lead to cerebral palsy or autism. It has also become common for a sample of cord blood to be taken at birth. However, it must be remembered that what is a small sample of blood for an adult represents a much greater proportion of the circulating blood in a tiny infant. Another reason for taking blood from the umbilical cord, which is gaining in popularity, is to harvest stem cells for possible use in the future. Nevertheless, some feel strongly that sampling cord blood is too risky a procedure and unjustified, as it is often not in the interest of the child.

Attempts to deny a link between birth events, especially cerebral palsy, with the problems during the delivery reflect claims for compensation, which are increasing at an alarming rate. Emotions are in turmoil when a child is born with problems; today there is little acceptance of imperfection, and we also live in a culture of blame. By the end of 1999, settlements totalling £200 million had been made in the UK and at the end of 2000 there were 1,500 claims as yet unsettled (*File on 4*, Radio 4, July 17, 2000). A 2011 action for brain damage admitted to have been caused by oxygen deprivation at birth was settled for over £6 million.

Reacting to this situation in the mid-1990s, obstetricians and midwives from 12 countries set up an international forum to reach a worldwide consensus on whether cerebral palsy (CP) was related to events at birth. Several international conferences were organised and were supplemented with discussions on the Internet. The consensus report, A Template for Defining a Causal Relation Between Intrapartum Events (during birth) and Cerebral Palsy: International Consensus Statement, was finally published in several journals, including the *British Medical Journal* in October 1999.[14] The bias of the group was obvious—by attempting to implicate events in the womb occurring antepartum, that is, during pregnancy and *before* birth to account for cerebral palsy. It is all too clear in the following statement:

Complications occurring in the antepartum period are common and important causes of cerebral palsy.

In other words, according to the contributors to the consensus statement, cerebral palsy is most commonly caused by events *during* pregnancy, and not by a problem occurring during delivery. However, this dogmatic statement is not supported by published evidence, and it is certainly incorrect to use the words "common" and "important." This leaves already emotionally fraught mothers to agonise over what they may have done during the pregnancy to cause the problem. The consensus statement goes further by stating the following:

Epidemiological studies suggest that in about 90% of cases intra partum hypoxia (lack of oxygen during delivery) could not be the cause of cerebral palsy.

This *cannot* be correct and here, as in studies of multiple sclerosis and trauma discussed later, the consensus group has fallen into the trap of attempting to use epidemiological studies to prove or disprove *causation*. The group went further in suggesting that the uncomfortable term "fetal distress" should actually be abandoned, and replaced by the banal expression "non-reassuring fetal status." The term "non-reassuring" applies to the reassurance of the medical professionals involved, because monitoring is unable to determine the status of the infant.

As clinical signs often poorly predict a compromised fetus, and continued use of this term [fetal distress] may encourage wrong assumptions or inappropriate management.

Unfortunately, the wrong assumptions are all too obvious. Fetal distress is real and is important because it may indicate a problem and should trigger immediate action. The cornerstone of the treatment of hypoxia is to give more oxygen. As we saw in Chapter 10, this may mean using a higher than normal atmospheric pressure in a pressure chamber, and the case report from Glasgow showed how effective and simple this can be.

It was acknowledged by those contributing to the consensus there is an observable correlation with a difficult birth in those babies who develop the severest form of cerebral palsy, *spastic quadriplegia.* This condition, in which the child is unable to move all four limbs, is often associated with global brain damage and subsequent failure of the head of the baby to grow, which is termed microcephaly. However, it should not be surprising that it becomes more difficult to find a correlation between lesser degrees of damage and an event occurring during labour, as the number of variables increases. Although epidemiological studies have shown a poor correlation for milder degrees of brain damage, babies actually delivered by elective caesarian section have been shown to have a *lower risk* of developing cerebral palsy.[15] In other words, it is less common for a child delivered by elective caesarian section than by normal delivery to develop cerebral palsy. Caesarian section can avoid much of the delay and trauma sometimes associated with a natural delivery. However, it must be remembered that caesarian section is most often an emergency procedure undertaken when it is clear that a baby would be at risk if delivered normally.

A consensus view was reached with some difficulty by the group in relation to the most critical area—that is, the use of imaging of the brain in the timing of events. The group questioned:

. . . the current validity of neuroimaging in the infant to retrospectively determine the precise perinatal timing, pathology or cause of the abnormalities seen on imaging . . . The task force awaits the publication of strong data.

This, as already discussed, is truly the crux of the matter: For the consensus committee to actually arrive at conclusions *without* this critical information, when the technology has been available and in use for many years, was ill-advised. Moreover, this is especially the case when imaging can determine a relationship between birth and brain injury almost in real time. This impasse appears to have prompted a study, which was finally published in

2003, some three years *after* the publication of the consensus paper.[16] Before discussing the paper, it is first necessary to examine the theories proposed to account for the brain damage known as cerebral palsy by those supporting the consensus view.

In the consensus statement it was suggested that events during pregnancy are responsible for brain injury; that is, problems occurring whilst the baby is in the womb. Incredibly, it was actually suggested without *any* supporting evidence, that auto-immune disease, or infection is responsible for 90% of cases of cerebral palsy. The parallel to the same allegations made in multiple sclerosis will be apparent later but, in this case, the blame is shifted to the mother, which is grossly unfair. To add to this distress without evidence is reprehensible, and there is certainly no evidence whatsoever that auto-immunity is involved in damaging the brain during pregnancy. Also, intrauterine infection is extremely rare. Crucially, there was no discussion in the consensus statement of how either of these processes can produce damage to the small area of the mid-brain of infants that gives rise to cerebral palsy.

The only concept discussed in the consensus document is simple *asphyxia*, a term that indicates that a baby is generally deprived of oxygen, for example, because the umbilical cord has been compressed, or the placenta has separated, reducing the transfer of oxygen. The consensus participants agreed a robust but unqualified statement that;

> *. . . to attribute cerebral palsy to prior asphyxia with reasonably certainty there must be evidence that a substantial hypoxic injury occurred.*

There is no attempt in the document to justify this assertion; in fact, for cerebral palsy to develop, there only needs to be damage to nerve fibres that control limb movement in a very small area in the mid-brain, or in the brainstem. The absence of such a substantial hypoxic event in most children who develop cerebral palsy is the basis of the mistaken claim that, in 90% of cases, lack of oxygen during birth cannot be the cause.

Although it is argued correctly that many, indeed probably most, children who have a significant lack of oxygen at birth do not develop cerebral palsy, as already stated, a relationship between spastic quadriplegia and severe birth asphyxia is accepted. This is because studies have shown a correlation to exist for this severe form of cerebral palsy. However, if a correlation cannot be found for lesser degrees of disability, for example when a baby has only the legs affected, it suggests that the sensitivity of tests for brain damage at birth is poor and, in fact, the lack of sensitivity is well known. A second factor is that the spasticity, the characteristic stiffness of the limbs associated with cerebral palsy, may not develop for many months after birth.

Another unfortunate allegation is that the brain injury that gives rise to cerebral palsy is fixed, that is, the damage does not change as the baby grows. This negative position, which becomes a self-fulfilling prophecy if no attempt is made to treat affected infants, was expressed by a paediatrician commenting on the use of oxygen treatment.

Any "good" paediatrician will point out to parents of a child with cerebral palsy (CP) that their child's brain damage is fixed and cannot be altered. This is not being over pessimistic but simply honest.

This is certainly refuted by clinical experience. Children often have some limb movement for months after birth, then experience loss of function, and may develop spasticity as late as two years later. In fact, delay in the onset of symptoms is properly documented and acknowledged in the *dystonias*, the brain disorders associated with muscle spasms, which neurologists have acknowledged is due to an injury at birth. From published reports, the symptoms of dystonia may appear as late as *11 years* after birth, and may continue to worsen for up to 28 years.[12] This, at the very least, is powerful evidence that a *window of opportunity* for treatment exists.

A global lack of oxygen denoted by the term asphyxia is unlikely to be the most important mechanism of injury at birth; in fact, it is well known that it is *not* essential for a substantial hypoxic event to have occurred in children who develop cerebral palsy. The mechanism that was studied after the treatment of Jessica covered in Chapter 9, known as reperfusion injury, which is caused when blood flow is stopped for a time and then restarted, was not considered by the international consensus group. The attraction of white blood cells and their release of free radicals contribute to the blood-brain barrier opening and to the tissue damage shown on MRI, as it does in the bubble damage of decompression sickness. However, it is now necessary to discuss this data in relation to the typical mid-brain damage evident in children with cerebral palsy.

Powerful evidence of a link between cerebral palsy and an event during delivery has already been mentioned; cerebral palsy is less likely to occur in children born by elective caesarian section. Delivering the baby this way avoids the compressive forces acting on the head of the baby during labour, that inevitably reduce blood flow in the brain. Ultrasound and MRI have both been used to follow the sequence of events from birth to the development of cerebral palsy. To establish the true role of birth events in neonatal brain injury required a full examination of events in the brain using both pathological studies and brain imaging as the Consensus statement admitted. Groups at the Royal Free Hospital in London and in the University of Amsterdam took up the challenge. Their stated aim was to determine if the encephalopathy that follows severe brain swelling after birth, which is often associated with convulsions, is really due to a problem during pregnancy. This was, of course, the opinion of those who contributed to the international consensus. The study was very comprehensive, with 351 children recruited and detailed clinical, radiological examinations were undertaken including, sadly, for some babies, post-mortem examination. The author's conclusions in the *Lancet*[16] *completely overturned* the consensus view.

> *Our findings show that more than 90% of full term infants with neonatal encephalopathy, seizures, or both . . . had evidence of perinatally acquired insults.*

In other words, in almost all cases the brain damage was not the result of infection or auto-immunity during the pregnancy; they were clearly caused by a *perinatal event*, around the time of birth. It is ironic that the figure stated of 90% is *just* the one suggested, but in the opposite direction, by the members of the international consensus. However, the MRI study merited just one publication and, in marked contrast to the multiple publications of the flawed consensus statement, press attention was minimal. The results have been confirmed. A study in California, published in 2010, showed that adverse obstetric events *are* associated with significant risk of cerebral palsy.[17] The study enrolled 7,242 children who had cerebral palsy and 59% of them had been delivered at term. Children without cerebral palsy acted as controls. It was found that 31.3% of the children with cerebral palsy had adverse events during birth, compared to 12.9% in the controls ($p<0.0001$). In fact, this observation held both for term infants at 28.3% controls 12.7% and preterm infants, 36.8% versus 15.9% in the controls— $p<0.0001$. So the consensus statement is *wrong* and it should be retracted.

The extraordinary techniques developed for magnetic resonance imaging, which have given us such astonishing pictures of the living brain, have been refined in the last few years to look at its chemistry in real time. Magnetic resonance spectroscopy can determine the molecules present in a cube of brain tissue. The key molecule adenosine triphosphate (ATP) has been discussed earlier in this book—it is the energy molecule of life. It exists in three forms: alpha, beta, and gamma. Their levels have been followed within the tissues of the brain of infants from birth to six weeks, using MRS.[18] The technique allows a measure of the quantities of the three forms of ATP in selected areas of brain tissue.

Figure 11.1 shows the MRS of an infant with obvious neurological problems scanned after birth, then at seven days, and 35 days. The paper was published in 1996, just as the international consensus forum was forming. The levels of the three forms of the energy molecule, ATP, at the first scan are very low, and the normal cadence of their values from the highest, gamma (γ), via alpha (α), to beta (β), the lowest, was not present on the scan on the first day or on seventh day but by 35 days the correct cadence was present, but the values were still only a third of those found in a healthy child. This indicates that because of lack of oxygen there was severe energy failure. However, the oxygen levels in the infant's blood would, of course, have been recorded as normal. It is not surprisingly, that the authors found that the ATP levels did not correlate with the babies' Apgar score, which is a rather primitive measure of vitality in common use to assess the newborn. The method was devised in 1952 by a paediatrician, Dr. Virginia Apgar,[19] and relies on a simple clinical evaluation of five factors at the bedside. The test is normally done at one and five minutes after birth. The acronym used is based on Dr. Apgar's name, the letters standing for appearance, pulse, grimace, activity, and respiration. Table 11.1 demonstrates a basic version of the scoring method. It is clearly a very crude assessment tool.

It is clear that the lack of oxygen due to lack of blood flow in the infant, termed hypoxic-ischaemic encephalopathy, demonstrated using advanced MRS, was present at birth and had not resolved over *a month later*. It is not stated in the paper how much oxygen this baby had been given, and it is possible that 100% oxygen may have been given, albeit briefly. It is most likely that the baby will have been kept in an incubator in an atmosphere of 40% oxygen for several weeks. Unfortunately, incubators are not capable of being pressurised, if they were, high levels of oxygen could be used intermittently, as was done in the diminutive hyperbaric chambers used in Glasgow in the 1960s.[20] Those who express any reservations at placing a newborn in a pressure chamber should remember that the infant whose MRS graphs are shown in Figure 11.1 would have been anaesthetised in order to be scanned three times. For the scan the baby would have been placed in the tunnel of the magnetic resonance imager, and each scan would have taken about 45 minutes.

The acceptance that all that is required for distressed infants is to establish that they have normal *blood* oxygen levels is evident in this statement made by a leading UK paediatrician in correspondence with the author in 2003:

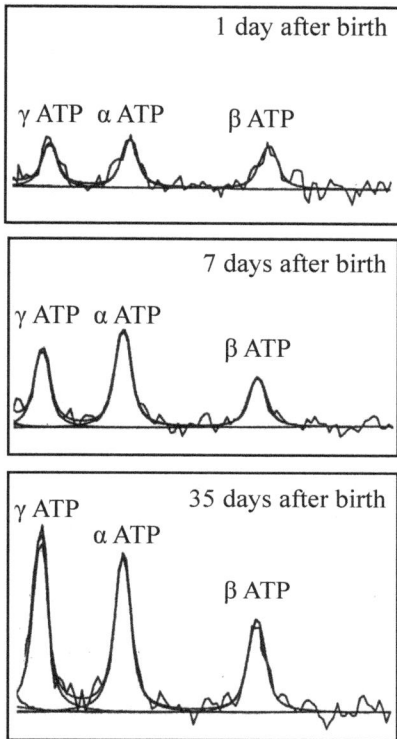

Figure 11.1:
MRS of a newborn, at one day, seven days, and 35 days after birth. The ATP levels at 35 days are still a third of normal values. (Redrawn from Martin E, Buchli R, Ritter S, et al. *Pediatric Res.* 1996;40:749-758.)

Table 11.1: The Apgar Score

	SCORE	SCORE	SCORE
	0	1	2
Appearance	Cyanosed (blue)	Feet and hands blue	Pink
Pulse	Absent	Less than 100	More than 100
Grimace	No response	Grimace or cry	Sneeze or cough
Activity	None	Some	Active
Respiration	Absent	Weak	Strong
The maximum score possible is obviously 10 when each assessment scores 2.			

All infants have their oxygen levels measured regularly from blood gases and continuously from O₂ saturations and levels are maintained within a normal range.

The letter continued with the implied but rarely stated inference that if *blood values are correct*, then it follows that tissue values are likely to be normal. Clearly, as already discussed, in conditions like stroke and heart attacks, areas of tissue in the body can suffer from severe lack of oxygen when blood levels are completely normal.

I don't think, however, during this time there is evidence for a lack of oxygen supply to the tissue. If there was a parlous supply of oxygen then, of course, one would increase it.

The evidence needed can be provided by measurement but, of course, the limit to increasing the supply would be the prevailing barometric pressure. However, it is clear from the letter that this paediatrician does accept that there is a window of opportunity to treat acute problems; it is the reason for research investigating cooling the head or the whole body, when there is lack of oxygen associated with low blood flow.

I do not, however, think that all pathology is fixed. This is the basis for the ongoing trials of very early hypothermia in perinatal asphyxia where it is thought, and there is certainly evidence to support this view, that there is a short window of opportunity for treatment before "secondary energy failure" and permanent damage becomes fairly established by about 6-12 hours.

The objective of cooling the brain is to reduce the demand for oxygen.[21] A major study of cooling babies with brain problems due to lack of oxygen was published in May 2012, and has shown a level of benefit that may justify the associated adverse effects, but whole body, rather than just head cooling, is needed, as it is in adults.[22] Clearly, inducing whole body hypothermia is a complicated procedure and is unlikely to be successful in avoiding brain damage in many infants. In contrast, placing an infant in a chamber and administering more oxygen using a hood, is simple and addresses the *primary issue*, which is lack of oxygen. Figure 11.2 shows a mother supervising the treatment of her baby in one of the charity hyperbaric chambers in the UK.

Real-time evidence from MRS shows that tissue oxygen values in the brain can be severely subnormal when *blood* values are normal. The relationship between the detection of lactate/lactic acid in the brain 18 hours after birth has been shown to correlate with adverse outcomes at one year of age.[23,24]

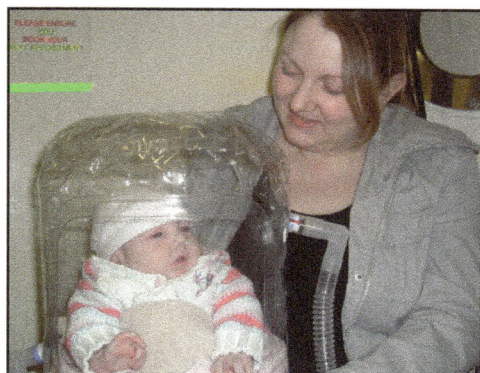

Figure 11.2:
An infant being treated in an oxygen hood in a multi-person chamber. (Courtesy of Mrs. Donna Ellington.)

Another study, published as long ago as 1997, compared the outcome of 36 infants with a variety of neurological problems, who had lactic acid/lactate peaks on MRS, with 63 who did not.[25] The results were entirely predictable: those infants with increased lactate were more likely to die (39% vs. 7%), or to be severely disabled (39% vs. 10%). The children without lactic acid were more likely to have had a good outcome (23% vs. 3%) or recover to a mild, (38% vs. 6%) or moderate level of disability (20% vs. 0%). The conclusions of the authors were that the data *suggests* that patients with elevated cerebral lactic acid/lactate levels are more likely to die acutely or are at greater risk for serious long-term disability, and MRS is useful in predicting long-term outcomes in children with neurological disorders. There was no discussion in the paper of the fact that lactic acid actually indicates lack of oxygen, or that the children would have benefited from being given oxygen as a treatment.

There could not be a clearer indication to use a high level of oxygen than in the treatment of a baby whose brain has been affected by lack of oxygen, but giving oxygen to infants has had bad press. Every medical student is taught that oxygen may cause blindness due to "toxicity." Supplementary oxygen using incubators came into widespread use in the late 1940s because of the association of lack of oxygen with brain damage, and it was seen to improve the survival of premature infants. Oxygen levels up to 80% were used in some cases for more than 100 days. There is no more graphic illustration of the tragic consequences of the failure to understand the use of oxygen in medical practice than the story that unfolds and, as will be seen, this applies to events before, during, and after birth. However, controversy about the level of oxygen used continues and even extends to the use of oxygen in the immediate resuscitation of newborn babies. A proper understanding of the use of oxygen is desperately needed as confusion still reigns; one paediatrician commented in 2002, more than 50 years after the problem surfaced, that the depth of our ignorance is really embarrassing. This is an emotional subject; those who care for desperately ill babies deserve our unstinting admiration, because the stress involved is often at high personal cost. But we need to focus our attention on the issues involved to determine what can and cannot be achieved. Fortunately, at long last, the very latest technologies are yielding answers, and a myth propagated for over 50 years has been shown to be wrong; oxygen does not make babies go blind, *withdrawing* it too quickly does because of lack of oxygen, that is, hypoxia.

It became obvious by the early 1950s that many of the children saved after a premature birth had damaged sight. It takes time to recognise blindness in babies because they obviously cannot tell us what they see. The characteristic sequence of damage in the eyes was soon detailed. The retina became swollen and then detached, eventually forming a mass of fibrous tissue in the centre of the eye. The condition was first called *retrolental fibroplasia*, which is translated as fibrous tissue behind the lens, and the use of oxygen was soon limited to 40%. Retinal detachment became rare, especially in full-term infants, and the name of the condition was then changed to retinopathy of the premature (ROP). However, the limitation imposed on the levels of oxygen used in incubators has not eliminated the problem, and lesser degrees of retinal damage still cause visual impairment.

It is fair to point out that there was great reluctance to blame oxygen in the 1950s; it was only after detailed investigations of many factors that it was accepted that oxygen was involved, although it was not understood how it caused the problem. The reason for the reluctance was because oxygen had been administered in good faith, and for good reason, as premature infants often had problems breathing. However, by the early 1950s it had been confirmed beyond doubt that oxygen was involved. A large co-operative multi-centre trial had been done in the US, and incubator oxygen levels were then limited to a maximum of 40%, and the use of 100% oxygen reserved for emergency resuscitation. Here is the essence of a tragedy; oxygen had been identified as being involved in the epidemic of blindness[26] without the reason being discovered. It was simply assumed that the problem was due to oxygen "toxicity"; in other words, that *molecular oxygen* itself was poisonous. It is ironic that, since the 1950s, the only risk factors that have been clearly identified for this type of blindness are those associated with *lack* of oxygen in the womb. Although the description retinopathy of the premature is now universally used, the disease may actually affect full-term infants and also many infants who have not received *any* supplemental oxygen. Even more confusing is the fact that it may only affect one eye. However, if the causes of retinopathy in adults are examined, it is clear that they are *always* associated with lack of oxygen as, for example, in patients with diabetes. In diabetes, damage to the wall of the blood vessels resulting from the very high blood glucose level causes damage which reduces the transfer of oxygen into the tissues of the eye. This is because the glucose binds to some of the proteins in the blood vessel wall, causing the wall to become thicker, and less oxygen than is needed reaches the retina. The response to a reduction in the level of oxygen is, predictably, an increase in the hypoxia-inducible factor proteins, which upregulates the gene responsible for the growth of new blood vessels.[27] The growth of new blood vessels simply compresses the sensitive light receptors in the retina and this results in blindness.

In the 1950s, one doctor did not accept that the blindness in infants was due to oxygen poisoning, an American paediatrician—Dr. Thomas S. Szewzyck. By 1951, he had conclusively shown that the developing pathology in the retina of a baby could actually be *treated* by returning the infant to a high level of oxygen, and that the key to preventing a recurrence was to slowly *wean* the child to the normal oxygen concentration in air.[28] In other words, taking a baby out of an incubator with an atmosphere of 80% oxygen to breathing just 21% is dangerous, being a severe physiological stress. Given the level of controversy caused by Szewzyck's observations, a controlled trial was needed, and it was published in 1954.[29]

The study followed 24 premature infants who were slowly reduced to a normal concentration and 26 who were abruptly withdrawn from a high oxygen concentration, meaning that they were simply lifted out of the incubator. Only two infants in the group that had been weaned slowly developed the retinal damage, compared to 13 in the second group in which the oxygen was withdrawn abruptly. This really does not need to be analysed statistically, but it is obviously highly significant ($p<0.001$), and even more significant biologically. Unfortunately, the study was dismissed in the US because the infants who were in the weaned group had received a little less oxygen overall. However, it is very clear that by this time clinicians had already decided that the retinal damage and blindness were definitely due to a still undefined mechanism of poisoning due to oxygen.

Further studies were done in the UK with, most importantly, direct monitoring of the infants by actually looking in their eyes; the blood vessels of the retina are the only vessels in the body that can actually be seen. The studies confirmed Szewzyck's contention that the lack of oxygen created by the abrupt reduction is responsible for the damage to the retina. Also in 1954, Dr. R.M. "Sam" Forrester and colleagues in Manchester described the effect of returning infants with developing retinal problems to a high level of oxygen as dramatic.[30] They developed a method to hold the eyelids of the infants open and, using an ophthalmoscope, they watched the early changes—engorgement of blood vessels and tissue swelling, rapidly disappear when the infant was returned to a higher oxygen atmosphere. The author discovered a letter by Dr. Forrester published in 1964, which highlighted the continuing failure to use oxygen properly in paediatrics, when looking for another reference in the journal.[31] In a meeting with the author at his home in Ambleside in 1999, Dr. Forrester confirmed that the improvement was truly *spectacular*, in each individual case the retinal vascular pattern, having shown gross abnormalities, returned to normal. As in the study in the US, weaning the infants off a high level of oxygen, regular examination of the retina using direct observation by ophthalmoscopy was used to control the rate of the reduction to a normal atmospheric oxygen concentration. In a series of 17 very premature infants, 12 recovered with normal eyes and five had minor permanent changes not causing blindness. Dr. Forrester recorded that two infants in the series needed a third period of exposure because the disease again became active. Many of the infants were exposed to high oxygen concentrations for very long periods (the longest were 93, 88, 85, and 83 days). Dr. Forrester tellingly commented;

> ... *if one believes that oxygen has a direct toxic effect on the infant's retina these surely would have been the infants who became blind, for they were all of very low birth weight, all had the early retinopathy and they were all subjected to intensive and prolonged therapy.*

The changes they witnessed were entirely consistent with lack of oxygen, which increases the leakage from blood vessels, even to the extent of allowing red blood cells to escape, because of gross failure of the normal barrier formed by the wall of the blood vessels and the sensitive tissues of the retina. Scientists are now certainly aware that a fall of oxygen levels provokes the blood vessel overgrowth that causes blindness. Drs. Pugh and Ratcliffe,[32] in a review of the role of hypoxia in new blood vessel formation published in 2003, wrote:

> *Pathological new vessel growth, causing blindness from retrolental fibroplasia, can be precipitated by hypoxia arising from a return to normal inspired oxygen concentrations.*

The benefits of giving oxygen in retinal conditions are slowly being recognised by eye specialists. Oxygen has been used in an experimental model of retinal detachment to preserve the retina on the premise that lack of oxygen is involved in the death of photoreceptors.[33] It was found that oxygen supplementation to the level of 70% reduced the death rate of the light sensitive cells in the detached retina and limited the proliferation of the cells responsible for the scarring. The authors suggested that supplemental oxygen should be used to preserve the detached retina in patients awaiting the cryosurgery needed for reattaching the retina.

In 1999, the author submitted a commentary to the *Lancet* about the tragic mistake of attributing the retinopathy of newborn to poisoning by oxygen detailing the evidence and pointing out that infants are still being deprived of sufficient oxygen. After considerable controversy, the paper was refused, although it was finally published in the Proceedings of the 3rd EPNS Congress by the European Paediatric Neurology Society.[34] A comprehensive collection of papers, which discussed the issues raised in the use of hyperbaric oxygenation for brain-injured children, was published in 2002.[35]

Retinopathy is still a very important problem in the premature and it also affects infants born at term. A new ophthalmic industry has been created based on retinal laser surgery. This painful technique is used to burn the new blood vessels that have grown in the retina, but the results are poor, with children often being left with defects in their visual fields. Drugs have also been ineffective. It is desperately important for it to be generally recognised that even the levels of oxygen currently in use should be reduced much more slowly to avoid retinal damage. Regrettably, it seems that most doctors still regard a reduction of the level of oxygen from the 40% normally used, to the 20.9% in air as trivial. As any chemist will confirm, halving the concentration of such a reactive metabolite is highly significant in a biological system.

There are growing concerns that the restriction of oxygen usage with target oxygen saturations is adversely affecting the death and disability rate of newborn infants. The fear is not new; in the 1950s, Dr. Alison McDonald at the Hammersmith Hospital in London had recorded a rise in the incidence of cerebral palsy when the restriction of the oxygen level to 40% came into force in the 1950s.[36] Of 16 children born from 1950 to the end of 1952, when 60–80% oxygen was used, only one developed the brain damage known as cerebral palsy, with four developing retinal problems. In the following three years, when incubator levels were reduced to 40%, 10 of 25 children developed cerebral palsy (p<0.05), and none developed retinopathy (p<0.02). McDonald's comment was that unfortunately, it may prove impossible to prevent spastic diplegia by increasing the ambient oxygen concentration without causing retrolental fibroplasia. She was not correct; it is possible, providing that oxygen levels are reduced slowly. The controversy

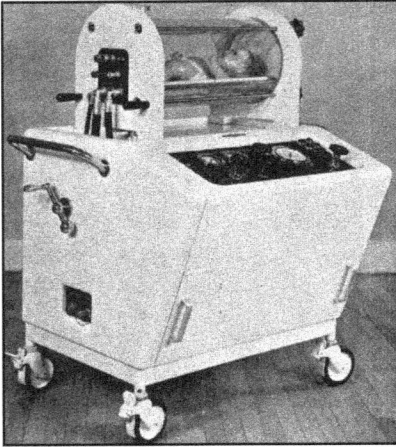

Figure 11.3:
The Vickers experimental chamber for neonates.

surrounding the restriction of oxygen levels based on target oxygen saturations for premature infants continues,[37] again with allegations that it is resulting in an increase in deaths.

Recent research suggests that *continuous* high levels of oxygen, albeit at normal atmospheric pressure, are not optimal, and premature infants may be better managed breathing room air, high levels of oxygen being used for emergencies. The Norwegian paediatrician, Dr. Ola D. Saugstad has campaigned for many years for the use of prolonged courses of oxygen in neonates to be reviewed.[38] In fact, what is needed is a *short exposure* to a high level of oxygen using hyperbaric conditions to correct a lack of oxygen after delivery, because it will resolve brain swelling and inflammation. Work undertaken in the 1960s in Glasgow has shown that higher levels of oxygen can certainly be used safely and without retinal problems. The Vickers Medical Company built a special chamber for a study of resuscitation of the newborn in Glasgow (Figure 11.3) and the preliminary results were published in the *Lancet* in 1963.[39]

The initial pressurisation was to 4 ATA for 10 minutes using an atmosphere of pure oxygen. This level was progressively reduced, giving a total time in the chamber of 15–30 minutes. Professor James H. Hutchinson, the distinguished paediatrician in charge of the study, saw the method as replacing intubation, that is, the placement of a tube in the throat, which often causes difficulties for inexperienced doctors when dealing with a tiny baby. If simply placing an infant in a chamber could achieve as good a result as intubation, then more babies could survive. This proved to be the case but, not surprisingly, the study proved to be very controversial and a critical and emotional letter was published in the *Lancet*,[40] which elicited a careful reply.[41]

Undeterred, Professor Hutchison obtained funding for a controlled study; hyperbaric oxygen treatment was compared to the standard treatment of intubation and ventilation on 100% oxygen. The study found that the mortality for the two groups was the same.[42] However, it is obvious that unskilled junior doctors would not have been allowed to participate in the trial. It is also obvious that it could not have been admitted that infants had been dying in Glasgow because inexperienced staff had not been properly supervised. Sadly, at no time was it ever suggested that infants should have the benefit of intubation, *and* the advantages conferred by treatment with oxygen under hyperbaric conditions. This would, of course, have required a larger chamber and a doctor present inside.

There were many accounts of startling results from using oxygen under hyperbaric conditions in the 1960s and 70s when powerful groups in medicine—cardiac and neurosurgeons—were experimenting with the technology. In Chicago, surgeons were learning to operate on children born with complicated congenital heart conditions, and, distressingly, there were many deaths on the operating table. The use of a pressurised operating theatre with infants given 100% at just twice atmospheric pressure—2 ATA *abolished* the mortality during operations—that is the intra-operative mortality.[43,44] However, the surgeons were clearly less than enthusiastic about operating in a chamber and they were almost dismissive of their astonishingly positive results (see Chapter 21). Many experimental studies have confirmed that energy status and mitochondrial function can be restored by hyperbaric oxygenation in even the two grams of tissue that constitute a rat brain.[45,46] Reference has already been made to the fact that lactic acid/lactate peaks found by magnetic resonance spectroscopy are associated with adverse outcomes in severely ill young children. So, although the risk of a child dying, remaining in a coma, or surviving with severe disabilities has been known for 25 years,[25] giving such infants more oxygen is *never* discussed, and this is simply because the level of oxygen in their blood is normal. Now, imagine explaining all this to the parents of a brain-damaged child.

In the next chapter, the trials of hyperbaric oxygen treatment for children with *established* cerebral palsy are discussed—which have shown improvements, often despite the lapse of years. Strange as it may seem, this has also proved highly controversial. This is because it strikes a raw nerve in medical practitioners who constantly allege that birth injuries are fixed. Indeed, the diagnosis given for a newborn child with brain injury is that they are suffering from a *static encephalopathy*. In other words, the damage has been done, cannot be influenced, and no treatment can help the brain to recover; parents are told that disabilities simply have to be accepted and managed. This self-fulfilling prophecy ensures that nothing will be done. However, the latest experimental evidence shows that, far from being fixed, recovery is possible from brain damage in the newborn—sustained growth of new nerve cells may occur and stem cells mobilised; the injury is *not* fixed.[47] However, treatment must be urgent; brain injury is an emergency.

CHAPTER 12

Cerebral Palsy and Oxygen Treatment:
A Tale of Trials

There need be no apology for tackling only a symptom rather than an aetiology; the misery of these patients cannot wait.

Jose Jorge Machado. Sao Paulo, April 26, 1989.

The term cerebral palsy, first used by the renowned physician and friend of J.S. Haldane, Sir William Osler, refers to disorders of motor function that is, of movement of the limbs and associated postural problems.[1] Cerebral palsy has achieved more attention than other consequences of brain damage, for example, the autistic disorders, because the disability can be easily seen and measured. Damage to areas in the centre of the brain may not only affect movement, it may involve critical structures which are involved with, for example, concentration, memory, emotional processing and even sleep. The number of children born with cerebral palsy has only shown a small reduction over the last 50 years although it is very likely that the numbers would have fallen more if it was not for improvement in the survival of the very premature infants who often have such disability. The emotional and physical burden on carers, and indeed the rest of society, of looking after children with brain damage is enormous and it is obvious that any treatment which can improve the burden should be made available. However, the suggestion that a little more oxygen may help brain-injured children has proved to be controversial. The public may find this difficult to understand but the actions of those who use oxygen treatment is, in effect, a criticism of those who do not and often generates emotional and illogical rebuttals. The facts that have generated the controversy must, therefore, be made available to the public; Dr. Machado's observation is correct; the misery of these patients cannot wait.

The use of hyperbaric oxygen treatment for problems both during pregnancy and after delivery was well established in the Soviet Union in the 1970s and many studies were done. In the 1980s and 90s, hyperbaric centres in Sao Paulo, Brazil and Fuzhou in China reported modest but, nevertheless, worthwhile benefits from hyperbaric oxygen treatment in children with severe cerebral palsy.[2] A study of children with epilepsy undertaken in China reported marked reduction of seizures which often allowed a reduction in their medication.[3] The drug treatment of epilepsy reduces seizure activity by general sedation of brain activity and, not surprisingly, children may underachieve educationally, especially when several drugs are used together.

In the mid-1990s, a UK national newspaper reported the benefits gained from a course of hyperbaric oxygen treatment by a boy of 14 called Doran Scotson, who had suffered brain damage after he developed severe jaundice shortly after birth. The improvement was even noticed by neighbours and his school teachers, as he stopped falling over and started to ride a bicycle. His mother, Linda Scotson founded a charity, the Hyperbaric Oxygen Trust, to enable other children to access the treatment. It is now known as Advance and is based in East Grinstead. A Canadian mother, Claudine Lanoix, who had twin boys with brain injury due to the twin transfusion syndrome during pregnancy was given a copy of a newspaper article from the UK and contacted the trust to investigate matters further.

Michel's and Mathieu's Story, Told by their Mother Claudine Lanoix

Smaller than most dolls, my boys weighed in at 840 and 1,065 grams and were just over 30 and 33 cm long. Due to their unfortunate early entry into this world and a lack of oxygen at the time of their birth they were found to have cerebral palsy and poor vision. This set us on a new path in life, one with many ups and downs, triumphs and great concerns. As a parent I vowed not to leave any stone unturned as I set out on a life quest to help "fix" my babies.

They were just a little over three years old when a friend that I had made on the Internet living in the United States sent me a newspaper clipping from an English newspaper, the *Daily Mail*, titled "Deep Sea Cure for Brain Injured Children." The headline caught my attention and I knew in an instant that I had to follow my gut instinct and look into this new approach called hyperbaric oxygen treatment (HBOT); it just sounded right.

I quickly discovered that the medical facilities in Canada that had hyperbaric chambers were not willing to treat children with brain injury or, in fact, patients with any other neurological injury, except divers. I was feeling defeated when I suddenly remembered that at the bottom of the *Daily Mail* clipping about the "deep sea cure" was the name of an American physician, Dr. Richard Neubauer in Lauderdale-by-the Sea, Florida.

After months of reading hyperbaric articles and research papers that had been sent to me by Julie Gordon of the MUMS parent to parent support network and several conversations with Dr. Neubauer himself, my research was done and the decision made; our family spirits lifted, our hope and faith restored. We decided to pursue hyperbaric oxygen treatment for our twins!

It was at this time that Dr. Neubauer suggested that considering the fact that we were Canadian and our currency was very weak against the US dollar it would be more cost effective if I would take the twins overseas to a charity centre in England rather than to pursue treatment in the US that was more than quadruple the price. He then gave me the phone number of his very good friend who was in Dundee, Scotland. He suggested that I should speak to Linda Scotson, whose son had featured in the *Daily Mail* article. Linda was a great help and put us in contact with a Multiple Sclerosis Charity Centre at Bradbury House in Bedford. In the next few days with the help of Valerie Woods, manager of the center, all the arrangements were made, we would go to England on May 18, 1998 for hyperbaric oxygen treatment along with my American Internet friend Debbie Nardone and her son Todd, who was the same age as my twins and also had spastic quadriplegia; the cerebral palsy had resulted from a birth injury.

Now all we had to do was figure out how to pay for it. We were a family of seven with only one small income to provide for us all, the answer, fundraising of course . . . Debbie and I shared ideas and encouraged each other all the way along and in just a few weeks we both had enough funding to cover the travel and treatment costs. A local Montreal TV news station broadcast our story and by the next day it had received attention coast to coast. Our phone was ringing night and day with parents of children with cerebral palsy wanting more information, what was hyperbaric oxygen treatment, how does it work, what are the results, can it help my child and where can we get it? We also had the attention of Mr. Jeffrey Williams of Perry Baromedical, a chamber manufacturer connected to the hyperbaric research facility at Montreal's, McGill University. He asked us to keep in contact with him and provide him with updates whilst we were in England.

There was so much to do, flights to book, accommodations, car rental, and then to make sure that everything was organised within our household for my husband and three older children, Tiffany who was 16, Justin 12, and Eric, who would turn six while we were away for our month long stay in the UK. Finally, with great excitement and anticipation I boarded the plane Friday evening with Michel and Mathieu and my mother Dorothy, who had taken a leave of absence from her work to help me with the twins while we were in England.

We quickly settled in to our new home away from home and tried to get accustomed to driving on the other side of the road! The hyperbaric sessions would start on Monday morning doing two one-hour sessions each day with a few hours in between each session for physiotherapy and to eat lunch. We were warmly welcomed by Val Woods and her staff at the MS Therapy Centre in Bradbury House and they took time to explain what could and could not go into the chamber and how to clear our ears during the pressurization period of the treatment.

I was as nervous as a mother could possibly be as I stepped into the enormous 10 person hyperbaric chamber for the first time, my imagination vivid with all that could go wrong, I kept having to tell myself that "everything would be OK." My heart pounded as they turned the latch on the door. As the pressure in the chamber was building I was working with the boys to help them clear their ears and forgot about mine until a painful sharp feeling struck on each side of my head. A sip of water was helpful but my ears were still blocked as I turned my attention back to Michel and Mathieu. Grandma was great and kept us all under control. The hour seemed long as we kept the boys occupied by stories and singing all the while trying not to disturb our chamber mates who were all adults with multiple sclerosis who were there for treatment. Our entire experience in England was fantastic, the people kind and helpful the countryside beautiful and our visits to London along with a little sightseeing full of history, beautiful architecture and culture. We loved every moment and returned to England a second time for follow-up later that same year and then were later successful in obtaining HBOT closer to home in Canada and the US.

The changes and progress Michel, Mathieu, and Todd experienced in just one month were incredible. Every day, another small miracle took place. I had to find a way to share this with other families, to spread hope and transform other children's lives.

I was energised and full of hope for our future, once back home I contacted McGill University asking for an interview with the hyperbaric department. I knew that Michel and Mathieu would need more treatments and other families like ours could also benefit from this amazing therapy. The University's Hyperbaric laboratory was dedicated to sports research so I needed to find a way to convince them to consider a new research direction and be able to continue our treatments here at home. With the help of the boy's rehabilitation physician, Dr. Pierre Marois, we were successful with our attempt and within a few months of our return from England a research pilot project was underway. The objective was to determine if hyperbaric oxygen therapy could alter spasticity in children with cerebral palsy.

This pilot study published in the journal *Undersea and Hyperbaric Medicine* was a success and led to a multi-center trial the next year. I was invited by Dr. David Montgomery, the head of the HBO department, to join the research team as a hyperbaric technologist in October 1999 and completed my formal training.

Fast forward to 2011 – Michel and Mathieu are now 17 years old and have been fortunate enough to have received over 800 HBOT sessions in three different countries, in seven different facilities over the past 13 years. In 2004, we opened our own hyperbaric center so that we no longer have to travel for treatments, and I have the pleasure and honour along with my husband, Thomas Fox, of providing HBO treatment to children just like mine. I am proud to say that I experience little miracles every day when a mom or dad says to us "my son took his first step yesterday," "my daughter said 'I love you' for the first time," "my child played, really played with their siblings last night."

Michel who uses a wheel chair for mobility is far more independent than we ever could have imagined. He speaks two languages and there was a time when we could not even get speech therapy because it was said that "he didn't have enough ability to work with." He loves music, cars, watching hockey games on TV, and girls, just like any other teenager.

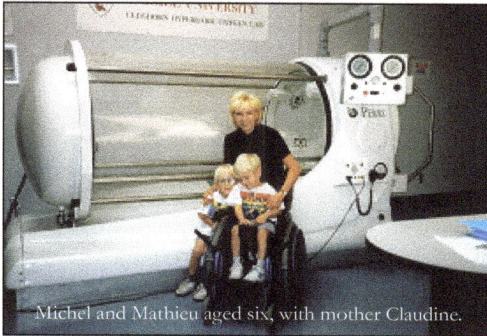

Michel and Mathieu aged six, with mother Claudine.

Mathieu is now integrated into regular high school studies, is a computer genius, and an aspiring photographer. He had the honour of giving a Power-Point presentation he had done himself, called A life Under Pressure, to 200 delegates at the Seventh International Hyperbaric Symposium in California, USA in 2010, and he received a standing ovation. He was just 16 years old. Mathieu wrote this in one of his slides:

> *I know first hand that our lives would not be the way they are today if it was not for HBOT and our family's drive to improve the destiny of our future. I believe that HBOT has helped me and my brother to overcome a physical disability and turn it into ability. This therapy has allowed me to begin a journey towards better health and physical well-being. I was three years old when I was at the beginning stages of learning to walk. This treatment has also helped me improve and accelerate in ways that my family was told were impossible and that I would be severely handicapped and "mentally retarded." Well, I completely defied the odds and I have improved so much due to the fact that I was able to have access to this treatment throughout my childhood and teen years. I've seen constant improvements in my school work and I am driven to the best that I can. I always try to prove anybody wrong who has underestimated me and also show them that anything can be possible. If I think I can do it then I can do it!*

Their mother says that she still sees improvement in both boys with continuing hyperbaric oxygen treatment. The improvements seen illustrate the astonishing powers of repair possessed by the body. However, it is inevitably limited by the degree of damage incurred. The lesson gained for using oxygen as a treatment is obvious; if hyperbaric oxygen treatment is used when the injury occurs it will be very much more successful and avoid much of the anguish suffered over the rest of a patient's life. In the words commonly used by the health care industry, it will be "cost effective."

The group formed to undertake a study in McGill University was led by Dr. Pierre Marois, who had monitored the progress of Michel and Mathieu. Funding was received from three private organisations and foundations for a pilot study of children with cerebral palsy. It should be noted that most of the doctors involved were highly sceptical of the treatment and certainly not convinced that "it" i.e. oxygen, could be of any benefit! The children recruited for the pilot study had a form of cerebral palsy, known as spastic diplegia, in which their legs were affected. The term diplegia is used to indicate that the problem lies in the brain, not the spinal cord; the paralysis of the legs associated with spinal cord damage being termed paraplegia. One leg may, of course, be affected if there is damage to either the brain or the spinal cord and in cerebral palsy a leg and an arm on one side may be paralysed, or all four limbs may be affected. In most children with spastic diplegia the damage is located in an area in the middle of each hemisphere of the brain known as the internal capsules. As discussed in Chapter 1, the blood supply to these areas is rather poor, indeed some of the nutrition depends on transfer from the veins which drain blood from the grey matter of the cerebral cortex. The zones around these veins are free of capillaries and the arteries supplying these areas, known as the lenticulostriatal arteries, do not connect to adjacent arteries to form the loops known as anastomoses, as other arteries do in the brain. This renders the tissues of the internal capsules vulnerable to disturbances of the blood supply and partly explains the frequency of hemiplegic stroke in adult patients.

The first McGill University study[4] was described as observational because it did not have a control group. However, the children recruited had been undergoing regular and intensive standard therapy at rehabilitation centres and so the only change was the inclusion of hyperbaric oxygen treatment. Most of the children showed clear benefits and some were very impressive. Of course, as with the multiple sclerosis patients, the treatment could not be said to cure; sadly it is obvious that for patients with long-established disabilities that the "sights have to be set lower." Unfortunately, despite the success of the pilot study there was no change in the acceptance of the treatment by the Canadian authorities.

Undeterred, the researchers who were convinced by the results of the pilot study, and the campaigning parents, maintained pressure on the government for further trials to be undertaken and eventually funding was made available. The group of investigators was expanded to conduct a much larger study of children albeit with much less well-defined disabilities.[5] The protocol was the same as that devised for the testing of pharmaceuticals in that an attempt was made to include a control group given a placebo. The children in the hyperbaric oxygen treatment group breathed oxygen at 1.75 ATA, whereas the children in the so-called placebo group, also went in a chamber, but breathed compressed air at 1.3 ATA. This level of compressed air actually causes a 50% increase in the concentration of oxygen in blood plasma. It is most important to be aware that all other therapies, *including all drugs and physical therapy*, were stopped six weeks before the study commenced. Both groups had 40 sessions of an hour, Monday to Friday, delivered over just eight weeks.

The doctors involved had been concerned that using air at hyperbaric pressures was an active treatment. For this reason in their original protocol they had suggested that a third group of patients who did not receive any treatment should be studied as controls. Unfortunately, the government appointed a medical statistician to be in charge of the project, who without the consent of the other researchers abolished this control group. The group receiving conventional hyperbaric oxygen treatment were compared to a group pressurised using air to 1.3 ATA.

In fact, this pressure, an increase of a third over normal atmospheric pressure has been widely used in supercharging cars. The graph in Figure 12.1 shows that the power output of an engine that dates from WW2. The maximum engine power of 54 b.h.p. (curve 1 STD) is almost doubled to 97 b.h.p. by the use of a supercharger (curve 2).

The benefit from a much more modest increase in atmospheric pressure, in fact, less than a tenth of an atmosphere, has been clearly demonstrated in a study of adult patients with advanced lung disease at the Dead Sea, in Israel.[6] The patients who were all receiving supplementary oxygen in Jerusalem benefited greatly and were able to walk considerably further. This derives both from the increase in the partial pressure of oxygen but also from the abrupt change of air pressure, which by changing the total gas concentrations in the blood causes another phenomenon, osmosis. Osmosis was recognised by Haldane from the work of James Waterston and is well known from school experiments but, in the case of a change in atmospheric

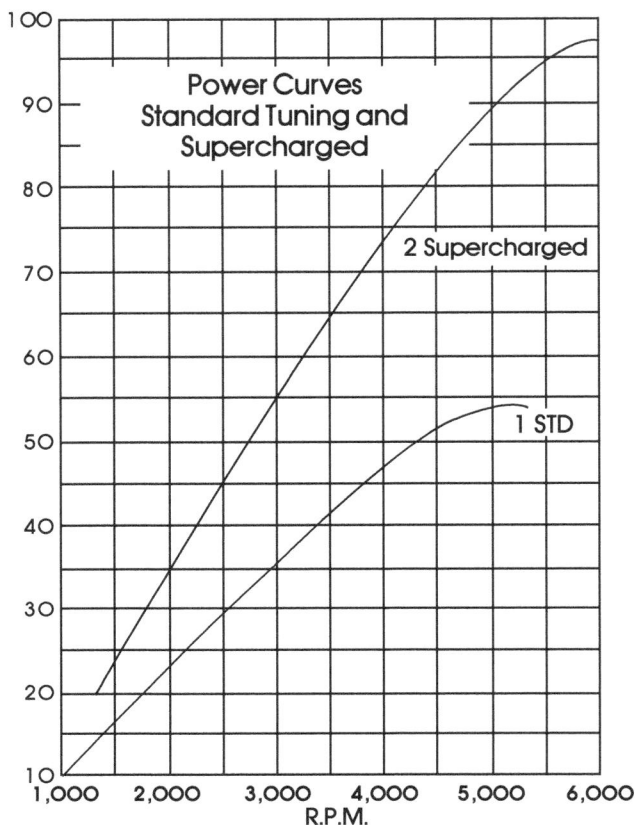

Figure 12.1:
Supercharging power increase over standard engine.

pressure, it is caused by dissolved gases. The late Professor Brian Hills suggested that it may contribute to the benefits found in routine hyperbaric oxygen treatment[7] and this has recently been supported by a theoretical analysis.[8] These phenomena are physical effects defined by the gas laws and can be measured. They accompany a sudden fall in atmospheric pressure due to the weather, as most of us senior citizens will testify from feeling the aches and pains of old age worsen!

So the second Canadian trial[5] simply compared the effects of two regimes, both using an increased dosage of oxygen at an increased ambient pressure. The emphasis was on changes in gross motor function and it is again important to stress that all other treatment the children were having, including anti-spasticity drugs and physical therapy, was stopped in both groups for the duration of the study. They were not resumed until six weeks after its completion. Despite this both groups showed clear and objective improvement from the 20 sessions but, unfortunately, it soon became clear that the Quebec authorities were keen to portray the trial in the worst possible light, fearing the cost implications if the treatment was generally recommended. Government doctors, who actually did not see any of the children, analysed the data statistically; incredibly, the results were withheld from the physicians who had collected it for the study and supervised the treatment of the children. Dr. Jean-Pierre Collet, in writing the report, attempted to refer to the study as a "placebo controlled trial" despite the placebo group being given an active treatment using compressed air. It was emphasised that the results did not support hyperbaric oxygen treatment over compressed air treatment. Nevertheless, it was firmly stated in the publication that the children in both groups showed *striking and significant* clinical improvement.

Many of the researchers and parents involved in the Canadian study reacted angrily when they realised that results were being presented in a negative light, because they had witnessed benefits from the treatment in most of the children. Many had undertaken years of conventional medical therapies with little improvement. In an unprecedented action, one parent wrote on behalf of the group to the editorial staff of the *Lancet* expressing their dismay:

> *We, as parents, were extremely disappointed in Dr. Collet's presentation and have since discovered that Dr. Collet acted under the orders of the government of Quebec, Canada to sabotage the study in order to find or, reportedly, to find that the government did not have to pay for this therapy.*

They also complained about the unique exclusion of the doctors who were actually responsible for the care and examination of the children, not only from the analysis of the data they had collected, but also from giving their personal experience. The first author of the paper, Dr. Collet, a medical statistician employed by the Quebec Department of Health, did not see any of the children. By this time, the physicians who had dealt with the children were convinced that the so-called control arm could not be regarded as a placebo and were fully aware of the tone of the manuscript submitted to the *Lancet*. Three of the main researchers were so upset at what had happened that they sent all the correspondence to the author by courier service and in a telephone conversation, Dr. Marois said he would not be able to look himself in the mirror in the morning unless he took action to correct the misinformation.

On receiving the correspondence from the representative of the mothers, the editor of the *Lancet* contacted Dr. Marois for an explanation. He then referred the matter to one of their senior editors with the necessary physiological knowledge, who agreed that compressed air at 1.3 ATA, was *not* a placebo. The result was that all reference in the manuscript to the use of a placebo, and also to the study being a *controlled* trial, had to be deleted. It was then described as a double-blind, randomised clinical trial and the pressurisation to 1.3 ATA was absurdly termed an exposure to slightly pressurised air. In fairness, the original paper did state that a possible effect of increased pressure could not be ruled out. However, compressed air at 1.3 ATA actually increases the concentration of oxygen in arterial blood from typically 95 mm Hg to about 148 mm Hg, which is an increase of 50%. Again, to increase the concentration of such a reactive substrate by 50% is certainly of major physiological importance, and the graph in Figure 12.1 shows just how dramatic such an increase can be to combustion efficiency.

A brief editorial under the heading "Hyperbaric Oxygen: Hype or Hope?" was included in the *Lancet* issue in which the Canadian study was published.[9] It called the results intriguing, but the use of the word hype illustrates the prejudice that still surrounds the use of increased pressure in treatment. However, the day after the publication of the article in the *Lancet* the Government of Quebec sent out a press release modifying the title and the conclusions of the article, stating that our research had proven, without any doubt, the inefficacy of HBOT in cerebral palsy and that the changes in the children were due to a placebo effect. Dr. Marois was so furious that the next day he invited journalists to a press conference and, with two colleagues, showed them the fraudulent change of the title of the paper and the inexcusable conclusion made by government officials.

The *Lancet* subsequently published three letters commenting on the study and it is essential to give the details here. The first was from the late Dr. Richard Neubauer[10] and it gave an account of the treatment of a young disabled boy who began to walk after a course of treatment. Single photon emission tomography (SPECT) imaging demonstrated dramatic improvement in blood flow through the brain. The second letter, from the author,[11] drew attention to the value of compressed air when used as a treatment for neurological decompression sickness. It recounted the story of a compressed-air worker who "fainted" during the final stage of decompression after completing an eight hour shift at 2.5 ATA in the Dartford tunnel workings in 1960.[12] Although he recovered quickly, paralysis of his legs developed overnight and he was recompressed in a chamber on site. The symptoms were quickly relieved but returned during the subsequent decompression. He spent nine days in the pressure chamber, losing consciousness several times and even developed limb paralysis. Small increases in air pressure reversed the symptoms on each occasion but oxygen was finally administered to resolve his problems. The second case referred to in the letter referred to a case which had been published in the *Lancet*[13] which graphically illustrates the value of a small increase in pressure. A girl aged 16 years trekking in Nepal became unsteady, a condition known as ataxia, during a descent from 11,392 feet altitude, which is 0.36 atmospheres less than sea-level pressure (an absolute pressure of 0.64 atmospheres). She steadily worsened and was placed in a soft hyperbaric chamber known as a Gamow bag, which was pressurised with a simple foot pump. After just 15 minutes of being pressurised to nearly sea level, that is one atmosphere, she recovered completely. The pressure was maintained for two hours and she was then decompressed. However, just one hour later, she worsened becoming semiconscious. She again recovered on compression and was kept in the chamber intermittently for four days. The third letter[14] from Drs. Gunnar Heuser and J. Michael Uszler, both respected physicians from UCLA, gave details of the treatment of an autistic child treated at the same air pressure used in the compressed air arm of the Canadian study. The improvement was demonstrated by high resolution SPECT images.

Despite the statement made in the *Lancet* paper describing the Canadian multi-centre study as finding no difference between the group treated at 1.75 ATA with oxygen and the group treated with compressed air at 1.3 ATA, the children in the two groups did differ: The children in the group given hyperbaric oxygen treatment were actually more disabled but, despite this, they improved faster than the children given hyperbaric air (personal communication, Dr. Pierre Marois). Overall the rate of improvement in both groups was *ten times* the improvement documented from other interventions, such as intensive physical therapy. Again it must be stressed that all such supportive therapies were *withdrawn* from the children for the whole period of the study. But some dramatic effects had also been seen in the children that were not mentioned. This may be less difficult to understand when it is recognised that the first author of the paper had not actually been involved in the treatment of any of the children. In 2003, Dr. Marois,[15] responding to an attack on the use of hyperbaric treatment for children from an English paediatrician in the journal *Developmental Medicine and Child Neurology*,[16] stated that "at an age when we did not expect to see any dramatic changes, some children started to walk, to speak, or to sit for the first time in their lives." He dealt in detail with allegations that the benefits found were due to a participation effect and commented that "The Government of Quebec, who funded the research, and some scientists chose to believe solely in this possible cause." The scientists he refers to includes those who had actually written the paper, but not the clinical doctors who had dealt with the children. Dr. Marois pointed out the subsequent positive studies undertaken by the US Army[17] and Cornell University,[18] which were carried out at the insistence of parents and they should ultimately be able to decide on their children's treatment.[19]

The controversy over the McGill University study was continued in 2005 by the publication of a paper entitled "The Neuropsychological Effects of Hyperbaric Oxygen Therapy in Cerebral Palsy," which listed Dr. Marois as a co-author *without* his permission.[20] Despite the independent ruling of the physiologist consulted by the editor of the *Lancet*, which led to the insistence that all reference to placebo be removed from the paper by Collett et al., this new publication of the *same data* again alleged that air at 1.3 ATA was a placebo, providing a "sham" treatment arm needed to support the claim that the study was actually a controlled trial. Again, the benefit, which were found in both groups, was downplayed as a participation effect. However, in 2007, Dr. Marois co-authored a paper in the *American Journal of Physicians and Surgeons*[21] pointing out that the study demonstrates that results from hyperbaric treatment in children with cerebral palsy are better than any currently accepted therapies, for example, surgery to the spinal cord which, of course, cannot be tested under controlled conditions and involves considerable risk. The paper details the political interference with the presentation of the data in the *Lancet*:

> *The funding organisation, the Fonds de Recherche en Santé du Quebec, (FRSQ) a government agency, has persistently misrepresented the results as negative. An official communiqué published by the FRSQ in 2001 even changed the title of the paper from "Hyperbaric Oxygen for Children with Cerebral Palsy: A Randomised Multi-Centre Trial" to "No Advantage of High Pressure Oxygen for Treating Children with Cerebral Palsy." The conclusion of the study was also changed as it was stated that "hyperbaric oxygen therapy produces no therapeutic effect in children with cerebral palsy."*

The adoption of this absurd position by the FRSQ comes as no surprise to those in the field of oxygen treatment and represents a continuing betrayal of the trust the public places in the profession. There has, nevertheless, been a curious development; a law was enacted in March 2005 by the Canadian government, which authorised the Department of Revenue of Quebec to grant tax credits to families in the province using hyperbaric treatment for their children suffering from cerebral palsy.

As discussed, the children in the group pressurised in compressed air to 1.3 ATA in the Quebec study received an increase in both the oxygen concentration and the total gas concentration, that is, the total gas pressure that they were breathing. The US Agency for Healthcare Research and Quality (AHRQ) reviewing the Canadian study[22] has admitted that the use of compressed air might have had a beneficial effect stating:

> *The results of the only truly randomised trial were difficult to interpret because of the use of pressurised room air in the control group. As both groups improved, the benefit of pressurised air and of HBOT at 1.3 to 1.5 ATA should both be examined in future studies . . . The authors of the trial thought that the children in both groups improved because participation in the study provided an opportunity for more stimulating interaction with their parents . . . This is speculative, however, because there was no evidence to suggest that the parents and their children had less time together, or less stimulating interaction, before the study began . . . The possibility that pressurised room air had a beneficial effect on motor function should be considered the leading explanation.*

In fact, the same increase in oxygen concentration can be obtained at normal atmospheric pressures by using the masks routinely used in hospitals with a flow rate of about 5 litres a minute. The authors of the paper recognised this but stated without explanation or, in reality, any justification that it must be assessed before it can be recommended. Despite the positive results recorded by the Quebec study and its publication in the *Lancet*, one of the most prestigious medical journals of the world, no trials have been undertaken in which children with cerebral palsy have been given 28% oxygen to breathe for an hour a day. The cost of such a study would be negligible. The author is aware, however, of studies being undertaken of brain-injured children using 100% oxygen supplied by hood and the results are proving positive (personal communication, Michael W. Allen).

A new study of 150 children with follow-up over eight months has been undertaken by a team led by Dr. Arun Muhkerjee in collaboration with a group in Quebec led by Dr. Pierre Marois.[23] It compared a control group given only intensive physiotherapy, to three groups of children treated under hyperbaric conditions. One group breathed compressed air at 1.3 ATA, one group breathed oxygen at 1.5 ATA, and one at 1.75 ATA. The sessions were of one hour and for six days a week to a total of 40 sessions and the results are shown in Figure 12.2.

The paper was submitted as an answer to the controversy created by the original article in 2001 but the *Lancet* has refused publication.

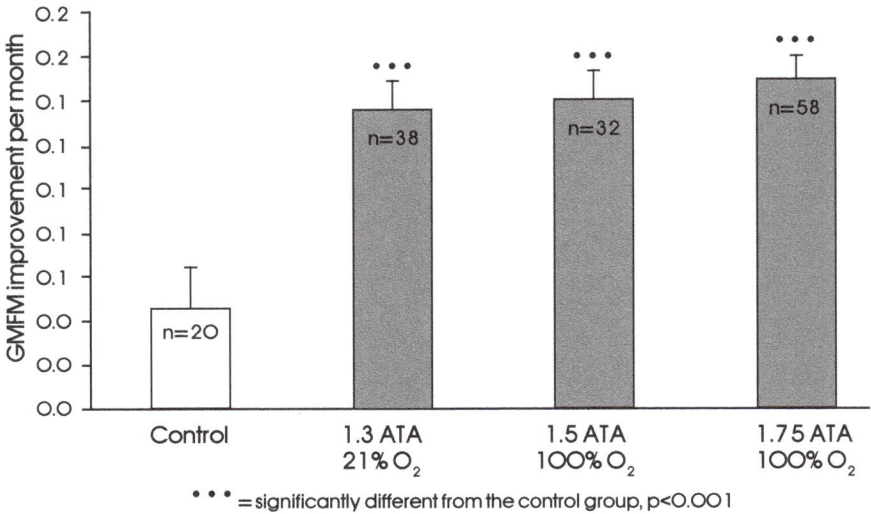

Figure 12.2:
Improvement in gross motor function measure per month of children with cerebral palsy in the UDAAN study. (From Mukherjee A. et al., 2014, New Delhi, India.)

This simple treatment using compressed air at a pressure up to 1.5 ATA could be undertaken in a commercial jet aircraft on the ground, treating 600 people at a time! Figure 12.3 shows the interior of a Boeing 747-200 retired from service with Lufthansa. The pressure bulkhead can be seen at the rear of the aircraft in the second picture.

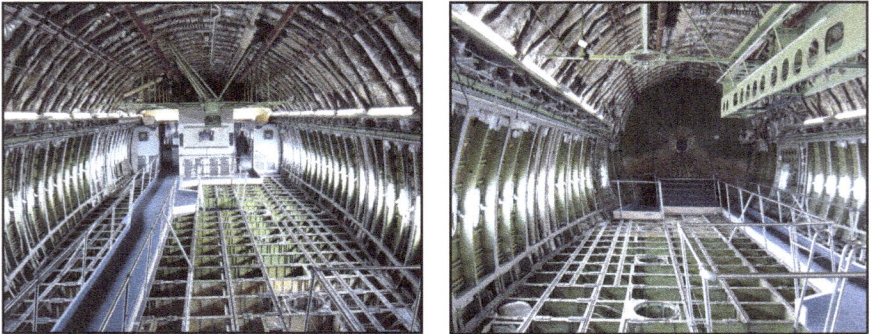

Figure 12.3:
Pressure hull of a Boeing 747-200. (Courtesy of Dr. B. Sostawa.)

Soft chambers have been available for sale in the US for some years, ironically limited by Food and Drug Administration policy to 1.3 ATA. They are usually supplied with an oxygen concentrator to increase the internal oxygen concentration to about 24%. The benefit of a modest increase in pressure has

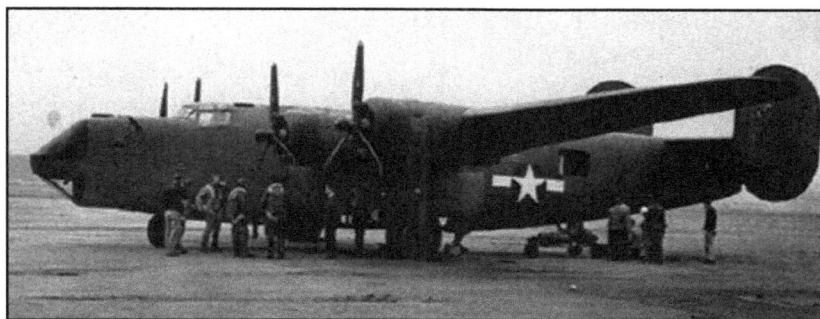

Figure 12.4:
The B24 Liberator used for high altitude research.

been well established by the use of a rapid descent in the treatment of altitude sickness in mountaineers. An expedition by Edinburgh University medical students investigated the effects of living at low atmospheric pressure on Mount Chacaltaya in Bolivia. The recovery of the producer of the BBC's *Horizon* television programme "Mountain Madness" on Mount Chacaltaya, detailed in Chapter 3, illustrates what climbers have known since British alpinists started the sport of mountaineering in the 1800s; a very small descent can produce dramatic benefit. The increase in pressure can be produced by a simple fabric pressure chamber and this soft chamber approach has been used in the treatment of divers for many years; the design is known as the Hyperlite. During WW2, a soft chamber was used in a B24 Liberator bomber by the US Air Force to study decompression sickness (Figure 12.4). It was stripped of its armour and armament to conduct high altitude flights. The subjects undertook exercise at altitude to study the recently recognised problem of altitude decompression sickness in the presence of a flight medical officer. A portable pressure bag was equipped with a mask and oxygen supply to treat subjects who developed symptoms at altitude immediately, to avoid the need for the aircraft to make a rapid descent.

The bag was capable of being pressurised to 3 psi, above ambient pressure in the aircraft (152 mm Hg), which is only a fifth of an atmosphere. When an aircraft is at an altitude of 35,000 feet, this increase in pressure is equivalent to a descent to about 25,000 feet, and it was found that this was usually sufficient to treat a crew member with decompression sickness. The chamber was placed on the floor of the aircraft and the casualty was loaded into the bag and zipped in. The pressure was increased using a foot pump with the casualty breathing oxygen by mask. A paper in the *Journal of Aviation Medicine*[24] in 1945 gives details of its successful use in the B24, but, however, it was not used when one subject developed severe shock:

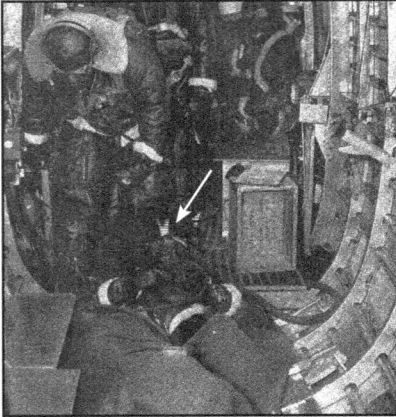

Figure 12.4:
An aviator (face arrowed) entering the pressure bag on the floor of the aircraft. (Courtesy of the Aerospace Medical Association.)

G.D.K., aged twenty-one, was classified as susceptible. He developed occasional shooting pains from the left hip down the anterior thigh to the left knee (at 35,000 feet altitude) but with no localization at the knee. After the eighth exercise he had a sudden sensation of nausea and slight dizziness. He started coughing when the next exercise was started. However, at no time did he have chest pain. Because of his extreme pallor and lack of response to questions and commands, the plane was sent into a fast dive. During the first five minutes of this dive, his respiration rate was 60 to 90 per minute. The cough did not improve during this time and he could not swallow. Later he had no recollection of the very rough air or any other events taking place during the dive. When his mask was removed at 12,000 feet, his color was ashen and his face was covered with perspiration. He was semi-comatose, for about 10 minutes. After regaining full consciousness around 10,000 feet, he was aware of extreme cold, and this was associated with perspiration. The cough continued for one-half hour after reaching the ground. He was taken to the hospital and given hot coffee and wrapped in hot blankets and hot water bottles and he fully recovered. The only residual symptom or sign was a very severe headache which started about three hours after the plane landed and lasted for eight more hours until he went to sleep. In summary, G.D.K. had severe chokes manifested by constant cough and accompanied by vasomotor collapse and moderate shock. The plane was sent into a dive at the rate of 5,000 feet per minute. The safe rate of descent for heavy planes is 1,500 feet per minute. Although an altitude pressure bag was available, the observers decided against its use because the subject might have drifted into a more profound shock.

The rapid descent of the Liberator was, astonishingly, at three times the safe limit and so risked the loss of the aircraft and the death of all on board.

It was feared that if the subject was placed in the bag he could have drifted into a more profound shock, but the increase in pressure from the descent of the aircraft was *precisely the same* as would have been achieved by using the hyperbaric bag. This decision would have been taken by the doctor on board and graphically illustrates the extraordinary reluctance to use hyperbaric treatment which is still so common today.

The principle of the USAF bag was developed by Professor Igor Gamow to allow climbers suffering from mountain sickness at very high altitudes to be treated on the mountain when a rapid descent is not possible. A simple foot pump is used to increase the bag pressure by a modest 2 psi (105 mm Hg) which at an altitude of 14,000 feet is equivalent to a descent of about 7,000 feet down a mountain. The effects can be dramatic; Chapter 3 discussed a climber on the North Col of Everest who had developed the acute lung swelling known as pulmonary oedema, in which plasma leaks out of the blood flowing through the lungs into the air spaces,[25] and whose life was saved by repeated use of a mountain bag. Imagine the reaction of doctors in a hospital intensive care unit to the suggestion that a patient in such a condition would benefit from pressurisation in a mountain bag! So compressed air is certainly a treatment, as any climber surviving altitude sickness from the use of a pressure bag can testify! Unfortunately, many physicians, even those involved in hyperbaric medicine, still claim that the use of compressed air at 1.3 ATA is an inactive placebo despite, as we have seen, in Chapter 1 compressed air having had a long history as a medical treatment in the US, in Europe, and especially in Germany. The increase of blood oxygen values above those typically found at sea level (Air 1 ATA) for the two regimes in the Canadian study are given in Table 12.1.

Table 12.1: Arterial Gas Tensions at Sea Level, Compressed Air at 1.3 ATA, and Breathing Oxygen at 1.75 ATA			
Gas breathed	Air 1 ATA	Air 1.3 ATA	Oxygen 1.75 ATA
Absolute Pressure (mm Hg)	760	988	1330
PO_2	159	207	1330
Sat. Vapour Press.	49	49	49
Max. Alveolar PO_2	110	158	1281
$PaCO_2$	40	40	40
$PvCO_2$	30	30	30
Maximum PO_2 (mm Hg)	100	148	1271

Today we are facing an epidemic of the disease labelled autism and many controversial theories have been postulated to account for the syndrome. There is no diagnostic test and the range of problems to which this label has been applied is very large. Many parents of such children when asked will confirm that they were aware of subtle problems at birth, such as floppiness or difficulties feeding, and many children labelled autistic have obvious neurological problems, that is, objective signs of brain damage. However, they fall short of the requirements for a diagnosis of cerebral palsy which, by *definition*, must involve a disorder of movement. Mid-brain damage may lead to subtle personality disorders and very bizarre presentations, but there are no simple bedside tests that can be used in their evaluation. Because children are still growing, the complex social interactions that form personality have not taken place and they obviously cannot understand or communicate their problems.

Studies have shown that there is reduced blood flow in areas of the brain in autistic children when compared to normal children,[26] and the vulnerability of the mid-brain has already been discussed. The blood supply of these areas depends on the draining veins where white cells cross from blood into the brain. The walls of these veins, although possessing a blood-brain barrier, are more permeable than other blood vessels in the nervous system. It seems likely that a minor birth event, not severe enough to give rise to obvious "objective" symptoms, such as weakness, may still leave the immature brain vulnerable and this may lead to cognitive defects.[27] The blood-brain barrier may remain more leaky than usual during the child's growth to adulthood. Many of the molecules present in blood, such as proteins, are toxic to the brain and it is also possible that some of the allergic responses seen in children labelled autistic, for example to some foods, result from a failure of the protection of a normal blood-brain barrier. If, in the presence of a damaged blood-brain barrier, children are challenged, for example, by vaccination, critical mid-brain structures may not be protected and chronic brain inflammation may follow. A study has demonstrated an active neuro-inflammatory process in the brains of autistic children, notably in the cerebral cortex, white matter, and cerebellum.[28] Given our knowledge of the role of oxygen in the control of inflammation, there could not be a more convincing argument for the treatment of children with hyperbaric oxygenation.

The possibility that acute brain inflammation, that is encephalitis, may follow vaccination is always acknowledged in the data sheets provided by the vaccine manufacturers. Parents in Warrington, Cheshire, were awarded £91,500 after an 18 year fight for compensation for their son, who developed brain injury after receiving the Measles Mumps and Rubella (MMR) vaccine (the *Sunday Times,* August 29, 2010). He was a healthy 13 month old who had begun walking and saying "Mummy" and also "Daddy here," but he suffered a fit 10 days after vaccination and further seizures followed. The suggestion by the parents that this was a reaction to the vaccine was initially dismissed, although this pattern of losing acquired skills, referred to as regression, is typical of such reports. His mother, who has two other children, found medical articles on the Internet detailing the side effects of the vaccine and involved a solicitor in her fight. She also began a support group for parents called Jabs (Justice, Awareness, and Basic Support). The UK government recognises that vaccines may cause brain damage and actually runs a *vaccine damage compensation scheme.* However, when contacted by a reporter from the *Sunday Times,* an official at the Department of Health was apparently unable to give details of any other children who had developed a vaccine reaction and it was simply stated that the MMR vaccine is safe. Clearly by safe they mean it is safe for *most* children, but clearly not *all.* As always, it is likely that there are subacute versions of a condition like encephalitis, in this case, vaccine-induced pathology, which may lead to unusual presentations. Since children have yet to develop formed personalities, it is hardly surprising that bizarre symptoms like those typical of autism occur when the brain is damaged.

Vaccination is important in disease control and has had a massive impact in some infectious diseases; smallpox has been eradicated and polio may soon be conquered. However, it has been at a cost; some children have died and others have been brain damaged by vaccines. Vaccines are given for two reasons; to improve the immunity of the child, but also for "herd" immunity, so that there is less chance of the transmission of an infectious disease in a population. It is obvious that parents trust physicians to do no harm; if there is an adverse reaction, doctors are likely to be defensive and continue to assert that the vaccine is safe. One of the key factors in establishing a link between vaccination and a subsequent illness is, obviously, the timing of events. It is common for both adults and children to get a slight reaction to a vaccine within 48 hours, and if an encephalitis does develop, it is usually within days. However, there *is* a neurological condition, the Guillane-Barre syndrome, which affects nerves in the limbs, that is known to follow swine influenza vaccination. Astonishingly, the reaction may follow a delay as long as 70 days.[29] The encephalopathy that may follow rubella vaccination may appear after a delay of 99 days.[30] Given such long intervals, it is easy to use statistics to discount a connection, which prompted this powerful statement from the late Dr. Charles M. Poser.

The dependence upon epidemiological statistics to establish causal relationships appears to be a new dimension in our clinico-pathological tradition. It sweeps aside the experience of clinicians and neuropathologists, it denigrates the work of the experimentalists, and it substitutes calculations of probabilities for the recognition that variability in the manifestations of disease reflects the diversity of humanity's genetic attributes.

It is clear that it is not possible to know the status of the blood-brain barrier in any individual prior to vaccination and, unfortunately, adverse effects will continue to occur. Society, therefore, has a responsibility to recognise and to treat vaccine reactions to prevent long-term disability. Oxygen is the only agent that can relieve hypoxia, reconstitute the blood-brain barrier and control inflammation. Hyperbaric oxygen treatment should be made available to treat vaccine encephalitis and lesser reactions. It is notable that a double blind multi-centre study of children with autism has now been published and it shows clear benefit which was identified both by doctors and parents.[31]

What can be learned from all of the studies that have shown that long-term brain damage can be ameliorated by hyperbaric oxygen treatment? It is simply that we are failing, failing to use sufficient oxygen to prevent the long-term consequences of injury. The proper place of oxygen treatment is in dealing with emergencies and, no doubt many readers will be astonished that this has not been grasped by those they must entrust with their care.

CHAPTER 13

An Anecdote: A Policeman's Story in the High Courts

In the last analysis, we see only see what we are ready to see, what we have been taught to see. We eliminate and ignore everything that is not a part of our prejudices.

Jean-Martin Charcot, 1825–1893

In 1990, Nicholas M. Dingley, a police constable in Strathclyde Police, developed symptoms typical of multiple sclerosis within days of being involved in a vehicle accident in the course of his work. It was not until 18 months later that he was told he had the disease, and Mr. Dingley felt that it had been caused by the injuries he had received. After taking legal advice, he claimed compensation from the Strathclyde Police Force. The story makes fascinating, but disturbing reading. No apologies are made for the copious detail; it is too important a subject to be economical with the facts. This extract from the court proceedings tells the story:

On the 11th of April 1990, Mr. Dingley was in the back of a police van with other officers when the driver lost control. The vehicle left the road, overturned and landed on its roof. Seat belts were not fitted in the rear of the vehicle and the officers in the back were thrown about violently. Mr. Dingley felt a "crick" in his neck and emerged dazed and bruised. He had sustained a blow to his head with a scalp abrasion and a whiplash injury. He was taken to hospital, but soon discharged as his injuries were regarded at the time as minor. It appears that within a few days, his wife and a colleague (P.C. McCreight) noticed that he had developed problems with his eyesight. Then, 17 days after the accident, after walking for a couple of miles, he started dragging his leg. His symptoms worsened intermittently over the subsequent months and he was eventually told, eighteen months after the accident that he was suffering from multiple sclerosis.

The case was heard in the Court of Session in Edinburgh in 1996 in front of Lord Dawson, who was clearly impressed by the appearance of the symptoms so soon after the accident. He ignored the opinion of several of the expert witnesses, who claimed that trauma could not cause multiple sclerosis, preferring his own common sense assessment. After reviewing the evidence, Lord Dawson agreed with Mr. Dingley's assertion that his illness was caused by the accident, and awarded him the substantial figure of £547,245. The Chief Constable of Strathclyde appealed against the judgment in a reclaiming motion two years later, again held in the Court of Session. Three judges heard the appeal, Lord Rodger as the Lord President, Lord Prosser, and Lord Caplan. Lord Rodger was moved by Mr. Dingley's plight in finding himself face-to-face with the onset of a disease that had transformed his life, stating:

> *This is an anxious case. Anyone who reads the evidence cannot fail to be struck by the frank and straightforward way in which the pursuer has conducted himself in the face of the onset of a disease which has transformed his life. Nor can one avoid feeling great sympathy for him.*

Lord Prosser made some rather pointed observations about Lord Dawson's judgment; the case he made rested on a connection made between the whiplash injury suffered by Mr. Dingley and the damage identified as typical of multiple sclerosis in the brain on MRI. The situation was complicated by the fact that some symptoms suggested that the spinal cord was also involved. Lord Prosser's observation, that it was necessary to establish if the whiplash injury to the neck could have caused damage to the spinal cord, was unfortunately overlooked.

It is sometimes difficult to be certain that the spinal cord is damaged on clinical examination, and in Mr. Dingley's case it appears that only the brain was scanned. Imaging of the spinal cord is time-consuming and technically difficult, so it is rarely done. It appears that the presence of damage to the spinal cord had not been established clinically and, to confuse matters further, one of the expert witnesses supporting Mr. Dingley's case, Dr. Charles Poser, pointed out that it was possible the damage to the brain found on MRI could mimic damage to the spinal cord. As he was keen to link the onset of Mr. Dingley's symptoms to his whiplash injury, the failure to ask for an MRI examination of the spinal cord is difficult to explain. The expert witnesses called by the defendant, the Chief Constable of Strathclyde Police, also do not appear to have reached a conclusion about whether the spinal cord was affected. Even more surprising was their failure to discuss the first symptom that Mr. Dingley had developed within days of his accident—he had a problem with his eyesight. This is most important, as problems with eyesight are the first symptom in about a third of patients who are eventually told they have multiple sclerosis.

In summing up the evidence in the reclaiming motion, the Lord President said that it was not possible to determine from Lord Dawson's analysis why, in view of the opposing arguments of the experts, he had arrived at his conclusions. The controversies aired in this case raise some uncomfortable questions about the quality of the proceedings.

There can be little doubt that this case is likely to have cost the UK tax-payer several million pounds, but a key paper was not produced, or even cited correctly. This paper, which was actually referred to as a mainstay of the pursuer's case, was not the paper discussed in the reclaiming motion. Both are by Gonsette et al., but the first paper referenced[1] relates to experiments in which detergents were injected into the carotid artery in an animal. The second paper,[2] which was the one actually discussed, relates to new areas closely resembling those of multiple sclerosis formed along needles inserted during neurosurgery in patients with an established diagnosis of multiple sclerosis. This was a serious error. The detailed summary of the proceedings of Mr. Dingley's case, by the Lord President, is reproduced in the blocked section.

> So far as the pursuer is concerned, it quickly became obvious that one of the mainstays of his case was an article by R. Gonsette, G. Andre-Balisaux and P. Demote entitled "La permeabilite des vaisseaux cerebraux. VI Demyelinisation experimentale provoquee par des substances agissant sur la barriere hemato-encephalique," published in *Acta Neurologica Belgica* volume 66 (1966), 247–262. It also quickly became clear that the precise findings of the paper were a matter of controversy between the pursuer's experts and defender's experts. Despite its importance, the paper was not among the pursuer's productions and, even though the proof required to be adjourned over a period of months, no attempt was made at any stage (by either party) to lodge the paper. Its precise terms were therefore never satisfactorily adduced.
>
> I must deal briefly with the Lord Ordinary's (Lord Dawson) finding that "not long after the accident, perhaps a week or two, the pursuer began to experience problems with his eyesight." This was the only part of his findings on the development of the pursuer symptoms which gave rise to controversy. It was suggested that the Lord Ordinary was wrong to say that this had happened perhaps a week or two after the accident, which would place it shortly before or around the time of the leg dragging episode. We were referred to the passages in the evidence of the pursuer, his wife and his colleague, P.C. McCreight. The evidence about timing is not particularly clear, but my impression is that, while conceding that he could be wrong, Constable McCreight was much inclined to put the first mention of this matter into a period within about two weeks of the accident that being so, and not having had the advantage of seeing or hearing the witnesses, I should not be inclined to differ from the Lord Ordinary's findings on this point.

On the other hand I do not attach any importance to it. It is plain that, at the time when this evidence was being led, counsel for the defender was concerned to suggest that the pursuer's eye trouble had occurred much later, perhaps months after the accident. His cross-examination was framed accordingly. At some later point in the proceedings, however, counsel for the defender became aware that there was another possible line of approach, viz that the eye trouble had occurred shortly after the accident and was indeed due to MS, but that the base showed that the first symptom of the pursuers was not associated with the spinal cord and could not therefore be associated with any damage to the cord in the accident. The late change of front meant, however, that the exact nature of the pursuer's eye trouble was not established. So the defender's own expert Professor Compston, who did not consider that the point was critical, was quite unable to say whether the problem from which the pursuer was suffering was actually a symptom of MS. (5/644-646;656; 10/1357 and 1364.) In any event, again presumably because the point was viewed differently at the relevant time, defender's counsel did not seek to clarify with the witnesses whether the evidence of any optical symptom of MS at around the time of the leg-dragging symptom would have affected their views about the way in which the pursuer's illness had developed. For these reasons I consider that the trouble with the pursuer's eyes should simply be ignored in the discussion of the pursuer's case.

The failure to discuss the eyesight problems experienced by Mr. Dingley was a matter of critical importance and the sequence of events is disturbing. The counsel for the defendant first attempted to say that Mr. Dingley had developed the eye problems *much later* than the leg symptoms. He then realised that an opportunity had been missed to make a positive point against Mr. Dingley, because, he thought, such eye symptoms could not have been caused by the whiplash injury. As it turned out, it was simply too late to change matters. The judges would not have been aware that disturbances of vision are so common in multiple sclerosis, and so the matter was quietly dropped which, to say the least, was reprehensible. But why is it so important? It is because the *key* question in multiple sclerosis; is it a tissue or a blood vessel disease, has been answered by looking in the eyes of patients, and this is discussed in Chapter 15.

There are two curious aspects raised by the former policeman's case. First, the acceptance by the two experts supporting his claim that the whiplash injury was the cause of *all* his symptoms, when it had not even been established if the spinal cord was damaged. The second relates to the usual diagnostic requirement imposed for a minimum of a month to elapse between attacks. As Mr. Dingley had visual problems within a few days of the accident and then leg weakness only 15 days, and not a month later, a diagnosis of multiple sclerosis was not possible *by definition*, until he developed other symptoms. The problem of the so-called diagnostic criteria for the disease needs further discussion and is far from academic—it is critical to the timing of an effective treatment.

The first committee to set out the criteria for the diagnosis of multiple sclerosis was convened in 1974 by Dr. George Schumacher,[3] and it was a stipulation that "dissemination both in time and in space" was a requirement. The two areas affected, however, must not be too close. For example, two areas affected in the *same* optic nerve would certainly not qualify under current criteria. In a debate in the *Annals of Neurology*,[4,5] one neurologist stated that he would not allow two affected areas, one in each optic nerve, to qualify, because they would not be discrete enough to be multiple. The decision that there must be a minimum interval between attacks—dissemination in time—is not based on science, it is entirely arbitrary. It is also unique; multiple sclerosis is the only disease requiring a minimum of two episodes separated by a minimum time for a diagnosis. The terms "multiple" and "sclerosis" simply translate as *many* and *scars*. A description is masquerading as a diagnosis; *the emperor has no clothes!* But, if more than one area is affected and the time interval between attacks is a few hours or at most days, the disease is given a different label; it is termed an acute disseminated encephalomyelitis or, in plain language, sudden-onset, scattered brain inflammation. It is a reminder that multiple sclerosis was once known as *disseminated* sclerosis, implying that it is spread by the bloodstream. So what if the two attacks are more than a few days and less than 28 days apart? There is no sensible answer to this question and an analogy is needed to put matters in perspective.

Imagine that we invent a new disease associated with scarring in heart muscle. Using the same logic used to describe multiple sclerosis in the brain, we can call it multiple *myocardial* sclerosis, or MMS for short; myocardial referring to heart muscle. We can also decree that a patient cannot qualify for the diagnosis of MMS unless they have a minimum of *two attacks* separated by *at least a month*. Sclerosis (scarring) of heart muscle is caused by a heart attack, but it is painfully obvious that many patients will never qualify for MMS because their first heart attack is fatal, and so leaves no prospect of a second episode. To debate this in front of sharp legal minds would have soon revealed the absurdity of alleging that the label multiple sclerosis can be a diagnosis. But we all accept words without examining them, especially when they are in common use. Unfortunately, medicine is riddled with archaic nomenclature and syndromes that often serve to obscure matters.

The terms multiple and sclerosis are simply a description of more than one area of damage in the nervous system. The requirement for "dissemination in time" is frequently used to delay telling patients they have the disease and this delay, as it was in Mr. Dingley's case, is often measured in years. Over this time, many patients fear that they have a brain tumour, or that they are actually losing their minds. Dr. James Le Fanu, a general practitioner who writes for the *Daily Telegraph*, shared a personal vignette with readers of his weekly column, Doctor's Diary (August 10, 2009, page 20). Ten years before, he had stepped into a bath and noticed the temperature in his left leg seemed substantially cooler than the right. He was immediately concerned that he had a brain tumour. Fortunately, after an MRI had been organised by a friendly neurologist, a tumour was excluded. Dr. Le Fanu was informed that something he presumed was a passing virus, must have damaged the temperature discriminating nerves to the leg. He was told that it would either get better, or not; he would just have to wait and see. So far, it has not changed.

Such stories are actually very common. In 1988, a neurologist at Cornell University conducted an anonymous survey of colleagues, asking if they had experienced transient neurological symptoms.[6] Of the 80 of 87 departmental members who responded to the questionnaire, 25 admitted to having such episodes over a five-year period. Fifteen of those were related to a disturbance of vision, but some experienced weakness, loss of balance or coordination, and some even had multiple episodes. The median age at the time of the first episode was 31. No residual neurological deficits were recorded, but MRI studies were not undertaken. Transient symptoms also occur in patients with established multiple sclerosis.[7,8] Curiously, the same edition of the *Daily Telegraph* with Dr. Le Fanu's story carried an article on the same page about a patient experiencing similar symptoms who also feared that she had a brain tumour. Investigations eventually revealed that she actually had multiple sclerosis. Interestingly, the article quoted a neurologist as saying that a new drug, based on a Chinese mushroom, was the best hope for multiple sclerosis sufferers, appearing to be slightly more effective in reducing attacks than the beta interferons.

It seems obvious that the dilemma posed by the so-called diagnosis of multiple sclerosis would be solved if a diagnostic test was found. However, despite the disease being clearly recognised over 140 years ago, there is still no such test and there are very good reasons to doubt that there ever can be. This needs further discussion and in Appendix 3 there is an account of such an unfortunate patient. She was effectively tortured for years, before being told she had multiple sclerosis by one consultant, only to have it questioned within months by another. The complexity introduced by successive committees examining the so-called diagnostic criteria for multiple sclerosis defies belief (see http://www.mssociety.org.uk/). After the latest deliberations, which brought 30 neurologists together from around the world, the consensus reached was that now only three categories are needed. They are 1) not multiple sclerosis, 2) possible multiple sclerosis, and 3) definite multiple sclerosis.[9] In fact, the only change that has resulted from this international meeting was that patients meeting *slightly* less than the strictest criteria would no longer be labelled as *probable* multiple sclerosis. One wonders what the loss of just this word actually cost.

It is very clear that there can be no escape from this absurdity for those locked into the industry created around the disease, whether they are patients or clinicians. It would be altogether too embarrassing to the profession to debate these issues publicly. Nevertheless, this is what *must* happen; a road map must be developed, or this sterile debate, and the misery it creates, will still be with us for another hundred years, and this despite the fact that MRI has already provided the necessary answers.

Although eyesight problems are common in multiple sclerosis, one of the expert witnesses denying Mr. Dingley's claim said he did not consider the point important. He was unable to say whether the eye problem Mr. Dingley suffered was actually a symptom of multiple sclerosis. It would seem that the matter became altogether too embarrassing and, probably after some "horse trading" between the counsels representing each side, the matter was dropped. Finally, in his closing speech, the Lord President told the court the following:

> *I do not find it proved, on a balance of probabilities, that trauma in general, or whiplash in particular, can trigger the onset of symptomatic MS . . . I am left with sufficient doubt about the pursuer's case that I am not satisfied that he has proved it on the balance of probabilities.*

Mr. Dingley's award was accordingly reduced from £547,245 to just £1,500.

The consensus view in neurology is, of course, that trauma does not cause multiple sclerosis, although, as with the late Dr. Poser and Dr. Behan, a minority of neurologists believe that trauma may cause a relapse in patients who already have the disease. At this point, the reader may question if similar stories to Mr. Dingley have been published—they have indeed. In 1964 the late Henry Miller,[10] a neurologist working in Newcastle upon

Tyne, gave details of seven patients he saw in his clinical practice in whom not only did symptoms typical of multiple sclerosis occur within hours of a significant trauma, they also tended to relate *anatomically* to the site of the injury. In other words, the symptoms reflected the site of the injury. Miller's approach was that of a careful, old-fashioned doctor who listens to the patient, and he took a meticulous history followed by a detailed examination. Case number six in his paper is reproduced below. Nystagmus refers to an oscillation of the eyes, scotoma to a loss of some of the field of vision of an eye, and parasthesia to a feeling of "pins and needles" in the skin.

Case 6

A 17-year-old merchant seaman on board ship received a glancing blow on the head with a steel cable. He was briefly dazed but not unconscious, and he had no residual headache. Five hours later he noticed blurring of vision in both eyes and some pain behind both eyes, especially on the left. The next day both hands became clumsy and unsteady. These symptoms persisted, but he continued his work until about a month later, when he noticed painful cramps in both legs during the night. Examination at this time revealed sustained nystagmus, a central scotoma on the left, and a paracentral scotoma on the right, with no abnormality in the optic fundi and no other abnormal signs in the nervous system except for increased reflexes in the lower limbs. During the ensuing five years, nystagmus has persisted, his visual acuity has varied but has never returned to normal, and he has had intermittent periods of unpleasant parasthesia in both legs.

Today, with the pressures of work and the proliferation of special investigations, it is rare for patients to be given time to tell their story. Miller was well aware of the resistance to the idea of a relationship between trauma and multiple sclerosis, not least because of the truly enormous legal implications. Patients often allege that their diseases, especially cancer, have been triggered by injury or, at the very least, by a traumatic event in their lives. In the case of cancer, despite professional denials, some may well be correct. It is now known that apparently simple tissue injury can lead to extremely complex gene activity resulting from a lowering of tissue oxygen levels. Miller mulled over this young man's case and came to the conclusion that, even though most injuries are not necessarily followed by multiple sclerosis and in most cases the onset appears to be unrelated to injury of any kind, it is perfectly possible that doctors are too reliant on an entirely statistical approach. This may well, as Miller wrote, "cause an occasional but conceivably significant relationship to be overlooked."

Miller, who was known for his sense of humour, then set about giving an example. He chose asphyxiation from eating a Yorkshire pudding, arguing:

. . . among ten thousand consecutive people who ate Yorkshire pudding there may indeed be no case of accidental choking but, nevertheless, people are occasionally choked by Yorkshire pudding and the validity of these statistics is unlikely to give much solace to the hapless victim or his bereaved family.

It would, of course, be established beyond *any possible doubt* at post-mortem examination if a piece of Yorkshire pudding was found obstructing the airway. However, what cannot be known from a single case is how common this form of asphyxiation is, and this can only be established by epidemiological surveys involving very large numbers of people over a very long time. Obviously, the less frequent the event, the larger the survey has to be in order to produce accurate numbers. Miller's point was that after failing to find a single death in ten thousand instances of the ingestion of Yorkshire pudding, researchers could well be tempted to conclude that it could not happen—they would be wrong.

After he reviewed the evidence of his seven cases where neurological symptoms had rapidly followed injury, Miller recognised that blood vessels were involved in multiple sclerosis, as both Rindfleisch[11] and Charcot[12] had done as long ago as the 1860s. However, unable to think of a mechanism to make sense of it all, Miller was forced to conclude that the patients he had seen *already had the disease*, and the traumatic injuries had simply triggered a relapse. Like most of his contemporaries, he did not consider *embolism*, or the importance of the protection given to the brain by the special construction of the blood vessels in the nervous system that form the blood-brain barrier. Despite being discovered by the Nobel Prize winner Paul Ehrlich in the 1870s, the importance of this structure had barely been acknowledged in neurology as late as 1960.[13] A detailed study of the integrity of the blood-brain barrier in 74 patients with the various forms of multiple sclerosis was published in 1993 from the National Hospital of Neurology and Neurosurgery in London.[14] It showed gross impairment of the barrier in acute relapses and worsening of barrier function across the spectrum of presentation, including patients with both primary and secondary progressive disease. The blood-brain barrier has, however, been of special interest to the pharmaceutical industry, in fact, one of the first questions asked about a new drug is whether it actually crosses the barrier. In September 2001, the author attended the first meeting that brought research biologists and neurologists together in Chicago to discuss the blood-brain barrier.

It was sponsored by the pharmaceutical company Merck Serono, who make one of the beta interferons used in the management of multiple sclerosis. The symposium was entitled Dysfunction of the Blood-Brain Barrier in the Pathogenesis of Multiple Sclerosis.

Cases similar to that of Mr. Dingley still come to court. One published in the *Lancet* on March 4, 2002[15] gave the details of a patient who also developed typical neurological symptoms soon after being involved in a road traffic accident. He was subsequently told he had multiple sclerosis, and became involved in a lengthy court case, claiming that the accident had caused his disease. One of the expert witnesses called, who had also been involved in Mr. Dingley's action, again claimed that whiplash injury could lead to the development of multiple sclerosis. The judge dismissed his "embellished" arguments and ruled that the patient was just a victim of an unfortunate coincidence. Unfortunately, the judge strayed well beyond his area of expertise by declaring that he found himself "unable to agree that trauma could precipitate the onset of multiple sclerosis in any circumstances."

In Chapter 8, the evidence was discussed that the brain and the spinal cord are vulnerable to damage caused by agents in the circulation; that is, by small emboli, such as bubbles. However, this concept, which was introduced by Haldane, has even come under attack in the world of diving because it has been claimed there is no disease where damage to the spinal cord is associated with small emboli—infections like syphilis were obviously discounted, as disease due to infectious emboli are now rare, at least in the West. Nevertheless, there is such a disease, and the details have been available for over 50 years. Inexplicably, the expert witnesses in Mr. Dingley's case failed to inform the judges that injury to a *spinal disc* can lead to brain and spinal cord damage. It is known as *fibrocartilagenous embolism* and occurs when material from the soft centre of a spinal disc, which is known as the *nucleus pulposus*, is squeezed into the circulation. It can certainly result from a whiplash injury, and it is covered in textbooks of neurology as one of the conditions that must be included in the list of possible diagnoses in patients with symptoms suggestive of multiple sclerosis. Despite this, it is commonly overlooked, as it was in Mr. Dingley's case. The case reports make for uncomfortable reading.

The first report of fibrocartilagenous embolism was published in 1961,[16] and gives the terrifying account of the death of a 15-year-old boy in the US who fell backwards onto the floor whilst playing basketball in school before class. Although the impact was sufficient to cause onlookers some concern, he was able to continue playing for the 10 minutes to the end of the game.

One hour later in class, he complained of severe pain in his abdomen and was taken to the headmaster's room. He requested a drink of water, but was unable to hold the glass. In the ambulance on the way to hospital, he lost consciousness. Just three hours after the fall, he stopped breathing and died. At the post-mortem examination, emboli, clearly identified as being fibrocartilage, were found impacted in the small arteries supplying the brainstem and 10 levels of the spinal cord. The material had been squeezed into the circulation as a result of compression of the spinal disc. Mr. Dingley had recalled striking his head in the accident and even feeling "a crick in his neck," and it was acknowledged by all involved that he sustained a whiplash injury. Despite this, the possibility of fibrocartilagenous embolism was not raised—it would certainly have drawn the attention of the judges to the importance of embolism as a mechanism causing damage to the nervous system, and led to some searching questions.

The neurologist Dr. Harold Klawans, well known for his popular books about neurology, gave an account of a nurse in his 1991 book *Trials of an Expert Witness*, who, like Mr. Dingley, sustained a whiplash injury.[17] In 1974, she had been travelling in a train on the high level system in Chicago that had stopped in a station when it was hit from behind by a second train. She suffered a whiplash injury and, as in Mr. Dingley's case, was seen in an emergency room. Both her physical examination and X-rays, etc. were normal. However, within hours of returning home, her neck became painful and she began to walk like a drunk. Her condition worsened with the development of double vision, and a night's sleep did not improve matters. Being a nurse, she realised a neurological opinion was needed, and rang Klawans. A careful history revealed that she had not experienced *any* neurological symptoms prior to the accident. An examination confirmed damage to the nervous system which, Klawans claimed, involved three sites, and so qualified as multiple. He then reveals in the text the dreadful dilemma created by the so-called diagnosis of multiple sclerosis that neurologists still face today:

> *So what did she have? In all probability multiple sclerosis. But only one attack. A puzzlement. What do you tell a patient? She might not have multiple sclerosis. And even if she did, she may not have another attack for fifteen or twenty years. Would it be fair to give her the label of multiple sclerosis.*

Note his use of the term "label" as opposed to "diagnosis." When the patient asked Klawans what she had, he replied, "Areas of inflammation in your brain and spinal cord." Her rejoinder was, "You mean multiple sclerosis," to which he replied, "Perhaps, but we're not certain." She was hospitalised and given steroids to decrease the inflammation. All seemed to be going well for a few days; her double vision disappeared and her walking was slightly improved. However, on waking on the morning she was scheduled to go home, she found that she could not see anything out of her right eye. Klawans' relief seemed almost palpable:

> That answered the question. She had now had a second episode separated in time. She now had multiple areas separated in space and time.

The diagnosis was now certain: She had qualified for the label multiple sclerosis by a second attack meeting the criterion for dissemination in time. However, fibrocartilagenous embolism should have been considered as a delay in the appearance of symptoms is a well-established feature associated with the release of small emboli trapped in the capillaries of the lungs.

The patient sued the train company, and Klawans was contacted by her lawyer and asked to be an expert witness. The lawyer asked if the accident had caused her multiple sclerosis. Klawans replied, "Not caused, brought on." Clearly, like Henry Miller, he could not think of any way in which her whiplash injury could have been responsible for the areas that were damaged in her brain, spinal cord and an optic nerve. They are, of course, all linked together by the circulation. Years later, Klawans was approached by the same lawyer about a similar case. His opinion had changed—he felt that epidemiological studies had disproved any link between injury and multiple sclerosis. He was mistaken.

Since the 1961 paper that described human fibrocartilagenous embolism for the first time, many more case reports have been published and over 34 fatal cases. It is obvious that many cases will be missed. Surprisingly, at least for those of us involved in human medicine, this form of embolism is regarded as a common cause of neurological problems in veterinary medicine. It has been found to affect dogs, cats, sheep, pigs, horses, and even turkeys. As in the case of the unfortunate schoolboy, the diagnosis has been established *beyond doubt*, because the animals have either died or been sacrificed because of their disabilities and subjected to post-mortem examination. The most dramatic case report gives the details of an 11-day-old lamb[18] that developed uncontrollable shaking and was sacrificed because of concerns about infection in the flock. Emboli were disseminated throughout the brain, including the cerebellum, and six levels of the spinal cord. Lambs are, of course, well known for jumping, which puts great strain on the spine and the discs.

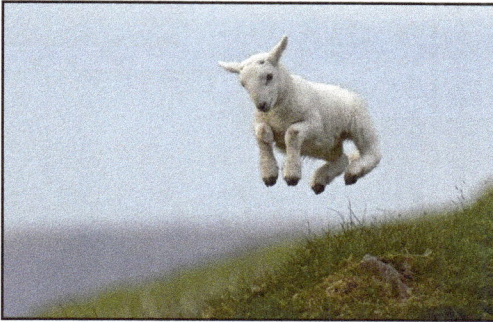

Figure 13.1:
A spring lamb springing.

The youngest fatal human case reported is a girl 13 years of age and the oldest a man of 63. In all cases, fibrocartilagenous material has been found at post-mortem examination blocking small arteries.

> The explanation given in the 1961 paper[16] was that the damage to the spinal cord was due to the entry of material from the damaged disc *directly* into blood vessels adjacent to the affected areas of the spinal cord. Two ways have been suggested to account for the presence of the fibro-cartilage in the arteries. The first is that the annulus fibrosis, the strong outer rim of the disc, is torn and the tear extends into a nearby artery supplying the spinal cord. It was postulated that this allows the fibrocar-tilagenous material to be forced into an artery and carried by the flow of blood to impact downstream within, or close to, the spinal cord. The second suggestion was that a tear had extended into a vein, and in some way material is forced against the normal direction of blood flow back through the capillaries into an artery. It is important to recognise that these explanations are not supported by any evidence and, in truth, are unlikely. Certainly no local bleeding, which would always occur in a tear of the tissues, has ever been described when the spinal column has been examined postmortem. Although there is no doubt that the fibrocartilag-enous emboli have been derived from the centre of a spinal disc, because they have been identified by staining, the route taken to reach the brain and spinal cord is still said to be controversial. Veterinary pathologists, unlike neurologists, are very familiar with the condition (see http://www.veterinarypartner.com), and have linked it to *Schmorl's nodes*, which are defects in the bony endplates of vertebra.[19]

The publication of a report in 1993[20] has established the route taken by fibrocartilagenous emboli beyond any possible doubt. A 17-year-old girl fell, also playing basketball, and several hours later she developed left-sided weakness. She was admitted to hospital and suffered a fatal heart attack the following day. At post-mortem examination, a 200 micron (0.2 mm) fibro-

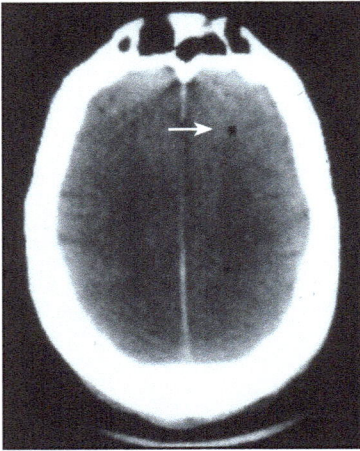

Figure 13.2:
Air (arrowed) in the right middle cerebral artery.
(Courtesy of Professor Brian Hills.)

cartilagenous embolus was found in the brain, lodged in the middle cerebral artery. An air embolus has been demonstrated in this artery by CT. Figure 13.2 shows air in the right middle cerebral artery of a patient.

In order for the fibrocartilagenous material to reach this artery, it must have been transported in the arterial blood from the left ventricle of the heart. The middle cerebral artery is known to be a *preferred pathway* for emboli reaching the brain. There is really only one credible explanation for such an event—there must have been a fracture of the endplate of the vertebra to allow the material access to the venous system. The veins within the body of the vertebra are sinuses that are kept open because they are supported by the bone structure. This allows the blood elements formed in the marrow of the vertebra to be released into the circulation. Having been forced into the veins, the fibrocartilagenous emboli must have been carried to the inferior vena cava, which drains into the right atrium. The embolic debris either escaped being trapped in the lungs and entered the general circulation, or bypassed the lung by transferring through a hole in the heart. The latter is known as paradoxical embolism, and is usually associated with the persistence of the hole present before birth in all of us, known as the foramen ovale. It should be noted that even fragments of bone marrow have been found to embolise the brain after fractures.

> The fibrocartilagenous emboli that have been found at post-mortem examination have measured between 20 and 200 microns, and emboli in this size range are known to occasionally escape being trapped in the lungs. There is no indication as to whether there was a hole in the heart of this 17-year-old girl. However, the presence of the embolus in this artery in the brain has firmly established that material from a spinal disc can damage the nervous system. The patient died from a heart attack, which

resulted from blood flow to an area of the muscle being stopped abruptly; the pain is triggered by lack of oxygen. Fibrocartilagenous emboli were found in the arteries of her heart, and again bone marrow emboli have also been found after trauma. These forms of embolism are, therefore, a cause of both stroke and sudden death in young people,[21] although they are rarely mentioned as a possible diagnosis, nor are they included on websites relating to sudden death syndromes. It is obvious that unless such a diagnosis is suspected, it will be easily overlooked at post-mortem examination. Extreme care must be taken to examine the arteries involved which is also the case for fluid embolism due to gas bubbles and fat.

There can be no doubt that embolism is rarely considered in the clinical diagnosis of spinal cord disease in humans, despite veterinary experience, although pathologists may find the evidence. One of the Case Records of the Massachusetts General Hospital, published in the *New England Journal of Medicine* in 1991,[22] gives details of a 61-year-old woman with a history of intermittent backache, who developed leg weakness over a period of just three hours. Fibrocartilagenous embolism was not included in the differential diagnosis by the clinicians, but it was found when a biopsy of the spinal cord was undertaken. The pathologist asked to comment, Dr. Ann C. McKee, added another case of such embolism. A 13-year-old boy had experienced the abrupt onset of neck pain, headache, and vomiting, minutes after doing somersaults. Six hours post-onset, he developed left-sided weakness, problems speaking, and difficulty in breathing. He died after a cardiac arrest, and fibrocartilagenous material was found in the arteries of the cervical spinal cord. Dr. McKee observed:

The evidence suggests that this condition is much more common than is usually recognised. Despite the few reports in the literature, it is possible that in many cases of undiagnosed transverse myelopathy it is due to this lesion.

Transverse myelopathy describes inflammation in the spinal cord, and is one of the many discrete conditions that occur in patients with multiple sclerosis. It is called transverse myelitis because the inflammation spreads horizontally across the cord causing it to swell. The fact that emboli, in this case of fibrocartilage, can cause transverse myelitis is further evidence that the underlying disease process in multiple sclerosis primarily involves the blood vessels in the nervous system.

The introduction of MRI has made the diagnosis of fibrocartilagenous embolism possible in non-fatal cases. In 2002, a seven-year-old girl developed acute paraplegia after minor injuries sustained when a car driven by her mother collided with a crash barrier.[23] She remained fully conscious and her only complaint was of chest pain when examined in hospital. It was attributed to the visible bruising of her chest wall. After an interval of approximately 24 hours, weakness of the legs began to develop, together with problems in bladder and bowel control. There was no obvious fracture or other bony abnormality on MRI, but there was clear enlargement of the spinal cord with an area of hyperintensity extending from the fourth thoracic vertebra down to the lower end of the cord—the equivalent in the spinal cord of an unidentified bright object in the brain. This eventually reduced over a period of several months to a small area just visible on MRI at the level of the twelfth thoracic vertebra. The patient made a partial recovery over the next year, but remained significantly disabled with continuing problems with bladder and bowel control. The author has been involved in a similar case where the tentative diagnosis was also the spinal cord problem transverse myelitis. The 21-year-old man had suffered back pain, lasting about 10 minutes, after falling backwards playing football. Three days later, he developed an acute headache with vertigo, followed by paraplegia on the sixth day postinjury. The MRI of his spine and brain (Figure 13.3) show that he had suffered a collapse of a spinal disc—the area indicated by the white arrow on the left image; the black arrow showing the area of hyperintensity. The arrows in the right hand image of the brain show the damage in the cerebellum that caused his vertigo. The diagnosis was changed to fibrocartilagenous embolism.

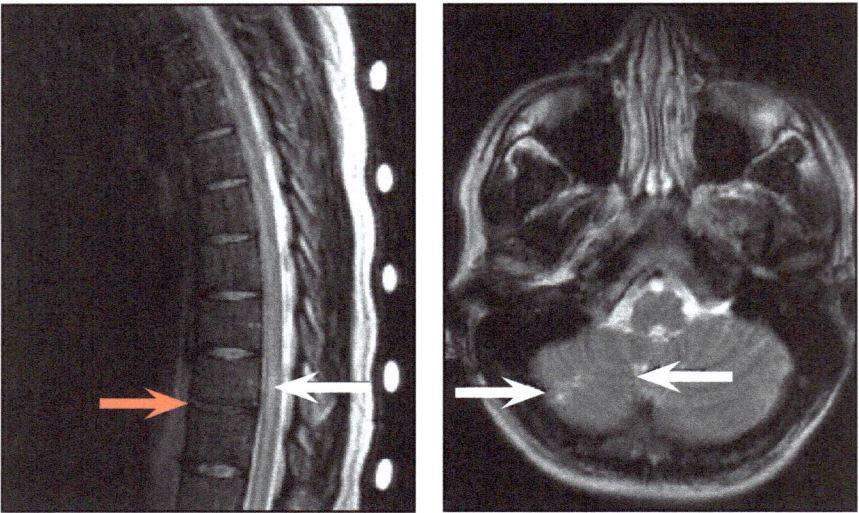

Figure 13.3:
MRI - left showing collapse of a vertebral disc (red arrow).
White arrow shows hyperintensity in the cord (left) and the areas of damage in the cerebellum (right) which gave rise to the vertigo.

Several features of these cases are important in discussing Mr. Dingley's history, as it has clearly been established that sub-acute fibrocartilagenous embolism can occur with survival, but only partial recovery.[24] Most importantly, this form of embolism may be associated with a *latent interval* between the trauma and the onset of symptoms. This delay in the development of the symptoms is typical of that associated with the transit of material through the circulation of the lung and is a well-known feature of a condition known as fat embolism. The MRI findings have been confirmed pathologically,[25] and, most importantly, embolism may also occur without evidence of spinal injury. These findings are very relevant to Mr. Dingley; if the judges had been made aware of fibrocartilagenous embolism, they would certainly have viewed his claim more favourably. It is also likely that they would have asked some awkward questions but, as we shall see, there is much more to the story of embolism.

On March 6, 1998, the judgment made in the reclaiming motion against Mr. Dingley featured in an article in the *Scotsman*. His lawyer was quoted as being confident that they could overturn the judgment, by winning an appeal in the House of Lords. Unfortunately, as will be seen in the next chapter, his confidence was misplaced.

CHAPTER 14

The Final Appeal to the House of Lords

Asking judges to rule on matters of scientific controversy would be to invite the court to become an Orwellian ministry of truth.

British Chiropractic Association vs. S. Singh.
Court of Appeals, Civil Division April 1, 2010.

The lawyers acting for Mr. Dingley were successful in their application for an appeal to the House of Lords, and five Law Lords were assigned to the case. Their remit was simple: to determine if there is any evidence that a remote injury, for example to the neck, arm, or leg could be associated with damage to the nervous system and give rise to multiple sclerosis. The judges were advised to consult undergraduate texts about the disease; in other words, to read the basic accounts written for medical students, so that they could assess the opposing evidence of the expert witnesses. However, they were certainly not in a position to arbitrate on the controversies that surround multiple sclerosis and an opinion recently aired in a different context by the UK Lord Chief Justice, Lord Neuberger, would appear to concur. Commenting on criticisms made of chiropractors by the journalist Simon Singh; he said that asking judges to rule on matters of scientific controversy would be "to invite the court to become an Orwellian ministry of truth."

The judges would have been aware that textbooks often enshrine fashionable ideas, even presenting them as established facts, and this is certainly true in multiple sclerosis. The affected areas are typically described as being white matter damage with loss of myelin, although this omits key pathological features, such as the loss of nerve fibres which was documented well over 100 years ago. The constant misrepresentation of the pathological facts is little short of disgraceful and this paragraph in the Final Judgment of the Law Lords[1] illustrates the problem.

> *The nerve fibres are covered in a sheath of myelin, which has an insulating effect on the electrical signals which they transmit. Damage to the spinal cord is liable to interfere with these signals and may cause paralysis. In it the myelin which covers the nerve fibres within the CNS (central nervous system) becomes depleted, although the nerve fibre itself remains intact.*

The myelin sheaths, which wrap around sections of nerve fibres, do not insulate—they increase the speed at which nerve impulses are conducted.

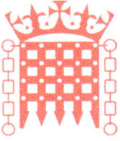

House of Lords

Judgments - Dingley v. Chief Constable of Strathclyde Police

HOUSE OF LORDS

Browne-Wilkinson Lord Nichols of Birkenhead Lord Steys Lord Hope of Craighead Lord Clyde

OPINIONS OF THE LORDS OF APPEAL FOR JUDGMENT

IN THE CAUSE

DINGLEY (A.P.)

(APPELLANT)

v.

CHIEF CONSTABLE OF STRATHCLYDE POLICE

(RESPONDENT)

ON 9 MARCH 2000

Figure 14.1:
The front page of the Appeal for Judgment as it appeared on the Internet.

Some fibres in the nervous system do not possess myelin sheaths and they work fine, although they conduct impulses more slowly, typically at about half a metre a second. The same size of fibre possessing a myelin sheath may conduct impulses two hundred times faster, at 100 metres a second. This speed is especially important for complex tasks, for example, those involving rapid movement, such as gymnastics. The sheaths are extensions of a parent cell, known as an oligodendrocyte, which resembles an octopus and its tentacles. The tentacle-like extensions, which may number as many as 40 for one cell, form the myelin sheaths, wrapping round a short length of a nerve fibre like a Swiss roll. The segments of myelin are interspersed by unwrapped sections of fibre, named after their discoverer—the nodes of Ranvier. A single oligodendrocyte may measure as much as 1.5 mm across their myelin sheath extensions which, as far as cells are concerned, is truly gigantic. Many think that nerve cells, which are known as neurons, are the cells most affected by oxygen starvation but, in fact, oligodendrocytes being more active metabolically are known to be much more vulnerable,[2,3] and this is true from birth.[4] There can be no doubt that myelin sheaths are damaged and destroyed in patients with multiple sclerosis and the parent cell, the oligodendrocyte, often dies. But glossed over in recent years is the fact that the nerve fibres within myelin sheaths may also be destroyed, a finding reported as long ago as 1868, by the French neurologist Charcot.[5]

In 1947, however, Drs. Tracey Putnam and Leo Alexander[6] quantified the loss of nerve fibres in a typical area of damage in the spinal cord in multiple sclerosis. They compared the nerve fibre count under the microscope between a normal and an affected area on opposite sides of a section of the same spinal cord. The loss of fibres in an affected area of the cord was found to be *at least 20%*, and as the cord is such a small structure, this will usually produce symptoms. Pathologists, as distinct from clinical doctors, always refer to the preservation of nerve fibres as relative in multiple sclerosis, indicating in other words that some fibres are always destroyed. In 1998, an MRI study published in the *New England Journal of Medicine*[7] demonstrated this finding in the brain and received worldwide publicity. Not surprisingly, Putnam and Alexander's paper was not cited, as it predates today's computer databases. Magnetic resonance techniques are being increasingly used to quantify brain tissue loss in multiple sclerosis patients,[8] but it is the loss of neurons and nerve fibres that is responsible for the disability not, as is usually claimed, damage to myelin sheaths. As the loss of myelin sheaths simply slows down the speed of nerve conduction, some function is often preserved. For example, most of the myelin sheaths may be lost from a section of the nerve to an eye in optic neuritis, without any loss of vision. However, a test of the speed with which nerve impulses are transmitted from the eye to the area responsible for vision at the back of the brain will be slowed—the visual evoked response. Unfortunately, in the severest areas of damage in multiple sclerosis, nerve cells are destroyed, especially when the disease involves the spinal cord.[9]

The conclusion of the Law Lords that injury does not *cause* multiple sclerosis was an opinion shared by both the experts who supported Mr. Dingley's claim, and those who did not. In an article written in 1994, the late Dr. Charles Poser,[10] who did support the action, went much further by declaring, "Injury to an extremity, that is an arm or leg, cannot cause damage to the nervous system." This is certainly wrong; indeed, the facts have been known since the 1870s, and are in every textbook of pathology. Poser was a highly regarded neurologist in the field of multiple sclerosis research and known for his strong views. He was very critical of the lack of progress made in finding the cause of multiple sclerosis. In this incisive statement, he emphasises the involvement of blood vessels in multiple sclerosis evident from the leakage of the blood-brain barrier seen by imaging the living patient:[11]

> *. . . nothing, regarding multiple sclerosis in terms of pathogenesis has been proved, nothing. The immunological theory is a theory. But, the only thing we know for a fact is there is an alteration of the blood-brain barrier and we know this because of the gadolinium-enhanced studies of MRIs. But you ask a neurologist to tell you what the mechanism is and . . .*

By reading textbook accounts of multiple sclerosis, the Law Lords were exposed to the auto-immune theory, a concept which dates back to the 1930s. The central tenet of auto-immunity postulates that the immune cells of the body attack normal tissue. Somehow, it is postulated, a component of normal tissue becomes an antigen in multiple sclerosis patients and is said to be responsible for attacking the myelin which forms the sheaths around many nerve fibres. However, it is usual for a trigger to be suggested that initiates the sequence of events, and it is usually claimed that it is a virus. However, no virus has ever been found, despite years of research, which has even included biopsies being taken from the brains of patients during acute attacks. Equally, no antigen has been identified in normal tissues. Despite the absence of any scientific evidence, the viral auto-immune theory is often presented as certain fact:

> *Multiple sclerosis . . . is an autoimmune process directed against myelin in*

the CNS which occurs as a consequence of a viral infection in a genetically predisposed individual.

Graham DI, Bell JE, Ironside JW.
Colour Atlas and Textbook of Neuropathology. Mosby-Wolfe Publishing, 1995.

The judges, as would be expected of such learned gentlemen, reproduced the auto-immune theory accurately in their examination of the issues. Their deliberations reinforce the impression that the mechanisms involved in multiple sclerosis are impossibly complicated. It is necessary here to examine the various components of this still pervasive theory. Their first statement about the role of immunity is undoubtedly correct and applies to foreign bodies, which, in infection, includes microbes.

The body is supplied with an immune system which responds to an attack by a foreign body by producing organisms known as lymphocytes. These are of two kinds. B-lymphocytes produce antibodies which react with the foreign body and render it harmless. T-lymphocytes attack the foreign body in various ways which complement the role of the B-lymphocytes.

The foreign proteins of microbes like bacteria are examples of antigens and, after they are identified, the body responds to them by producing antibodies. When the antibodies produced find the appropriate antigen they lock together, and the resulting complex is engulfed and removed by white cells, the neutrophils also known as *macrophages*, the big eaters. The theory of auto-immunity alleges that these primary defences of the body initiate an attack on *normal* tissue. It is a concept that has been applied to many diseases where no cause has yet been found, such as rheumatoid arthritis and diabetes. While it may seem strange to include a section in this chapter about diabetes, it illustrates the slow recognition that auto-immunity is *not* a primary disease process, and the latest research can, finally, allow the true story to be unravelled. The claim was made as long ago as the 1920s that insulin-dependent diabetes is an auto-immune disease although, as in the case of multiple sclerosis, the caveat has since been added: in a genetically susceptible host.

The era of auto-immune theory appears to be finally ending. Dr. Jens Nerup, an eminent and respected researcher of diabetes, together with colleagues, have expressed reservations about the role of auto-immunity as the first event in the disease.[12]

However, if the term pathogenesis defines the earliest events and mechanisms involved in beta cell destruction . . . there is ample evidence to support . . . that

Chapter 14: The Final Appeal to the House of Lords ~ 241

> *a series of distinct events takes place well before the invasion of the islets by T-lymphocytes and beta-cell destruction by cytotoxic T cells is possible.*
>
> The evidence, therefore, indicates that in diabetes auto-immunity is also a secondary process responding to damage from another cause. Nerup and his colleagues continue:
>
> *To us this suggests that beta cells are not destroyed because islet proteins are antigens in their native form. Rather, these proteins become antigens when and because beta cells are destroyed. This means that auto-antibodies are secondary in importance and time in the pathogenetic process and that the islet proteins are probably made antigenic through a common mechanism.*
>
> Clearly, the breakthrough here is that the idea that normal cells become antigens is questioned; in fact, no evidence has ever been produced that they can be. It should be noted, however, that no explanation is offered by Nerup and his colleagues for the common mechanism, there is just the vague suggestion of "toxic" or "viral" factors. It is interesting to speculate that, like the tissue of the nervous system, the insulin-producing islets of Langerhans are a vulnerable tissue where a disturbance of the microcirculation produced by micro-embolism would have severe consequences. The key question for researchers, therefore, is the following: Is there a blood-tissue barrier in the pancreatic islets that is the equivalent of the blood-brain barrier?

It must be emphasised that there is a need for the body to be able to identify *damaged* normal tissue and then remove it to allow healing to take place; it is obvious, of course, that damaged tissue is no longer normal. Clearly, this is a more difficult process than the identification of the proteins in microbes, because they are foreign. Some years ago, an investigation of a possible role for auto-immunity in cancer was halted because it was eventually recognised that most patients had undergone surgery, which of necessity involves trauma to tissues, and this had caused profound immune changes (personal communication, Dr. C.R. Gillis).

After studying the texts they had acquired, the judges gave their understanding of auto-immune theory:

> *The immune system can however work in an incorrect way. This results in its failure to distinguish between foreign bodies and other bodies from within the body against which it reacts. When the system is in this condition the activated T-lymphocytes may behave in a deranged manner in a way that is associated with the development of plaques.*

Incredibly, although the judges could not possibly have known, there is no evidence to support this statement. There is certainly evidence that the immune system is active in multiple sclerosis patients, but it is most likely that its actions and the damage are secondary to *inflammation*. This is a most important theme that will be explained in detail later. There can be no doubt that if normal tissue becomes damaged, the body must recognise the changes to be able to remove self material that is beyond repair, a process of deconstruction. This is essential for recovery after every form of tissue injury, whether it is caused by trauma or infection. However, it is obvious that once damaged, a tissue is no longer normal, whereas auto-immune theorists postulate that attacks are directed against normal tissue. Since WW2, and the growth of science as an industry within the world of medicine, multiple sclerosis research has accounted for the expenditure of billions from both governmental and charitable sources. Despite this, there is still no diagnostic test for the disease. As the professor of neurology at Oxford, George Ebers, observed in an article in the *British Medical Journal*,[13] there are also no adequate measures of disease activity or, even disability. It would be difficult to find a more damning indictment of the failure of medicine over more than a century. In fact, it has been research into an animal model that has consumed most of the billions raised for multiple sclerosis since WW2.

The auto-immune hypothesis has held centre stage in multiple sclerosis since the founding of the National MS Society of America in 1946. The society was started by Mrs. Sylvia Lawry after her brother developed multiple sclerosis. In 1945, she placed an advertisement in the *New York Times* appealing for contact with other patients. The following year she brought together 20 of America's most prominent medical scientists, including Dr. Tracy Putnam, who had moved to New York from Yale University. Putnam had conducted some outstanding research during the 1930s, confirming the importance of damage to blood vessels in causing multiple sclerosis, which will be discussed later. Unfortunately, the catastrophic events of WW2 intervened, the thread was broken, and research into this aspect of the disease ground to a halt. Sadly, a family tragedy in New York severely curtailed Putnam's brilliant career and, despite being a founder member of the National MS Society of America, he received little support for his ideas from other members (personal communication, Dr. Roy L. Swank). This blunted research into the role of blood vessels in multiple sclerosis, although after WW2, two investigators in the UK continued his work—Drs. Lumsden in Aberdeen,[14] and Woolf in London.[15] The latter's experiments, like those of Putnam, reproduced the earliest damage seen in multiple sclerosis; an observation relevant to embolism which will be discussed in Chapter 16.

The newly formed US National MS Society needed to initiate a research programme, but faced a serious problem: no other animal, with the possible exception of the gorilla, actually develops multiple sclerosis. It was noted in the 1930s, when investigators were attempting to develop a vaccine for tuberculosis, that some of the animals injected with killed tubercle bacilli included in an emulsion with mineral oils developed patchy areas of inflammation in the nervous system. This became the basis of the animal model experimental allergic encephalomyelitis (EAE), which is now studied in many countries. The details are disturbing—it involves injecting brain tissue removed from a healthy animal, mixed with Freund's adjuvant.[16] The term adjuvant which translates as "helper," refers to a mixture of mineral oil and killed tuberculosis bacteria developed in the 1930s as a vaccine for tuberculosis. Mineral oils cannot be broken down in the body and have been used to increase the effectiveness of drugs. Although they are still used in veterinary medicines, adjuvants have been banned from use in human pharmaceuticals, although squalene has been allowed to be used in a new H1N1 (swine flu) vaccine. The reason for the ban in their use with drugs is obscure, but almost certainly relates to official governmental recognition that they work by damaging blood vessels causing inflammation, which itself may cause tissue damage. In the early 1990s, the UK government also banned the use of mineral oil as a coating for the plastics used in food packaging, perhaps because a large post-mortem study published in 1984 had shown that droplets of mineral oil are common in human tissue.[17] The UK Veterinary Medicines Agency seemed curiously suspicious of attempts by the author to obtain information about mineral oil adjuvants. The extraordinary ability of mineral oil based emulsions to cause gross inflammation was shown by the accidental self-injection of a veterinary vaccine containing a mineral oil adjuvant by a farm worker.[18] A severe chronic inflammatory reaction developed, and extensive surgery was required to remove the mineral oil. The authors stated that "very small quantities of oil are required . . . there appears to be enough on a dirty needle to cause local inflammation." It is not surprising that adjuvant is needed for the putative animal model of multiple sclerosis; it is so effective in promoting inflammation. In fact research workers have also suffered from accidental injection, but the disease they develop does not resemble multiple sclerosis.[19]

MRI studies of the animal model EAE[20,21] have shown that the first event is opening of the blood-brain barrier—exactly the same as in patients with the onset of an acute attack typical of multiple sclerosis.[22] In fact, in a research study many years ago, blood-brain barrier leakage was actually found before the patient went into the attack.[23] It is clearly a seminal event in EAE, but it has been largely ignored. But how does the material injected, for example into a foot pad or the skin at the back of the neck, reach the nervous system in the model EAE, and how does it open the blood-brain barrier? It is impossible to find this discussed in the thousands of publications. However, droplets of the mineral oil used in Freund's adjuvant in the circulating blood are certainly capable of opening the barrier, and acting with the tubercle bacilli will cause inflammation. The only reasonable explanation is that droplets of mineral oil enter the circulation from the injection site and transport the antigen directed to attack nervous system tissue. In other words, the mineral oil droplets are embolising the nervous system *just like bubbles* do in divers. There is more evidence; it has been found that the mineral oil adjuvant can be replaced in the production of EAE by tiny *micro-spheres*. In order to be successful, the microspheres must be in the size range of three to eight microns, and must also be capable of binding the antigenic tissue to their surface.[24] Microspheres of a similar size have been developed for use in routine ultrasound examinations, such as the heart. They are injected intravenously, and so must go through the lungs in order to allow an examination of the chambers of the left side of the heart. It is not surprising that it has been found that the size range of microspheres required for EAE to be successful is from three to eight microns, which means they will readily pass through the capillaries of the lungs, just as Haldane suggested small bubbles may do in divers. However, a detailed letter published in the *Lancet*[25] drawing attention to the possibility that the droplets of mineral oil and the microspheres act as *micro-emboli* and vehicles in EAE, failed to elicit any response from the enormous industry researching the model.

Criticism of EAE has been increasing and, because the word allergic links it to a pre-war era, it has been renamed "experimental *autoimmune* encephalitis"—a tribute to the power of the fashions that influence medicine. But EAE cannot be an auto-immune disease, simply because the brain tissue injected that is used to provoke the immune response is from a *different* animal. It is therefore simply an immune disease and the response of the animal injected is the same as the immune response to the transplant of an organ like a kidney, which, again, is triggered by the presence of foreign proteins. The injected material *must* reach the nervous system via the *blood supply*, because no other route is possible. It has been clearly established that the lymphatic circulation of the body, which drains away the fluid that leaks from blood vessels, does not communicate with the fluid that surrounds the brain and spinal cord. The model EAE, therefore, *must* use embolism, and this begins the sequence of events in the nervous system.

> Fortunately, the value of EAE is, at long last, being challenged. A paper published in 2005 entitled "Experimental Allergic Encephalomyelitis: A Misleading Model of Multiple Sclerosis" may signal the beginning of the end.[26] Unfortunately, the scale of activity is still growing—there were over 1,600 articles on EAE published between 2001 and 2005. Sadly, although there is no question that the research is of good quality, it is simply not relevant: EAE *cannot* be regarded as a model of auto-immunity for multiple sclerosis.

The judges were not made aware that the auto-immune theory in multiple sclerosis is underpinned by an animal model. Imagine their reaction if they had been told that the model depends on an animal being injected with brain tissue mixed with mineral oil and killed tubercle bacteria into a foot pad, or the back of the neck, or the abdomen. In other words, the model of multiple sclerosis used by the research industry is actually produced by a *remote injury* to the animal. The doctors involved in Mr. Dingley's case would probably have known that the model EAE uses *remote* injection, although this research is generally undertaken by biological scientists, not doctors. There has been, however, one positive outcome from this research. Studies have shown the effectiveness of hyperbaric oxygen treatment in both *preventing* animals from developing the disease after being injected, and also in *treating* the symptoms, once it has developed. This demonstrates the key role of oxygen in treating inflammation, and the blood flow changes leading to blood-brain barrier breakdown in patients labelled as having multiple sclerosis.[27]

Auto-immune theory is now being seriously questioned, as it is in this text. In 2008, a neurological editorial[28] asked, "Is the immune system of multiple sclerosis patients so easily fooled?" It pointed out that "despite 60 years of research, the mechanism still eludes researchers." It is important to note that an immune response always follows tissue injury from any cause, even the tissue damage caused by surgery, simply because the response is essential to healing. A perceptive colleague once remarked about auto-immune theories that "if we do not know the cause for a condition, we usually blame the patient" (personal communication, Dr. K.G. Wormsley). It was not original; Plinius the Elder observed in 400 A.D. that doctors "make the patient responsible: They blame him who has succumbed." The tradition continues today with the inclusion of genetic factors which, of course, extends blame to the parents. So, not only did Mr. Dingley fail in his attempt to implicate his injuries in causing his multiple sclerosis, he had the ignominy of being blamed for developing the disease.

Despite most popular accounts of multiple sclerosis implying that auto-immunity is proven, there is now solid evidence of the involvement of neutrophils, not lymphocytes, as the first event and this is where the role of oxygen is pivotal. The question, then, is: What is the first event, the trigger? The later immune activity which involves lymphocytes actually appears to be involved in repair. In other words, it is an important component of *recovery*. It has been found to be active in other conditions that affect the nervous system such as strokes, or even head injuries. The evidence that follows produced by neurologists in Scandinavia has had very little publicity.

The so-called diagnostic criteria for multiple sclerosis drawn up by successive committees include some laboratory tests. One such test examines the fluid that surrounds the brain and spinal cord, known as the cerebrospinal fluid, and it requires patients to undergo a lumbar puncture. The fluid is examined for proteins by the presence of what are called oligoclonal bands. The bands, demonstrated by electrophoresis of the fluid, are frequently used as supporting evidence for the diagnosis, despite the fact that by no means all patients who have symptoms typical of multiple sclerosis test positive, and positive results are *not* restricted to patients with multiple sclerosis. In 1982, Kostulas and Link[29] reviewed 998 patients with a variety of nervous system diseases for the presence of oligoclonal bands and listed 26 different diseases in which they can be found. The list even includes patients with head injury. So, using the same logic as for multiple sclerosis, head injury must be an auto-immune disease! The bands are, therefore, a *non-specific* marker of damage to the tissues of the nervous system. Note that the term non-specific actually applies to *every other test* used to label patients as having multiple sclerosis. Work has continued in this area investigating the T cell activity that has so captivated researchers in multiple sclerosis. They have extended their research to include patients with cerebro-vascular disease— blood vessel diseases of the brain—which, of course, includes patients with a stroke. It is difficult to overstate the importance of this paper published as long ago as 1992.[30] It states:

> ... *the autoimmune changes described in multiple sclerosis occur in patients with cerebro-vascular disease and at the same level.*

It is, of course, universally accepted that strokes are due to thrombosis or embolism, *not* auto-immunity; survivors of stroke tend to improve, sometimes making an excellent recovery from serious disabilities. This clearly indicates that these immune changes are evidence of repair, and not a disease process. This one sentence puts the final nail in the coffin of the auto-immune theory as the cause of disease or derangement in multiple sclerosis, and indicates that more than half a century of research and billions of dollars have led down a cul-de-sac—it seems unlikely that there is room for it to turn around. It is notable that this seminal paper on the immune findings in stroke, now more than two decades old, has been cited *only once*, by a senior neurologist in a general article about multiple sclerosis, which can be easily verified by an invaluable search feature available online. However, no one involved in the merry-go-round of research and grant funding wants to challenge the status quo and, as usual, if it is difficult to see a reason, look for the financial interest. The immune trail is coupled to immune suppression by drugs and they have been touted since the early 1960s. There are *some* features of EAE that are similar to multiple sclerosis, as discussed above, the second event that occurs after the animals have been injected involves blood vessels. MRI has shown that some of the animals that do not develop symptoms develop another feature seen in patients, known as unidentified bright objects—UBOs.

To account for the disease process that underlies the formation of areas of sclerosis, it is necessary to first determine what may cause damage to blood vessels in small areas of the nervous system, compromising the barrier they form. Actually, the pathological evidence allows us to be more specific about the type of blood vessel involved—they are *veins*. The damage surrounds veins like a sleeve. As the area extends, this relationship is lost with the development of the characteristic scar tissue of sclerosis. Astonishingly, there appears to be only one proper reconstruction of the early lesion (Figure 14.2), and it was published in 1942.[31]

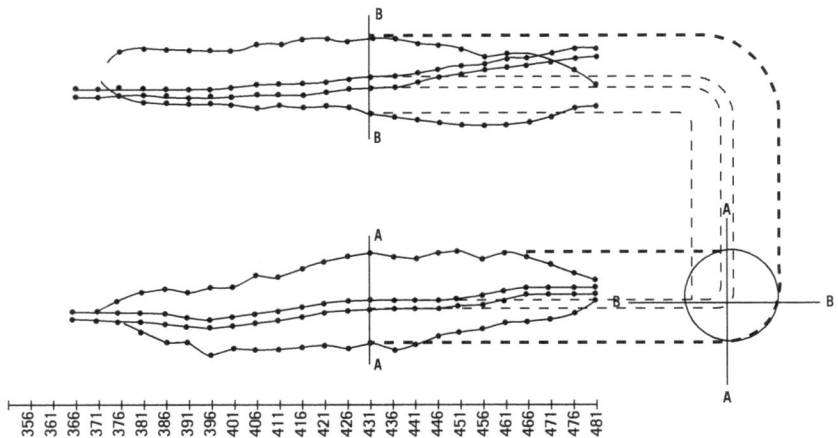

Figure 14.2:
Reconstruction of a multiple sclerosis plaque by Dow and Berglund, 1942.

The sections shown in the next figure illustrates the end and longitudinal views of similar areas of damage in the brain (left) and spinal cord (right).

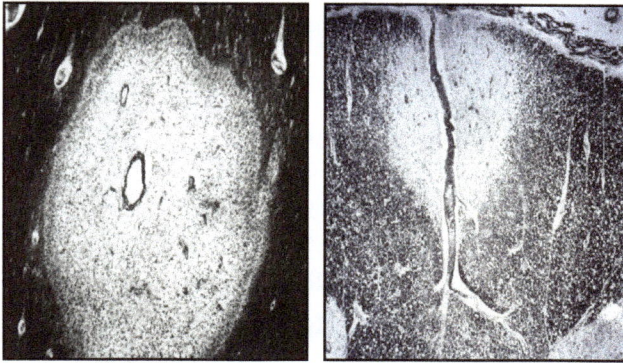

Figure 14.3: Plaques in the brain and spinal cord from patients with multiple sclerosis. (Courtesy of Dr. D.R. Oppenheimer.)

It is perfectly obvious from these pathological sections that the tissue damage *surrounds the vein*, and that the patterns suggest the diffusion of damaging substances from blood. There could not be a more convincing explanation that plaques are due to breakdown of the blood-brain barrier. The evidence of blood-brain barrier failure from the leakage from the blood vessels in the brain readily shown by MRI was actually produced by a much less sophisticated imaging system, using injected isotopes, as long ago as 1965. In the intervening years, it was demonstrated by three more forms of imaging, the last being computed tomography (CT).[32] It is critically important to note that the auto-immune theory offers no explanation *whatsoever for the location* of the typical areas of damage in patients with multiple sclerosis. The development of MRI has continued to provide dramatic confirmation of this relationship to veins in living patients as the strength of the magnetic fields used has increased dramatically,[33] but it has not extended our understanding beyond microscopic studies that date back to 1863.

In the report of the second committee formed in 1984 to revise the diagnostic criteria for multiple sclerosis,[34] chaired by Dr. Charles Poser, there is the report of a relevant case where CT was used.

The second example who would be so diagnosed was described as being a young man who, following an automobile accident, is found to have several contrast-enhancing periventricular lesions on CT scan.

Note that the term "contrast enhancing" refers to leakage of the iodine containing dye used as a highlighter in CT images of the brain. It is *unequivocal* evidence of damage to the blood-brain barrier. Curiously, despite his support for Mr. Dingley's assertion that his symptoms were caused by his injuries, Poser did not refer to this case, which would have provided great support for the allegation that trauma can be involved in multiple sclerosis. Since the time the Poser committee deliberated, CT has largely been replaced by MRI, where the use of another contrast agent, which contains gadolinium, may also show enhancement associated with leakage across the blood-brain barrier. As will be seen in Chapter 16, MRI has revealed even more about the changes in the brain, which can follow trauma in the living patient. Also omitted from consideration by the judges in Mr. Dingley's case was supportive evidence from neuropathology, that has been available for many years, and it is discussed later.

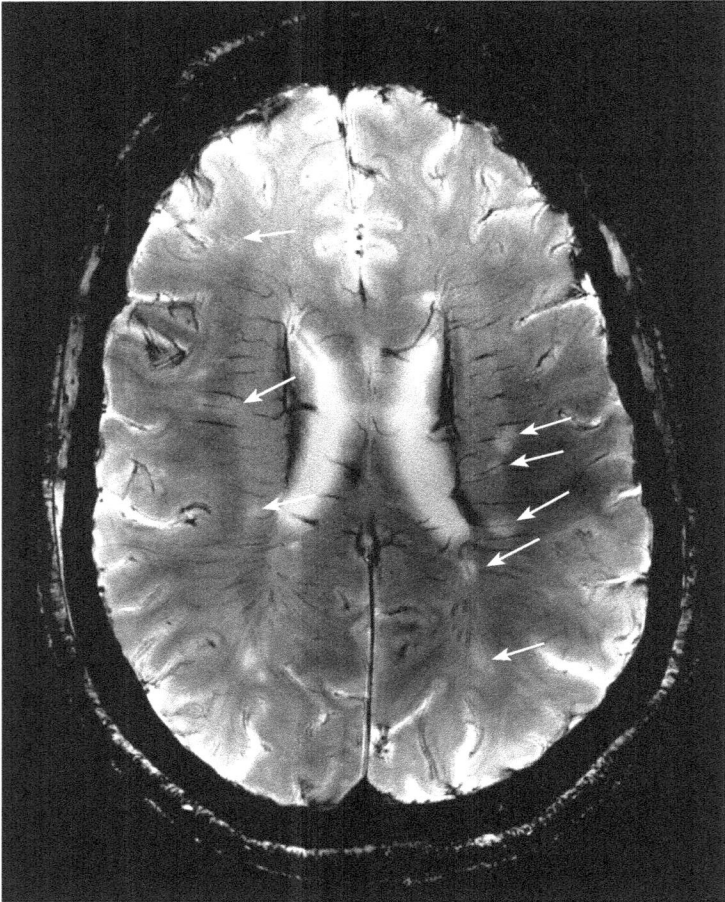

Figure 14.4:
MRI of the brain of a 54- year-old MS patient acquired using a 7 Tesla magnet.
(Courtesy of Dr. Y. Ge.)

The Law Lords were made aware of the importance of the blood-brain barrier in the protection of the sensitive tissues of the nervous system from dangerous components present in blood. Their report states:

The organs of the CNS require to be supplied with various nutrients which are delivered by means of the blood stream. But the brain could be damaged if harmful substances were to be allowed to pass into the brain. A structure exists between the blood and the brain whose function it is to prevent this. It is known as the blood-brain barrier (BBB). It consists of a layer of cells, each of which is opposed to the other by a tight junction.

Although the central importance of blood-brain barrier damage in multiple sclerosis was actually accepted by both sides in the case, it was common ground that the reason for the disruption of the barrier is said to be unknown.

The starting point of Dr. Poser's theory is that trauma may cause alteration of the blood-brain barrier. That is accepted by both Professor Compston and Dr. Sibley. Dr. Poser and Dr. Behan [two of the expert witnesses called by the defendant] would say that the breach of the blood-brain barrier might be at a site remote from trauma. Dr. Poser also points out that the earliest sign of the development of a new plaque which is detectable on MRI scans is indeed an alteration of the blood-brain barrier. As he emphasised, it is not known how alteration in the barrier occurs, or how the substances pass through it . . . While therefore there are doubts about the mechanisms involved, it should be emphasised that the experts who gave evidence all agreed with Dr. Poser that alteration of the blood-brain barrier is the earliest detectable sign of the development of a new plaque.

This is an *extremely* important statement, because standard textbooks rarely draw attention to blood-brain barrier damage in multiple sclerosis and, when they do, give no indication as to how the barrier is damaged. The author suggested in 1989 that multiple sclerosis should be known as "blood-brain barrier disease," awaiting agreement about the cause.[32] However, typical textbook accounts of multiple sclerosis continue to endorse the auto-immune theory, linking it to a still-unknown virus and, of course, genetic susceptibility, and fail to mention the established changes to the blood vessels.

It is not surprising that early investigators thought that multiple sclerosis was due to an infection because the hallmark of the disease is a patch, a discrete area, of *inflammation*. The search for an infective agent began in the late nineteenth century, and by 1908 it was claimed that an organism had finally been demonstrated in multiple sclerosis patients.

It was termed *Insularis spheroidis*, but the evidence was found to be flawed, and eventually the hypothesis was discredited. Since then, much effort has been expended looking for a bacterium or virus, and it is obvious that the absence of a diagnostic test for multiple sclerosis has allowed great freedom for speculation. Some claims have proved embarrassing as, for example, a publication in the *Lancet* in 1979 claiming that an organism had been isolated which, on further investigation, proved to be a laboratory contaminant. New bacteria have been discovered in the last few decades, such as *Legionnella pneumophila, Helicobacter pylori,* and *Borrelia burgdorferi*—in fact, the latter causes an infection of the nervous system. However, there are insurmountable obstacles to the postulation that an infection causes multiple sclerosis, based upon first principles and no bacterium or virus has ever been found, despite an intensive search over the last 100 years. Contrast this with the rapid detection of the virus responsible for AIDS, the human immunodeficiency virus (HIV), and the speed with which the bird flu (H5N1) and swine flu (H1N1) viruses were isolated.

The main argument against multiple sclerosis being a bacterial infection actually derives from the pathology because, as was observed by the pathologist Charles Lumsden[35] in the 1970s, bacteria known to cause infections of the nervous system, for example the spirochaete of syphilis, actually arrest in *capillaries*, before invading the surrounding tissue. In contrast, the damage in multiple sclerosis occurs around veins. No consistent evidence of an infectious agent has ever been found in the surrounding tissue at post-mortem examination or, indeed, when biopsies have been taken from patients during life. The symptoms and some pathological features of nervous system diseases caused by bacteria, such as the spiral bacteria responsible for syphilis and Lyme disease can certainly mimic multiple sclerosis; for example, they may cause the eye nerve condition optic neuritis. However, other clinical features and changes detectable in the blood are used to confirm the presence of the infecting organism. Nevertheless, in 2002 the *Lancet* published a commentary with the surprising title "Bacterial Infections as a Cause of Multiple Sclerosis."[36] It discussed the possibility that *Borrelia burgdorferi*, the causative organism of Lyme disease, may also be one cause of multiple sclerosis. However, it can be stated with certainty that the great majority of multiple sclerosis patients have *not* had any exposure to this organism.

Whether infection with B. burgdorferi is a cause of multiple sclerosis or whether it is merely a result of heightened susceptibility of multiple sclerosis patients to infection due to damage to the blood-brain barrier remains one of the enigmas of multiple sclerosis research. Indeed this caveat applies to all infectious pathogens that have been associated with multiple sclerosis.

> The authors appear to be unaware of Lumsden's powerful arguments ruling out a bacterial cause for multiple sclerosis. It is notable that the authors raised the possibility that infection may highlight pre-existing areas of damage to the blood vessels of the nervous system. There can be little doubt that their observation is true—why else would a barrier be present? They also draw attention to vulnerability of the brain if there is damage to the blood-brain barrier.

Infection is most unlikely to be the cause of a first attack typical of multiple sclerosis, simply because most patients do not feel feverish, or ill, in any way. There is also no evidence that the disease is infectious. However, once a patient has sustained the characteristic areas of damage in the nervous system, infection associated with fever is certainly capable of causing a *relapse*, as most patients will readily confirm. As we have seen, MRI has shown that the initial damage to the blood-brain barrier in multiple sclerosis patients is often silent, and associated with the formation of unidentified bright objects. The onset of neurological symptoms at the time of an infection may then be wrongly interpreted as the initiating event of the disease, because infections are often associated with the generation of fever due to circulating toxins. If the blood-brain barrier is already damaged, the toxins may cross from blood into brain tissue and cause symptoms.

The induction of a fever, simply by using a hot bath, has been shown to cause relapse in patients who have had symptoms typical of multiple sclerosis. There is, obviously, no infection involved. The "hot bath test" was first used in patients suspected to have multiple sclerosis in 1937 in the US. It was promoted as a diagnostic test for those patients where the symptoms and signs had resolved by the time the patient was seen by a specialist. The test, therefore, was devised to allow *objective* evidence to be found to corroborate a patient's story. At the time, a diagnosis of hysteria was common, and patients were often not regarded as reliable witnesses. The symptoms could be provoked by immersion in the hot bath, and normally disappeared when the patient cooled down. However, in 1983, Berger and Sheremata[37] at the University of Miami gave details of four patients in the *Journal of the American Medical Association*, where disabilities induced, unfortunately remained. The last patient they described was a 28-year-old man with a two-year history of difficulty in walking, following an episode of brain inflammation (acute encephalitis), who was suspected of having multiple sclerosis. Initial examination revealed poor vision, a squint, and weakness in his right leg and he was placed in a hot bath.

Whilst in the bath, flaccid quadriparesis (weakness of all four limbs) and visual blurring developed. By the next day, his vision had returned to normal but his weakness persisted during the course of the next week. Subsequently a gradual stepwise deterioration in his gait and lower extremity strength during the ensuing five years resulted in a spastic paraplegia.

Following their experience, Berger and Sheremata issued a plea for caution in its use, but a tepid bath is clearly of no diagnostic value. Equally, it is not possible to predict which patients will recover from the test after being cooled. Fortunately, the test is no longer used because of the availability of other objective methods, especially brain imaging. However, multiple sclerosis patients and those suspected of having the disease should always be warned to avoid exposure to high temperatures. It is not difficult to see how infection has appeared to be a credible mechanism in multiple sclerosis, when neurological symptoms often appear when a patient develops a fever. However, the hot bath test, in producing dilatation of the blood vessels and symptoms without infection, indicates the continuing presence of blood vessel damage—that is, damage to the blood-brain barrier. A high body temperature developed during exercise may also be a factor in relapse.

As we have seen, it is now usual to point out the importance of genetic susceptibility, and many studies have attempted to determine if certain genetic factors are involved in patients with multiple sclerosis. However, genetic factors are obviously involved in some way in *every* disease, simply because susceptibility and our reaction to disease are determined genetically. However, there is an important difference between a genetically *caused* disease, such as haemophilia, and diseases where genetic *susceptibility* plays a part. It would seem absurd at first sight to assert that there is a genetic susceptibility to head injury, but the logic is actually inescapable. Tall parents generally have tall children, because there are genetic factors involved in determining height. The world is designed for people of average height and so, for example, the height of door lintels caters for the majority of people, but not for the few who are significantly taller than normal. Very tall people must bend in order to pass under most door lintels, but if they forget, which is likely at some time, they will bang their heads. The death of a very tall man, also a former diplomat, who purchased an old house with low ceilings and suffered a fatal brain haemorrhage from striking a door lintel, was reported on November 24, 1988 in the UK *Daily Mirror*. The headline read: "Tiny Home Kills Tall Diplomat." This does not, of course, mean that *all* tall people will consistently sustain more head injuries than shorter people, because some will learn to be very careful. It just means that *as a group*, very tall people will bang their heads more frequently than very short people. Despite all the expensive research, genetic studies have not helped in unravelling the mystery of multiple sclerosis—they have simply stated the obvious.

The report of the Law Lords continued,

A key question in the case is whether, and if so in what circumstances, trauma may also alter or open up the BBB so as to allow activated and deranged T-lymphocytes to enter the brain.

There is no evidence that the lymphocytes are deranged in patients with multiple sclerosis; based on the evidence from stroke patients, they are involved in attempts to repair. However, another white blood cell is certainly involved in the attacks typical of multiple sclerosis where the blood-brain barrier fails—the neutrophils. The loss of the protection afforded by this exquisitely constructed barrier is clearly a very serious matter.

Despite the absence of evidence, auto-immunity remains fashionable and, as a consequence, the research using the putative animal model continues to receive very substantial funding. It is particularly bizarre that it still holds centre stage, because it provides no explanation for the *location* of the areas typically affected in patients with multiple sclerosis. For example, it does not attempt to explain why the *optic nerves* are so frequently affected in the condition labelled optic neuritis. It should be noted at this juncture that every known cause of optic neuritis, from syphilis to leukaemia, involves damage to the blood vessels of the nerve.

Today, with investigators obsessed with the molecular pathology, it is rare for autopsy studies of the basic pathology to be undertaken, despite the fact that it is still alleged that little is known about the very first events in the disease. However, a group working in the University of Sydney have examined patients who have died following an acute relapse. They have found that there is no evidence of an initial invasion of the white cells responsible for the immune response; the myelin damage is evident first, and the immune cells then move in to repair the damage. Their paper in 2004[38] questioning the auto-immune concept was so newsworthy that it was covered in a worldwide press release from Reuters (Figure 14.5) and they have continued the research.[39]

As we have seen, a laboratory model is not needed: In marked contrast to the myths and legends of auto-immunity, we have a human model, a well-established cause of UBOs that results from decompression sickness. The areas affected in multiple sclerosis are known to be associated with reduced blood flow and this has recently been reviewed,[40] emphasising the role of inflammation and the hypoxia-inducible protein systems. Despite details of the effects

NEW YORK (Reuters Health)

Findings from an autopsy study by Australian researchers question the theory of multiple sclerosis (MS) that holds that an auto-immune attack on myelin is the inciting event for the disease. Instead, it appears that myelin-producing cells die first and then immune cells show up to clear out these dead cells and their myelin, lead author Dr. John W. Prineas, from the University of Sydney, said in a statement.

- The results, which are reported in the February 23rd online issue of the *Annals of Neurology,* are based on the clinical and pathologic findings noted in 12 patients with relapsing and remitting MS who died during or soon after a relapse episode.

- In seven of the cases, the researchers observed pathologic changes that had not previously been observed in newly formed multiple sclerosis lesions. Specifically, the lesions showed extensive oligodendrocyte apoptosis and microglial activation, but little or no lymphocytes or myelin phagocytes.

- The authors believe that the current findings could have a profound impact on MS research, which is largely focused on determining why the immune system attacks myelin.

- "The important point, at this stage of our investigation, seems to be that we have no laboratory model for this sort of pathology," Dr. Prineas said.

Figure 14.5:
Reuters press release featuring the 2004 paper from the University of Sydney.

of lack of oxygen, there is no mention of giving more when there is simply no substitute. Hyperbaric oxygen treatment as used for decompression sickness is effective in both preventing and treating animals affected by EAE, and in treating patients with multiple sclerosis. The evidence is discussed in Chapter 17.

It is time to return to Mr. Dingley's appeal: The judges were not made aware of an important condition that every doctor should know from their basic training in pathology. They should have been told that the brain *can* be damaged by a remote injury—it is called fat *embolism* and the condition can actually be seen in the eye.

CHAPTER 15

Evidence Overlooked, but "The Eyes Have It"

Scholars who with all this written and practical evidence before them chose to see none of it; their learning seemed like a bandage round their eyes.

A Short History of the Gout and the Rheumatic Diseases.
WSC Copeman, 1964.

It will be recalled that Mr. Dingley's problems with his eyesight were noticed by his wife and by the colleague he drove to work within a few days of his accident, although there is no reference to it being investigated by the neurologist who first examined him. However, in the Court of Session hearing for the Reclaiming Motion, the counsel acting for the Chief Constable of Strathclyde, the defendant, was at first keen to establish that the symptoms occurred sometime *after* the weakness of his leg. This raises some uncomfortable questions about the legal process, and the language used belongs to a different age.

It is plain that, at the time when this evidence was being led, counsel for the defender was concerned to suggest that the pursuer's [Mr. Dingley's] eye trouble had occurred much later, perhaps months after the accident. His cross-examination was framed accordingly.

When it became apparent that the eye trouble occurred within a few days, the counsel suddenly realised that the information may be useful to his case because he thought that the visual symptoms could not be attributed to the whiplash injury. The expert witness's support for Mr. Dingley rested on establishing a connection between his symptoms and spinal cord damage caused by the whiplash.

At some later point in the proceedings, however, counsel for the defender became aware that there was another possible line of approach, viz that the eye trouble had occurred shortly after the accident and was indeed due to MS, but that the base showed that the first symptom of the pursuers was not associated with the spinal cord and could not therefore be associated with any damage to the cord in the accident. The late change of front meant, however, that the exact nature of the pursuer's eye trouble was not established.

The visual problems suffered by Mr. Dingley were simply not included in the examination of the evidence; indeed, it is not clear if they were investigated at all. The implication was that they were simply not important. One of the expert witnesses stated that he could not even be sure if the symptoms were those typical of multiple sclerosis. The judges would not, of course, have been aware that a disturbance of vision is the first symptom in a third of patients who are eventually told they have multiple sclerosis.[1] The matter was, therefore, quietly dropped which was, to say the least, reprehensible. Why are the effects on the eye so important? It is because they can solve the central question in multiple sclerosis already raised in Chapter 14: Is it a disease of the blood vessels, or of the tissues of the nervous system? The disturbance of vision is most commonly due to inflammation of the optic nerve and so is known as optic neuritis,[2] but the disease process often involves the retina.

Unlike the rest of the nervous system, the nerve tissue of the retina and the blood vessels that supply it can be seen through the pupil using an ophthalmoscope. They can also be photographed through the pupil. Figure 15.1 shows the wonderful array of blood vessels that allows us to see the world around us. A branch of the single artery supplying the eye, the ophthalmic artery, passes into the centre of the optic nerve as the central retinal artery. It emerges into the globe of the eye through the optic disc. The arteries that branch from the central retinal artery supply the capillaries in the quadrants of the hemisphere. The capillaries drain into veins, which then unite to form the central retinal vein, which leaves the globe through the optic disc.

Changes in vision are, of course, easily noticed because we observe events through our eyes. It is little known that hearing loss also occurs in patients who develop multiple sclerosis,[3,4] and it is due to inflammation in the

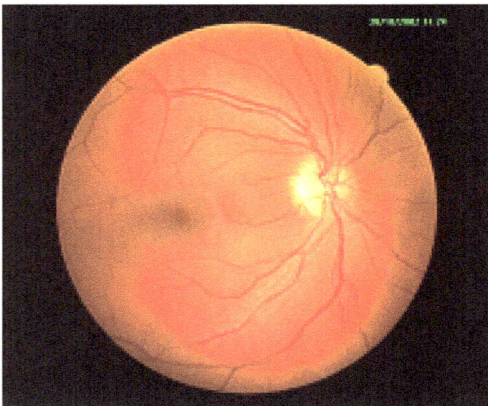

Figure 15.1:
The blood vessels of the retina of a normal human eye.
(Courtesy of Dr. John Ellis.)

cochlea.[5] A reduction in hearing, or mild weakness of the power of muscles, say in an arm or leg, is more easily overlooked by patients than a disturbance of eyesight. Sudden deafness may immediately follow cardiac surgery and is most likely due to embolism.[6] Unfortunately, the complications that affect the eye in patients with multiple sclerosis are rarely discussed in textbooks of neurology. This is because patients with eye problems are usually referred to ophthalmologists, rather than neurologists. To conduct a detailed examination of the retina it is necessary to use drops to dilate the pupil, which is a task routinely undertaken by ophthalmologists. This is yet another example of the problems created by the fragmentation of medicine into specialties.

The eyes are isolated spherical capsules held in the bony orbits of the skull by the muscles responsible for their movement. The eyeballs are not physically connected; their synchronised movement is coordinated by nerves which have their control centres in the brain stem. The accuracy of this control is truly astonishing; even a tiny deviation from synchrony results in double vision. The eye may be damaged by an object penetrating the globe; for example, a high velocity metal fragment, or by infectious agents, such as viruses or bacteria, which are delivered via the blood supply. The globe of the eye is a strong capsule, known as the sclera, which is continuous with the cornea, the transparent tissue in front of the iris and pupil, which is itself covered by a very thin membrane, the conjunctiva. The optic nerves join together forming the optic chiasm, and the nerves transmit the impulses created by the photoreceptors of the retina, to the grey matter at the back of the brain, known as the occipital cortex. It is here that the nerve impulses are processed and perceived as images, but it must be remembered that the brain can produce images without the input from our eyes—they form our dreams.

The image formed on the retina is actually upside down, and the images we perceive are constructed by the brain based on logging our surroundings using faculties like touch. There is obviously no film screen at the back of the brain in the occipital cortex! In a famous experiment, a subject wore specially constructed binoculars that turned the images seen by the eye upside down. The subject wore them every day. At first he had great problems, for example in reaching up for objects that were in fact down. However, at the end of 10 days the brain had learned to reverse the image perceived so that objects and his environment appeared the correct way up. When he removed the binoculars, he again saw everything upside down and went through the same uncomfortable period until the brain was able to reverse the image again. This inversion can actually be produced by damage to the visual tracts in the mid-brain from swelling involving the basal ganglia.[7] Perception of shape and form can be processed in other areas of the brain, an example of what is strangely called plasticity, a term that seems to have been introduced by the late Dr. Paul Bach-y-Rita. In a groundbreaking, but little known experiment published in 1967,[8] he used the image from a camera to produce signals to activate multiple stimulators placed in a grid on the back of six blind subjects. They learned to perceive objects and even recognised Twiggy, a model famous in the 1970s. Given the advances made in micro-electronics over the last 40 years, it is time for this work to be revisited.

It is necessary to know the basic anatomy of the blood supply to the eye and the optic nerve to understand the conditions that often affect patients with multiple sclerosis. Visual problems can be the result of damage to the eyes, to the optic nerves, or to the grey matter of the occipital cortex of the brain's hemispheres. Damage to the centres in the brainstem that control the muscles can lead to double vision. The arteries supplying the optic nerves and the eyes are known as the ophthalmic arteries. They are derived from branches of the internal carotid arteries, whereas the posterior cerebral arteries supply the imaging processing area at the rear of the brain. They are derived from the basilar artery, which is formed by the connection of the two vertebral arteries. The basilar artery supplies the brainstem and the organ of coordination and balance, the cerebellum. The right carotid artery derives from the brachiocephalic artery, which arises from the arch of the aorta. After passing through the base of the skull, the internal carotid artery curves around the outer margin of the sella turcica, (the "Turkish saddle") where the pituitary gland is located. On the apex of its turn through about 180 degrees, the carotid artery gives off a branch, the *ophthalmic artery*. This relationship is similar to that of the brachiocephalic artery, which is the first artery on the curve of the aortic arch. In both situations there are important implications for blood flow, because it is known that they are preferred pathways for any small particulate matter—that is, micro-emboli present in blood.[9] The ophthalmic arteries are very unusual because they not only supply blood to the optic nerves and the connection that exists between them, known as the optic chiasm, they continue on to supply the tissue of the choroid behind the retina and finally the tissues of the retina itself. The blood supply to the choroid is actually many times greater than that of the retina, through large diameter vessels, which ensures that a constant supply of oxygen is available for diffusion even if a branch of an artery in the retina is blocked.

In order to access the globe of the eye and the retina, the ophthalmic artery has to enter the optic nerve and pass down the centre of the nerve in order to emerge through the optic disc. The branches that provide the nutrition for the beginning of the optic nerve arise before the artery enters the nerve, but the part of the nerve immediately behind the eye is supplied from internal branches of the artery after it has actually entered the nerve itself. The ophthalmic artery emerges through the optic disc at the back of the eye to become the central retinal artery, and it usually divides into four branches to supply the hemisphere of the retina. The retinal blood supply to each eye derives, therefore, from a single artery, which emerges from the centre of the optic nerve at the optic nerve head and then branches over the surface of the retina to supply each quadrant.

> Four conditions may affect the eye itself in multiple sclerosis that relate to structures within the globe of the eye. In all four, localised inflammation is present which is, as usual, denoted by the suffix "itis" and they are *papillitis, iritis, uveitis,* and *retinal periphlebitis.*[2] Each may occur in one, or in both eyes as an isolated condition. As myelin is not present in any location within the eye, these conditions provide further evidence that the changes in blood vessels are the first event in the disease that underlies multiple sclerosis. Even more compelling is the fact that they occur in many other conditions where the agent responsible is spread in the blood supply, as for example, in cancer. Papillitis is a swelling of the optic disc area of the retina where the nerve fibres fan out across the retina. It is usually associated with inflammation and swelling of the section of the optic nerve immediately behind the globe of the eye, sometimes called retrobulbar neuritis. Inflammation of the optic nerve itself appears to be more common than the inflammatory conditions occurring within the eye or, at least, it is reported more frequently in patients with multiple sclerosis.

Evidence of optic neuritis can be found using nerve conduction studies in about half of multiple sclerosis patients,[2] and MRI has confirmed that it is very common: The question is why. Optic neuritis is often associated with significant swelling of the optic nerve, which may become so enlarged as to fill the hole in the bony skull, known as the optic foramen, through which the nerve passes out of the skull to the eye socket. The terms "optic" and "neuritis" simply describe inflammation of the optic nerve, and so like multiple and sclerosis—are not a diagnosis; they are yet another label. The patient may then feel pain when looking from side to side, and pain is also felt if pressure is exerted on the eyeball. In some patients, the severity of the pain has required surgery to *decompress* the optic nerve by opening the aperture in the bone. The eyes move over a considerable arc, which means that the optic nerves move slightly in the hole in the skull they pass through in the socket of the skull known as the orbit. The nerves are covered by membranes, which are the extension of the membranes that cover the brain and spinal cord, known as the meninges. They are liberally supplied with pain nerve endings, and so inflammation of the optic nerve is usually associated with pain. If the segment of the optic nerve within the bony aperture of the socket swells, it may occupy the whole of the available space. The pressure in the nerve will then rise because it is trapped. This inevitably reduces the blood supply and also, of course, oxygen delivery, causing the blood vessels to try to open more widely. The blood vessels leak causing further swelling and thereby create a vicious cycle. Any movement of the eye causes pain, which triggers more inflammation. Steroids are frequently prescribed for optic neuritis, which may help by limiting the permeability of the blood vessels, relieving inflammation, allowing the swelling and pain to subside.[10]

The most common cause of inflammation is infection, and infection *external* to the nerve may cause optic neuritis. For example, infection of the sinuses may spread to include the surrounding bone and soft tissue of the eye socket and the optic foramen. The inflammation causes the optic nerve to swell, which is limited by the surrounding bone and the nerve fibres become compressed. External tumours may also cause compression. In all these examples, the symptoms may be much the same as in the optic neuritis of multiple sclerosis with patients complaining of blurring of vision and eye discomfort on moving the eye. On rare occasions, optic neuritis may be associated with viral infections, such as varicella, the virus responsible for chickenpox and shingles. Bacterial infections may also be responsible for the condition. For example, both tuberculosis[11] and syphilis[12] may produce optic neuritis, although they are now rare causes of the condition in the developed world. The lodging of such bacteria in capillaries is not generally viewed as embolism, but the mechanism is essentially the same because they are foreign particles carried in blood.

However, inflammation can also occur without infection and, logically, it is then called *aseptic* inflammation. Direct trauma is an important cause of inflammation and, as discussed, micro-emboli such as bubbles may cause inflammation internally by damaging the lining of the blood vessels. Cancer cells are carried in the blood and may cause optic neuritis[13,14] as they do in leukaemia where cells have actually been found blocking a vessel in the optic nerve.[15] Cancer cells may also cause both iritis and uveitis, as may bubbles in decompression sickness,[16] reinforcing the link between small emboli and multiple sclerosis. Unique confirmation of this has come from cardiac surgery.

Optic neuritis occurs in 10% of patients who have been connected to a heart-lung machine for heart surgery.[17] Cardiac bypass, as it is known, is associated with micro-embolism from a variety of particles, from marrow and fat released by splitting the sternum to open the chest, to plastic debris from the tubing used in the blood pumps. Emboli have been visualised during cardiac surgery using heart bypass machines[18] and some patients suffer loss of hearing.[19] Most importantly, patients who have been investigated by MRI immediately following cardiac surgery have been found to have UBOs in the mid-brain.[20] The changes in the mid-brain after cardiac surgery in children—evident by an increase in the size of the ventricles in the hemispheres due to loss of the myelin sheaths, have been followed by CT[21] and found to be reversible. This is powerful evidence that dramatic recovery from brain damage can occur, especially in children, because, of course, they are still growing.

Optic neuritis may also be caused by particles breaking off the fatty deposits that can accumulate in the carotid arteries in the neck in older people and clots.[22] It is then called ischaemic optic neuritis, which means that it is recognised to be associated with a reduction of blood flow. This very remarkable story of a patient with this problem begins and ends with episodes of loss of consciousness, both of which were immediately preceded by an extraordinary out-of-body experience.

> *Mr. X had his first episode at the age of 50. One morning when he was just about to leave the house to drive to work, he suddenly felt himself floating up to the ceiling and watched his body crumpling onto the hall floor before everything went black as he lost consciousness. He woke up with his family doctor at the foot of his bed who was unable to find a cause for the blackout, and referred the bemused patient to hospital. The investigations proved negative, and seven years passed until the next event.*
>
> *It was a Friday afternoon, and Mr. X noticed on looking up that his wall calendar seemed somewhat incomplete. Closing his left eye, he realised that his right eye was completely blind, with not so much as a glimmer of light visible. As he had been treated some months before for mild glaucoma and had an outpatient appointment the following Monday, unperturbed, he went home to rest and eventually to bed. On waking the next morning he was somewhat relieved to be aware of a little light with the affected eye and, as there was no pain, he saw no reason to bother his doctor. The eye specialist who saw him on the Monday was unable to see any reason for the loss of vision, but recommended an urgent consultation with a general physician. This was arranged through the family doctor, and Mr. X was fortunate enough to be seen that afternoon. Examination of the right side of his neck revealed the characteristic noise, called a bruit, associated with partial blockage of the artery. An appointment was made for him to be admitted to hospital later in the week for further investigations.*

On the Wednesday afternoon he was at home watching a television programme about Africa using, of course, his good right eye. It featured a spectacular sunrise and as the flaming orange globe rose on the screen, Mr. X experienced a blinding flash of light in his good eye and realised to his consternation that he had now gone completely blind. An urgent phone call was made to his hospital consultant who, rather surprisingly, felt able to reassure Mr. X that all would be well and reminded him that in any case, he was due to be seen in hospital in two days' time! The consultant even agreed that tickets bought for a performance at the local amateur operatic company that evening should not be wasted. The patient attended the performance and enjoyed the music despite being only aware of a dim kaleidoscope of colours.

Subsequent investigation in the hospital confirmed the presence of obstructions in both his carotid arteries, and operations to clear the debris were undertaken over the following months. By this time, his vision was steadily improving. The patient, anxious to go on holiday, was reassured that he could go and "would be fine." However, the morning after arriving at the resort Mr. X, about to get into the shower, again found himself floating up to the ceiling and observed his body crumpling to the floor before he lost consciousness. Waking up some 12 hours later, none the worse for the experience, he carried on with his holiday waiting to report the incident until he returned home. Further investigations showed that the artery in the right side of the neck was completely blocked.

The loss of vision was caused by an identical event in each eye. On both occasions, tiny particles of material from the fatty deposits in the carotid arteries had flowed into the ophthalmic artery blocking most, but fortunately not all, of the blood supply to the eye. Enough blood, or at least plasma, continued to flow to prevent death of the tissues of the eyes, but not enough oxygen reached the retina to allow vision. Almost certainly the particles of fatty material had stopped where the branch of the ophthalmic artery, which forms the central retinal artery, enters the optic nerve. It is arrowed in Figure 15.2.

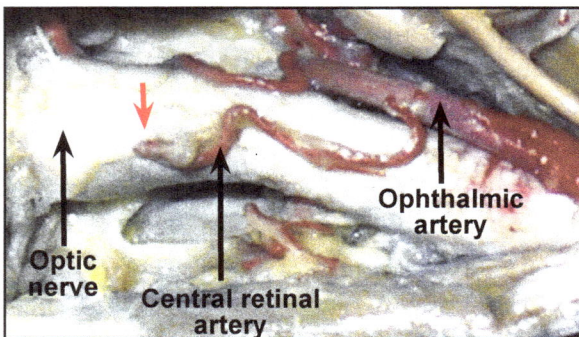

Figure 15.2: Diagram drawn from a dissection showing the ophthalmic artery and the central retinal artery which enters the optic nerve (red arrow). (Redrawn from Kocabiyik N. et al., 2009 Turkey.)

The central artery of the retina is an *end artery* just over half a millimetre in diameter. To have a critical sense such as sight reliant on such a small blood vessel would seem rather cavalier, but we have two eyes and can manage very well with just one. However, there is a very special arrangement that undoubtedly came into play in Mr. X's situation. Behind the retina is a zone of the globe of the eye, which has a much larger blood supply—estimated to be about 200 times that of the retina. It is called the *choroidal plexus* and acts as a reservoir of oxygen to support the supply of the retinal arteries, especially for the macula, which is the area where the maximum visual acuity is needed. It is said to provide about half of the oxygen needed for sight. Fortunately, Mr. X's eyesight was almost completely restored, because most of the nerve cells in the retina did not die. This means that they had enough oxygen to survive, but not enough to function and allow sight. In time, flow was restored in the retinal artery as the material causing the obstruction would eventually have been removed. By increasing the dissolved oxygen content of blood under hyperbaric conditions, vision can be restored in patients who have a blockage of the central retinal artery at the point where it enters the optic nerve. If the blockage is due to a clot, this can extend the window of opportunity for vision to be restored by using a *thrombolytic*, a clot-busting agent. This principle can also apply to the brain itself, and will be discussed in more detail in Chapter 20.

These events, as we shall see, together with other causes of optic neuritis, occur because the hydraulics of the internal carotid artery allows material carried in the blood vessels to enter the ophthalmic artery and reduce the blood supply. The symptoms may be caused in two ways: either the material lodges in the artery, or it damages the wall of the vessel and leakage then causes the nerve to swell. Excluding local traumatic injury, tumours and bone infections, *every* identified cause of optic neuritis involves emboli carried in the blood supply and, as discussed earlier, this includes bacteria like *Treponema pallidum*, which is responsible for syphilis and the spirochaete, *Borrelia burgdorferi*, which causes Lyme disease. Of course, in the days before antibiotics when bacterial infections often spread throughout the body, the dissemination of bacteria in the blood was in the forefront of medical consciousness, and this included the infection responsible for childbed fever.

When the many known causes of optic neuritis have been excluded it is clear that, in the great majority of patients (at least in the Western world), attacks of optic neuritis are *not* associated with an infection. Nevertheless, the local symptoms of inflammation, with discomfort on eye movement and impairment of vision in multiple sclerosis patients are much the same as those from other clearly identified causes. Use of the term *local* raises the question of *distant* factors, because when optic neuritis is associated with more generalised diseases, like tuberculosis, syphilis, and septicaemia, the patient is usually ill, or at least has other symptoms which allow a diagnosis to be made.

Patients with optic neuritis typically notice some blurring of vision, often with some loss of part of the field of vision. The eye may be tender to touch and often painful on movement. A disturbance of colour vision is common, but may not be noticed by the patient. This is, like so many textbook descriptions, a generalisation, because the optic nerve may be found to be damaged by using special tests in patients described as having multiple sclerosis who have never suffered the typical symptoms of optic neuritis. In other words, the other symptoms developed by the patient have been more noticeable, whereas the damage to the optic nerve has been silent. The damage to the myelin sheaths of the optic nerves themselves can be detected by delays in visual evoked response testing. A light is shone into the eye, and the time interval measured when the response can be detected at the occipital cortex at the rear of the brain. At the other end of the disease spectrum, there are patients who have an attack of optic neuritis so devastating that they lose the sight of the eye permanently. The author recalls a young man in his twenties who had two such attacks and was left totally blind—nothing emphasises more the critical need for immediate treatment. The tremendous range of both the pathological changes and clinical effects in multiple sclerosis is not just seen in the patches of damage which occur in the optic nerve—other sites in the nervous system affected in patients with the disease may show a similar spectrum. However, the answer to the central question in multiple sclerosis can be seen in the eye—the veins of the retina may become inflamed. It is known as retinal periphlebitis, which is translated as "inflammation around veins of the retina" and it is also detailed in the book *Optic Neuritis*.[2] The text provides a fascinating insight into the conflict between fact and fiction and the beliefs that have arisen in multiple sclerosis. A chapter by the late Professor Ian McDonald discusses the changes in the retinal veins in multiple sclerosis and stated that:

> *It seems likely that the retinal vascular changes are the visible manifestations of the pathological process which occurs in the white matter of the optic nerve in optic neuritis and elsewhere in the central nervous system in multiple sclerosis.*

He continued with this astonishingly controversial statement which confirms that the changes in the blood vessels in multiple sclerosis come first and are not secondary to auto-immune attack on myelin. There is no myelin in the retina.

The retinal nerve fibres are, of course, unmyelinated. The occurrence of vascular lesions provides support for the view that the vascular changes are primary, not (as some have suggested) secondary to myelin breakdown.

The phrase "provides support for the blood vessel changes" should read, "shows conclusively," but it is very rare to see such firm language used in medical texts. It is also curious that the phrase "as some have suggested" is in brackets, because the belief that loss of myelin, that is, myelin breakdown, is the first event in multiple sclerosis has dominated neurological thinking for the last 70 years; so "some" is the vast majority of clinicians. McDonald also muses as to whether an attack involving the optic nerves followed after a month by changes in the retinal veins would allow a diagnosis of multiple sclerosis because it would meet the requirement imposed for dissemination in time. There could not be a better example of the mindset that has benighted the field of multiple sclerosis.

At least 25% of patients who are eventually told they have multiple sclerosis at some time develop inflammation of the veins of the retina.[23,24] The sequence of three images shown in Figure 15.3 from a patient, show the arterial, capillary, and venous phases of a fluorescein angiogram. The dye fluoresces—that is, it produces visible light when irradiated with ultraviolet light. It is injected into a vein in the arm and flows to the heart and through the lungs to reach the arterial circulation of the eye. It first fills the blood vessels of the dense network of blood vessels behind the retina, known as the choroid *plexus*, and then the dye fills the arteries of the retina.

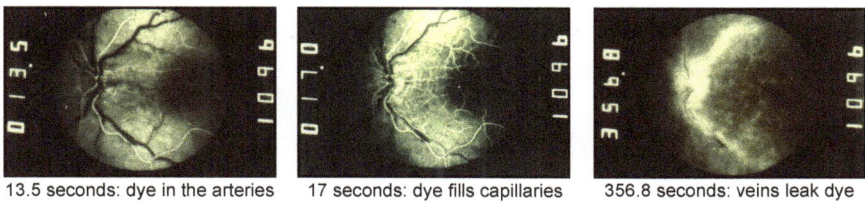

13.5 seconds: dye in the arteries   17 seconds: dye fills capillaries   356.8 seconds: veins leak dye
Figure 15.3:
The eye of a patient with retinal periphlebitis. (Courtesy Dr. W. Haining.)

The first picture timed at 13.5 seconds after injection of the dye into an arm vein shows the arteries. The dye then passes through into the capillary bed as shown in the second frame at 17 seconds. Finally, the third frame timed at 356.8 seconds shows the dye is leaving the retina via the veins. Fluorescein, being a large molecule which binds to the proteins present in blood, should not leak out into the tissues, but the leakage from the veins can be clearly seen and is arrowed. Some red blood cells have also escaped—a small haemorrhage. A film of embolism in the eye of a patient with intermittent

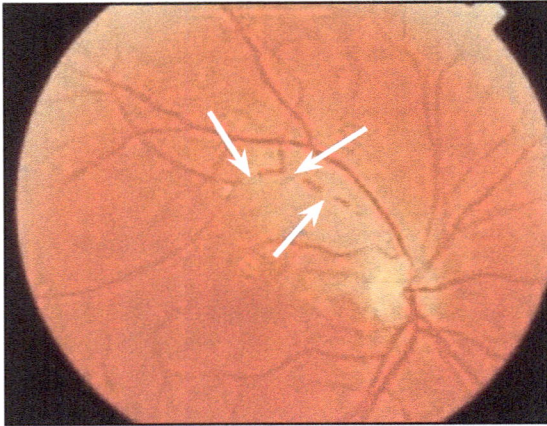

Figure 15.4
Emboli in a retinal artery.
(Redrawn from Wijman CA,
Babikian VI, Matjocha ICA
2000.)

disturbances of vision was made in 1967 by Dr. William Haining, who was on a sabbatical to Yale University from Dundee Royal Infirmary.[25] Figure 15.4 is a photograph of multiple emboli in an artery in the retina, showing the preference for emboli to enter one branch.[26]

What this data from direct observation of the eye provides is a *proof of principle* for micro-embolism. Despite being a major factor in a host of diseases, it has yet to be recognised in medicine, and it dictates the need for using oxygen in treatment. It is most important to recognise that exactly the same sequence of events begins the formation of one or more areas of sclerosis in the brain or the spinal cord and it has been shown by MRI. So research has demonstrated how the damage that surrounds veins is produced, beginning with the work of Haldane investigating bubbles in divers. It has solved the critical question in multiple sclerosis first posed in the 1860s; multiple sclerosis is a blood vessel and not a tissue disease and the evidence that, in most patients, it is due to micro-embolism is overwhelming. As long ago as 1947, changes in vision were investigated by Franklin and Brickner,[26,27] who were aware of the work on blood vessels by Putnam in the 1930s.[28] They pointed out that patients need to be asked about visual symptoms because they are usually mild often lasting for only a few minutes. The question raised is: How can trauma possibly be linked to blood vessel damage in the eye and the nervous system? The answer is by a "mechanism," ironically first described in the 1860s—fat embolism. The emboli can be seen in the blood vessels of the eye of patients, and may damage the retina.[29] Fat embolism can result from the simple bruising suffered by Mr. Dingley in his accident and trauma may cause multiple sclerosis.

CHAPTER 16

Trauma *May* Cause Multiple Sclerosis

There is no proof of what causes multiple sclerosis, but it is common ground that trauma never causes the disease.

The Law Lords, 2000

This dogmatic statement from the Final Judgment in the case of Dingley v. the Chief Constable of Strathclyde contains a startling contradiction, and it should have been obvious to sharp legal minds. It is simply this; if, as stated, there is no proof of what causes multiple sclerosis, how is it possible for experts to be *so certain* that trauma is not involved? As will be seen, published evidence indicates that trauma can indeed cause multiple sclerosis and is probably responsible for most cases, but even the expert witnesses who supported Mr. Dingley's claim failed to convince the judges that an injury may exacerbate the symptoms of patients already affected by the disease. If Mr. Dingley had sustained a fractured skull, or a dislocation of his neck, such a link would have appeared more plausible. As the vehicle had turned over it is very likely that he had banged his head and so may have sustained a "mild" head injury, and a laceration of the scalp was found when he was examined in hospital. He had also reported that his neck was sore from a whiplash injury. But the judges were also not told that MRI has shown that mild head trauma without loss of consciousness may cause the changes in the brain already referred to as UBOs—unidentified bright objects. It is ironic, in view of Mr. Dingley's accident being in Glasgow, that the first report of these MRI findings in mild head injury was in 1986 from neurosurgeons at the Southern General Hospital in the city.[1]

In 1997, the *Lancet* published an MRI study of players of contact sports which showed that many had UBOs and the authors suggested that they were caused in footballers by the trauma involved in heading the ball.[2] As these changes are part of the range of abnormalities seen using MRI in multiple sclerosis patients, then a link to trauma, including head injury, would seem likely. However, the central nervous system also includes the spinal cord, but, for technical reasons it is rarely imaged. There are mounting concerns about head trauma in the National Football League in the US with players suffering problems often years after retirement. In 2012, The NFL awarded a group of retired players who were pursuing a class action $765 million but without admitting liability. The question raised is then obvious: What causes the UBOs seen on MRI after trauma?

Mr. Dingley also sustained the inevitable bruising from such accidents, but none of the expert witnesses suggested that simple bruising may be associated with brain damage. But suggesting that such injuries may initiate the events that lead to multiple sclerosis raises a second and obvious question: Why would the symptoms be delayed? Clearly the longer such a delay, the less likely a connection would seem likely or, indeed, possible. With no evidence available to the Law Lords linking any of the injuries sustained by Mr. Dingley to the onset of multiple sclerosis, their decision was inevitable. The final judgment came 10 long years after Mr. Dingley's fateful accident; their conclusion was that "on the balance of probabilities" that trauma could not have been involved in the development of his multiple sclerosis. They were wrong.

Only the neurologist involved in Mr. Dingley's diagnosis in 1991 and Lord Dawson, who presided over the first hearing in 1996, felt that, despite his injuries being regarded as minor, they could have caused him to develop multiple sclerosis; in other words, that it was more than a coincidence. However, even the two expert witnesses who supported a link in the reclaiming motion failed to mention the possibility of fibrocartilagenous embolism as discussed in Chapter 13. MRI has now shown that there is a *subacute* version of this condition and it may also involve the spinal cord.[3] Moreover, these cases confirm that there may be a latent interval between the release of the fibrocartilage into the circulation after the injury to the spinal disc, and the onset of symptoms. The symptoms may also be, at least, partly reversible.[4] This delay is well known to be associated with the passage of material through the capillaries of the lungs. Nevertheless, it is very unlikely that Mr. Dingley had this form of embolism, as fibrocartilagenous debris contains solid material which tends to block arteries and cause the death of tissue. Also, the symptoms usually appear more suddenly; his illness developed gradually with only the disturbance of vision appearing in the first few days and the weakness of his leg over two weeks later. Nevertheless, many patients with multiple sclerosis do report the abrupt onset of their symptoms, although it is often disregarded in taking a medical history. An indication of the unreality that surrounds the disease is evident in this statement by an eminent neurologist: "The symptoms of multiple sclerosis provide no clue as to its pathogenesis," which is obviously true if the details are ignored!

All the expert witnesses agreed that Mr. Dingley had suffered a whiplash injury and no one doubted that he had sustained a head injury with a scalp wound and he also had considerable bruising. However, none of the expert witnesses suggested that *bruising* could have been in any way responsible for

Mr. Dingley's symptoms. Imagine the consternation of the judges, having reached their verdict, becoming aware that a simple bruise may cause damage to the brain, which may be so severe as to kill the patient. Their discomfort would be compounded if they had also been told that the first account was published as long ago as the 1860s and that the details are in *every* textbook of pathology. A bruise is caused by trauma damaging the tissues in and under the skin, and it is always accompanied by tearing of blood vessels. The rupture of tissues not only causes bleeding, it may also allow the debris of fat and other damaged cells to be squeezed into veins thus becoming emboli. It is, in fact, common to find such material, including fat, trapped in the lungs at routine autopsy if they are examined microscopically. The emboli follow the route taken by bubbles in divers detailed by Haldane, that is, from the veins to the right side of the heart to be, hopefully, trapped in the lungs. Note that the disruption of tissues by gas in the tissues of divers may cause fat droplets as well as gas bubbles to enter the circulation.

Figure 16.1 shows fat trapped in the capillaries of the lung. As already discussed, entrapment may sometimes fail to stop material, including bubbles, from the blood flowing through the lungs, and so emboli are allowed to reach the arteries of the left side of the circulation, which includes those supplying the brain and spinal cord.

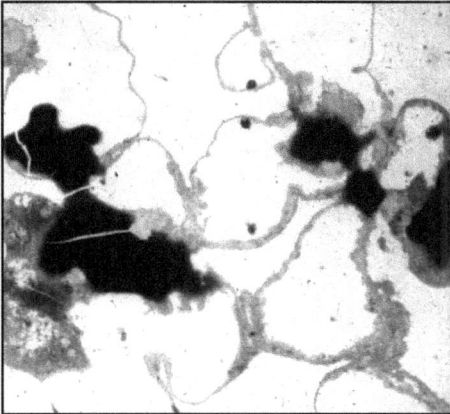

Figure 16.1:
Fat trapped in the capillaries of the lung.
(Courtesy of the late R. Alistair Bennet.)

Sometimes such emboli may also enter the left side of the circulation through a hole in the heart, a defect between the right and left atria. As we have seen, most of these defects are due to the persistence of the hole, known as the foramen ovale which allows blood to bypass the lungs during life in the womb. If it does not close after birth, then some blood may pass through in the wrong direction from the right atrium to the left and it may carry emboli which may reach the brain. It is known as paradoxical embolism and is a risk factor in diving and aviation. Normally, because the pressure in the left atrium is higher than the right, blood moves through such a hole from left to right. Other types of defect may occur in the wall separating the two atria, but the net effect is the same. As about 25% of the "normal" population have either an obvious hole, or an atrial flap that can open, it is clear that paradoxical embolism to the brain is likely to be much more common than currently recognised. Fat,[5,6] or any other small emboli, such as bacteria, or even cancer cells,[7,8] present in blood reaching the right side of the heart may travel to the brain via such a hole in the heart, just as bubbles do in divers and aviators with the same problem.[9] As debris is routinely found trapped in the lungs at post-mortem examination it makes sense to question if it may, on rare occasions, embolise the spinal cord, and also if some patients with multiple sclerosis actually have a hole in the heart. A 39-year-old nurse with a history of migraines was seen in a neurology department after colleagues noted she was strangely subdued and was unable to recall her home address. Her symptoms had begun with a headache on waking 48 hours earlier and, astonishingly, her vision "flipped" 180 degrees for several hours, which had happened 12 years before. MRI showed symmetrical areas of damage in the mid-brain in each hemisphere (thalamus). It was found that she had a large hole between the atria of her heart.[10] Micro emboli are well known to be a cause of migraine headaches.

But there is another dimension to fat embolism; unlike bubbles, fat may be broken down by enzymes present in the lining of the blood vessels to release fatty acids, which may be highly toxic. The fatty acids released from body fat represent the spectrum of fats in our diet, introducing yet another variable into an already complex story.[11] These emboli can not only open the blood-brain barrier, there is a subacute presentation in the barrier that may be permanently damaged[12,13] and areas of loss of myelin sheaths may also occur;[14] these features are obviously typical of the areas affected in patients with multiple sclerosis and Appendix 2 lists the pathologists who have made the connection to the disease. Fat embolism, like bubble embolism, is well established as a mechanism by which remote injury can cause brain damage and is a much better fit to Mr. Dingley's symptoms than fibrocartilagenous embolism. It should be noted that what are usually described as bubbles in blood are more correctly described as *droplets* of gas. Fat is liquid at normal body temperature and so is in the form of oil droplets; both gas and fat are examples of fluid embolism and a report recently published showed pictures of the retina of a patient who had his own fat injected into his forehead to reduce his wrinkles.[15] Millions of people will have died from fat embolism, as it is an inevitable consequence of fractures. However, fractures are common whereas fatalities from fat embolism are very rare. Nevertheless they do occur and soft tissue trauma, even without a fracture, may also cause fat embolism of the brain, and even be fatal. It is possible for this to affect any one of us, because we all have body fat, that is, adipose tissue; some more than others. It is, of course, a store of energy as an insurance against starvation, and so tends to be significantly greater as a percentage of body weight in women.

Over the last hundred years there has been an enormous increase in the number of patients told they have multiple sclerosis and it parallels the increase in human obesity and trauma from warfare and civilian accidents. Fractures are *always* accompanied by the entry of fat and often bone marrow into the circulation and the quantity usually, but not always, depends on the degree of violence involved. When the level of violence is high, fat embolism is inevitable. In 1979, an Air New Zealand DC10 crashed into Mount Erebus in Antarctica on a sight-seeing flight and lung tissue was available from the post-mortem examination of 205 of the 231 victims.[16] Evidence of fat and bone marrow embolism in organs was present in 194, despite death occurring very soon after impact. A degree of fat embolism always occurs when bones are fractured and has been produced experimentally without fracture by repeated impacts to the tibia. It has also been detected using ultrasound during operations on bones, for example, in hip replacement surgery where a prosthesis is hammered into the bone marrow cavity of the femur.[17] It is likely to be a factor involved in the brain damage sometimes seen after such operations. Again, like bubbles, the fat present in cells in the bone marrow is squeezed into veins and transported to the lungs during surgery. The danger is that a significant quantity may then escape into the general circulation and reach the brain.

What is little known is that fatal fat embolism may occur after a simple soft tissue injury, even without evidence of bruising. It is unlikely to be thought of clinically if the patient has minor neurological problems but, if the patient dies, its demonstration at post-mortem examination leaves no room for doubt. In 1981, a pathologist in Manchester writing in the *British Medical Journal* gave details of three patients who died from fat embolism after very minor injuries, and one had no evidence of bruising.[18]

Case 1

An 80-year-old man was found semiconscious in the toilet of a local lodging house. Chest radiography showed a "snowstorm" appearance, which is a well recognised feature of fat embolism. He died five hours later, after admission. At necropsy, a bruise eight centimetres in diameter was noted in the scalp, but there was no skull fracture.

Case 2

A 23-year-old girl with spina bifida was dropped when being carried, bruising her ribs. She became progressively breathless and was admitted to hospital 24 hours later. She died three hours after admission despite 35% oxygen.

Case 3

A 62-year-old man who had suffered from atypical multiple sclerosis for 15 years fell and hit his head in the bathroom. He became progressively breathless and, despite 35% oxygen, died five hours after admission to hospital. At necropsy no skull fracture or bruise was identified.

All three patients were found at post-mortem examination to have severe fat embolism in the brain, kidneys, and lungs.

There is an obvious question in relation to fat embolism: If is so common, why does everyone not develop multiple sclerosis? The answer is that many of us probably do develop some minor abnormalities in the brain, over a lifetime, associated with blood vessel damage from embolism and they can be identified as UBOs on MRI, but they normally repair without even intruding on our consciousness. We are likely to ignore very fleeting symptoms, and this includes neurologists, who are most aware of their significance. As discussed earlier, the survey of 87 members of the neurology department of Cornell University indicated that such events are, in fact common, as they are in patients labelled as having multiple sclerosis.[19] It is, therefore, those in whom the damage is more severe and affects the spinal cord who actually develop disability, and so they represent the tip of a pathological iceberg. Many studies have shown that UBOs are common in the general population[20] and their frequency increases with age. By the eighth decade of life they are ubiquitous and typically appear, like the damage of multiple sclerosis, in the central areas of white matter in the brain.[21] The suggestion that Alzheimer's disease is due to embolism[22] has been reinforced by a controlled study using ultrasound.[23] Not surprisingly, the study also showed that emboli are associated with so-called vascular dementia. Logic also suggests that the competence of such a complex structure as the blood-brain barrier will decline with age,[24] and there is evidence to suggest that the *amyloid* protein deposition in Alzheimer's disease is due to protein leak from the subtle blood-brain barrier dysfunction. Micro-embolism over the many years that the hydraulic system has to function into old age could readily account for this pathology. The way has been opened for using oxygen treatment to improve these conditions.

Today, because the fat embolism syndrome is so well-known medically most cases are simply not published, but there are exceptions; this remarkable story appeared in the *Daily Telegraph* on July 4, 1997 entitled, "Bruise Led to Death of Woman." It reported the findings of a coroner's inquest in Swindon (Figure 16.2).

THE DAILY TELEGRAPH

Bruise Led to Death of Woman
By Sean O'Neill

THE WIFE of the bursar of Marlborough College died from a rare condition that developed after she bruised her arm while applying her car's handbrake.

Simon Eveleigh said yesterday that the death of his wife Philippa, 49, three days after going into hospital was "the loss of a soul mate."

Mrs. Eveleigh is also survived by their two daughters, aged nine and eight.

Dr. Albert Goonetilieke, Home Office pathologist, told an inquest in Swindon this week that the cause of death was a fat embolism.

"It is very, very rare. I have only seen it three times in 30 years' practice."

Mrs. Eveleigh's arm was bruised after she noticed her car rolling forwards in a car park in Marlborough. Wilts, and leaned in to apply the handbrake.

The bruise became painful after a few days. She was treated with painkillers and her arm put in a sling, but her condition deteriorated.

David Masters, the Wiltshire coroner, recorded a verdict of misadventure.

Mr. Eveleigh said: "It is hard to believe that she died as the result of a bruise. It seemed like such a little thing that we took no notice of it."

Figure 16.2:
Daily Telegraph article published on July 4, 1997.

In securing the handbrake the lady bruised her forearm. The bruising was not extensive, as her husband indicated, and, despite being admitted to hospital, she died several days later. There was no possible doubt as to the cause of death, because it was found at the post-mortem examination. Droplets of fat had been released into the circulation from the bruised tissue of her forearm and travelled in the blood to the lungs. After a delay of some hours passing through the lung capillaries, the emboli entered the left side of the heart and were then transported in the arterial blood around the body. Some reached the brain causing fatal swelling. It is, of course, exceptionally rare to die of a simple bruise, but the fact that this well-established mechanism of injury to the brain was not discussed by *any* of the expert witnesses in Mr. Dingley's case illustrates the gross neglect of embolism as a concept in medicine. Ironically, all the experts had agreed that there needs to be a defect in the blood-brain barrier to cause multiple sclerosis but none offered an explanation. There can be no conceivable doubt that fat emboli can damage blood vessels in the brain and open the barrier. Fat accumulates in fat cells as an energy store for periods of famine. Many tissues have such cells which are known as "adipocytes" and Figure 16.3 shows them within a muscle.

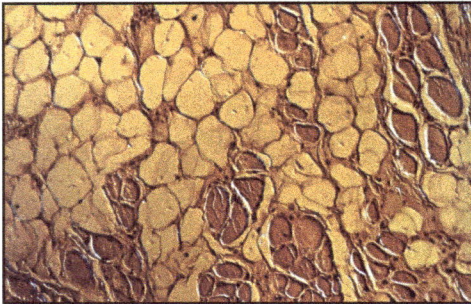

Figure 16.3:
Fat cells associated with obesity in a muscle.

Severe forms of fat embolism are often fatal, leaving the questions; do patients survive lesser forms and may they also develop neurological problems after a delay? They certainly can and, although it is now unusual for them to be reported, 12 cases were described in the journal *Neurology* in 1986.[25] All followed fractures and the delay in presentation ranged from eight hours to at least a week. Again, it is obvious that the longer the delay, the less likely a connection will be made between the trauma and the development of symptoms. Mr. Dingley had his first symptoms within days of his accident and so fat embolism should have been considered as a possibility, but it was many weeks before he was eventually seen by a neurologist. Many more cases have been published since this paper, using MRI rather than CT to examine the brain. Most cases of fat embolism resolve clinically, that is, the patients appear normal on bedside neurological examination, but the tell-tale changes often remain on MRI, especially in the white matter of the brain.[26–28] This has established *beyond any doubt* that there is a subacute version of the disease and that fat embolism is one cause of UBOs found on MRI. In fact, since the cause is *known*, they should actually be termed *identified* bright objects, that is, IBOs. Like the areas of damage found on MRI in divers and compressed-air workers from decompression sickness,[29] they cannot be distinguished microscopically from typical areas found in multiple sclerosis patients. The blood

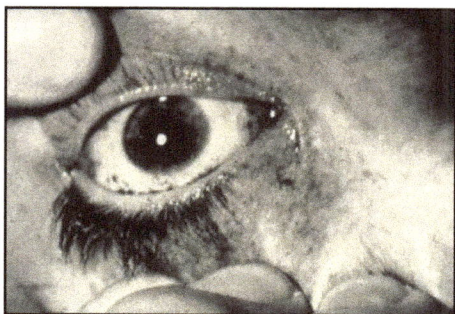

Figure 16.4:
Haemorrhages due to fat emboli in the skin and the conjunctiva.

vessels in the eye and in the skin are often involved in fat embolism evidenced by the petechial haemorrhages shown in Figure 16.4.

The haemorrhages are due to the presence of fat emboli in blood vessels[30] and are visible proof of exactly the same process that occurs in the brain and spinal cord. This means that the emboli damage the blood-brain barrier allowing the leakage of water, proteins, and red blood cells from the blood into the tissues of the brain. This is responsible for the bright areas on MRI associated with swelling and, inevitably, hypoxia. The fat emboli derived from adipose tissue can also cause inflammation from the release of a wide range of fatty acids.

So can trauma *cause* multiple sclerosis and can the disease start from an episode of fat embolism which damages the blood-brain barrier? The answer is simply yes. Those who require more detail will find the detailed evidence brought together in the *Lancet* in 1982[31] entitled "Evidence for Subacute Fat Embolism as the Cause of Multiple Sclerosis." It is supported by 70 peer-reviewed references. No claim is made for priority; much of the credit is due to the pioneering work of Drs. Tracey Putnam,[32] Roy Swank,[33] and Alan Woolf.[34] It is important to recognise that the evidence has not been refuted, indeed it has been greatly strengthened by the referenced MRI studies of patients with fat embolism, an investigation not clinically available in 1982. Probably more has been written about multiple sclerosis than any other human disease and yet only one letter was received by the *Lancet* about the paper.[35] It was from the two pathologists at Guy's Hospital responsible for the UK MS Society sponsored Brain Bank, which contained the donated brains of multiple sclerosis patients. They commented that they had not found fat emboli in any of the brains they had examined. It is only too obvious why; by definition patients *cannot* die from a first attack; two attacks are required with dissemination *in time* for it to be called multiple sclerosis, and so none of the brains could possibly provide evidence of the initial causative event. The disease is rarely a cause of death and it is absurd to expect to find emboli present years after the first attack which signalled the onset of the disease.[36] The case for subacute fat embolism has been further strengthened by the use of injected dye in a patient reported in 2003 who recovered.[37] All the hallmark features of the onset of multiple sclerosis were present in this patient, with localised blood-brain barrier failure causing oedema, changes which have been studied in an experimental model.[38] The emboli are too small to block the larger arteries but, nevertheless, they are able to cause the typical damage to veins, which has been called the perivenous syndrome.[39]

In the last century, nine pathologists commented on the close resemblance of the affected areas found when death has been delayed in cases of fat embolism to those of acute multiple sclerosis and the details are listed in Appendix 2. It is truly astonishing that these observations have been overlooked when they are from *human* pathology, not from animal experiments. Much of the blame for the current situation can be attributed to the events of the WW2, because it broke the continuity of the research into the role of blood vessels in the disease begun by Dr. Tracey Putnam.[32] Two forms of *fluid* micro-embolism, gas and fat, can, therefore, open the blood-brain barrier and reproduce the typical plaques of multiple sclerosis in the brain and spinal cord.

The brain shown in Figure 16.5 is of a 36-year-old male pedestrian, who died from fat embolism associated with a leg fracture after being hit by a car. The dark red spots arrowed are due to the accumulation of red blood cells which have escaped through the vessel wall to cluster around the vessel. They are known as ring or ball haemorrhages. It is clear that they are almost exclusively in the white matter, although a few are in the grey matter of the areas known as the basal ganglia in the centre of the brain and some are also in the cerebellum. The bulk of the white matter is due to the presence of the myelin sheaths and when fluid leaks from the blood plasma in oedema, and haemorrhage occurs, the tissue damaged is myelin. The crevices between the convolutions of the brain, known as sulci, and the liquid filled cavities in each hemisphere, the lateral ventricles, are almost completely obliterated by the swelling of the tissues. As the brain swells, the pressure inside the head rises reducing the blood flow, because bone cannot expand. The reduction of blood flow worsens the oxygen deficiency, and the blood vessels attempt to enlarge further so increasing the pressure. As in this patient, the vicious spiral often leads to death. A microscopic examination of the brain would reveal many fat emboli, curiously, despite the damage being almost exclusively in the white matter, there are many more emboli in the grey matter of the cortex. This is a paradox that has been noted many times and it also applies to the spinal cord. However, the spinal cord was not removed in this case, simply be-

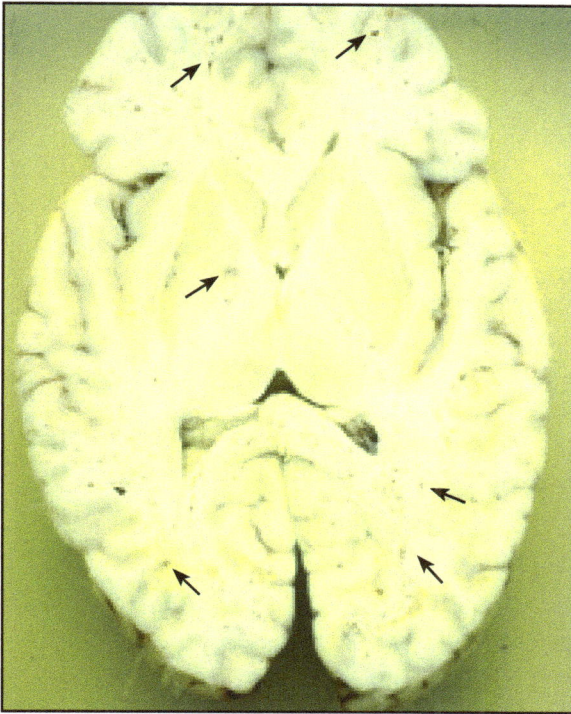

Figure 16.5
Section of the brain from a patient who died from fat embolism. Some of the many tiny haemorrhages are arrowed.

cause damage to the cord did not contribute to the death of the patient. Had he survived, however, it may well have contributed to continuing disability.

The appearance of the brain in Figure 16.5 closely resembles the illustration of a similar case that a pathologist, the late Professor Charles Lumsden, included in his second contribution to the 1970 *Handbook of Clinical Neurology*.[40] It has the intimidating title "Pathogenetic Mechanisms in the Leucoencephalopathies, in Anoxic Ischaemic Processes, in Disorders of the Blood, and in Intoxication." The patient was a 23-year-old man who died of fat embolism after sustaining several compound fractures. The illustration in the chapter is accompanied by this astonishingly relevant observation.

> *The vast numbers of lesions attending classical instances of fat embolism are always very striking and one cannot help feeling that sporadic and clinically silent lesions (in the brain) must commonly be associated with many non-fatal fractures and soft tissue injury of minor, even trivial degree.*

There is no discussion of the importance of the lung as a trap for material in blood in protecting the nervous system. As for the "clinically silent lesions," which obviously occur in survivors, Lumsden actually states:

These minor traumatic lesions can simulate early multiple sclerosis plaques quite remarkably but their occurrence within a very few days of a traumatic episode or associated with a recent subarachnoid haemorrhage gives a clue as to their nature.

In other words, the damage from fat emboli in the nervous system following minor trauma reproduces the areas which are typical of those in acute multiple sclerosis patients. Why Lumsden and, indeed, the other investigators listed in Appendix 2 failed to grasp the importance of this disease process to finding the cause of multiple sclerosis is truly a mystery. It is obvious that such lesions may, or may not be, silent and the question raised is: What if only one area of damage was present, would the patient die and if not, would it leave an area of damage? Such patients do indeed survive with the damage and, of course, they are classified on MRI as UBOs.

Obviously the patient discussed above who died from fat embolism could not, by *definition*, qualify for a "diagnosis" of multiple sclerosis; he only had one event and, although multiple areas were affected, they were not *disseminated in time*. Fat embolism is then pathologically, an acute disseminated encephalomyelitis (ADEM). This translates simply as a sudden onset, widespread inflammation involving the myelin of the brain. Like the terms "multiple" and "sclerosis," it is simply a *description* of the pathology and not a diagnosis. Fat embolism is certainly one cause of this disease but, curiously, is not actually classified as such in textbooks of pathology. This is almost certainly because the history of injury will be known to the pathologist at the time of the post-mortem examination and, on finding fat globules in blood vessels, a definitive diagnosis of fat embolism can be made. Equally, in discussions of the causes of acute encephalitis, or encephalomyelitis, in neurological texts, fat embolism is never cited.

The relationship between acute disseminated encephalomyelitis and multiple sclerosis has been argued over for many years and it is now recognised as often being the first presentation of multiple sclerosis in children. The pathology of ADEM was also discussed by Lumsden, but again without reference to fat embolism. The key difference is said to be that the encephalomyelitis is always fatal but in discussing this with a pathologist in the author's own hospital many years ago, the only patient he remembered with the condition was a young man who recovered from the first attack and died after the second some months later (personal communication, Dr. John Anderson). As the condition is very rare, most pathologists, including those who write textbooks, will perhaps only see a single case in their professional lifetimes. However, some patients with the acute disease undoubtedly recover, but will have tell-tale UBOs detectable on MRI in the brain.

Death from bone marrow and fat embolism is rare and, obviously, after minor trauma exceedingly rare, although there will undoubtedly be many cases that have not been published and many others that will have gone unrecognised. Deep venous thrombosis and pulmonary embolism after aircraft flights were thought to be rare but, with publicity, emergency departments close to major airports reported that they have seen such patients regularly over many years. This is known as the finder effect. Nevertheless, the odds against death from minor trauma are, of course, extremely large. The examination of many millions, or even billions, of cases of minor injury would in all likelihood not find a single death from such a cause and so such a mechanism may be readily discounted by those who argue from epidemiological and statistical data. This is, of course, just the argument used by Henry Miller about asphyxiation by Yorkshire pudding (see Chapter 13). In fact, it is the *only* argument open to those who discount a link between trauma and the development of multiple areas of sclerosis. However, the cause of the lady's death following the forearm bruising covered by the *Daily Telegraph* was established beyond question, simply because droplets of fat were present in the lungs and in other organs, including the brain, at post-mortem examination. As the level of trauma increases, so does the likelihood of fat embolism. Fat embolism can also provide a solution to a puzzling feature of multiple sclerosis; it affects twice as many women as men and women generally have twice the body fat content of men. Each feature of fat embolism is subject to a normal or Gaussian distribution, from the release of fat into the circulation, to trapping in the lungs, to finally sustaining damage in the nervous system. In other words, some people will be more likely to have such an event, others very unlikely, with most of us having an intermediate risk.

Dr. Poser, the senior expert witness supporting Mr. Dingley's case has been adamant for many years there is a link between trauma and multiple sclerosis. Despite this, he was prepared to state in 1993,[41] that "there is no way that injury of a limb could cause injury to the nervous system" when fat embolism from such an injury, even a simple bruise of the forearm, may cause extensive brain damage and death. Dr. Poser invited the author to his home in Boston and he was certainly aware of subacute fat embolism and the importance of trauma.[42] The patient whose brain is shown in Figure 16.5 had a large number of areas affected in the brain, but this mechanism is clearly capable of producing any number from one upwards, that is, from a single lesion to multiple lesions. The most evident damage is also in the white matter of the brain, although the basal ganglia and the grey matter of the cerebellum are also involved.

Finally, embolism is able to make sense of the range of conditions that surround multiple sclerosis, from the clinically isolated syndromes, with only one area affected, to an acute disseminated encephalomyelitis, where there may be hundreds present and patients often die. It is also possible to reconcile the common MRI finding in patients with a first attack typical of multiple sclerosis with only one area detectable on clinical examination, for example, optic neuritis, but who have multiple areas evident on MRI.[43] This is actually true on initial imaging of most patients who are eventually told they have multiple sclerosis. By definition they have a *subacute disseminated encephalomyelitis*, although this label would never be used by a neurologist. But patients who have multiple areas on MRI present after their first attack cannot have multiple sclerosis by *definition*, because the patient would not meet one of the criteria required for the diagnosis; dissemination in *time*. Faced with this quandary, the late Professor of Neurology, Dr. Ian McDonald, was even prepared to commit this statement to paper:[44] "Although it may be tempting to diagnose multiple sclerosis in the presence of multiple lesions, it is inappropriate to do so." This is constantly defended in practice by the assertion that the diagnosis of multiple sclerosis must be clinical and made by an expert, that is, a neurologist.

The case for embolism as a cause for multiple sclerosis would clearly be strengthened if there were cases where proven embolism was confused with the disease. Misdiagnosis is not often admitted and even more rarely published, but a case report published in 1987[45] illustrates one such example. A 30-year-old man had relapsing and remitting neurological symptoms over nine years and had attracted the label of multiple sclerosis. It had apparently been confirmed by imaging, which at the time was CT. Eventually a thorough examination discovered a heart murmur and on investigation it was found that he had a tumour in the left ventricle. His symptoms were due to embolism of blood platelets which stick on the surface of such growths. Removal of the tumour ended his attacks. This unusual case must not be taken as indicating that all of the attacks experienced by patients who have multiple sclerosis are due to embolism associated with a tumour. However, it does demonstrate that the time course of attacks and remissions seen in multiple sclerosis patients is perfectly consistent with embolism.

Mention has already been made of the recent studies of Dr. Paolo Zamboni in Ferraro which has renewed interest in blood vessel problems in multiple sclerosis.[46] Another discovery, which again drew attention to the importance of blood vessels was the discovery of the anti-phospholipid syndrome, named after its discoverer, as the Hughes syndrome.[47] It may be confused with multiple sclerosis and is sometimes responsible for strokes in young people. It is also an important cause of miscarriage and the diagnosis of this condition for patients presenting with symptoms typical of multiple sclerosis is very important because it can be treated with aspirin.

So far this discussion has centred on the brain and not the spinal cord. It is commonly alleged that embolism only affects the brain, but as already discussed, decompression sickness and fibrocartilagenous embolism also affect the spinal cord and cord damage is more likely to cause disability than damage to the brain. Fat emboli were found in the spinal cord by Courville[48] who commented on the similarity of the damage he found to that of multiple sclerosis. In 1994, a case was reported where a patient suffering from fat embolism developed paralysis of all four limbs associated with damage to the spinal cord in the neck.[49] But the principal reason for the paucity of accounts is probably because an examination for emboli is problematic; removal and detailed microscopic examination of the spinal cord is both difficult and time consuming. The primary reason for conducting a post-mortem examination is to determine the cause of death and conditions affecting the spinal cord are rarely fatal. In contrast, the greatest disability in patients with multiple sclerosis is from damage to the spinal cord; an area of damage to the spinal cord in the neck may cause paralysis of all four limbs, whereas one further down may produce paraplegia. Unfortunately, bladder control is usually affected in both cases.

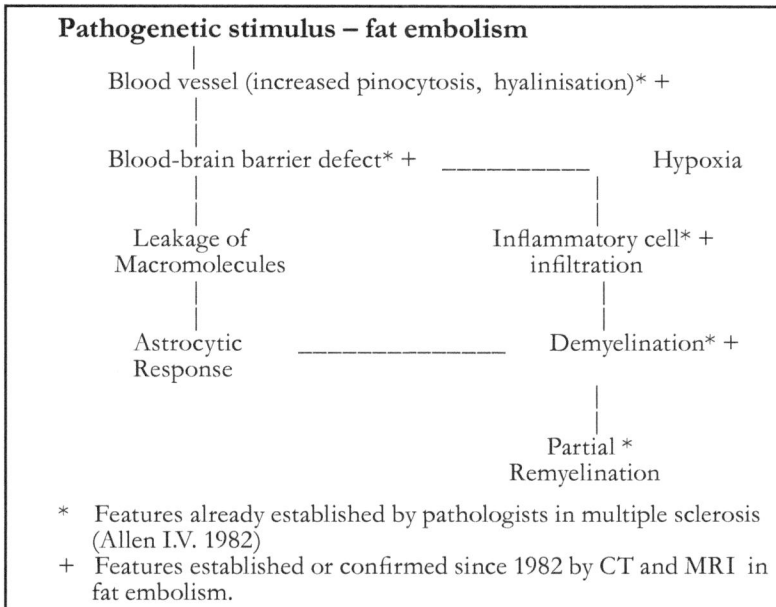

Pathogenetic stimulus – fat embolism
|
Blood vessel (increased pinocytosis, hyalinisation)* +
|
|
Blood-brain barrier defect* + _____ Hypoxia
| |
| |
Leakage of   Inflammatory cell* +
Macromolecules   infiltration
| |
| |
Astrocytic   _____ Demyelination* +
Response
                                               |
                                               |
                                         Partial *
                                        Remyelination

   *   Features already established by pathologists in multiple sclerosis
      (Allen I.V. 1982)
   +   Features established or confirmed since 1982 by CT and MRI in
      fat embolism.

Figure 16.6:
Redrawn from the schematic by Dr. Ingrid Allen.

Chapter 16: Trauma May Cause Multiple Sclerosis ~ 283

We are now in a position to review the evidence that trauma and fat embolism may cause multiple sclerosis and it is useful to refer to the paper by Dr. Ingrid Allen[50] published in 1982 entitled "The Pathology of Multiple Sclerosis–Fact, Fiction, and Hypothesis." It was a truly astonishing castigation of the lack of direction in multiple sclerosis research. Although deriding attempts to construct hypotheses, she brought together the pathological abnormalities that *have* been established in multiple sclerosis in a valuable schematic which provides a perfect fit with the concept of micro-embolism. It should be noted that the nebulous term "pathogenetic stimulus" simply includes every relevant factor; we are only a product of our genes and the environment! Fat embolism can be substituted for this term in the schematic and *all* the features listed are known to be associated with the disease. "Fat embolism" and "hypoxia" have been added to the original schematic.

Note that the word inflammation appears and it is the one feature that is *universally agreed* to in multiple sclerosis. It also provides a key link to the putative animal model EAE, which will be discussed again in the next chapter, because of its critical importance to oxygen treatment. It is clear that micro-embolism due to fat can provide the required pathogenetic stimulus without difficulty and all the features required are already well established by human pathological and imaging studies.

Table 16.1:
Some Unsolved Problems in MS Pathology

- The "geographical" distribution of the areas of damage
- How the first changes occur and how myelin is removed
- The significance of mildly affected areas
- How the changes in the chemistry relate to the pathology
- The significance of the increased number of the cells known as astrocytes
- How changes in the number of cells and their position relate to the disease and
- How changes in the fluid surrounding the brain relate to the nervous system damage

---

Professor Allen then gave a long list of all the features of multiple sclerosis that, despite more than 150 years of research, are still said to remain unexplained. Table 16.1 is translated from the medical jargon used in table 1 of her paper.

The list is so all-encompassing that it is difficult to find anything that is not included and, despite the passage of more than 30 years since the article was written, little has changed. The world of MS is truly in a MESS.

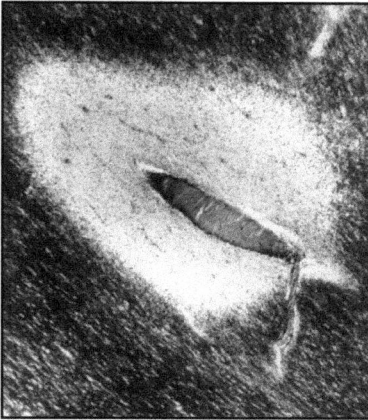

Figure 16.7:
Brain lesion around a vein.
(Courtesy of the late Dr. D. Oppenheimer.)

The evidence that it is a blood vessel disease is beyond doubt; all of the known data fits. However, the most important confirmation has been provided by five different methods imaging living patients in real time. The most obvious fact is that the multiple sites typically affected in multiple sclerosis patients can *only* be connected by the circulation. The universal relationship of the early lesions to veins is rarely mentioned in clinical texts and the author cannot recall an instance in which the painstaking reconstruction by Dow and Berglund[51] shown in Figure 14.2 in Chapter 14, has been reproduced, or even discussed, since its publication in 1943. Figure 16.7 shows another example of the damage around a vein under the microscope.

The relationship of the areas of damage in multiple sclerosis to veins is, as Lumsden stated, a historical fact, and it will be seen that this feature is especially important to using oxygen in treatment. The viral/auto-immune hypothesis has *no explanation* for this finding, indeed no explanation is ever offered for the venous involvement, nor one to account for the general dissemination of the areas affected. There are times that it would appear that no progress has been made since Charcot[52] wrote: "The cause of the very singular mode of arrangement under which the sclerosed islets are distributed in different parts of the central nervous system is, at present, completely unknown to us." After more than 60 years of auto-immune research, the absurdity of this is all too obvious and the evidence for micro-embolism discussed here, underpinned by a human model—decompression sickness—is overwhelming. The restatement of the primary role of blood vessels in multiple sclerosis barely impacted on medical consciousness in 1982, but the controversy was noticed and studied in detail by sociologists.[53]

The auto-immune theory has stifled the progress of treatment and its legacy is now that patients are consigned to the management of their disease with long-term and toxic drug use. The UK risk sharing scheme has now shown that many of the drugs, far from benefiting patients, actually do more harm than good.[54] It beggars belief that the UK Department of Health is continuing this flawed scheme, which has already cost over *half a billion* pounds. A better approach to treatment is desperately needed, especially because each of the attacks typical of multiple sclerosis may cause permanent disability, and must, therefore, be treated as an emergency. As will be seen in the next chapter, there is conclusive evidence, from the demonstration of lactic acid in affected areas by magnetic resonance spectroscopy, that this has to include giving more oxygen; breathing air simply does not provide enough. In the next chapter we will see that multiple sclerosis patients may still respond to oxygen treatment, despite suffering years of chronic disease.

In 1981, during the gestation period of the author's paper in the *Lancet* giving the evidence for fat embolism as the cause of multiple sclerosis,[31] a young man working for a diving contractor in Scotland was involved in a car accident. He developed symptoms typical of embolism when undergoing an X-ray investigation of his head. His improvement with hyperbaric oxygen treatment was dramatic. After discussions, Ian Munro, then editor of the *Lancet*, kindly suggested that it should be incorporated as an addendum to the main paper. Reproduced herein, it encapsulates all the arguments presented in this chapter. It should be noted that the reference numbers have been changed from the original text in the *Lancet*.

Addendum

A 21-year-old man became briefly unconscious following a car accident and sustained a scalp laceration in the left parietal area. Two hours later he had a severe headache, momentary loss of vision in both eyes, and loss of sensation in the distribution of the left trigeminal nerve. Two weeks later he had slight swelling of the left optic disc associated with poor visual acuity and he complained of double vision, persistent headaches, and lassitude, although the facial numbness had resolved. No other neurological abnormality could be detected, but petechial haemorrhages, which had appeared on the anterior aspect of his thighs several days after the accident were still visible.

The delayed (by two hour) onset and clinical features are very compatible with subacute fat embolism, and so is the fact that the ophthalmic artery is a preferred pathway for emboli.[55] The efficacy of oxygen in fat embolism[56] and the proximity of a compression chamber suggested a trial of hyperbaric oxygen. The immediate improvement in visual acuity from 6/18 to 6/6 as pressure was increased to 2.8 bar confirmed the presence of hypoxia. Three sessions using a procedure from diving practice[57] continued the improvement and the patient reported that the double vision, which had prevented him from watching television, had gone and he felt generally much better.

Over the past year his condition has remained stable, although he has had two very brief episodes of whole-body tingling, which may be due to the presence of small lesions in the posterior columns. It may be argued that this man did not have multiple sclerosis but, in view of the clinical features, what other diagnosis is possible? Hyperbaric oxygen is an effective agent in the treatment of animals with experimental allergic encephalomyelitis (the experimental model for multiple sclerosis),[58,59] and a preliminary report of a favourable response in patients with established multiple sclerosis[60] has prompted a clinical trial. The relief of hypoxia by hyperbaric oxygen in acute multiple sclerosis should minimise the extent of the demyelination and neuronal damage and prevent the development of the progressive disease, whilst the stabilisation of the blood-brain barrier in chronic lesions may slow or even arrest further deterioration. Computerised tomography using contrast enhancement[61] will allow both these assertions to be tested in individual patients. Few therapeutic agents have the proven value and intrinsic safety of oxygen.

At the time of the paper's publication in February 1982, the clinical trial of hyperbaric oxygen treatment referred to in this addendum had already been completed. It had been undertaken by the late Dr. Boguslav Fischer and colleagues in New York University Medical Center and the paper had been submitted to the *New England Journal of Medicine*. It was finally published in the journal on January 27, 1983[62] and the author was given a copy by Dr. Fischer at a meeting in the Bronx Hospital in New York on that day. It was the beginning of a controversy that, sadly, has still not been resolved. Why giving just a little more oxygen to patients with multiple sclerosis should generate such extraordinary hostility needs to be explained.

CHAPTER 17

A Tale of Trials and the
New England Journal of Medicine

In truth, what is needed to achieve a cure, is a treatment which deals with the first attack and any subsequent attacks of the disease.

Byron H. Waksman, National MS Society of the US, 1983

The treatment of patients with multiple sclerosis has been surrounded by more controversy than that of any other disease, but anyone who has made even a cursory study of the pathology of the plaques typical of the disease will know that Dr. Waksman's statement above is true. Nevertheless, nothing has proven more controversial than the suggestion that patients may benefit from being given more oxygen. This seems difficult to understand, after all everyone knows that the brain requires a great deal of oxygen and it would seem eminently logical that giving more should assist its recovery from injury, or from disease. The logic is, in fact, impeccable; recovery or as it is usually called *remission*, in multiple sclerosis cannot take place without sufficient oxygen in an affected area. However, there are times when human behaviour defies logic and professional attitudes are often shaped by emotion, probably more so in medicine than in other disciplines. The neglect of the obvious, that *pressure* is important to the delivery of oxygen, has already been discussed, but many of the suppressed fears about oxygen treatment centre on the equipment, the technology of pressure chambers, and not on the gas itself. It has also been obvious within the profession and government administrations that, if trials of hyperbaric oxygen treatment proved successful, it would have profound implications for medical practice.

The assessment of patients has improved dramatically with the introduction of brain imaging, especially MRI, which, as we have seen, has steadily improved to the point where it can show the pathology in a living patient. Unfortunately, despite being capable of revealing astonishing detail, as yet MRI cannot determine if an abnormal area in the brain is a scar, that is, sclerosis, or an area of inflammation with swelling; in both cases the water content of the tissue is increased. Successful recovery from the attacks typical of multiple sclerosis depends on limiting the extent of the scarring; the swelling may respond to treatment, but sclerosis will not. Sclerosis is the lowest common denominator of healing *in any tissue* and it is patently absurd to suggest a cure for healing. The first objective of treatment in patients must, therefore, be to ensure the best possible recovery from attacks, but especially the first one, because MRI has shown that in the first attack *multiple* areas may be affected even though the patient has only one symptom. However, as discussed, this does not mean that the patient qualifies for the so-called diagnosis because another one is required and it must be separated in time—by at least a month. In 1974 Dr. George Schumacher,[1] who chaired the first committee to determine the diagnostic criteria for multiple sclerosis, tellingly wrote:

> *Obviously any treatment capable of eradicating or providing long-term prevention of multiple sclerosis automatically will serve the additional purpose of allowing a current acute episode to subside as rapidly as nature will permit the lesion to repair itself.*

The term "nature" could not be more appropriate to the use of oxygen; it underpins all *natural* recovery. The controlled trials of hyperbaric oxygen treatment undertaken in the 1980s only recruited patients with long-established disabilities and typical disease durations measured in years. The reasoning used was simple; these patients would not be likely to have a natural, "spontaneous" remission, which neglects the obvious; remission *cannot* occur without correcting an oxygen deficiency. Professionals, and even patients, often appear to have great difficulty in grasping this logic, but it is certainly compounded by the use of the word "hyperbaric." On Saturday the August 14, 2010, the *Palm Beach Post* quoted a Florida neurosurgeon as saying that technical trials of hyperbaric oxygen treatment are needed in brain injury because: "There is no other way to be sure if it is natural recovery or real; nobody knows how oxygen works, and it's very hard to do the research."

Many of the patients recruited in the multiple sclerosis studies would have had damage in vulnerable areas of the brain stem and spinal cord, where there is little spare capacity; the structures are small volumes of tissue and the blood supply to both is relatively poor. Unfortunately, it is difficult to imagine any current treatment will produce substantial benefit to the spinal cord when it is seriously damaged. Although rarely discussed openly, these factors limit medical expectations for any treatment.

Early in the disease multiple sclerosis is usually characterised by attacks from which patients often get better without any treatment; they have a spontaneous remission. Whilst this may imply that they have escaped any permanent damage, MRI has shown that this is often not true. Unfortunately, despite the dramatic developments in imaging, there has been little research of the treatment of acute attacks. Jack Haldane, in one of his many essays entitled "The Time Factor in Medicine," summed up the problem brilliantly.[2] Nothing has changed, especially the huge emphasis on diagnosis rather than treatment, although the medicine bottle has now been replaced by a box of pills.

> *The average man or woman goes to the doctor to be cured of some disease or injury, and for this purpose expects either surgical treatment or something out of a bottle. And the critics of modern medicine complain that while the surgical treatment is often unduly violent, the medicine is usually ineffective, except as a generator of faith. They also point out that in medical teaching enormously greater stress is laid on diagnosis than on treatment. Fortunately for the medical profession, its critics commonly support some therapeutic system such as faith-healing, osteopathy, or herbalism, which is quite demonstrably less efficient than that of ordinary medicine. Again, the study of immunity has fallen into some disrepute because, although immune sera are often potent prophylactics, they are not of much value in curing diseases other than diphtheria. The reason for this is a simple one. The doctor is generally called in to cure a scar.*

When the trials of oxygen treatment were planned, doctors were still talking about a cure for multiple sclerosis; today the word cure is rarely mentioned by professionals, discussions are centred on "disease management." So the goalposts have been moved; treatment, for example with the beta interferons, is only aimed at reducing the number of relapses to, hopefully, slow the progression of the disease, rather than improving existing disability, or effecting a cure. This change of neurological focus has meant that treatment has the potential for the generation of vast revenues by the pharmaceutical industry. The beta interferons were initially promoted because controlled trials showed that the drugs were able to reduce the number of attacks from three to two over two years. This modest change, produced at a cost of £10,000 a year, obviously cannot be regarded as a major advance, especially when a single attack may lead to permanent disability. But the real question raised by the use of these drugs is; why do they only prevent some of the attacks and not all? The answer relates to the cause of the relapse. Judged by both pathological studies and by imaging, the first attack suffered by a patient leads to damage to the blood-brain barrier and this may not fully heal leaving the area vulnerable to any stress which causes the damaged blood vessels to leak. The complexity of the blood-brain barrier has developed for a critical reason; it is essential to the protection of the sensitive tissues of the nervous system. A barrier is not just present in higher species like mammals, a blood-brain barrier is even present in insects. Once the barrier is damaged, any toxic or infectious agent in blood, such as a virus, may be able to cause an attack. This is confusing as a virus infection, such as influenza, in causing a relapse may produce exactly the same symptoms that were caused by the first episode, despite being due to an entirely different cause. An example of this, already discussed, is a relapse in multiple sclerosis produced by a hot bath,[3] because heat dilates blood vessels causing increased leakage, allowing constituents normally retained in blood, such as plasma proteins, to escape and cause inflammation.[4] It is most unlikely that any of the drugs used in "managing" multiple sclerosis would prevent a relapse caused by a hot bath, but it is equally true that the disease is not actually caused by a hot bath.

As discussed in Chapter 10, the same approach used to test drugs has been applied to trials of hyperbaric oxygen treatment, which implies that there is no proof that oxygen is needed for the brain to repair. It was first suggested that giving oxygen to multiple sclerosis patients may be beneficial in the 1950s, when two doctors in the US suggested that patients suffering an acute attack should breathe oxygen at normal atmospheric pressure.[5] Unfortunately they gave no indication either of the apparatus they used, or of their results. However, after independent reports of improvement from hyperbaric oxygen treatment from four countries, the first double-blind, placebo-controlled, randomised controlled trial was undertaken at New York University with the results being published in the *New England Journal of Medicine* in 1983.[6]

The events that led to the funding of this trial began with a small open study in Czechoslovakia by Drs. Boschetty and Cernoch.[7] In 1970, they reported short-term improvement in the symptoms of multiple sclerosis from hyperbaric oxygen treatment in a study of 26 patients. In 1978, the late Dr. Richard Neubauer of the Ocean Medical Center, in Lauderdale by-the-Sea, Florida, in a paper published by the *Journal of the Florida Medical Association*,[8] found benefit in 70 patients from a course of treatment. In 1974 he had been intrigued by seeing the improvement in symptoms in a multiple sclerosis patient having a course of hyperbaric oxygen treatment for a bone infection. He then collaborated with a neurologist in a study in which patients were examined before and after a course of treatment, and objective measurements were made of improvement of bladder function. There were reports of the treatment used for multiple sclerosis patients from other countries, Dr. Formai[9] and Dr. Pallotta[10] in Italy, both reported improvement, as did the late Dr. Henri Baixe in France.[11] They had compared the symptoms of multiple sclerosis to those of decompression sickness in divers where, as we have seen, hyperbaric oxygen treatment is well established.

Dr. Neubauer continued to treat multiple sclerosis patients, but it was press publicity given to his outstanding work that led to pressure from patients for the National MS Society of America to investigate the treatment. The society first funded studies of the animal model experimental allergic encephalomyelitis[12–14] which showed that if, after being injected, the animals were given hourly sessions of oxygen under hyperbaric conditions each day they would remain healthy. After an arbitrary 34 days, the daily sessions of treatment were stopped and many of the animals then developed symptoms. In another series of experiments, animals were allowed to develop the disease and it was found that oxygen treatment ameliorated their disabilities.[15] It was suggested that the mechanism involved was immunosuppression.[16] In 1980, Neubauer published a second report also in the *Journal of the Florida Medical Association.*[17] It was prefaced by an editor's note, some of which is reproduced in Figure 17.1. Many of the referee's comments beggar belief, especially when the treatment simply involves giving patients just a few hundred grams more oxygen a day. Contrast this with the continued use of exotic and dangerous immune-suppressing drugs, none of which are evidence based. It is absurd and telling that the use of oxygen should generate enormous controversy.

All of the first studies were "open," that is, they did not incorporate controls. They reported improvement in patients with very long-standing symptoms, but the authors did not offer an explanation for the changes. After some publicity and patient pressure, the National MS Society of America gave $250,000 to New York University Medical Center to fund a double-blind study. It was undertaken by three neurologists, Drs. Boguslav Fischer, Morton Marks, and Theobald Reich in a chamber that had been installed in the Rusk Rehabilitation Center in New York University (NYU) many years before. The modifications made for the trial included elaborate arrangements for blinding, that is concealing the pipework from both the patients and the investigators. Gas switching codes were also devised to prevent patients knowing whether 100% oxygen, or the placebo gas which contained 10% oxygen in nitrogen was in use. The codes were only known to the technician in charge. The second gas containing only 10% oxygen gives the same concentration of oxygen at twice atmospheric pressure—2 ATA, as is in air at normal atmospheric pressure. Much care was given to ensuring that the masks fitted well. In fact, the masks used known as the Acme Scottoramic No. 707 had been devised for use in nuclear installations to prevent workers inhaling dangerous radioactive gases. The two groups were then randomly allocated to either the treatment or the control groups for 20 sessions, which were undertaken at 2 ATA for 90 minutes, five days a week for a total of

Editor's Note

In the tenure of every Editor, several articles will surface that engender enormous controversy. The following paper entitled "Exposure of Multiple Sclerosis Patients to Hyperbaric Oxygen at 1.5–2 ATA; A Preliminary Report" is one such manuscript. This document has been reviewed by 12 different physicians both within and outside the state of Florida. The review covered a panorama of opinions including:

1. It should be published as a preliminary report—even in the absence of a vigorous therapeutic and controlled trial of therapy.

2. Represents but another form of therapy for a very remission-prone disease.

3. Do not publish—very speculative—no scientific basis.

4. Must be published: It may well turn out to be the most important paper ever published in our search for the understanding of multiple sclerosis. To have its wealth of clinical experience wasted, and its impressive results unknown for any length of time, would be comparable to the fate that befell Fleming's delivery of penicillin.

5. Cures for multiple sclerosis—reported as "possibilities"—or "preliminary" are ubiquitous. They range from snake venom to lettuce diet. All show preliminary improvement based, in large measure, on subjective patient reaction. Publication of this paper would lead to false hopes It is based on no convincing evidence.

6. Contents of this paper are of considerable scientific interest. This preliminary report is conservatively presented.

7. Broad claims without statistical calculations.

8. OK as an informative provocative article. Double blind study going on in other centers will either substantiate or deny effects.

9. No controls—no placebos. This is poorly explained—conclusions are unjustified.

Figure 17.1:
Journal of the Florida Medical Association: Portion of the editor's note.

four weeks. The follow up was for eighteen months without the codes being broken to ensure that the rigorous blinding was kept in force and the results were kept secure. The author, on a visit to Dr. Fischer at NYU in September 1981, saw that the papers were being kept in a large combination safe in his office. He confirmed then that the funding from the National MS Society had been to demonstrate that hyperbaric oxygen treatment was *not* of benefit to multiple sclerosis patients. An important reason for the introduction of scientific methods in the assessment of treatment was to avoid such malignant prejudice and bias.

However, the results were actually positive, with many patients showing clear benefit from the treatment, despite disease durations averaging nearly 10 years. This needs to be put into perspective; there are 168 hours in a week and breathing more oxygen for just 7.5 hours a week, to give a total of 30 hours in a month, was able to ameliorate symptoms of a disease present for very many years. Because of the importance of their results, the authors were keen to publish the study in the *New England Journal of Medicine*. Following the strictures of a former editor, Dr. Ingelfinger, the journal will not accept papers which have been published elsewhere. Being aware of this, Fischer and his co-authors requested permission from the editorial staff of the *NEJM* to give an oral presentation to a meeting of hyperbaric physicians at Long Beach Memorial Hospital in the summer of 1982. The permission granted included the publication of an abstract. A tape of Fischer's presentation was made and transcribed for the patients who wanted to start a self-help hyperbaric centre in Scotland. It opened in August of 1982 and was affiliated with a UK charity known as Action for Research into Multiple Sclerosis (ARMS).

The abstract of the paper, finally published in the *NEJM* on January 27, 1983,[6] differed from the abstract from the Long Beach meeting in one critical respect; a final paragraph was added which states:

> *These preliminary results suggest a positive, though transient, effect of hyperbaric oxygen on advanced multiple sclerosis, warranting further study. This therapy cannot be generally recommended without longer follow-up periods and additional confirmatory experience.*

This is a travesty; the second paragraph within the *NEJM* abstract actually refers to the *long-term benefits* in many of the patients which were still present at the end of a year of follow-up. Not surprisingly those opposed to the use of hyperbaric oxygen treatment have constantly referred to the authors being, apparently, unwilling to endorse the treatment. But, Dr. Fischer and his colleagues were obviously *required* to add the paragraph to the abstract in order to have the paper published; a betrayal of the hopes of many thousands of long-suffering patients. Also at the time it was rumoured that the publication of the New York University study was being delayed to await the results of a Boston study on immune suppression by drugs, so that both could appear in the same issue. This was later confirmed by Dr. Fischer; the results of the study had been available and the paper written at least six months prior to their publication. The fact that the paper on immune suppression, an *uncontrolled* study, was published in front of the hyperbaric oxygen trial in the *NEJM* is again clear evidence of medical bias. Dr. Fischer was quoted by Dr.

Sheldon Gottlieb, in his book *The Naked Mind,*[18] as saying:

> *The National Multiple Sclerosis Society has to be credited with funding the research project, although there was an undercurrent, though never publicly expressed at that time, of the inefficiency of this particular approach to treating MS. When we [Dr. Fischer et al.] found HBOT to be effective, they instituted a campaign to discredit our work. They even went so far as to attempt to prevent its publication.*

The controlled trial by Drs. Fischer, Marks, and Reich was probably the most thorough in the history of medicine, combining matching of the patients before allocation into treated or control groups, close supervision of the sessions in the chamber, with detailed evaluations during, and immediately on completion, of the course of treatment. For the first time in the long history of multiple sclerosis, a treatment had shown benefit to patients with chronic disease. But the results were not received well by neurologists and their disinterest was transmitted to patients. This was a betrayal of trust; after all, which patient could countenance that a successful treatment would *not* be endorsed by their physician?

The patients had first been matched in pairs according to their disabilities and the duration of their symptoms, before being randomly allocated to either the treated, or the control group. All had moderate disability, and all had been suffering from multiple sclerosis for an average of at least five years; the average disease duration was, in fact, greater than 10 years. Assessments were done blind to the allocation of the patients immediately before, during and immediately on completion of the month of treatment. Follow up was then undertaken monthly and the code was not broken until more than 18 months after the completion of the study (personal communication, the late Dr. Fischer). The results at the end of the month were *unequivocally* in favour of the treated group (p< 0.0001). Each nervous system function was independently scored, and again, with the exception of mobility, there were high levels of significance in each category in favour of the hyperbaric oxygen-treated patients. At the end of a year of follow up, the patients in the hyperbaric group had significantly less deterioration than the control group, (p< 0.0008), despite no further treatment being given. If this had been a drug trial, the share price of the drug company involved would have soared and it would have been rigorously marketed.

The cover of the issue of the *New England Journal of Medicine* provides a remarkable insight into the influence of fashion in medicine and the intransigence of its practitioners. The journal featured two articles on the treatment of multiple sclerosis, the first by Hauser et al.,[19] the second the study by Fischer et

Original Articles

Intensive Immunosuppression in Progressive Multiple Sclerosis: A Randomized Three-Arm Study of High-Dose Intravenous Cyclophosphamide, Plasma Exchange, and ACTH 173
STEPHEN L. HAUSER, DAVID M. DAWSON, JAMES R. LEHRICH, M. FLINT BEAL, SHERWIN V. KEVY, RICHARD D. PROPPER, JOHN A. MILLS, AND HOWARD L. WEINER

Hyperbaric-Oxygen Treatment of Multiple Sclerosis: A Randomized, Placebo-Controlled, Double-Blind Study 181
BOGUSLAV H. FISHER, MORTON MARKS, AND THEOBALD REICH

Editorials

Treatment of Multiple Sclerosis 215
DALE E. MCFARLIN

Multiple Sclerosis and the Ingelfinger Rule... 217

Figure 17.2:
Redrawn from the front cover of the *NEJM* (1982;386:180-186).

al.,[6] and they were followed by two editorials. The paper by Hauser et al. from Harvard Medical School in Boston was, therefore, given precedence in the journal as shown in Figure 17.2.

The first paper on intensive immunosuppression gave the results of a three arm study comparing the use of the immunosuppressive drug cyclophosphamide with and without adreno-cortical hormone (ACTH) and a technique of plasma exchange known as plasmapheresis. The investigators in this study were not blinded; it was impossible because of the obvious side effects, nor did the study have a control group. In contrast, the report by Fischer et al. was a randomised, placebo-controlled, double-blind trial which, for the first time in the history of multiple sclerosis, provided *unequivocal* evidence of benefit to patients with established, chronic disease. But reading the two editorials in the *NEJM* commenting on these studies, readers could be forgiven for missing this crucial point. The editorial[20] entitled "Treatment of Multiple Sclerosis," was invited from a neurologist, the late Dr. Dale E. McFarlin. The second[21] was contributed by the deputy editor of the journal at the time, Dr. Marcia Angell. It refers to the *NEJM* Ingelfinger rule, invoked to prevent the results of a study accepted by the journal being published elsewhere.

McFarlin first reviewed the current status of trials in the treatment of patients with multiple sclerosis, observing that ACTH is the only agent to have demonstrated a favourable effect under controlled conditions in the acute disease, by reducing the duration of symptoms of patients with the eye condition known as optic neuritis. Discussing the trial methods necessary, McFarlin then stated:

> *It is obviously essential to have control groups of patients who are matched for age, sex, type of disease, and clinical course. Patients in various groups should be evaluated by the same methods, preferably by examiners who are unaware of the treatment being given.*

Despite this stricture he states, disarmingly and incorrectly that:

> *In both studies, efforts were made to follow the guidelines for valid clinical trials mentioned above. Patients were matched and randomised, criteria were established, and both short term and long term (one year) evaluations were conducted.*

The fact that the Boston trial comparing cyclophosphamide, ACTH, and plasmapheresis did *not* use a control group was ignored; again the negative bias is blindingly obvious. In contrast, the hyperbaric study was not only controlled, it used double-blinding and the patients were matched in pairs before being randomised to either the treated or the control group. Matching is critically important because of the enormous variation, not only in the severity of the sclerosis, but also because of the duration of the disease in the multiple areas affected. A patient, who may have had leg weakness from spinal cord disease 10 years before a course of treatment, will be much less likely to improve than a patient who developed the same symptoms 10 days before. The enormous variations in multiple sclerosis were acknowledged by Dr. George Schumacher in 1974,[1] who went as far as stating that there are 1,457 forms of the disease! We are all different when we are healthy and we become even more different after suffering the ravages of disease.

McFarlin raised questions about the lack of placebo effect in the hyperbaric oxygen therapy study but could not, of course, do so in relation to the trial of immune suppression, because a placebo treatment had not been used. He then asks in relation to the hyperbaric oxygen treatment:

What of the other findings? Five of seventeen did maintain some improvement for one year. The restoration of bladder control and the disappearance of nystagmus each for varying periods cannot be ignored.

Why would any doctor *want* to ignore positive results? Unfortunately, this is precisely what has happened; they *have* been ignored. But he selected only two of many features recorded as improving in the study, and certainly did not emphasise the fact that just 30 hours of oxygen breathing at twice atmospheric pressure, spread over one month, reduced the *rate of deterioration* in the group receiving hyperbaric oxygenation for a further 12 months. Despite this omission, McFarlin stated that he found the differences between the groups in the *immune suppression study* convincing. Statistics are usually only applied in placebo controlled studies but, despite this, statistics were compiled just as if there was a control group, and the figures look deceptively impressive. McFarlin then questions the clinical implications of the results from the two studies, as if the benefits and side effects were actually comparable, using emotive language:

These are preliminary reports of experimental treatments that should be studied further. What do these reports mean for the future? Should all patients with multiple sclerosis be treated with hyperbaric oxygen, cyclophosphamide, or both. Absolutely not! These are preliminary reports of experimental treatments that should be studied further.

There really could be no greater contrast between two agents; oxygen, is the substance most essential to human life, but cyclophosphamide is a highly toxic man-made drug which has no counterpart in living organisms. Patients did indeed worsen in the cyclophosphamide study, but no patient was recorded as worsening at the end of the course of hyperbaric oxygen treatment. Nevertheless, McFarlin denigrated the proven improvement derived from oxygen treatment, stressing the cost and complications of using the equipment needed to use hyperbaric conditions. He even warns of side-effects not seen in any patient in the study; they relate to the very high oxygen pressures in divers. The balance is redressed only slightly by the admission that there are indeed risks associated with the use of cyclophosphamide. Nevertheless, incredibly, the authors of the immunosuppression study were allowed to claim, under the subtitle "Complications and toxicity of therapy," that:

. . . there were no major complications in any of the treatment groups.

The patients given cyclophosphamide suffered the indignity of losing all their hair and bouts of severe vomiting, which are both well-recognised side effects of the drug. In fact, several of the patients in the three groups in this study worsened considerably. Even more importantly, patients given cyclophosphamide have been found to suffer a reduction of brain volume, which is thought to be due to a direct toxic effect of the drug. Other, more long-term risks include inflammation of the bladder wall, bladder cancer, and leukaemia. Astonishingly, McFarlin placed oxygen and cyclophosphamide in the same category of risk, stating that he regarded both treatments as "experimental":

> *Woe be it unto the physician who fails to explain that these approaches are experimental and that they entail risks.*

So a safe and effective treatment, which simply uses more oxygen, is rated as being as dangerous as the administration of a highly toxic poison. This is a travesty and yet another example of the influence of pseudoscience and fashion. The only positive comment from McFarlin about the hyperbaric oxygen treatment was the improvement in patients' bladder function but, strangely, it is not properly aligned to it in the text:

> *Quantitative assessment of bladder function is indicated because improvement in the latter was a major finding in the current report.*

Dr. McFarlin's editorial then discussed at length the need for controls and double-blind techniques for trials in multiple sclerosis stating *categorically* that no trial should be accepted for publication if it does not conform to this standard. But he makes no comment about the failure of the Boston group to apply this gold standard to the immune suppression study. Using his criteria, it should not have been published. In contrast, there is the absurd allegation that minor temporary changes in vision experienced by some patients in the oxygen study may have compromised the blinding of the investigators. Some patients given cyclophosphamide suffered from disabling bleeding from the bladder; ironically, oxygen under hyperbaric conditions is an effective treatment of this condition.[22] In contrast, the dosage of oxygen administered in the trial by Fischer et al. does not carry *any significant risk*, indeed patients are safer inside the chamber than they are outside! The only side effects encountered with the treatment when it is properly administered are not from the oxygen, they are from the change in pressure and involve the ears and, very rarely, the sinuses.

None of the treatments used in the immune suppression study, which carry very significant risks, have subsequently been shown to be of any value in treating multiple sclerosis patients, and there is now considerable evidence that they make patients worse. Certainly, in the case of cyclophosphamide, the results of further studies indicated that patients with chronic progressive disease were worse at the end of two years of treatment than if they had not had any treatment at all.[23] The obsession with immune suppression was clearly evident in the UK in a British Medical Research Council trial based in London, which used the drug azathioprine (Imuran). The preliminary results of the study, published in the *Lancet* in 1980[24] reported that two of the immune suppressed patients had died from a well-known complication of this approach—infection; they died of pneumonia. However, in the final report in the journal published two years later,[25] the patients were actually included in the statistical table of the results having been given a disability score; they had been classified with a Kurtzke disability rating of 9, which is dead. The desperation of the authors to confirm the validity of immune suppression for multiple sclerosis patients is all too obvious in their discussion of the results.

Despite being out with the normal limits of statistical significance our results suggest that the principle of immunosuppression is valid.

In other words the results were *not* statistically significant. Reading this paper no one should doubt the coercion still exerted by the myopic fads and fashions of medicine.

The trial of hyperbaric oxygen treatment in New York had followed public pressure on the US National MS Society generated by the work of Richard Neubauer. As already discussed, the New York University results were presented by Dr. Fischer to a meeting of hyperbaric physicians in Long Beach in the summer of 1982 and, not surprisingly, the news that they were positive soon spread, although the author has been unable to trace any press coverage. The patients, however, were desperate to have them published and voiced their concerns. In the second editorial in the *NEJM* entitled "The Ingelfinger Rule," the deputy editor, Marcia Angell, wrote;

Even before this paper was submitted to us, both the authors and the Journal's editors began to receive pressure from a number of sources to publish the manuscript rapidly and to release the details of the study to the news media.

She went further, stating that:

. . . the article in question deals with the use of hyperbaric oxygen in the treatment of multiple sclerosis. As Dr. McFarlin's editorial makes clear, the data in this study in no way indicate that this is a cure for multiple sclerosis.

It is obvious that at the time the profession at large appeared to believe in a cure for multiple sclerosis, but there are no illusions about the latest drugs, for example, the beta interferons, being a cure. The article by Fischer and his colleagues about what amounts to the use of just a little more oxygen was subject to an extraordinary degree of scrutiny. According to Angell it was:

> . . . *reviewed by no fewer than five experts on multiple sclerosis, it was twice reviewed by our statistical consultants, and it underwent two revisions, during which the authors were asked to supply additional information and further analysis of the data.*

No such rigour appears to have been encountered by the authors of the paper on the immune suppressive therapies, despite their well-known dangers and they have all proved to be ineffective. Dr. Angell, later appointed editor of the journal, subsequently wrote a controversial exposé of the pharmaceutical industry.

The publication of the results of the first clearly successful treatment for multiple sclerosis patients received very little publicity and there was no correspondence published by the *NEJM*. The trial which had cost $250,000 was not actually completed as it was funded to continue the follow-up for a total of three years. No further studies were commissioned by the National MS Society of America. By June 1983, by order of the administration of New York University Medical Center, the hyperbaric chamber was removed from the building and all work on the treatment of multiple sclerosis ceased. Figure 17.3 reproduces the letter sent by Dr. Fischer to Dr. Neubauer in 1983. When the author visited Dr. Fischer in September 1982, the chamber was rusting in the parking lot; it was obviously too dangerous to leave it in the building.

Further trials were sponsored by the MS Society in the UK and were undertaken in London[26] and Newcastle. The London study was reported as negative by the authors, but, nevertheless, showed positive results, especially in bladder function. Measurements of bladder volume, (cystometry) were made which confirmed a similar study in the US.[27] Some sensory functions also improved to a level that was statistically significant in the oxygen group. The Newcastle study was the only one of the two that was actually completed, and it demonstrated improvement in bladder and bowel control.[28] At the end of the year of follow up, after just 20 sessions in the first month, it was found that there was less deterioration in the oxygen treated group from just 20 sessions.[29] However, the treatment was poorly supervised; the techniques used caused many cases of ear pain with one patient even suffering a ruptured ear drum. The reports, which are discussed in more detail in the next chapter,

BOGUSLAV H. FISCHER, M. D.
NEW YORK UNIVERSITY MEDICAL CENTER
400 EAST 34TH STREET
NEW YORK, NEW YORK 10016

Dr. Richard A. Neubauer
Ocean Medical Center
4001 Ocean Drive
Lauderdale-by-the-Sea
Florida 33308

New York, 5-31-83

By administrative decision of the New York University Medical
Center the Hyperbaric Oxygen Facility has been dismantled.
It is with deepest regret to inform you that at this Center
all further research concerning the use of hyperbaric oxygen
in the treatment of multiple sclerosis has been discontinued
for an indefinite period of time.

truly yours

B. H. Fischer
Boguslav H. Fischer, M.D.
Asst. Professor of Clinical Neurology

Figure 17.3:
Letter from Dr. B.H. Fischer to Dr. R.A. Neubauer regarding the
closure of the chamber at NYU.

were also clearly biased towards a negative result which, because the use of "controlled" trials is to avoid bias, is cruelly ironic. There can be no doubt that, as Schumacher[1] stated:

Far more realistic as an indicator of therapeutic effect than the lessening of symptoms or signs is the halting of progression of neurological deficit. The sole criterion of efficacy should be the prevention of downhill progression or recurrent exacerbations.

Much new information has been discovered to confirm the use of hyperbaric oxygen treatment since the trials of the 1980s; scientists have detailed the key role of oxygen in the control of inflammation, although this is not quite how it is usually stated. Their emphasis has been on studying the involvement of lack of oxygen in inflammation, rather than the importance of using oxygen as a treatment. The key protein involved, hypoxia-inducible factor 1 alpha, has already been discussed in Chapter 1. There has been increasing interest in the phenomenon of inflammation generally, and this is certainly true in relation to multiple sclerosis. There is also much less emphasis on the use of immune suppression in the disease and more on the control of inflammation. In the UK, research into multiple sclerosis in the National Hospital for Neurology and Neurosurgery in London is based in a new department of neuroinflammation, and its head, Professor Kenneth Smith, is not a neurologist; he is a biological scientist. He now leads a team that is again researching the use of oxygen under hyperbaric conditions in the animal model EAE, beginning, inexplicably, with studies to establish its safety.

Inflammation has long been recognised as a central feature of a host of diseases and always complicates injury. The migration of white blood cells from the circulating blood into the nervous system across the blood-brain barrier of the veins is the key to the control of infection in the brain. For this reason, the venous barrier is less secure and it is no coincidence that the areas affected in multiple sclerosis surround veins, just as they do in divers who suffer from decompression sickness. As discussed in Chapter 8, the research from the University of Pennsylvania demonstrating the role of white blood cells in decompression sickness has provided further evidence for the validity of the comparison of decompression sickness to multiple sclerosis, both in its causation and its treatment.[30] The need for hyperbaric conditions to provide the additional oxygen in treatment can now be explained and it is not a matter of biological plausibility or clinical opinion, it is physics and based on measurement.

In the 1960s, when interest in the clinical use of hyperbaric oxygen treatment was of interest to senior figures in medicine and surgery, Sir Charles Illingworth's group in the University of Glasgow conducted the defining experiments presented earlier in which the oxygen levels in the arteries and veins of the brain were measured. The experiments were undertaken in the large hyperbaric surgical operating room on the roof of the Western Infirmary.[31] The details bear repetition; anaesthetised animals were used and measurements taken, first breathing air and then 100% oxygen at normal atmospheric pressure, 1 ATA. Finally, measurements were repeated at twice atmospheric pressure, 2 ATA. As expected, the level of oxygen in the arteries was about 100 mm Hg with the animals breathing air and rose to about 500 mm Hg breathing 100% oxygen at normal atmospheric pressure because, of course an increase from 20–100% is multiplying by five. At 2 ATA it was over 1000 mm Hg, that is, 10 times the level breathing air. This means the *concentration gradient* for the transfer of oxygen from blood to cells was 10 times greater. What would not, however, be as obvious is that the increase in the concentration of oxygen measured in the blood leaving in the *veins* of the brain was modest; from 40 mm Hg breathing air at 1 ATA to only 70 mm Hg breathing 100% oxygen at 2 ATA.

So what is the explanation for this effect? It is simply due to the poor *solubility of oxygen in water*; the additional dissolved oxygen in the plasma is used before oxygen is detached from the molecules of haemoglobin carried by red blood cells. What physics would not predict is that from normally breathing air to breathing pure oxygen in the chamber, the blood flow through the brain fell by a truly enormous 20%. To increase the delivery of oxygen to the tissues whilst reducing blood flow is unique to oxygen administration and can *never* be achieved by a drug. The reduction in blood flow is associated with a reduction of the diameter of blood vessels, because this is how blood flow is controlled and leakage from veins is largely related to their diameter and porosity. Note that the 20% reduction of blood flow through the brain also reflects a 20% reduction in the output of blood from the heart, again illustrating the central importance of oxygen to the control of the circulation.

Fortunately, the professional disinterest that followed the publication of the controlled trials of oxygen treatment did not end the matter, at least in the UK and Ireland, where the patients' interest in oxygen treatment continued to grow. A detailed new study using two years of follow up was undertaken in the MS Therapy Centre in Glasgow,[32] ironically a stone's throw from the site of the dismantled chamber at the Western Infirmary. Now, after more than 30 years, thousands of patients in the UK and Ireland continue to provide their own hyperbaric oxygen treatment in dedicated community-based charity centres. In fact, their right to do so is now enshrined in UK legislation. Control of the most powerful treatment in medicine has gone from a sceptical medical profession into the hands of patients. The next chapter covers their remarkable story.

CHAPTER 18

The UK Multiple Sclerosis Therapy Centres: Self-Help in Action

The MS National Therapy Centres have pioneered the use of low pressure barochambers in the community and this simple treatment has given improved quality of life for thousands of patients.

The late Right Hon. Lord Whaddon, 2003

In the autumn of 1981, patients who had taken part in a small study in Dundee based on the publications of Dr. Richard Neubauer[1,2] and monitored by a local neurologist, decided that they wanted to continue their treatment. They formed a "self-help" group and, being keen to be involved with an existing charity, they approached the committee of an organisation called Action and Research into Multiple Sclerosis (ARMS) in London. It had been formed in 1974 by MS Society members who had been concerned that not enough was being done to address the practical day-to-day needs of sufferers, or encourage some of the less mainstream research. A number of discussion groups had formed around the country to look at the evidence of improvement from graded exercises with physiotherapy and the low fat diet pioneered in Canada by the distinguished neurologist Dr. Roy Swank. In the summer of 1982, the Dundee patients called a public meeting which was attended by John Simkins from the ARMS management committee, and it was agreed that the patients could form a group to be known as Friends of ARMS. A chamber was purchased and operations began in August 1982 in an industrial unit in Scotland, in Peddie Street, Dundee. The street, which would have been known to Haldane, is close to the University and city centre. The chamber had been built during WW2 for the Institute of Aviation Medicine in Farnborough to study altitude sickness, providing an interesting link to an earlier theme in this book. After demobilisation from the Institute, it had been acquired by a diving contractor and used offshore in the gas fields of the southern North Sea and finally on a diving contract at an oil terminal in Milford Haven, before being "retired" to a farm in Bedfordshire.

A pilot study of the first 30 patients attending the centre was undertaken and all were assessed by the same neurologist, Dr. Duncan Davidson. The results, published in 1984,[3] clearly confirmed the findings of the New York University trial by Fischer et al.[4] The neurologist questioned how patients who would benefit significantly from the treatment could be selected, as it was likely to be expensive in the NHS. This would obviously mean the unacceptable exclusion of many patients and the charity centres had shown that the treatment could be provided at minimal cost. Following press publicity over the following year, several hundred patients attended the centre to have the recommended 20 sessions. Many travelled long distances, some from as far as Brazil, Australia, and Canada. When they saw the simplicity of the chamber and its operation in Dundee, not surprisingly, some patients decided to acquire their own chambers and start their own centres. This initiative was not welcomed by other Multiple Sclerosis organisations and one even issued a press release, alleging a fire risk. Fortunately, most of the newspapers made enquiries clearly suspecting that it was scaremongering; all but one decided not to publish the release. More oxygen is only a risk if there is a fire, but a fire *cannot* be started without a source of ignition and, of course, a fuel to complete the "fire triangle." No lighters, matches, or other sources of ignition are now allowed to be used in pressure chambers, although many years ago the Royal Navy allowed smoking in diving decompression chambers. It was stopped after a serious incident when a fire was caused by a diver who spilled petrol from a cigarette lighter. It is important to recognise that the cabins of aircraft pose a similar risk—being confined spaces, and there is the added complication that occupants obviously cannot be evacuated at altitude. Many passengers have died in aircraft fires but, thankfully, there is now an almost total ban on smoking in commercial aircraft. Smoking is also banned in public buildings in many countries, which must have significantly reduced the number of deaths from fires.

The professional response to the double-blind controlled study published in the *New England Journal of Medicine* reporting the benefit from hyperbaric oxygen treatment in patients with multiple sclerosis was almost universally negative. This was graphically illustrated when the chairman of the UK MS Society medical advisory committee was interviewed for the *Medicine Now* programme on BBC Radio 4 in 1983 by the reporter Geoff Watts. Strong support was voiced for the paper reporting the Boston study of immune suppression,[5] despite its lack of success, imperfect trial design, and the dreadful side effects of cyclophosphamide. It was "felt" that the way forward in the treatment of multiple sclerosis was sure to be improvement of immune-suppressing drug regimes, despite their well-documented dangers. In fact, *none* of the immunosuppressive drugs trialled from the 1960s to the 1980s remain in use today, at least not in the US or the UK.

Following the publication of the successful trial and the interest generated among patients, the UK MS Society funded the two studies, one in Newcastle upon Tyne, where there was already a multiple occupancy hyperbaric chamber in the Royal Victoria Infirmary, and one in London. The London study[6] used two single person oxygen chambers. One was based at Whipps Cross Hospital in North London, and the other at St. Thomas' Hospital. The methodology was poor in both studies; patients were not matched in pairs to be randomised, nor did they use a proper chamber control with a "placebo" gas as Fischer et al. had done in New York. Both studies also used much more disabled patients, with an average disease duration of 12 years, not 10.

The Newcastle group released a preliminary report which was published in the *Lancet* on February 9, 1985.[7] It was clear that there were serious problems with the techniques used. In an attempt to secure "blinding," the investigators had simulated the increase in pressure for the "placebo" group by using the noise of compressed air for 10 minutes without actually pressurising the chamber. The patients in the treated group were pressurised to 2 ATA in the same time of 10 minutes, regardless of whether or not they were able to clear their ears. This led to 19 patients suffering severe trauma to the ear drum; in fact the drum was actually ruptured in one patient. Apart from causing the patients severe distress, which may have contributed to worsening of their illness, the pain prevented "blinding" of the physicians involved in their assessments. Their bias against the treatment became all too obvious with the publication of the paper, when the authors derided their own clearly positive results. The patients were not examined immediately before, during and on completion of the treatment, which was the meticulous routine that had been used in the New York trial. It was also clear that the Newcastle study report was hurriedly submitted to the *Lancet* in what certainly appeared to be an attempt to stifle the growth of the self-help movement, which aimed to provide hyperbaric oxygen treatment in community based centres. Despite being a preliminary report and showing that there *were* positive effects, especially, on bladder and bowel control, regrettably, the *Lancet* allowed the authors to actually include a conclusion:

> *The short term results of this trial do not support the claims made for hyperbaric oxygen in the management of multiple sclerosis.*

In fact, Fischer and his colleagues in New York had not made any such "claims," they had made two very logical recommendations; that long-term studies should be undertaken and, crucially, that further studies of the treatment should be of patients with *acute attacks* and relapses.

Unfortunately, in contrast to lack of coverage of the positive report by Fischer et al. in the US, which almost unreported by the press, the *Lancet* paper was given wide publicity through a release by Associated Press. This was probably instigated by the New York trial funding agency, whose chairman had already indicated his opposition to the treatment. It would need some investigative journalism to discover the background to this press release; the details were carried by the *Houston Post* on Sunday February 17, 1985.

BOSTON (AP) – A major new study contradicts the findings of a widely publicised report two years ago that sparked a burst of demand among multiple sclerosis victims for an expensive and controversial form of treatment… In the United States, the study's results were embraced by experts who had already doubted the worth of oxygen treatment.

Although the article did acknowledge "modest improvements in bladder control," it tellingly reveals the relief felt by doctors that the trial was, allegedly, negative. The results of the *NEJM* study by Fischer et al. were certainly not "widely publicised" and it is a sad reflection on experts that they admit to *embracing* a negative result. One professor of neurology, who is still active in Houston, actually stated in an unguarded moment, "unfortunately we cannot yet say that hyperbaric oxygen treatment is of no value." It is not surprising that the Associated Press release had a major impact in the US; after all it was *doctors* who were saying that the treatment was ineffective and most patients must trust that their doctors will not deny them a treatment that has shown benefit. The author commented in a letter to the *Lancet* about the Newcastle study in June 1985,[8] that this must be the first time in the history of medicine that doctors undertaking a trial have denied their own positive findings.

The Newcastle trial had been funded to allow the patients to be followed for a year after the completion of the 20 sessions, although they were not allowed any further treatment. The authors published their final report in another journal, the *Journal of Neurology, Neurosurgery and Psychiatry* two years later.[9] It indicated that the benefit to bladder and bowel function which, it must be remembered was from just 30 hours of hyperbaric oxygen treatment, actually lasted for six months. Also, it was found that patients in the treated group had less deterioration in balance evident at one year. With obvious reluctance, the authors actually called for *further studies*, but with no press release of the conclusions of the final report, it went unnoticed. One other study was undertaken in Italy and again it found evidence of benefit using tests of nerve conduction.[10] However, the funding body, the MS Society in the UK, has continued to tell patients that this and other trials have shown that giving oxygen is of no benefit ("Fresh Air Relief for MS Patients," *Daily Express*, January 7, 2014). Fortunately, matters have begun to change, evident from the funding of the animal disease. It is notable that, as in the case of the patients involved in the studies at Duke University, some of the Newcastle patients continued treatment in the chamber in the University of Newcastle for many years until it was eventually closed (personal communications, Professor Peter Bennett, late of Duke University, North Carolina, and Mr. John Cook, formerly hyperbaric technician in the University of Newcastle).

The results of the trials conducted at Whipps Cross and St. Thomas' Hospitals in London were published together in the *British Medical Journal* on February 8, 1986.[6] However, the journal editors actually allowed the authors to withhold the patient data. With the exception of results from a sub group of patients with severe bladder dysfunction, just tables of statistical data were published. This is unprecedented and reprehensible, because it does not allow the results to be analysed independently. The authors argued that the positive results, which were statistically significant, were simply due to chance, despite their use of controls. Patients with severe bladder problems were selected for study from the patients attending St. Thomas' Hospital. Tests of bladder function were conducted in nine of the multiple sclerosis patients who received oxygen under hyperbaric conditions and 11 controls who received hyperbaric air. The paper states:

> *In the group given hyperbaric oxygenation, bladder capacity increased in five patients and was unchanged in four; in the group given air it improved in one, was unchanged in nine and was worse in one.*

It is obvious that this is, indeed, a positive effect, especially important in view of the deliberate choice of patients with the most severe bladder problems. However, the statistical analysis used by the authors only allowed for patients remaining the same or improving, not for them getting worse. The statistical probability value published ($p < 0.07$) was said to only indicate "a trend in favour of the group given hyperbaric oxygen" which is consistent with the negative tone of the paper. However, if a statistical test is used that allows for the possibility of deterioration, the result is statistically significant ($p < 0.05$). Again the doctors demonstrated their bias by playing down their own results, just as those responsible for the Newcastle study had done. It is clear that if these papers were read, even by open-minded neurologists, they would dismiss oxygen being used as a treatment. Another study of bladder function with positive results had also been reported from a group in New Orleans.[11]

Several other studies were undertaken in other countries which deliberately chose patients with *chronically stable*, long-term disease and, not surprisingly, they again showed little or no benefit. This raises the question; why was the trial by Fischer et al. so different? The reason is simple; the patients in the New York study were examined on the day they started treatment, then each week during the treatment, and on the day they actually completed the 20 sessions, when the benefits were most obvious. The improvements were also carefully monitored at follow up examinations done at six months and one year. By the end of the year, some of the improvements had disappeared, but the major finding, as it was in the Newcastle study, was *less deterioration* in the treated group and it was still statistically significant at the end of the year of follow up. However, some of the patients attending the centre in Dundee soon found that if their benefits started to regress, a single treatment would often restore them and so they started to use the treatment regularly, as many of Dr. Neubauer's patients had done in the 1970s. Their expectations had changed from cure to managing the disease. MRI can be used to follow the results of treatment. The author was involved with Professor John Mallard in Aberdeen, the co-inventor of the technology, in scanning a patient before and after a session of hyperbaric oxygen treatment. Although the resolution of the water-cooled magnet machine was not optimal, it demonstrated improvement.[12] This approach was continued by Dr. Neubauer with Dr. Robert Kagan in 1984 using an imager with a superconducting magnet. The images in Figure 18.1 show a baseline scan in a 58-year-old man who was told he was suffering from multiple sclerosis four years before the treatment. The second image is one hour after the session of hyperbaric oxygen treatment in a Vickers monoplace chamber at 1.5 ATA, and the third on completion of 20 sessions at the same pressure. His hand co-ordination, walking, and fatigue all improved.

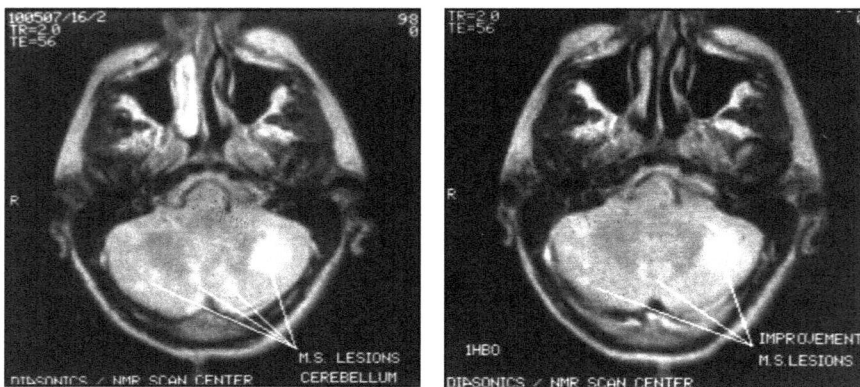

Figure 18.1:
Improvement (arrowed) in cerebellar lesions with HBOT in a 58-year-old man.

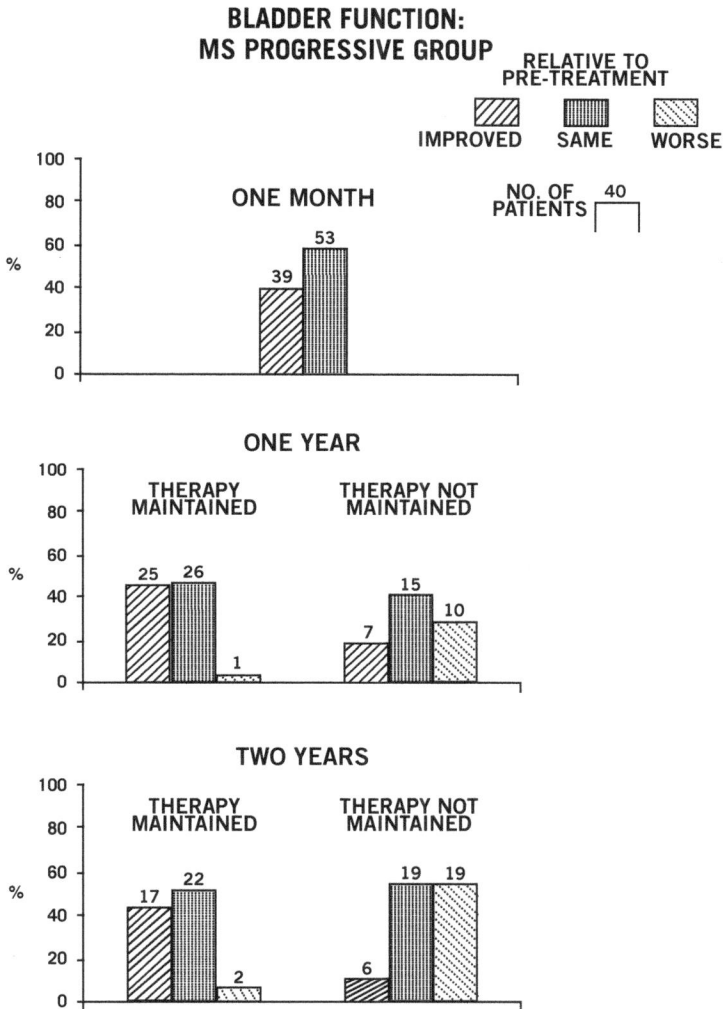

Figure 18.2:
Results of hyperbaric oxygen treatment on bladder function in patients with chronic progressive disease.

In 1985 the chairman of the Glasgow self-help centre, Dr. Colin Webster, himself a patient, raised funding for a detailed study of 128 patients, which again confirmed the benefit of continuing treatment. The publication, which was discussed in the *Lancet* in 1989,[13] allowed a comparison between patients who were able to continue treatment and those who were not. Figure 18.2 shows the deterioration over two years in bladder function in patients with progressive multiple sclerosis who were not able to continue treatment.

The trials had found unequivocal evidence of benefit from hyperbaric oxygen treatment in patients with multiple areas of sclerosis, despite disabilities having been present for many years. In fact, they had to have clear, objective evidence of disability, and symptoms that were constant on neurological examination to be included in the studies. Inevitably, these patients are the least likely to benefit. It is obvious that oxygen treatment should be used for acute conditions, not for disabilities that have developed over many years. Imagine telling a diver who has lost the use of his legs surfacing after a dive that his treatment must be postponed for 10 years, to ensure that it is only given when spontaneous improvement is unlikely!

At the time of all this activity in the 1980s, the crude advertising slogan being used to raise money for research into multiple sclerosis in the UK was; "give us the money and we will find the cure." One doctor, himself a sufferer, actually complained to the MS Society about the grim black and white advertisements. As usual, the campaign gave the mistaken impression that there will, eventually, be a drug, a magic bullet, to cure the scars of multiple sclerosis. Today, there is much less emphasis on cure; agencies like the National Health Service only talk about "disease management." This is largely because the drugs for long-term use to manage the symptoms of multiple sclerosis are heavily marketed by drug companies. As many of the patients who have accessed hyperbaric oxygen treatment have found, regular treatment is also required with these drugs, in fact, they must be prescribed for the life of the patient. The need for continued treatment is because of the persistence of the blood-brain barrier dysfunction and chronic inflammation. These aspects of the disease are, at last, receiving research funding. A programme in the series *The Material World*, broadcast on April 17, 2008 on BBC Radio 4, highlighted the stark contrast in the approach taken by a neurologist and a biologist to the importance of the blood-brain barrier. The neurologist wanted to find a way of breaking the barrier down to allow drugs to access the brain, whilst the scientist emphasised the critical importance of maintaining the protection it affords, to ensure the continued health of the brain.

It is clear today that, despite the use of controlled studies and the adoption of evidence-based practice, doctors are still very prone to bias. In the UK, NICE, the National Institute for Clinical Excellence was set up to evaluate treatment as objectively as possible. NICE is a "quango," that is, a quasi-autonomous government organisation. To be politically correct, it has added the word "Health" to its title to indicate a broadening of its scope, but the acronym NICE remains resolutely in use. Why has it been necessary to create this very expensive organisation? It is because there are many powerful speciality groups in medicine representing the professional interests of their members. The formation of NICE confirms that because each speciality fights for its share of the "cake" and cannot be relied on to provide unbiased opinions about medical practice. However, the principal function of NICE is to produce national clinical guidelines for NHS management in primary and secondary care, through consultation with "stakeholders." Experts are invited to contribute and interested parties can apply to be included in the stakeholder groups. Not surprisingly, the drug industry has been strongly represented in the debate about the treatment of multiple sclerosis, because the potential for profit generated by long-term treatment in such a common and chronic disease is truly enormous. The guidelines for the management of multiple sclerosis, published by NICE in November 2003, state that hyperbaric oxygen treatment should only be used in the NHS for patients with multiple sclerosis

---

NICE Multiple Sclerosis – National Clinical Guidelines for NHS Management in Primary and Secondary Care, March 2003

Hyperbaric oxygen

A systematic review (Level 1a) and one additional RCT (Level 1 b) met inclusion criteria. The review included 14 RCTs but the results were restricted to eight studies which were judged to be of reasonable quality. The review reported that only one of eight trials reported results in favour of hyperbaric oxygen therapy, the others found no clear positive effects. Side effects were generally minor with ear and visual problems predominating. The additional RCT, which was of good quality, reported a positive effect of treatment for all five outcomes investigated and reported only minor adverse events associated with treatment.

The agents listed by NICE that should not be used, or only used in controlled studies is as follows:

- Cyclophosphamide
- Anti-viral agents (e.g. acyclovir, tuberculin)
- Clabribine
- Linomide
- Hyperbaric oxygen therapy
- Whole body irradiation using radioactivity
- Injections of myelin basic protein (any type)
- A wide range of oral drugs (see evidence statements)

Figure 18.3:
Excerpt: the 2003 NICE guideline which mentions a hyperbaric oxygen treatment.

in the context of clinical trials. By this time the charity centres had completed *more than 20 years* of successful operation. The guidelines are based on the last draft of the consultation document reproduced in Figure 18.3. Note the grammatically incorrect use of the term "hyperbaric oxygen," instead of hyperbaric oxygenation.

So, again, the substance *universally accepted* as being essential to life, is ranked alongside poisons like cyclophosphamide and whole-body radioactive irradiation with its well-known dangers. The recommendation of NICE was that *within the NHS* the use of hyperbaric oxygen treatment should be restricted to randomised controlled trials. It is true, as stated, that only one of the three studies publicised *reported* benefit, but all three actually found benefit. No representative from the MS Therapy Centres using hyperbaric treatment had been present at the stakeholder meeting, nor were any of the authors of the UK studies present; normally, doctors want to "talk up" their findings. The press have recently discovered that the common practice for doctors to allow drug company marketing people to "ghost write" their papers; a chilling example of "the ghost in the machine."

The NICE report about hyperbaric oxygen treatment comments that "side effects were *generally* minor." The use of the word "generally," of course, implies that there were more serious problems, which is patently not true. Contrast this with the deaths of two out of just twenty patients from the drug azathioprine (Imuran) in the UK Medical Research Council funded study[14] and the dreadful side effects of intravenous cyclophosphamide,[15] both discussed in Chapter 17. Fortunately, with no evidence of benefit, NICE has included cyclophosphamide in the list of agents that the NHS should *not* use. The reader may remember the same ritual denial in the late Dr. Dale McFarlin's editorial from the *New England Journal of Medicine*[16] quoted to in Chapter 17; "Woe be it unto the physician who fails to explain that these approaches are experimental and that they entail risks."

There is actually no particular clinical expertise in an organisation like NICE; reviews are based on the published research of specialists with all bias that this often involves. The review about hyperbaric oxygen treatment used by NICE as their main source of information was a paper by two Dutch public health specialists, Drs. Kleijnen and Knipschild, which was published in 1995 in the journal *Acta Neurologica Scandinavia*.[17] Most of the trials of hyperbaric oxygen treatment had been completed by 1987 and this Dutch review was apparently provoked by multiple sclerosis patients in Holland still demanding the treatment from the health services in Holland. Again, these authors did not have any experience of hyperbaric oxygen treatment; they are simply involved in epidemiological and statistical studies. However, it is important to note that this paper actually discusses the importance of the various oxygen dosages used in the studies and the only trial in which the oxygen "dosage" the patients achieved was actually measured was the meticulous study undertaken at New York University.[4] It was shown that, at a constant pressure of 2 ATA, the blood oxygen tension varied from 860 mm Hg, (equivalent to 1.11 ATA), to a maximum value of 1,140 mm Hg (equivalent to 1.59 ATA). However, just a *single measurement* was made in each patient during the 20 sessions of their treatment. From a scientific standpoint the variation seems unacceptable, but the problem pales into insignificance when compared to the variation in blood levels of drugs taken by mouth. Figure 10.1 in Chapter 10 shows that the plasma concentrations of a drug taken by mouth may vary between patients by over 700%!

The author does not disagree with the NICE statement that hyperbaric oxygen treatment should not be provided for chronic multiple sclerosis patients in NHS hospitals; not because it would not be helpful, but because it would simply be impossible to provide the level of service needed at reasonable cost. The charity centres have shown that it is far better for such patients to organise their own treatment; as recent events in a health authority in England have shown, the NHS is far from perfect in managing patients with chronic disease. The MS Therapy Centre in Dundee, is not the largest of the 65 charity centres, but it treats an average of 160 patients a week Monday to Friday, including evening sessions, and three sessions on Saturdays. For this standard of care to be provided in the NHS would be inordinately expensive. Patients in the charity also have the freedom to organise and book their own treatment when they feel they need it, without having to convince a doctor! Actually, there are no tests that doctors can use to determine if a patient feels fatigued; a very common symptom in multiple sclerosis. The centres also organise other important services, like physiotherapy, which, despite lacking of evidence from controlled trials, are essential for many patients to maintain their mobility.

The drugs currently used for the management of multiple sclerosis are three forms of *beta* interferon (Avonex, Betaseron, and Rebif) and glatimer acetate, whose trade name is Copaxone. The marketing of these drugs was based on the reduction of attacks in patients with relapsing remitting multiple sclerosis. The reduction in their frequency was said to be from three to two over a two-year period.[18] NICE opposed the introduction of these disease modifying drugs (DMDs) in the UK on the grounds of cost effectiveness, as the prevention of one attack in two years would cost about £20,000. Lobbying by MS groups led to the creation of a "risk sharing" scheme in which the government agreed to bear the cost of the drugs prescribed, provided the drug companies agreed to reduce their cost if effectiveness judged in two yearly assessments was less than the drug companies claimed. Although the scheme was started in 2002, it proved to be very much more difficult to monitor, mainly because of disagreements about the methods used, and it was heavily criticised.[19] The first assessments were not published until 2009 in the *British Medical Journal*.[20] The results indicated that the patients were actually *worse* than if they had not received any treatment at all based on historical controls.[21] The controversy extended to the use of the disability assessment derived from the much-derided Kurtzke disability scale. It says much about the quality of multiple sclerosis research that more than 140 years after the comprehensive description of the disease by Charcot, the methods used to assess patients, to quote Professor George Ebers,[22] "are not fit for purpose." He goes on to point out in his analysis of the results of the risk sharing scheme, that the use of MRI of the brain to determine disease activity does *not* predict the progression of disability. Unfortunately, the reason is rather obvious, disability in multiple sclerosis patients is mainly related to areas of damage in the spinal cord, which is rarely included in MRI studies. The resolution of the spinal cord using MRI is poor because it is surrounded by liquid, and small areas of damage, for example to the long nerve fibres controlling muscles, readily cause weakness or paralysis.

Of the five commentators invited by the *British Medical Journal*, only one defended the risk sharing scheme, Professor Alistair Compston,[23] although he admitted that disease progression was not only worse than predicted, it was worse than in the untreated control group and well above the 20% tolerance for price changes. He pointed out that the funding had provided more dedicated nurses and, in fairness, disclosed that his department is involved in drug trials. The composition of the scientific advisory committee has rightly been criticised; far from being "independent," the drug companies were represented on the committee and it is actually admitted that they "gave permission" for its publication. Little doubt why the drug industries association office in London is in Whitehall opposite the Department of Health building. Astonishingly, in view of the greater deterioration of the patients being given the drugs when compared to the natural course of the disease, the Department of Health has indicated that it is still determined to continue the exercise. Nearly half a billion pounds has been spent on the scheme, despite the evidence indicating that the drugs are actually making patients worse. They were licensed for 20 years in 2002. The Multiple Sclerosis

Society in the UK, which campaigned hard for the drugs to be made available, has withdrawn its support for the scheme.

A second consequence of the disease management approach has been the reluctant approval by NICE of the drug natalizumab (Tysabri) which is a monoclonal antibody. It was withdrawn in the US in 2005 when it was found to be associated with progressive multifocal leucoencephalopathy, (PML) which is a chronic viral disease of the brain that is often fatal. However, after intense lobbying by the manufacturers the drug was reintroduced a year later, although restricted to severely-affected patients. The drug reduces the body's defences against the common "JC" polyomavirus responsible for PML, which was named after the first patient in whom the disease was identified, John Cunningham. In 2009, 24 patients had already developed the disease. This risk is common to other monoclonal antibodies because they suppress the immune system by removing lymphocytes from the circulation compromising resistance to infection. However, it is a particular problem in patients with multiple sclerosis, because of the damage present to the blood-brain barrier. The risk of PML increases with time, doubling from one per thousand in the first year, to two per thousand in the second. The dangers in pregnancy are so great that women must not conceive for *at least one year after* the last dose of the drug. If monoclonal antibodies are stopped and the immune system begins to recover—which takes months—the patient risks another serious complication, immune reconstitution inflammatory syndrome (IRIS). This may also occur after the withdrawal of other drugs that suppress the immune system. There are times when Einstein's quotation from 1917 seems appropriate: "Our entire much-praised technological progress and civilisation generally could be compared to an axe in the hand of a pathological madman."

On October 29, 2009 the results of a study of another drug in this class, rituximab (Rituxan), in patients with primary-progressive multiple sclerosis were published in the *Annals of Neurology*.[24] This drug also did not slow disease progression when compared with an inactive placebo. However, MRI had "suggested" some benefit in younger patients based on regular monitoring. But as pointed out by Dr. Ebers, the problem is that the level of disease activity in the brain followed by MRI does *not* correlate with the progression of disability in patients with multiple sclerosis. This is especially the case when sight is affected by damage to the optic nerve. It also applies to the spinal cord and it is not difficult to see why; it weighs a mere 50 grams in contrast to the 1,350 grams of a typical human brain. So not only are the clinical measures used to assess patients not fit for purpose, the use of MRI does not predict disability. But the failure of drugs highlights that the key problem in multiple sclerosis is not auto-immunity it is *inflammation*. What is clearly needed for the treatment of patients is an agent that reduces inflammation, but does not compromise the immune system; we have already found it; it is *oxygen*.

The contrast of drug therapies with the use of oxygen in treatment could not be more dramatic. After more than 30 years, no patient attending the UK charity centres has developed the deterioration seen after a course of the drugs used to suppress the immune system. As oxygen is essential to the activity of the body's defences and central to the control of microbial infections this should not be a surprise. The Department of Health in the UK has acknowledged the excellence of the community-based MS Therapy Centres, through the Healthcare Commission, now renamed the Care Quality Commission. It is important for NICE to endorse the provision of this treatment *in the community* as, after controlled studies and more than 30 years of experience by unbiased patients, it is certainly evidence-based. Successive governments in the UK have endorsed the concept of the expert patient. This now proven model can be adopted in other countries, although the continuing controversy generated by simply providing a little more oxygen with a modest increase in pressure is still astonishing. The response of many doctors asked about the use of oxygen for patients with multiple sclerosis is still, "There is no evidence that it works . . . and trials have not shown any benefit." It, of course, refers to oxygen and the statement is therefore absurd; the oxygen used in a chamber is no different to that in the air we breathe. This is, in fact, where it comes from; so-called "medical" oxygen is made by liquefying air. Remission is critically dependent on the level of oxygen in affected areas of the brain and obviously *cannot* take place in the absence of sufficient oxygen. It is difficult for patients to refute apparently authoritative opinions from doctors, but the facts are there for those prepared to study them.

A review of the controlled trials of the use of hyperbaric treatment was submitted to the Cochrane Collaboration; named after a public health doctor, Dr. Archie Cochrane. It collates evidence of the effectiveness of treatments. Cochrane actually ran into problems with his own methods in supporting the drug Atromid; despite seemingly adequate controlled trials, long-term studies showed it was ineffective! A drug-based approach was used in a Cochrane review of the hyperbaric oxygen treatment trials in multiple sclerosis patients, undertaken by a group in Australia. It gave equal credence to the trials, when even a cursory examination of the methods used shows that they were gravely flawed. This is very misguided;

the only properly undertaken study was the one undertaken in New York University[4] and it is certainly not invalidated by the poorly-conducted and biased studies that followed.

In the late 1990s the charity centres came under scrutiny with the formation of the National Care Standards Commission, which was rebranded under the title of the "Healthcare Commission" in 2001. This is another quango, which has been renamed, yet again, under the more "PC" title of the Care Quality Commission. The body was originally formed to enforce the requirements of the Private and Voluntary Healthcare Regulations 1999, and the Care Standards Act of 2000. It brought the use of hyperbaric oxygen treatment in England and Wales into the category of a "prescribed technique." Fortunately, after representations from the charity, it defined three types of chamber. The simple chambers used in the community centres were classified as "Category 3" and they are now called *barochambers*. They are only capable of being pressurised to twice atmospheric pressure, (2 ATA), leaving the term "hyperbaric" to be applied to chambers used for diving and intensive care as Categories 1 and 2. In 2003, a code of construction and working practice for low-pressure barochambers, based on the standards used for aircraft, was accepted by the UK government.[25] A letter from the late Lord Whadden, an industrial chemist, who was a patient at one of the MS Therapy Centres, and formerly a pilot, introduced the standard. It was the result of detailed consultations with the Healthcare Commission, the Health and Safety Executive, and the UK Fire Services. It is now backed by over 30 years of safe operation and well over 2.8 million sessions have been completed without a significant incident. As already discussed, aircraft are pressure vessels for human occupancy which are also equipped with oxygen breathing apparatus. Being aligned to aircraft, the standards for their construction and operation are, of course, accepted by every country in the world. The pressure vessels were termed barochambers

---

STATUTORY INSTRUMENTS

2008 No. 2352

PUBLIC HEALTH, ENGLAND

The Private and Voluntary Health Care (England) Amendment
Regulations 2008

Figure 18.4:
The Act of Parliament by which MS Therapy Centres were deregulated.

Chapter 18: The UK Multiple Sclerosis Therapy Centres: Self-Help in Action ~ 321

to escape from any connection to diving; the complex high pressure facilities needed for divers certainly require the expert supervision of professionals. In 2008, the use of hyperbaric oxygen treatment in MS Therapy Centres was formally deregulated by Act of Parliament (Figure 18.4). The patient-led hyperbaric movement continues to grow after more than 30 years and Figure 18.5 shows the locations of the 64 centres in the UK, Ireland, and Gibraltar.

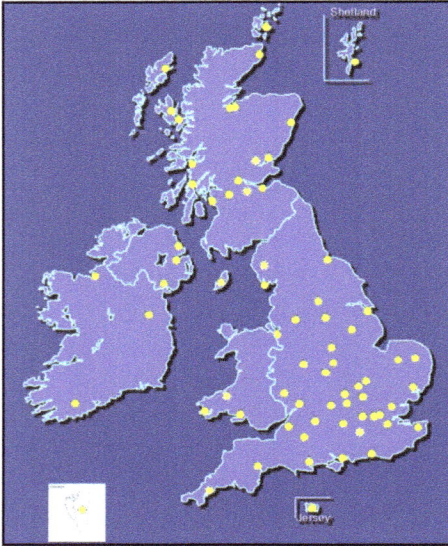

Figure 18.5:
The MS Therapy Centres of the UK and Republic of Ireland with inset the chamber in Gibraltar.

In their *New England Journal of Medicine* paper, Fischer and his colleagues called for studies of the treatment of acute attacks typical of multiple sclerosis and long-term follow up of patients with chronic disease. Acute attacks have yet to be studied, but a cohort of 705 patients has been followed over 15 years in the MS Therapy centres and the results published in the *International Journal of Neuroprotection and Neuroregeneration*.[26] The paper was rejected by many journals because historical controls were used, although this approach was, of course, accepted for the UK risk sharing drug scheme. The reduction of the number of relapses made by oxygen treatment was reported by Dr. Raphael Pallotta as long ago as 1980.[27] Both groups of his patients had undertaken an initial course of 20 sessions, but of the 22 patients, half did not continue and they had a greatly increased relapse rate (Figure 18.6).

The initiative to provide chambers in a community setting has required a truly enormous effort by patients, their loved ones, and carers. It has provided an impressive body of evidence showing beyond doubt benefit from hyperbaric oxygen treatment even in established disease. The movement has

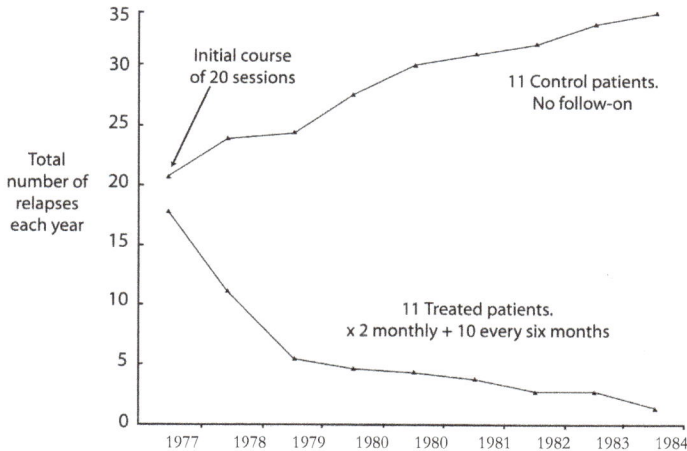

Figure 18.6:
Results of study of HBOT on yearly MS relapse rate by Professor Rafael Pallotta.
Controls show an increased relapse rate (upper line).
The relapse rate falls in patients using HBOT (lower line).

destroyed claims that the equipment must be run by expert teams with the patients supervised by highly qualified doctors which would result in the treatment being withheld from needy patients with chronic disease. The charity sessions are supervised by lay workers and volunteers who are, of course, trained to an appropriate level. The safety of these chambers can only be described as legendary and is determined by the quality of the engineering. The facilities are very simple and in 3 million sessions there has not been a significant incident.

In 1985 this patient-led movement was attacked by a Glasgow neurosurgeon. Quoted in an editorial in the *British Medical Journal*,[28] he referred to the use

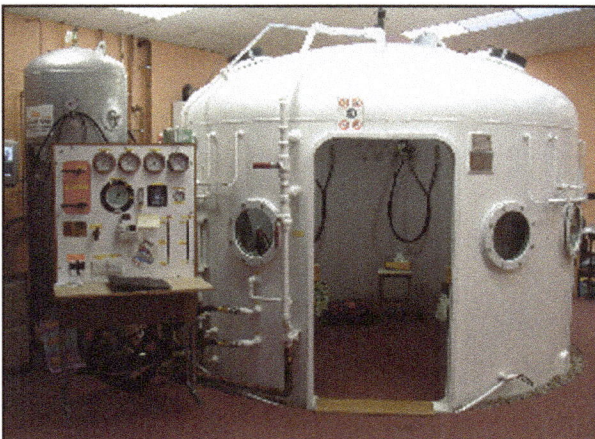

Figure 18.7:
A typical MS Centre barochamber.

Chapter 18: The UK Multiple Sclerosis Therapy Centres: Self-Help in Action ~ 323

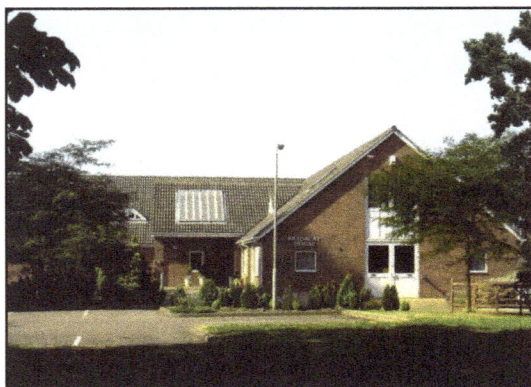

Figure 18.8:
The MS Therapy Centre in Bedford, England. (Courtesy of Mrs. Valerie Woods.)

of the chambers for multiple sclerosis patients as an example of the "inappropriate use of high technology." The high technology myth is still perpetuated in the US, where the author has seen a bill for $3,588 sent to an insurer from a Miami hospital for a *single* session of hyperbaric oxygen treatment in a multi-person chamber. The patient was being treated for a simple pressure sore. The insurers would in all likelihood not have actually reimbursed this cost and probably paid out only half of the amount demanded. This still generates a massive profit as the treatment can be provided for about $50 an hour, even in a hospital-based, single person chamber.[29] However, it is usual for hyperbaric centres to charge $50 per patient per session just for physician supervision, despite patients being safer inside a chamber breathing oxygen than outside breathing air! The Food and Drug Administration in the US (FDA) has been convinced that hyperbaric chambers and hyperbaric treatment must be highly regulated and inspected, an attitude obviously promoted by the owners of expensive hyperbaric facilities, and by many of the doctors involved. The attitude of the FDA, or at least advisers, to oxygen beggars belief. In an article on an FDA site, posted in 2002, advisers even warn of the risk of breathing oxygen for even a few minutes in an oxygen bar.[30]

The MS Therapy Centres are represented by a central group www. msntc.org.uk and a support line run by the Hyperbaric Oxygen Treatment Trust, www.hyperbaricoxygentherapy.org.uk. Nevertheless, when patients join a centre they join others in the group to provide their *own* treatment, which is the basis of the self-help concept. The shared experience is invaluable to many patients who experience the nightmare and isolation waiting for the so-called diagnosis, to be labelled as having multiple sclerosis. The story of one patient, reluctant to take the drugs offered who found one of the MS Therapy Centres on the Internet, shows how patients should use the treatment to manage their disease.

In 2001, when the patient was 48, he had what was said to be his first attack of multiple sclerosis, although he recognised that all may not have been well for some years as he occasionally had problems controlling his bladder and curious episodes in which his scalp itched. The attack in 2001 began when he became aware of some deafness in his right ear and then the right hand side of his face drooped. The deafness worsened and he developed vertigo, finding that when he moved his head quickly he would fall to his left side. At the time he was a farmer in Kent and during lambing he found he could not pick a lamb up without falling over.

He suspected that he had a brain tumour and his family doctor organised an urgent private consultation with a neurologist. An MRI was arranged and revealed a number of unidentified bright objects which he was told were areas of inflammation in the brain. When he asked the neurologist what had caused them, he was told that they could be due to "a virus" and there was a 70% chance of them happening again. Later he asked to see the letter written to his family doctor and read the word "demyelinating." He found that sometimes when he closed his eyes it was "like watching a firework display." He went on the Internet and became concerned that he had multiple sclerosis. With the finance for a move to a property in Scotland being organised, it was a worrying time. However, on a second visit to the neurologist he asked if he had MS and was told that it was "categorically not MS." The neurologist referred to the areas found on MRI as "holes in the brain" which led the patient to question if he actually had Mad Cow disease – new variant Creutzfeld Jacob disease or CJD. The doctor produced some scans of a patient with CJD to show that it was quite different. The patient was obviously relieved to be told that he did not have a brain tumour. He told the specialist that he was moving to Scotland and that he would be under the care of a teaching hospital.

Arrangements for the move to Scotland progressed and he found that his symptoms steadily improved. Over the next five years he only suffered occasional problems, such as some difficulty focusing which prevented him seeing objects clearly. At times he also felt a band developing across his chest, like wearing a seat belt and, again, his scalp itched. Both bladder and bowel control at times were difficult and caused him some embarrassment.

In 2002, the patient made a long trip from Scotland to the Midlands and on his return he had to stop close to home because of extreme fatigue and his eyes felt very heavy. He was able to eventually complete the journey, but the following morning he woke with double vision and he was unable to drive. He was still suffering from severe fatigue and his feet had become numb as if enclosed in bubble wrap. When matters did not improve he went to see his family doctor and *was referred to a neurologist who arranged his admission to hospital. A lumbar puncture was undertaken. Later at an outpatient appointment he asked the consultant why he had been admitted explaining that he only had double vision. The reply was "it is to be expected when you have MS." For the patient this came as a bolt from the blue. His specialist wanted to start a course of steroids and then beta interferon but, after reading about the side effects, the patient was very reluctant to embark on drug therapy. He was already on daily drugs for arthritis and a bowel complaint.*

Searching again on the Internet, putting "MS" into a search engine, he found entries describing a charity using hyperbaric oxygen treatment. He realised there were centres using the treatment in Scotland and one was only a few miles away. After calling the centre and speaking to the nurse he arranged to attend for a course of treatment. He recalls feeling hesitant when he arrived at the centre; "it was nerve wracking standing at the door." However, that soon passed once inside when he was made welcome. After the first session in the chamber he felt less fatigued and after completing five sessions he slept through the night for the first time in years. He had grown used to getting up to visit the bathroom three or four times a night. Over the course of 20 sessions, his double vision and the numbness in his feet disappeared. However, one year after his initial course of 20 sessions he found the double vision returning. Sensibly, he had five consecutive sessions in the chamber and recovered.

He now attends the centre once a week or sometimes more if he feels "under the weather." At Christmas 2009, he developed a cold and did not have treatment for three weeks. His bladder problem returned and he again found he had to get up three to four times a night. After three sessions on consecutive days his bladder control was restored.

The use of drugs in managing the disease of patients with multiple sclerosis will never be satisfactory as they cannot address the fundamental problems—damage to the blood-brain barrier, inflammation, and lack of oxygen. However, the key to using oxygen effectively must be for the *emergency* treatment of the first symptoms to prevent progression to sclerosis; it certainly makes no sense to withhold giving more oxygen whilst waiting for "objective" evidence of disability and MRI evidence of scarring. The professional actions necessary are discussed in the last chapter. Nevertheless, for those patients who already have multiple areas of sclerosis, the object of treatment must be to maintain remission and reduce the unfortunate deterioration that occurs with advancing years.

For the first time in the long history of multiple sclerosis, a safe, effective treatment based on sound science is available for patients, and it is supported by the most thorough trial ever undertaken in the history of medicine.[5] The basis of the control of the inflammation is now understood; oxygen controls the genes involved. Moreover, oxygen is also the *only* agent that has proved successful in the treatment of both the putative animal model and patients. For any treatment to produce improvement in chronically ill patients with disease durations of years, verges on the miraculous. It only needs a moment's reflection to recognise that to be truly successful oxygen should be used at the beginning, not at the end of the disease, especially when the organ involved is the brain. A high level of oxygen used within hours of the first symptoms developing may offer the prospect of a cure, at least for that attack, although, of course, it cannot prevent others. We already know that the oxygen level in air is often sufficient and so the question raised is: What is the appropriate dose of oxygen?

It is ironic that patients with *acute* symptoms were excluded from the "controlled" trials, because the benefits would have been not only immediate, but also very obvious. So what remains to be done are studies of oxygen treatment for patients with the first symptoms, to *prevent* disability, because this may even produce a cure by restoring the integrity of the blood-brain barrier, just as it has done in divers for over a hundred years. Such patients cannot by *definition* have multiple sclerosis, because that label requires more than one attack. It is also most important to recognise that the dose of additional oxygen needed may not actually require a chamber; a mask delivering 100% oxygen at the ambient atmospheric pressure may well be sufficient, and the use of MRI with spectroscopy can easily allow this to be studied *in real time*.

The disease that underlies multiple sclerosis is characterised by damage evident on MRI that, as we have already seen, is far from being specific to the disease and may even be caused by tiny bubbles in compressed-air workers and divers. But the same changes have also been shown to occur following head injury, and the next chapter discusses the importance of using oxygen treatment for such patients.

CHAPTER 19

Head Injuries—the Curse of Life in the Fast Lane

The decrease in mortality and improved outcome for patients with severe traumatic brain injury over the past 25 years can be attributed to the approach of squeezing oxygenated blood through a swollen brain.

Jamshid Ghajar. *Lancet*, September 9, 2000.

On a quiet Saturday morning on the 8th of January 2011 in Tucson, Arizona, a US congresswoman was meeting the people in the parking lot of a Safeway supermarket. It was not safe; a 22-year-old man shot her through the head with a 9 mm Glock pistol. In just 20 seconds he proceeded to kill six people, including a little girl just nine years old. It seemed for a time that the congresswoman would join the long list of US political assassinations, and, indeed, her astronaut husband was told she had died. Despite being shot at point blank range, she survived to undergo surgery and was on an operating table in just 38 minutes. With the eyes of the world focussed on Tucson it would be expected that the latest techniques would be used to save her life, and so it proved; the surgeons removed a large piece of the bone from the left side of her skull. Following well-established practice, a tube was inserted into the brain to drain away excess fluid, and the skin flap was replaced. It was not long before she delighted everyone by regaining consciousness, and a helmet was fitted to protect the brain. And there is a reason for including her story.

On the 26th of January, the congresswoman actually used a hyperbaric chamber equipped with an oxygen breathing system; she was flown 900 miles to Houston in a private jet, and admitted to the Memorial Hermann-Texas Medical Center. The journey was to allow her to be close to the Johnson Space Center, where her husband was training to command the space shuttle *Endeavour* on its final mission. The Hermann hospital group has a large hyperbaric chamber, but it is only used to treat wounds in the skin, not for wounds of the brain. Ironically, the shuttle had a hyperbaric oxygen chamber because, as discussed, astronauts risk "the bends" when they decompress to undertake EVA —extra vehicular activity. But would hyperbaric oxygen treatment have helped the congresswoman? Before discussing the controversies raised by this crucial question, it is important to understand the scale of the problem of brain trauma.

Worldwide, at least 1 million people die each year from a head injury, and head injuries are the leading cause of death and disability in young people in the Western world. Most are "closed" head injuries from motor vehicle accidents. In the US, with a population of around 275 million, about 1.7 million people have a serious head injury each year. Of these, over 50,000 die and 80,000 survive with very severe neurological problems. Many patients remain in persistent coma for years at prodigious cost to their families and to society. Over 275,000 brain-injured patients in the US require hospital admission each year, and over 3 million are left needing help with daily tasks. It is common for head injuries without loss of consciousness to be dismissed as mild concussion, but many such patients often have subtle neurological problems that are difficult to detect. They may be all too obvious to the patient and their relatives, but are almost invariably denied compensation, largely because our assessment of brain injury is grossly inadequate. The financial cost to society of head injuries, and the human cost to individuals and families are incalculable. Obviously, prevention will always be better than cure, but there are many difficulties; even imposing road speed limits is unpopular, and they are often ignored. However, lower speeds reduce the risk of an impact and give more time for avoidance. For car occupants, seat belts and airbags, together with major advances in safety engineering, have greatly reduced the number of casualties, but pedestrians lack such protection and it is only in the last few years that vehicle design has improved to reduce their risk of injury.

We have always been liable to head injury from falls and falling objects and when man started to ride animals, like camels and horses, both the height of the rider from the ground, and the velocity of movement greatly increased the risk of impacts to the brain. With the development of even faster mechanical transport, like the train and the car, impact levels increased again, and the numbers at risk has been increasing year on year; car ownership in China alone is increasing by thousands every day. Reducing speed lowers the forces involved, and will inevitably contribute to reducing accidental injury both to passengers and innocent bystanders. The skull provides only limited protection against weapons; even a stone from a sling may prove fatal, but modern munitions often have devastating effects, as the event in Tucson has shown. Curiously, the skull is also a liability because the brain is subjected to internal compression and decompression forces from a violent impact, and it can oscillate and rotate within the bony cavity.

If the skull is fractured, arteries and tissues within the skull may be torn and the brain may be lacerated by fragments of bone. Objects, like a bullet, that penetrate the skull destroy brain tissue causing bleeding, and severely head-injured patients often have damage simply incompatible with survival. In fact, about two thirds of patients with open skull fracture and direct injury to the brain die. In closed head injury, the shearing forces resulting from the impact may cause internal tearing, swelling and bleeding. In patients with lesser degrees of head trauma, it is the brain swelling and the damage which develops *after* the injury that is responsible for much of the residual physical and, unfortunately mental disability.

Head injury may also result in prolonged coma, which places enormous demands on relatives and society. Sometimes patients awake after many years: A patient, who made world headlines in 2003 was in coma for weeks and then in a minimally conscious state, unable to speak, for 19 years. He woke up and asked his mother for a soda. Detailed studies of the brain fibre damage were published in 2005.[1] Another patient also received extensive press coverage; on June 3, 2007, the UK newspaper the *Sunday Telegraph* (www.telegraph.co.uk/news) reported the case of a Polish man who was struck by a train in 1988 during the Communist era, who woke also after 19 years in coma. He was quoted as saying: "What amazes me today is all these people who walk around with their mobiles and never stop moaning. I've got nothing to complain about."

The spectacular advances made by brain imaging unfortunately contrast with the lack of progress made in treating head injury. In 2004 the front cover of the *Lancet* carried a stark message:

The administration of corticosteroids to brain-injured patients has seemingly caused more than 10,000 deaths during the 1980s and earlier.

Comment: *Lancet* 2004;364:12.

A report of a 32-year-old patient with a traumatic brain injury, in 2012 (Figure 19.1), used MR imaging to show the loss of nerve fibres deriving from the motor cortex.[2] The same technology was used to provide the image on the book cover. The green shows the normal concentration of nerve fibres which control movement and pass down in the areas known as the "internal capsules" in the mid-brain. These areas are supplied by end arteries that do not connect to other arteries which accounts for their vulnerability in conditions in cerebral palsy, multiple sclerosis and strokes.

Surgeons will always be faced with the need to help patients with head injuries resulting from a wide variety of causes, and neurosurgery will continue to be technically and emotionally demanding; indeed it is a speciality that deserves our respect. Currently, surgeons can either try to control brain swelling with drugs, or remove a substantial amount of the skull to allow it to swell unhindered. Most drugs act by reducing blood flow, inevitably, reduc-

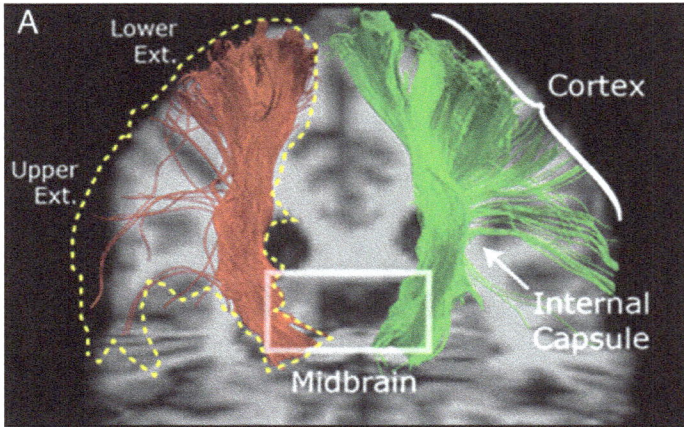

Figure 19.1:
The nerve fibres on the damaged side shown in red are clearly reduced when compared to those in the opposite hemisphere in green. (Courtesy of Prof. W. Scheinder.)

ing oxygen delivery. In the quotation at the head of this chapter[3] Dr. Ghajar refers to "squeezing oxygenated blood through a swollen brain." This may seem to be advocating the use of a pressure chamber to increase the dose of oxygen; sadly, this is not the case.

Perhaps it will not come as a surprise that using oxygen as a treatment for head-injured patients is controversial, and it reflects the desperate need to teach the science involved in our medical schools. But it is a terrifying indictment of the medical industry that doctors actually cannot agree on the level of oxygen to give head-injured patients. In 2008, a National Institute of Health public access paper "Hyperoxia – Good or Bad for the Injured Brain," discussed some of the factors involved.[4] It was published in its final form in *Current Opinions in Critical Care*.[5] Positron emission tomography (PET) was used in head-injured patients and the author indicated that:

> … *direct measurement of the ability of the brain to utilise oxygen indicates that hyperoxia does not increase oxygen utilization.*

The incorrect inference is that giving more oxygen is, therefore, not beneficial in head-injured patients. The spectre of oxygen toxicity at normal atmospheric pressure is also raised, despite the fact that oxygen delivered under *hyperbaric* conditions has been shown to improve outcome in acute head injury.[6] The term "hyperoxia," is also *not defined*, but can refer to a raised level of oxygen in *blood*, or in the *tissues*. The focus is simply on the role of oxygen in metabolism, and not on the powerful physiological mechanisms, especially the control of blood flow by oxygen,[7] and the immense complexities of gene regulation by the gas.[8] It is also clear that the factors influencing oxygen transport from blood to the tissues are not understood.

The three components which determine the outcome of head injury after the initial mechanical trauma are obviously interlinked; they are brain blood flow, the pressure in the skull associated with swelling, and the lack of oxygen, that is, hypoxia. The principal reason for giving more oxygen is to ensure that brain cells have enough to survive, but it is also critically important in the control of swelling. However, it is the flow of blood that produces brain swelling, when water from plasma leaks into the tissues, because of an increase in the permeability of blood vessels, that is, the blood-brain barrier. If tissues become waterlogged, oxygen transport into the cells is reduced, simply because the gas is poorly soluble in water. The lack of oxygen induces low-grade inflammation which, as will be discussed later, may continue long after the patient has apparently recovered. So the "key to the door" in treatment is to find a way to *reduce* blood flow whilst *increasing* the delivery of oxygen to the tissues and the *only* agent that can achieve this is oxygen itself.

As an impact to the head often causes damage to the brain from the mechanical forces involved, the prevention of accidents should be our greatest priority. However, it is also important to introduce measures to reduce the risk of an impact, hence the use of seat belts and airbags. Medical attention must be focussed on the prevention of the secondary damage, which may take place over many hours after head injury. It would appear that the lack of oxygen itself is not responsible for the damage, and it is here that the importance of the Dutch post-mortem studies published in the *Lancet*,[9] and discussed in Chapter 2 is clear. A brief reminder of the details of this extraordinary research will be helpful; the brains were removed eight hours after death under normal post-mortem conditions and tests were undertaken with slices of brain tissue that were provided with oxygen and glucose. It was shown that the nerve cells were still alive by the progression of a tracer. There is, in fact, no obvious reason why a brain cell should need more oxygen than a skin cell to remain *viable*, although brain cells obviously need significantly more to function, that is, to generate nerve impulses. The brain cells in the Dutch experiments were kept alive for up to 18 hours. It must be stressed that this does *not* mean the continuation of consciousness; the cells would not have been capable of functioning; they were "not dead, but sleeping." Nevertheless, this study has shown beyond any shadow of doubt that brain tissue will survive the arrest of blood flow for many hours, and that only very low levels of oxygen and glucose are needed to preserve the viability of nerve cells. And, to state the obvious; there can be no doubt about the extent of the head injury in this study; the brain had been removed from the skull.

What then is responsible for secondary brain damage? At least three mechanisms are involved. The first is bleeding, the second is leakage of proteins from blood, and the third invasion of the area by white blood cells. Bleeding occurs when red blood cells pass from damaged blood vessels into the substance of the brain. Their membranes then rupture releasing haemoglobin, which is broken down in the tissues, releasing free iron. This generates highly toxic hydroxyl radicals by the Fenton reaction, and damage to the walls of blood vessels *opens the blood-brain barrier*, causing severe inflammation and tissue destruction. The leakage of water, proteins and other toxic molecules from blood, causes further brain swelling by osmotic forces. The proteins escaping into brain tissue also trigger the complement cascade of inflammatory proteins. Finally, the lack of oxygen in the tissues attracts neutrophils—the white blood cells programmed to fight infection, which release free radicals.[10] Swelling is a severe threat to the brain, because the pressure in the head rises, and the tissues have only one place to go—to squeeze down through the large hole in the base of the skull, the foramen magnum. However, before this happens, a potentially catastrophic reduction of blood flow will have occurred with increased pressure within the skull. This rise in the internal pressure in the skull reduces the blood pressure difference needed to maintain blood flow. In fact, the pressure in the head may eventually rise to equal the blood pressure, stopping blood flow altogether. As already discussed many times in this book, it is still not recognised in medicine that swelling inevitably reduces oxygen delivery causing tissue hypoxia. This urgently needs to be acknowledged and taught as a "principle of disease."

In the 1970s, the invention of X-ray computed tomography (CT) revealed the gross changes in the brain that may follow head injury, but cannot be seen on an ordinary X-radiograph of the skull. CT is still in common use because it can readily show bleeding and has the advantage of taking only a few minutes to image the head. In the early 1980s, the first magnetic resonance imagers came into use alongside CT scanners and they soon showed that even in so-called "mild" head injuries, where the patient is said to be concussed and consciousness is not lost, there may be significant swelling and brain damage. Figure 19.2 shows the CT image and the MRI of a 36-year-old man published in the *Annals of Neurology* in 1984.[11] He was clubbed across the back of the head and briefly lost his speech, but did not lose consciousness. Following admission to a New York hospital, he was combative, had loss of memory for events around the time of the assault, and continued to suffer from a severe headache. On the third day

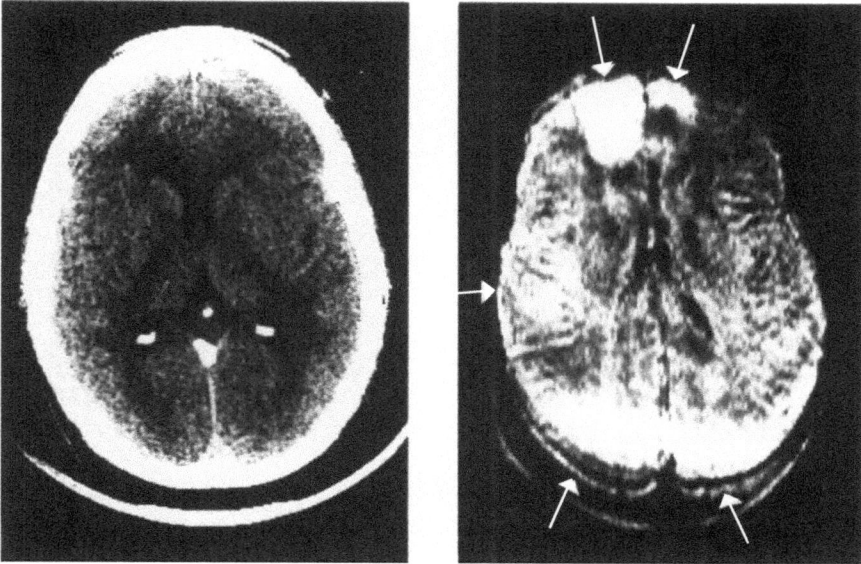

Figure 19.2:
CT and MRI of a patient who had been struck on the head. The CT is normal but the MRI (right) shows the oedema – arrows. (Courtesy of *Annals of Neurology.*)

post-injury, he was imaged with X-ray CT which showed a hairline fracture, but no brain swelling. A new MR imager had just been installed and his scan showed tissue selling in several areas of the brain. The patient would be described as having "mild" concussion as there was no loss of consciousness, but it is clear that the forces of compression and decompression in the skull had opened the blood-brain barrier to cause the swelling.

The clear white areas shown on MRI at the rear and the front of the brain (arrowed) are due to an increase in the tissue water content. They were caused by the brain bouncing back and forward in the skull. The brain also rotated, as the area on one side—also arrowed, is swollen. Again because of the poor solubility of oxygen in water this means that the brain cells in the area will be hypoxic and giving more oxygen constricts blood vessels reducing their leakage "buying" time for the extra tissue fluid to resolve.

It is important at this juncture to point out that using hyperbaric oxygen treatment does not replace other management strategies in head injury, for example, the need for surgery. However, every possible drug treatment has been tried to improve outcome; steroids are still used largely because they proved successful over 40 years ago in reducing the swelling around brain tumours. But more than 16 clinical trials of patients with head injury have shown that steroids are not effective, either in reducing death, or disability.

Similar reservations apply to the intravenous injection of *mannitol*, a complex sugar to draw water from the tissues back into the blood using osmosis. Its action cannot be confined to the brain and it may have adverse effects. The depressing situation was summed up by an article in the *Archives of Neurology* in 2001[12] entitled "Neuroprotection and Traumatic Brain Injury; the Search Continues": Nothing has changed and will not until the importance of oxygen is discovered.

It is also important to note that patients with head trauma often have other injuries, for example, injuries to the chest, and so may not breathe properly. There may also be associated injury to the capillaries of the lungs due to embolism by clot and bone marrow entering the circulation from fractures. Their blood may then contain considerably less oxygen than normal. As already discussed, when fat embolises the brain it damages the lining of the blood vessels and opens the blood-brain barrier which, if it persists, may leave telltale UBOs on MRIs in the central white matter of the brain, pathologically identical to those found in multiple sclerosis. There is no doubt that the brain swelling in head injury relates to breakdown of the blood-brain barrier and Chapter 13 highlighted an MRI study of contact sports where the high prevalence of UBOs are likely to be the result of minor head trauma.[13]

> The routine management of severe head injury introduces many problems; the key reason for an "endotracheal" tube, to be inserted in the throat is to prevent regurgitated material, or spasm from blocking the airway. However it requires a patient to be sedated, otherwise they will resist, often violently. The sedation must be continued once the tube is in place, which makes the assessment of the degree of brain injury from the level of consciousness impossible. A very frank statement about this approach was made by Dr. Mervyn Singer in an interview with Dan Jones in the *New Scientist* in 2010.[14] It was prompted by a study of the outcomes of amputation in soldiers who fought at Trafalgar and in the American War of Independence;[15] "We haven't evolved to cope with being sedated, put on a ventilator, and pumped full of drugs." He is right.
>
> There can be no doubt that maintaining the airway is important; it is not surprising that there is good evidence that it reduces mortality in head-injured patients. However, to be attached to a ventilator—a breathing machine adversely changes the dynamics of breathing. In normal breathing, the pressure inside the thorax falls below the surrounding air pressure, and atmospheric pressure is responsible for forcing gas into the lungs. The sedation of a patient means that positive pressure must be used to expand and ventilate the lungs. This increases the resistance to blood returning in the veins to the heart which, of course, includes the veins draining blood from the brain. Ventilation, therefore, despite improving

the oxygenation of a patient, may actually worsen brain swelling. It is also common for an increased breathing rate to be used to reduce the level of carbon dioxide in the blood. This is because carbon dioxide dilates the blood vessels of the brain and so "washing out" carbon dioxide results in their constriction. Unfortunately, it also causes the blood to become more alkaline, and oxygenated haemoglobin is less able to release its oxygen into the plasma. Together with the reduction of blood flow by vessel constriction and the change in the dynamics of oxygenation, over-ventilation may actually reduce the level of oxygen reaching the tissues of the brain. Unfortunately, there are also the mechanical problems that cause damage increasingly recognised as "ventilator lung."[16] Nevertheless, the use of hyperventilation is rarely questioned, largely because it is considered that there is no alternative. The author has had considerable experience of treating moribund patients in chambers who, despite having few reflexes, continue to breathe. The additional oxygen breathed in a chamber gives an enormous safety margin—the underwater breath-hold world record is held by Peter Colat who, at the age of 38 and after 10 minutes of pure oxygen breathing, achieved a time of 19 minutes 21 seconds—and, of course, he was still conscious!

A depressingly long list of drugs has been researched for head-injured patients, but not one has been found to be effective in controlling brain swelling. Cooling, an old remedy used for soft tissue injury, which has been investigated for brain injury in the newborn, is also being trialled in traumatic brain injury. Everyone knows that the pain and swelling of a sprained ankle is reduced by an ice pack; it works because cold causes blood vessels to constrict reducing their leakage and this interrupts the complex cascade of events associated with inflammation. Cooling the skull has the added benefit of reducing the brain's demand for oxygen. Another recent technique which was used for the US congresswoman is removal of part of the skull to allow the brain to swell. A tube known as a shunt is often placed in one of the fluid cavities—the lateral ventricles of the brain, and passed under the skin down into the abdomen to relieve pressure by draining excess fluid—cerebrospinal fluid. Both are drastic measures which, unfortunately, expose the patient to the risk of infection. Both interventions contrast starkly using the non-invasive use of the high levels of oxygen possible with a modest increase in pressure.

If current neurosurgical practice is to be changed to include hyperbaric oxygen treatment, it is necessary to present the evidence for its use in head injury. It has a surprisingly long history; neurosurgeons became interested in the use of hyperbaric oxygen treatment in the halcyon days of hyperbaric medicine in the 1960s when the technique was being used for cardiac surgery. The central figure in the story is Dr. Michael Sukoff, who began working with

Dr. Julius Jacobson, a surgeon who had been the driving force behind the acquisition of a large hyperbaric operating theatre in New York's Mount Sinai Hospital. It eventually ceased to be used for hyperbaric treatment and when the author visited the unit in 1982 it had become Dr. Jacobson's office. It was dismantled and removed from the building in the 1990s. Dr. Sukoff began with experimental models in which balloons or psyllium seeds were implanted into the brains of animals to induce swelling.[17] The results of hyperbaric oxygen treatment were very positive; oxygen was shown to be able to reduce the swelling and improve outcomes.

Unfortunately by the 1970s, enthusiasm in New York and the other active centre in Glasgow had waned, and the units fell into disuse. Several centres in Europe, however, continued to study using hyperbaric oxygen treatment in head-injured patients; Professor Holbach's group in the University of Bonn[18] and addressed the key issue of the correct oxygen dose, as had Dr. Ingevar earlier in Stockholm.[19] Unfortunately, this early pioneering work failed to establish the use of hyperbaric oxygen treatment in head injury and the research momentum fell away. By this time the large and expensive hyperbaric operating theatres had also fallen out of favour for cardiac operations, and the already muted enthusiasm of surgeons for what was regarded as an expensive and inconvenient technology, evaporated. No attempt had been made to incorporate the importance of pressure into teaching in medical schools and free radical research was gaining momentum, spurred on by research into rejection mechanisms in transplant surgery.

Michael Sukoff left New York for neurosurgical practice in the sunny climes of California, settling in Santa Ana and he installed a single person chamber in his unit. The chamber, made by Sechrist Industries, uses a clear plastic cylinder and was based on the design pioneered by the Vickers company in the UK in the 1960s. However, Sechrist engineered a suitable ventilator for use in their chamber and Dr. Sukoff developed techniques to allow the procedures normally used in an intensive care setting to be used. Together with an anaesthetic colleague, Dr. R.E. Ragatz, Dr. Sukoff published their experience of using hyperbaric oxygen treatment in severely head-injured patients in the prestigious journal *Neurosurgery* in 1982.[6] They used a pressure transducer to measure the internal pressure in the head and were able to observe the effect of giving oxygen actually in real time in 50 patients with serious head injury. As the chamber pressure increased to twice normal atmospheric pressure (2 ATA) with the patient breathing pure oxygen, the pressure within the skull reduced dramatically within minutes and treatments lasted 45 minutes. It was found necessary to repeat the treatment until the pressure stabilised. Not surprisingly, it was found that if the injury was too severe there was less response, or no response at all. A typical response is shown in Table 19.1.

Table 19.1	
Treatment 1	Intra-cranial pressure (mm Hg)
Immediately before HBOT	19
During session in chamber	3
1 hour post-treatment	4
4 hours post-treatment	4

Dr. Sukoff continued to use hyperbaric treatment and present the data at conferences. In 1995 he was invited to address a meeting of physicians involved in hyperbaric medicine, which the author attended in Columbia, South Carolina. He expressed his extreme frustration at their failure, and that of the medical community in general, to use this simple and safe intervention for head-injured patients. Again, the absurd demand from sceptics and detractors is for controlled studies to be undertaken; objective and *scientific*, measurements are dismissed in favour of statistical data from a group of patients, with the many confounding variables this inevitably involves. The experimental studies already referred to in Chapter 8, in which oxygen measuring electrodes were inserted into the tissue of the spinal cord,[20] had already shown as long ago as 1972 that, not surprisingly, tissue oxygen levels rise when the concentration of oxygen breathed is increased under hyperbaric conditions. The injury to the spinal cord was produced by the impact of a weight dropped on the exposed tissue and the results can readily be extrapolated to brain injury. Indeed, *this one study* answers all the questions and objections raised about using hyperbaric oxygen treatment for patients with head injury.

Not all the patients treated by Sukoff and Ragatz responded and here it is necessary to state an obvious but neglected principle. Although we use the one label, "head injury," for all affected patients, the extent of the damage to the brain can vary greatly, even when the symptoms and signs may appear to be much the same. A scale was developed by neurosurgeons in Glasgow in the 1960s, known as the Glasgow Coma Score, to try to grade the damage. The severity of head injury is assessed by the allocation of points based on three parameters, speech, movement, and eye opening, but it is a crude tool that can record only gross changes. In Dr. Sukoff's study, hyperbaric oxygen treatment reduced the measured pressure in the head, that is, the *intracranial pressure*. Predictably, the effect was less and not persistent, or even non-existent, in the patients with the most severe head injury. This should be expected, but it certainly does not counter the value of treatment for less severely-affected patients. To actually reduce the swelling affecting the brain and at the same time improve the delivery of oxygen is the Holy Grail still being sought by those caring for head-injured patients. What is needed is an apparent impossibility; a way of *increasing* oxygen delivery whilst *reducing* blood flow. There is only one agent that can achieve this objective, oxygen itself, and the futile search for an alternative will continue until the importance of value of pressure to oxygen delivery is understood.

It was the data produced in the hyperbaric chamber installed by Sir Charles Illingworth in Glasgow, already detailed in Chapters 10 and 17, that first demonstrated the unique ability of oxygen to reduce blood flow through the brain and simultaneously improve oxygen transport.[21] The first author of the paper, the late Dr. Ivan Jacobson, who was known to this author, became a neurosurgeon and practiced in Dundee. Close to the end of his career he expressed great interest in using hyperbaric oxygen treatment for head-injured patients. In the Glasgow research, the effect of breathing normal air was compared to breathing oxygen at double atmospheric pressure, 2 ATA, which of course, requires a chamber. It was found that at 2 ATA the blood flow through the brain reduced by 20% with, of course, the concentration gradient for the delivery of oxygen to the tissues increasing tenfold. The values were halved breathing 100% oxygen at normal atmospheric pressure which is important because it will never be possible to have hyperbaric chambers in every location they may be needed. It is comparatively simple to provide equipment to give the patient 100% oxygen at the scene of injury. As we have seen, Haldane had developed the necessary equipment in WW1[22] and it is notable that the distinguished respiratory physiatrist, Dr. John Nunn, endorsed the importance of 100% at normal atmospheric pressure in a letter to the *British Medical Journal* in 1994.[23] However, this was simply based on the *arterial* values achieved, whereas it is the *venous* values that are so important. This is a critical aspect of the physiology of oxygen which must be restated at this juncture; the leakage in head injury is mostly from the *veins* within brain tissue that are the capacity vessels and so, despite the tenfold increase in the oxygen concentration in the arteries at 2 ATA breathing 100% oxygen, there is only an increase of 1.5 times in the blood in the veins draining the brain. Increasing the oxygen percentage breathed at normal atmospheric pressure induces vasoconstriction with little increase in the dissolved oxygen concentration. This is why hyperbaric conditions are needed and are *so critical*, because they are essential to correct lack of oxygen in the tissues and constrict the leaky blood vessels at the *venous* end of the microcirculation whilst significantly increasing the plasma concentration. As we have seen in Dr. Zamboni's experimental studies of reperfusion injury, a reduced level of oxygen in tissue and veins is responsible for the attraction of white blood cells.[10] However, even when breathing 100% oxygen at twice normal atmospheric pressure at sea level, the increase in the oxygen tension in blood flowing through the veins of the brain is still very modest; from about 50 mm Hg to 70 mm Hg is an increase of just 40%.

After the publication of the superb study by Drs. Sukoff and Ragatz,[6] which was given six pages in the journal *Neurosurgery*, a group headed by the neurosurgeon Gaylan Rockswold in Minneapolis began a painstaking, long-term trial of hyperbaric oxygen treatment for patients with acute head injury.[24] Their final report was published in the *Journal of Neurosurgery* in 1992.[25] They also used single person chambers, and to fulfil the criteria required for advocates of evidence-based medicine, the trial included a control group. In all, 168 patients were recruited over nine years, half receiving oxygen under hyperbaric conditions; 1.5 ATA for an hour every eight hours, whilst patients in the other half of the study received standard care. The reason for the choice of this low oxygen pressure was not given. Hyperbaric treatment was continued until the patients were awake, or declared brain dead, resulting in an average of 21 sessions being used. This study was extraordinarily demanding and, although the dedication of the investigators was beyond doubt, it was fundamentally flawed. The protocol *prohibited* the use of hyperbaric oxygen treatment in the first six hours following injury because, it was argued, that patients may improve spontaneously during this time. The time was also needed to allow the comprehensive evaluation of each patient to allow proper randomisation to the two groups. The patients, therefore, were denied the benefit of early treatment on so-called "scientific" grounds, when it is universally acknowledged that the window of opportunity for effective treatment of the brain is *less than four hours*. In fact, it is recorded in the paper that one patient had their first treatment *34 hours post-injury*, and so would be likely to be in a much worse state than those patients treated earlier. So by its very design, this study was unlikely to show much benefit, especially as the patients were selected on the grounds that their head injury was *severe*.

Unfortunately, the trial was also very unsatisfactory for another reason; the failure to use *tympanotomy* in the first 38 patients allocated to the hyperbaric treatment group. This is simply the creation a hole in the ear drum and is essential in unconscious patients to allow equalisation of pressure in the middle ear cavity to prevent pain and rupture of the ear drum during compression. It had been noted early in the study that some patients occasionally showed a rapid increase in pulse rate and blood pressure during the pressurisation and it was eventually realised that they were suffering ear pain. Semiconscious patients cannot assist in clearing their ears, nor can they complain about ear pain, so tympanotomy should have been routinely used for every patient. The authors analysed the results of oxygen treatment in the last 46 patients *after* the introduction of routine tympanotomy and found the results were very much better. The need for the ear drum to be punctured in unconscious patients was highlighted as long ago in 1974 by the journalist, Vance Trimble, in his excellent book *The Uncertain Miracle: Hyperbaric Oxygenation.*

Despite the delay in treatment and other problems in the Minneapolis study, the mortality rate in the hyperbaric group was *half* that of the control group but then, incredibly, it was stated that "hyperbaric oxygen treatment did not increase the number of patients in the favourable outcome categories." To a casual reader, it would seem that there was no difference in outcome between the treated and control groups when, in fact, the mortality *had been halved.* This sentence in the paper guaranteed that it had no impact on neurosurgical practice, and it remains for us to speculate if the referees of the paper were responsible for its inclusion. The authors actually meant that there was no difference in the neurological status of the *survivors* in both groups. It should also be noted that four patients were included in the results of the treated group who did not receive *any* hyperbaric treatment. The inclusion of these patients was on the basis of a piece of statistical nonsense called *intention to treat*, said by statisticians to be necessary to avoid bias on the part of investigators. Sadly the bias in this publication appears to be *against* the positive results. Not surprisingly, the inclusion of these patients reduced the statistical difference between the treated and control groups, further diluting the impact of the study.

This was not the first such study undertaken; the neurosurgical team led by Professor Holbach in the University of Bonn had done it all before, and found even greater benefit from hyperbaric oxygen treatment.[18] In total, 49 of 99 head-injured patients were treated and the mortality in this group was 33%, whereas the mortality in the 50 patients in their control group was 74%. However, these researchers found that the outcomes in the oxygen group with continued treatment were *much better* than the controls with 33% making a good recovery compared to 6% of the controls.

Strangely, the group in Minneapolis still do not seem to be convinced that hyperbaric oxygen treatment is beneficial; a second study is comparing oxygen used with and without an increase in pressure, in other words with and without a chamber. Unfortunately, again it appears that no patient will be treated in the critical first hours following injury and so studies of hyperbaric oxygen treatment for head-injured patients tragically continue, with patients still unable to benefit from oxygen treatment even at normal pressure, let alone under hyperbaric conditions.

But, there is change in the air; in December 2011, a group of lawyers in San Francisco, at Walkup, Melodia, Kelly, & Schoenberger, who specialise in claims for brain and spinal injury, issued a press release covering a study which highlighted lack of oxygen as being a critical factor in recovery. This is hardly surprising and accords with the quotation that heads this chapter. Curiously, the release did not cite a reference for the study; it only indicated that it was from a group in the University of Pennsylvania.

Research Uncovers Critical Factor in Traumatic Brain Injury Recovery

New medical research finds brain oxygenation is key indicator for recovery of patients suffering traumatic brain injury

Press release service provided by http://www.24-7pressrelease.com

When a patient is admitted to the hospital for a traumatic brain injury, medical staff members monitor intracranial pressure (pressure which builds up in the brain from trauma infarction, swelling or bleeding into the brain) and blood flow to the brain.

Too much pressure or too little blood flow may be a sign that additional treatment is needed or that the patient is in danger. Swelling can prevent normal oxygenation by restricting blood flow. As a result, the volume of well-oxygenated blood is decreased.

Now, researchers at the University of Pennsylvania Medical Center have published new findings related to brain oxygenation that call into question old treatment assumptions.

"Cerebral hypoxia" is the medical term for reduced oxygen supply to the brain. The longer a person's brain is without adequate oxygen, the more cell death occurs, ultimately leading to the death of the injured person.

The study followed 103 patients with traumatic brain injury who were monitored for all three factors. The researchers then looked at the relationships between each of the measurements and the health outcome of the patient. A poor outcome was severe disability, vegetative state or death.

High intracranial pressure had previously been regarded as the most significant predictor of a poor outcome, but the study found that 81 percent of patients with high pressure but no hypoxia had good outcomes. Only 46 percent of patients with both high intracranial pressure and hypoxia had good outcomes.

Blood flow to the brain (cerebral perfusion pressure) was not an adequate indicator of oxygen getting to the brain. Some patients had good oxygen levels, but reduced blood flow. And currently recommended levels of blood flow were not always sufficient to avoid hypoxia and injury.

The greater the drop in oxygenation and the longer the patient went without sufficient oxygen, the worse the outcome. The researchers found that patients with a poor outcome experienced an average of eight (8) hours of reduced oxygen levels, while those with good outcomes experienced just under two (2) hours of hypoxia. (For each hour a patient suffers reduced oxygen levels, the risk of severe damage or death increases by 11 percent.)

The research supports a recent change in the medical guidelines for treating brain-injured patients with TBI. Medical staff should now monitor patients with severe head injury for brain oxygenation during the intensive care period.

The study referred to by the lawyers had also been published in the journal *Neurosurgery* in November 2011[26] and came from the departments of neurosurgery, neurology, radiology, anaesthesiology, and intensive care of the University of Pennsylvania. The lengthy title was "Brain Hypoxia is Associated with Short-Term Outcome After Severe Head Injury Independently of Intracranial Hypertension and Low Cerebral Perfusion Pressure." The phrase "associated with short term outcome" is meaningless, simply because a word *was omitted*—poor. The title wording was taken from the conclusions of the abstract, where the word poor is included. Translated from the jargon, the message of the paper is that lack of oxygen in the tissues of the brain after head injury is associated with poor recovery. This is hardly surprising, but it is claimed that lack of oxygen, hypoxia, was a *predictive factor*, independent of both blood flow and the pressure in the cranium. However, this is misleading because it is painfully obvious that oxygen can only be delivered by blood flow, and blood cannot flow into the brain if the pressure in the cranium is too high.

As the 2011 press release states, the University of Pennsylvania study reviewed the outcome of 103 patients who had suffered severe head trauma and had their brain oxygen levels monitored. The hypothesis being "tested" was that lack of oxygen in the brain is associated with worse short term outcome and, not surprisingly, it was found to be true. Despite the publicity given to this latest research, the finding that lack of oxygen is associated with a poor outcome has been known since the late 1990s. The brain is, of course, in a box which begs the question: How were oxygen levels measured deep in the tissues? What follows makes rather uncomfortable reading, but it is now an accepted protocol and, in the US, is *reimbursable*. Probes are surgically inserted at the bedside through a hole drilled through the patient's forehead. This invasive procedure will itself cause brain damage and is associated with significant bleeding in 1% of patients. Figure 19.3 shows the CT of a head-injured patient with the oxygen sensor (arrowed) inserted close to the area of damage and a pressure catheter some distance away close to the tip of the left lateral ventricle. A section of the skull bone has been removed to allow the brain to swell.

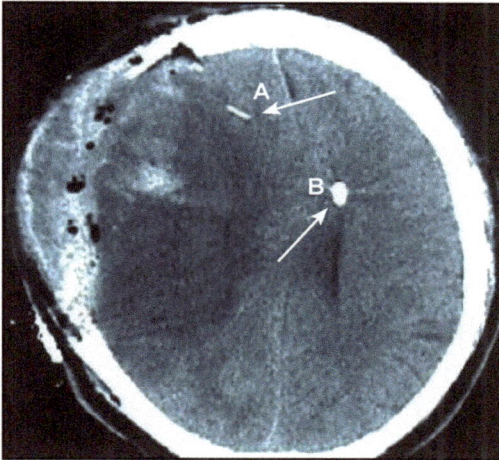

Figure 19.3:
CT of the head of a brain-injured patient showing where the bone has been removed on the right side. The oxygen (A) and pressure (B) probes are arrowed.

The stated justification for inserting the probes in the 2011 paper is that they allow a "diagnosis" of hypoxia, which can then direct the patient's treatment; "Efforts to Maintain Adequate Interstitial Partial Pressure of Oxygen in Brain Tissue may Play an Important Part in the Management of Severe Traumatic Brain Injury." A paragraph is included on the management of brain oxygen, which mentions increasing the level of oxygen administered to the patient to a heady 60% as one of the strategies for improving tissue oxygenation; another is, mistakenly, the use of hyperventilation. The lawyers in San Francisco do not seem to have noticed that several of the authors had contributed to a similar publication on monitoring brain oxygenation in the *Journal of Neuro-*

surgery[27] in 2010. This paper includes a table of therapies used to treat compromised brain oxygen and, curiously, mentions increasing the oxygen level to 100%, albeit only transiently and as a "challenge"; it is not clear what this actually means. Again, adjusting the settings of the ventilator is recommended "to improve oxygenation" and the target haemoglobin saturation at just 93%, regarded as acceptable in head-injured patients, represents an oxygen tension of only 70 mm Hg. The normal arterial tension is 100 mm Hg and so a value of 70 mm Hg means that there is a very significant reduction in the gradient available to transport oxygen into the tissues. Reference 53 in this second paper refers to research on tissue hypoxia in traumatic brain injury published in the same journal in 2004,[28] which clearly demonstrated that *100% oxygen improves outcome* in severe head injury. Astonishingly, this paper was not even discussed, despite the obvious relevance of the findings. A total of 52 patients were given 100% oxygen for 24 hours starting within six hours post-injury, with the results compared to a closely matched group of historical controls. Many measurements were made of biochemical changes and the benefit of giving the patients more oxygen was clearly demonstrated. No side effects were reported, but the authors did not suggest actually implementing the use of 100% oxygen; in line with the fashion of the day, they called for a prospective randomised controlled trial. It is, nevertheless, clear that there is a growing acceptance, at least by neurosurgeons, that restoring tissue oxygen levels is critical and, surprisingly, a value is even suggested in the 2004 paper for the minimum oxygen concentration necessary for cell survival.

The move to measure tissue oxygen levels in the brain actually dates from the 1990s and was a European initiative. One of the first reports showed, predictably, that both an increase in pressure in the skull, and a decrease in blood flow, caused the tissue oxygen level in the brain to fall. A clear relationship between the risk of brain-injured patients dying and lack of oxygen in brain tissue was well established from measurements in studies published by 1998,[29] but others had also shown that some of the procedures used actually risked *reducing* oxygen levels in the brain. None of the papers mention *barometric pressure* in relation to brain oxygenation, or reference the many papers on hyperbaric oxygen treatment already discussed; it is as if they did not exist. Unfortunately, the body which oversees hyperbaric oxygen treatment in the US, at least in relation to reimbursement, the Undersea and Hyperbaric Medical Society (UHMS), still refers to the use of hyperbaric oxygen treatment in head injury as off label!

The UHMS, originally called the Undersea Medical Society, was founded in 1974 to support research into deep diving. It was renamed the Undersea and Hyperbaric Medical Society in 1987 to attract physicians involved in hyperbaric oxygen treatment, as funding for deep diving research was declining dramatically. No other medical group in the US had become involved in hyperbaric medicine, and so the list of conditions developed by the committees responsible for hyperbaric oxygen treatment in the society has become by default the "approved" list reimbursed by US insurers. However, acute cerebral oedema, that is, acute brain swelling, which was endorsed in the early Hyperbaric Oxygen Treatment Committee Reports of the UMS, was dropped and emphasis changed to the less controversial treatment of problem wounds. There were, however, a few doctors who refused to accept this stance, who believed that wounds in the brain could indeed be helped. Dr. Edgar End had begun to treat stroke and dementia patients in Milwaukee in the 1950s, and mentored the late Dr. Richard Neubauer, who pioneered the use of hyperbaric oxygen treatment in patients with multiple sclerosis in the US. In 1990, Dr. Neubauer and colleagues had a seminal letter published in the *Lancet* entitled "Enhancing Idling Neurons."[30] It described the use of SPECT—single photon emission computed tomography, which images blood flow, to demonstrate dormant brain tissue in a stroke patient, cells that are "not dead, but sleeping." The patient was 60 years old and had suffered the stroke 14 years earlier. With a course of treatment she became able to look after herself after years in institutional care. In 1995, Dr. Neubauer resigned from the UHMS over the failure to endorse the use of hyperbaric oxygen treatment for neurological indications and took the far-sighted step of founding the American College of Hyperbaric Medicine.

The second US pioneer is a much younger man, Dr. Paul Harch. Working in New Orleans, he gained experience of diving medicine working with Dr. Keith van Meter in the support of commercial diving operations in the Gulf of Mexico. Dr. Harch started using SPECT imaging to follow the effects of hyperbaric oxygen treatment for commercial divers who had residual damage to the brain after diving accidents. He had access to the latest 3-D head scanner manufactured by the Picker Company and had been located in the West Jefferson Medical Center. The divers often had long courses of treatment and so it was unfortunately implied by some in the UHMS that Dr. Harch was profiteering, despite the reimbursement charges for the imaging and treatment going to the institutions involved. The divers were often involved in litigation and the evidence from imaging challenged the views of expert witnesses. It is notable that there have been only two prior investigations of divers following neurological decompression sickness. One was undertaken in the University of Texas Medical Branch in Galveston,[31] and the other—one of the very few clinical reports ever published by the US Navy.[32] Both found clear evidence of residual damage.

Dr. Harch also treated non-diving patients and used long courses of treatment, for example for survivors of carbon monoxide poisoning. Again he followed the improvement with hyperbaric treatment using SPECT imaging of the brain to provide objective evidence of benefit. In 1997, he was summarily called to a tribunal by the UHMS after a complaint from a committee member. After a two hour long hearing, it was accepted that his research was not experimentation, was properly conducted, and had generated unique data. He was asked, as one of 26 invited experts, to give a presentation at the 45th UHMS Workshop on the Treatment of Decompression Illness on August, 1995, in Palm Beach, Florida. It was, nevertheless, clear that his work dismayed some members of the Hyperbaric Oxygen Committee; using low pressures was clearly viewed as an implied criticism of US Navy procedures, which use very high oxygen pressures, despite the recognition that high oxygen pressures can actually be harmful. In fact, as was discussed in Chapter 8, a warning about the deterioration of neurological symptoms from using oxygen at the very high pressure of 2.8 ATA, has been included in every issue of the *US Navy Diving Manual* published since 1970, although no explanation has ever been offered for the phenomenon. Unfortunately, today some of the younger military diving medical officers with little hands-on experience actually deny that the US Navy treatment tables using oxygen at 2.8 ATA may cause deterioration. The investigations by Dr. Harch also opened an old wound; they endorsed the work of Dr. Neubauer, and several long-standing committee members had criticised Dr. Neubauer's use of hyperbaric oxygen treatment for patients with chronic neurological conditions, especially for patients with multiple sclerosis. Also, operating in a free-standing clinic, he provided treatment at a fraction of the cost levied by most US hospital -based facilities and often did not charge patients.

Despite the evidence that Dr. Harch had carefully documented both by clinical examination and SPECT imaging, his findings were still resisted and, faced with continued attacks from the UHMS executive board, he resigned from membership of the society. Courageously, he continued work in the field, following the clinical improvement from hyperbaric oxygen treatment using SPECT and extending his studies to patients with the residual effects of traumatic brain injury. In 1999, Dr. Harch gave a presentation at a hyperbaric meeting held in Columbia, South Carolina, which included brain SPECT images of a 29-year-old female patient he treated in 1994. This author still remembers the impact of these extraordinary images. The patient had attempted suicide by shooting herself in the right temple and underwent three surgical procedures in her first week in hospital. The first was to clean the wound, the second to remove the bullet, and the third to place a shunt, that is, a valve and tubing, to relieve a build-up of pressure in her brain. She was eventually discharged, profoundly disabled, after three weeks in intensive care. Many years later her physician recommended hyperbaric treatment to her desperate family and she duly underwent a course of hyperbaric oxygen treatment with Dr. Harch in New Orleans. SPECT scans were undertaken before, during, and after the course of treatment. The images are reproduced below and show the dramatic improvement, despite the lapse of six and a half years.

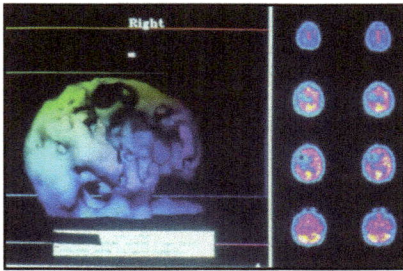

Pre-treatment scan 6.5 years post-injury.

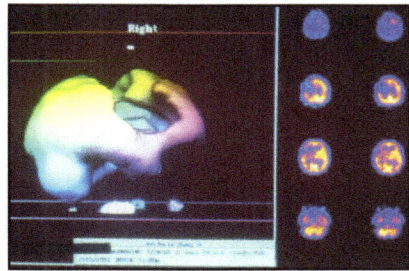

Scan post-80 hourly HBO treatments.

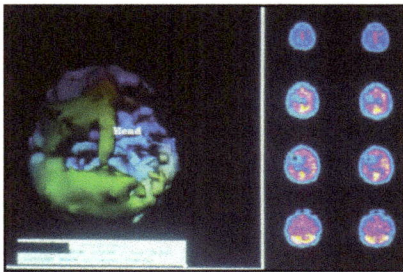

Pre-treatment scan 6.5 years post-injury.

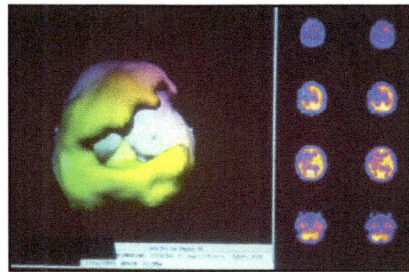

Scan post-80 hourly HBO treatments.

Figure 19.4:
SPECT images of a patient with a gunshot wound pre and post-treatment.
(Courtesy of Dr. Paul Harch.)

SPECT scans image blood flow, not the actual tissues, and so the absence of an area on a scan means that there is little or no blood flow, although not necessarily loss of tissue. There is obviously a threshold of blood flow below which the tissue cannot be visualised using SPECT. Given the trauma associated with the entry of the bullet, there must have been considerable loss of tissue but, nevertheless, it can be seen that after the course of treatment the blood flow has increased in the margins of the wound and the rest of the brain. Although the 3-D reconstructions are very striking the really important information is in the cross sections on the right hand side (Figure 19.5) which show that blood flow through the whole brain is greatly improved, as it was in the patient described from the paper published by Dr. Neubauer and colleagues in the *Lancet* 10 years after a stroke.[30]

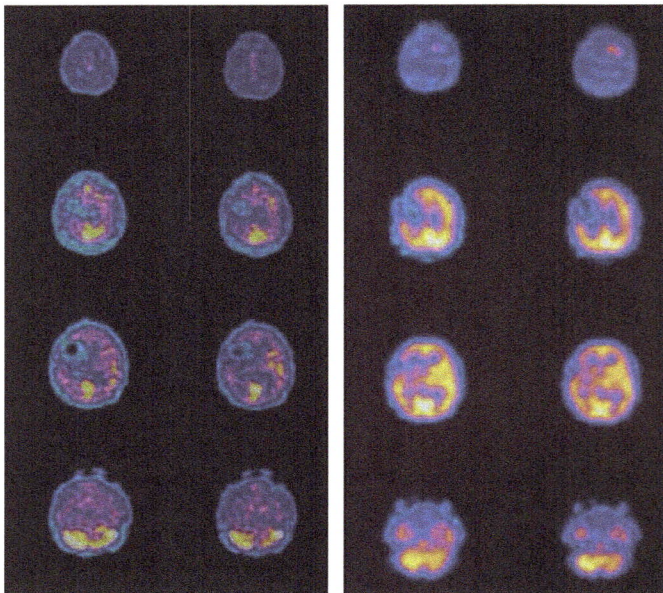

Figure 19.5:
Sagittal SPECT images before (left) and after treatment. (Courtesy of Dr. Paul Harch.)

Professional and independent assessment of Dr. Harch's patient indicated that there was a generalised reduction in spasticity, with improvement in both trunk control and left hand function. The patient reported that the severity and frequency of her headaches had greatly reduced; her speech and sleep was markedly improved. The improvement of movement of her left arm and hand, together with the resumption of normal bowel action, greatly added to her quality of life. The benefit was sustained, despite the delay to treatment. The inescapable logic must, of course, be to use this immensely powerful agent sooner rather than later. Astonishingly, the reason for the improvement demonstrated by SPECT in this patient can actually be explained by the results of an autopsy undertaken in 1934.[33]

In 1934, Dr. Cyril Courville, a distinguished pathologist, and a colleague, Dr. T.S. Kimball, examined the brain of a 57-year-old patient who died in the Los Angeles County Emergency Hospital from lobar pneumonia. The man had been shot in the head 22 years before whilst hunting, and the bullet had not been removed. Their detailed account occupies 11 pages of the journal *Archives of Pathology*. One paragraph uniquely confirms the persistence of recoverable brain tissue.

HISTOLOGIC OBSERVATIONS IN A CASE OF OLD GUNSHOT WOUND OF THE BRAIN

CYRIL B. COURVILLE, MD

and

T.S. KIMBALL, MD

It is natural to assume at the outset that a wound of the brain would become quiescent, as is the case of other wounds of other tissues. This study seems to indicate that this is not the case for after an interval of 22 years, the processes of disintegration, of phagocytosis and probably also of repair were still taking place . . . nerve cells persist in the margins of wounds of the brain for many years.

The persistence of nerve cells indicates that the oxygen present in the cerebrospinal fluid bathing the cells was enough to maintain their viability despite the passage of 22 years, which reflects the very high level of blood flow to the brain. More than 70 years after this paper was published, the sequence of SPECT images undertaken by Dr. Harch revealed the same findings in a living patient and, crucially, they have demonstrated how oxygen treatment can improve recovery, despite long intervals. The explanation is simple; at no time in normal life can we have a greater oxygen pressure than about 100 mm Hg from breathing air, and this applies from birth to the grave. However, this value may simply not be enough to allow the oxygen level in an injured tissue to approach the value needed for recovery. Increasing the oxygen concentration, in this case six and a half years after the injury, revived tissue that was "not dead, but sleeping," to initiate a more complete recovery. A similar case report was published in 2009 and the paper and images can be viewed online.[34] Dr. Harch and his colleague, Dr. Keith van Meter, have done many animal studies of oxygen treatment, and the latest to be published used an animal model of *chronic* brain injury.[35] It showed unequivocal benefit from hyperbaric oxygen treatment under the most carefully controlled conditions, and received very positive press coverage.

A change is now evident in the position of the UHMS, and this has much to do with the appointment of Dr. George Mychaskiw as editor-in-chief of *Undersea and Hyperbaric Medicine*.[36] In 2009, the journal published a remarkable account of two USAF special forces soldiers injured by roadside improvised explosive device (IED) when driving a truck in Iraq in 2008.[37] There was no direct impact to the head and no loss of consciousness, but they were both dazed and suffered tinnitus. They were given drug treatment for headache and light duties. Two weeks post-incident they returned to full duties. A week later, both airmen reported the return of headache, but drug treatment was ineffective. They developed sleep disorders, were quick to become angry, and reported that they stayed angry from trivial provocations for several hours. The also reported that their attention spans had shortened, that they were forgetful, and had inappropriate fatigue. Beginning insidiously at three weeks post-injury, the symptoms progressed for about two months and thereafter remained constant. The soldiers were *flown*(!) back to their home base in the US and attended a clinic for investigations still complaining of the same symptoms. A neurological examination was, predictably, normal, as was a CT scan and other investigations. To be accepted into the special forces, the soldiers were required to pass tests which included reaction time, procedural reaction time, code substitution learning, code substitution, delayed mathematical processing, and matching-to-sample tests. It was decided to repeat the tests, now six months post-injury. Both men showed significant decrements from their pre-injury scores and were still having difficulties at work.

Hyperbaric oxygen treatment was then undertaken in a private Florida clinic at 1.5 ATA for one hour a day, five days a week. Despite the lapse of eight months, improvement was rapid. One airman reported that his headaches stopped by the fifth treatment and did not return. He also found that he was able to sleep seven to eight hours per night uninterrupted. The second airman reported a reduction in the severity of his headaches; they lasted only one to two hours instead of eight to 10 hours. He was also able to sleep eight to nine hours per night uninterrupted. Both reported that they felt more mentally alert and were less forgetful, although they still did not feel completely normal. The airman who was less affected, having been further from the blast, felt that his symptoms had resolved. Repeat testing confirmed the improvement, the scores having returned to the baseline values and he returned to full duties. Although his colleague reported much improvement, he had lingering irritability and forgetfulness, and the decrements in his test scores returned. He was treated with a second course of hyperbaric treatment and the tests showed improvement at, or exceeding his pre-injury scores, and he reported feeling much better. It is the opinion of the author that such case reports with their corroborating measurements provide all the evidence needed to introduce the use of oxygen treatment especially when it is recognised that there is no other treatment for mild traumatic brain injury. Patients are "managed," which is "watch and pray," with rest, mental exercises, and drugs for the relief of symptoms. Although recovery normally takes three to 12 months, patients with persisting symptoms at one year rarely recover. Importantly, patients who have suffered mild traumatic brain injury are at increased risk if they have a second injury. This is termed the second impact syndrome. Leaving aside the suffering of patients, the costs of caring for patients with traumatic brain injury are truly astronomic.

It seems unlikely that medical officers in the USAF will agree that mild traumatic brain injury should be treated with more oxygen. A new study undertaken at Brooks Air Force Base claims to have shown that hyperbaric treatment does not benefit such patients.[38] The study used as controls patients who breathed compressed air in a chamber at 1.3 ATA, whilst the test group were given hyperbaric oxygen treatment on a wound healing protocol at 2.4 ATA, which studies have shown is too high a dose. Both groups were, therefore, treated under hyperbaric conditions but, despite alleging that hyperbaric treatment is not beneficial in chronic head-injured patients, it is, nevertheless stated that "both groups improved significantly."

The similarity of the USAF results to the Canadian study of hyperbaric treatment for brain damaged children, published in the *Lancet* in 2001, is startling.[39] This study also found benefit from both oxygen at 1.75 ATA and hyperbaric air at 1.3 ATA. The *Lancet* refused to allow the use of compressed air at 1.3 ATA to be called a sham, or a placebo. The children in both groups were also described as having "significant benefit." At 1.3 ATA the plasma oxygen tension increases not by 27%, as claimed, but by 50%. This is because the contribution of the partial pressures of carbon dioxide and water at alveolar level remain constant. An abrupt increase in ambient pressure also induces a net transfer of water from tissues to blood due to gas-induced osmosis.[40] It has been known for over 100 years in compressed air work that an increase of pressure to 1.3 ATA is often sufficient to treat decompression sickness when it affects the nervous system.

However, the authors of the USAF head injury study actually admit that their so-called "sham-controlled" group may have derived benefit, but then, inexplicably, state "it seems very unlikely such a minimal dose of oxygen *and nitrogen* could influence brain function favourably." This is truly astonishing, especially for physicians involved in aviation; pressurisation and oxygen are critical to aircraft operations. In Chapter 12, the USAF tests in a stripped Liberator bomber at 35,000 feet using a pressure bag to save aircrew stricken with neurological decompression sickness were highlighted.[41] The pressure increase in the bag that produced dramatic benefit was just 3 psig, that is 0.2 ATA. There has been little discussion in any of the clinical papers studying brain injury that changing levels of oxygen regulate genes via the HIF protein system and control inflammation. This provides a solid scientific basis for using more oxygen; the dose from air is often simply not enough to ensure recovery, as witnessed by the fact that many patients take years to recover from traumatic brain injury, if they recover at all. Unfortunately, the authors revealed their negative bias; alleging, despite its acceptance by neurologists,[42] and demonstration by SPECT imaging, that the concept of the idling neuron is "unproven."

However, persistence of the effects of brain injury was demonstrated in a unique study undertaken in New Zealand, published as long ago as 1980.[43] Ten university students who had sustained a head injury between *one and three years previously*, were matched with 10 students who had not had a head injury. Careful measurements of vigilance and memory were made at sea level and no differences were found between the two groups. However, when the tests were repeated at a pressure equivalent to 12,350 feet altitude using a *hypobaric* chamber, the post-head injury students were clearly less capable. This suggests that a persistent reduction in blood flow post-injury was present limiting oxygen delivery and full recovery. We now know why—low blood flow is associated with chronic inflammation. Hyperbaric oxygen treatment attenuates inflammation and stimulates the growth of new neurons and the blood vessels they need.[44] But these patients are at risk of serious deterioration if they sustain another head injury and the associated brain swelling has been termed "malignant." It is known as the second impact syndrome.[45]

A case report in the *Journal of Neurosurgery* in January 2013[46] describes a desperate sequence of events in a 17-year-old US high school football player. He had a violent helmet to helmet contact which left him dazed, and told a team mate that he "felt dizzy and could not see straight." Although he continued to play for 15 minutes to the end of the game, he experienced the onset of a persistent and severe headache. He was examined at a local hospital; no abnormalities were found and a CT scan was normal. Five days after the impact he was still complaining of a headache and he appeared to have difficulty concentrating but, nevertheless, returned to practice football hitting drills. On the fourth drill he was slow in getting up and several plays later he complained of dizziness, and said he could not feel his legs. He lost consciousness upon leaving the field, and had a generalised seizure. On admission to the local A & E department he was sedated and intubated. A CT scan showed brain swelling and bleeding within the skull. He was *flown* to a tertiary care facility, where his condition was managed with mannitol, drugs, and induced coma. Despite developing kidney failure, ventilator pneumonia, and suffering a cardiac arrest, he survived. The paper reports that after three years he had only regained limited verbal, motor, and cognitive skills.

Over the last 50 years, researchers in many countries have studied hypoxia in animal models and patients, and there is a veritable mountain of evidence that bears silent witness to the fact that lack of oxygen is of primary importance in head-injured patients. Despite increasingly sophisticated techniques to demonstrate the problem, some of which contribute further injury, there is still no consensus on the level of oxygen needed when no one will deny that there is no substitute and the fact that oxygen has actions beyond simple metabolism is slowly dawning.[47–49] Pressure is building for action in the US because of the long-term effects of blast trauma in military personnel.[50] The damage is, of course, associated with UBOs on MRI. An excellent crossover study of the use of hyperbaric oxygen treatment which has demonstrated amelioration of the chronic symptoms that commonly follow head injury has now been published from Israel.[51] What is now needed is political pressure to ensure that oxygen treatment is made available and used; the dreadful problems posed by head injuries will not go away. The initiative can only be driven by the public because the resistances raised by a sceptical medical profession are not easily resolved, although they are emotional not scientific. Many of the challenges faced in treating head-injured patients are also present in the treatment of stroke and, as will be seen in the next chapter, with one exception, drugs have a similar record of failure.

CHAPTER 20

Stroke and Hyperbaric Oxygen Treatment

When we have a stroke, our brain is starved of oxygen, causing the catastrophic death of nerve cells and leaving us paralysed and unable to speak.

Colin Blakemore, neuroscientist quoted in the
Daily Telegraph, March 2010.

Before the advent of the railways and the roads needed for motor vehicles, rivers were used for transporting goods and people. As we see all too often today, river banks can fail and, although the damage may be contained, flooding can blight the countryside. In contrast, a major obstruction to the flow of a river can be disastrous and needs immediate action to restore the flow of water. The hydraulic system of the body, the blood vessels and blood they transport, is affected in similar ways. As we have seen in multiple sclerosis, the brain may be damaged by minor leakage; waterlogged tissues impede the delivery of oxygen to cells and, if proteins and if white blood cells escape through the wall of a blood vessel, they trigger damaging inflammation. The blockage of an artery in the brain is a worst-case scenario and the symptoms are usually called a stroke, emphasising that the symptoms may be sudden in onset. As obstructing blood flow reduces, or may even prevent, the delivery of vital oxygen to an area of the brain, the reader may feel that this is surely one case where doctors will insist that patients are given oxygen treatment? Not so; oxygen administration has yet to be recommended for stroke and, in fact, many doctors discourage it, claiming it would be harmful. This means, of course, that they consider the dosage of oxygen we gain from air to be optimal. A discussion of stroke brings together all the concepts introduced in previous chapters, from the disruption of blood flow, to the complex genetic changes that take place in cells deprived of oxygen.

The first event a patient is aware of in a stroke is due to lack of oxygen because of a reduction of blood flow, and it causes the upregulation of the hypoxia-inducible factor proteins already discussed. The hypoxia attracts neutrophils to the affected area and, if the lack of oxygen is not relieved, they release free radicals, damaging the walls of blood vessels. This may lead to the most serious complication, bleeding into the tissues of the brain, and is known as a *haemorrhagic* stroke. The red blood cells are broken down and the iron released from their haemoglobin generates the most toxic of free radicals, the hydroxyl radical, causing the death of cells in the vicinity. The brain is uniquely vulnerable to these events although, as we have seen, they also take place in other organs of the body. Sometimes a tear can occur in the wall of a small artery in the brain damaged by atheroma—the same disease that damages the coronary arteries, which is commonly, but not always, associated with high blood pressure. In young people, a small bulge known as a Berry aneurysm may also rupture. Tears lead to haemorrhage under the delicate covering membrane of the brain known as the subarachnoid membrane. There is usually a headache, but other symptoms range from minor disturbances, such as pins and needles and numbness in limbs or the face, to loss of consciousness and coma. The author has treated a diver, who suffered a haemorrhage from a Berry aneurysm upon leaving the water, using hyperbaric oxygenation. He was later transferred for neurosurgery and made a remarkable recovery. The value of hyperbaric oxygenation in subarachnoid haemorrhage has been demonstrated in animal models[1] and was successfully used, with the improvements followed by imaging, in a 48-year-old patient.[2]

Stroke is an ill-defined lay term that has forced its way into general use in medicine to describe a variety of neurological symptoms resulting from a reduction of blood flow. It is usually to an area of the brain but, much less commonly, may involve the spinal cord. The symptoms of a stroke are usually sudden in onset and the most easily recognised form involving the brain is known as a hemiplegia. Half of the body, most commonly the left side, develops weakness or paralysis and it may include the muscles of the face, causing drooping of the mouth. The reduction of blood supply responsible is usually the result of material obstructing flow along one of the middle brain arteries supplying the motor cortex of the hemispheres or the nerve fibre pathways passing through the centre of a hemisphere. This may be due to the local accumulation of clot, known as thrombosis,[3] or to an embolism. The term stroke may also be applied to areas of damage to structures in the middle of the hemispheres of the brain and involve the basal ganglia and the central white matter. The arteries supplying the brain stem, the rear of the brain, and the cerebellum, which nestles above the nape of the neck, may also suffer blockage and very rarely the spinal cord may be affected by a stroke. An example, highlighted in Chapter 13, was due to fibrocartilagenous embolism. The lack of oxygen from the reduction of blood flow may lead to disruption of the blood-brain barrier.[4,5] In both location and the extent of the tissue destruction, the white matter damage is essentially the same as in the most severely affected areas in patients with multiple sclerosis. As discussed, the passage of small emboli damage the blood-brain barrier directly and there is increasing recognition that this mechanism underlies the development of dementia and Alzheimer's disease in the elderly.[6,7]

Strokes are the scourge of the Western world and the UK NHS Information Centre has reported that patients admitted to hospital with a stroke are now more likely to die than those who suffer a heart attack. In England and Wales, about 53,000 patients die from a stroke each year, with over 450,000 surviving with severe disability. They need long-term care and the annual cost is about £7 billion. Strokes most commonly affect older people who have arteries affected by the fatty deposits known as atheroma, which are linked to high saturated fat intake, obesity, diabetes, and lack of exercise. It is important, however, to note that strokes may still occur in the absence of these risk factors. Stroke may also complicate cardiac surgery, often associated with embolism;[8] cardiac surgery units should always have immediate access to a hyperbaric chamber. It makes sense to treat patients routinely post-surgery, not least because areas of the brain may suffer from low blood flow.[9,10] In the elderly, the key process is atheroma with patchy damage to the surface lining of arteries, which is clearly caused by substances actually carried in blood; the disease does not affect veins unless they are used to replace arteries, as they are in coronary bypass surgery. The veins used in "bypass" surgery rapidly assume the appearance of an artery; the muscle in the wall develops and they become liable to arterial disease, which sometimes develops very rapidly. This clearly shows the importance of the higher internal pressure present in arteries to the development of atheroma, and high blood pressure is known to be an important risk factor for the disease. Post-mortem information gained from young US servicemen dying in Vietnam showed the presence of early surface damage to arteries and subsequent studies established that the typical fatty streaks may form in very young children. Traditionally, fat, bouncy babies have been regarded as a picture of health in the West, a legacy perhaps from the days when infants died of malnutrition, as they are still prone to do in many countries in the developing world.

The location of atheroma is determined by the hydraulic factors which influence blood flow in arteries. It is well known that shear forces are important in their formation and the damage to the lining induces *inflammation*, again, by attracting white blood cells which cause damage by releasing free radicals. The damaged area then attracts the deposition of fat from the blood and the wall slowly thickens with fibrous connective tissue—essentially the same process that occurs over many years in multiple sclerosis. Later in life the hardening of the arteries, known as arteriosclerosis, is accompanied by the deposition of calcium. Platelets carried in blood often stick to the areas, especially in the arteries of the heart—the coronary arteries and it is termed coronary thrombosis. This also occurs, although to lesser extent in the arteries in the brain. The process may eventually block the flow of blood along an artery and, whilst this may seem catastrophic, if it takes place very slowly, the body creates new blood vessels to compensate for the reduction of blood flow. Again, this is controlled by genes upregulated by the hypoxia-inducible factor proteins. The same fatty deposits often occur in the carotid arteries in the neck and tiny pieces may break off, forming emboli which may flow along the arteries supplying the brain. Strokes may also occur when material breaks off damaged heart valves and when clots form in the heart. This is most commonly associated with stagnation of blood in the left atrium in patients suffering from the irregularity of contraction known as atrial fibrillation.

Strokes are rare in young people, but as we have seen in Chapter 13, if the endplate of a vertebra is damaged, fibrocartilagenous material from the centre of a spinal disc may enter the circulation and embolise the brain, or spinal cord, causing a stroke, as it did in the 17-year-old girl discussed earlier, who died in 1987.[11] Fibrocartilagenous embolism must always be suspected when a young person suffers a cardiac arrest, especially during sporting activity. The coronary arteries must be examined carefully at autopsy, otherwise small emboli will not be detected. It is notable that this form of embolism is not listed as a cause of sudden death (see www.suddendeath.org). Equally, it is rarely mentioned as a cause of nervous system damage in man, although it is well known in veterinary practice and affects a wide range of animals.

The route taken by emboli is determined by the hydraulic factors which influence blood flow, especially the angles at which arteries branch and, of course, their diameter. The size of emboli is also very important in determining the route taken. Reference has already been made in Chapter 15 to the artery to the eye being a "preferred" pathway for very small emboli, which accounts for the frequency with which the optic nerve is affected in optic neuritis and in conditions as diverse as syphilis and fat embolism. Small emboli that reach the brain can cause a wide variety of seemingly minor symptoms, from weakness of a limb, to small changes in sensation, even, for example, paralysis of just a thumb.[12] Again, the middle cerebral arteries which supply key areas in the brain hemispheres are preferred pathways for large emboli, not only in man, but also in other mammals.[13] Most of the arteries in the brain connect with other arteries forming a supply ring which can minimise the effects of a blockage as can be seen in Figure 20.1.[14]

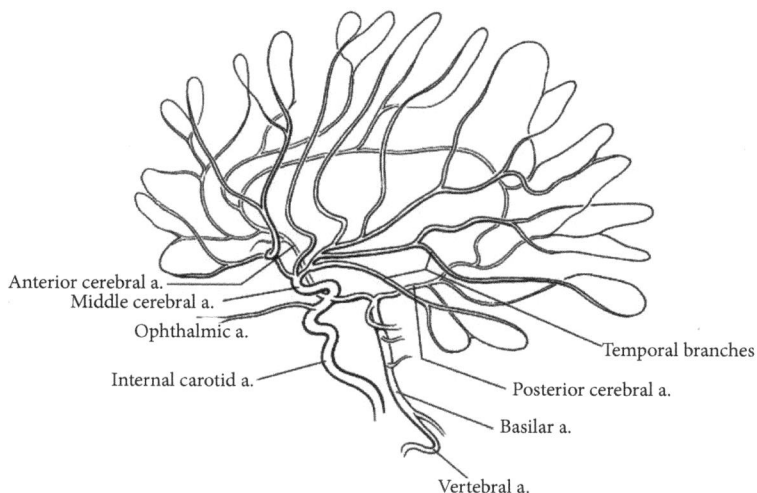

Anterior cerebral a.
Middle cerebral a.
Ophthalmic a.

Internal carotid a.

Temporal branches

Posterior cerebral a.

Basilar a.

Vertebral a.

Figure 20.1:
The anastomoses of the arteries of the brain. (From
Cerebrovascular Disease, courtesy of Dr. James Toole.)

The best known of the artery to artery connections in the brain is the
Circle of Willis, which connects the blood supply from the internal carotid
arteries to that derived from the basilar artery. Unfortunately, as discussed
in Chapter 2, the lenticulostriatal arteries do not connect to other arteries
and so are known as *end arteries*. The areas of the mid-brain they supply are
uniquely vulnerable and include the internal capsules, where the fibres that
control movement pass from the nerve cells in the grey matter of the motor cortex to the brain stem and onwards down the spinal cord. Damage to
these fibres means that the connection between the brain and limb muscles
is impaired or lost and weakness or paralysis develops. Because the nerve
fibres crossover in the brain stem, it is the right hemisphere that controls
the left side of the body.

The blockage of blood flow in a brain artery causes a major problem if
the surrounding blood vessels cannot compensate for the reduction in blood
flow and flow must be restored to allow the transport of critical oxygen to
resume. As stroke is commonly associated with clotting, it makes sense to
use an agent to dissolve clots and, in fact, the only agents that are approved
for use in the treatment of stroke are "clot-busting" drugs, principally, tissue
plasminogen activator (tPA). To be properly effective it must be used within
an hour of the onset of symptoms; after four hours, it is not beneficial and
increases the risk of bleeding. Its use is effectively restricted to just 5% of
stroke patients because of this complication. Curiously, seizures may precede
the onset of recovery during the administration of the clot-busting agent.[15]

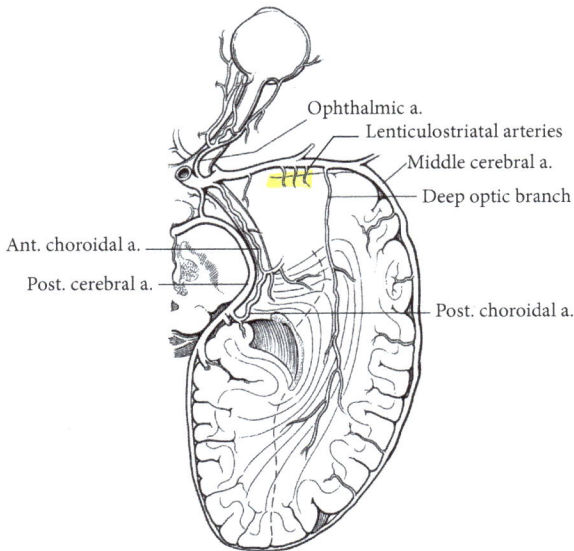

Figure 20.2:
The lenticulostriatal arteries (highlighted) of one brain hemisphere.
(From *Cerebrovascular Disease*, courtesy of Dr. James Toole.).

The treatment of stroke is widely recognised to be unsatisfactory; in 2001, a commentary in the *Lancet*[16] that followed the publication of yet another failed drug study, referred to the "plethora of recent negative trials." There has been intense research over the last 50 years attempting to find a drug that can protect the brain from oxygen deprivation in a stroke, but it has failed. Faced with an aging population, those in government certainly recognise the need to improve stroke treatment; the enormous costs involved in caring for stroke patients are a major concern. In the West, of those who survive to 85 years old, one in four will suffer a stroke.

In 2005, a report was published by the UK Department of Health[17] entitled Reducing Brain Damage: Faster Access to Stroke Care, in which it was estimated that stroke costs society about £7 billion a year, with the direct costs to the National Health Service being about £2.8 billion. The report argued for specialised stroke units and faster access to appropriate medical care, stressing that as a stroke must be regarded as a "brain attack" and emphasising the need for urgent treatment. For many years, a sense of nihilism has accompanied the treatment of stroke, which has been reinforced by the failure of most drug-based approaches. In Scotland, cards have now been distributed by the charity, Chest, Heart & Stroke Scotland, advising of the symptoms of stroke and the need to gain help by dialling the emergency number, 999.

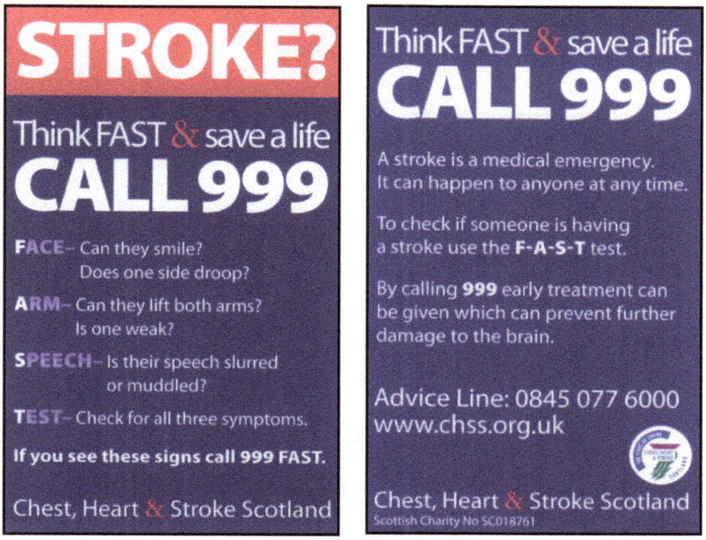

Figure 20.3:
Alert cards issued in Scotland for the symptoms of stroke.

However, the emphasis in the 2005 UK report is not on treatment, but simply on faster access to brain scanning. The first investigation recommended is a CT scan in order to detect bleeding; if bleeding is present, the outlook is grave and clot busters, the thrombolytic drugs discussed, are contra-indicated. The implementation of CT scanning is said to reduce death and disability because it allows treatable complications to be identified not, of course because it is itself a treatment. The UK target, announced in December 2007, was for an MRI to be undertaken within 24 hours in patients with "minor" strokes. It has been claimed that this will allow the prevention of 6,800 deaths a year in the UK (*Daily Telegraph*, December 6, 2007). An investment of £100 million was promised to provide the latest MRI technology by the last UK government. The money has not been provided and a more recent press report suggests that patients will only have access to MRI within a week of a stroke, which renders the investigation academic. It is notable that the word oxygen does not actually appear in the UK Department of Health report, despite the *universal* recognition that strokes are associated with oxygen deprivation from a reduction of blood flow. There can be little doubt that if a fraction of this massive financial investment was directed to the provision of oxygen treatment it would have a major impact in reducing deaths and disability. This includes the use of 100% oxygen at "normal," that is, the prevailing atmospheric pressure. There are many who would raise objections to confining a patient with an acute stroke in a hyperbaric chamber, but it is a place of safety for such a patient. The use of MRI renders patients inaccessible but, nevertheless, it is now common for it to be used for acutely ill patients. Ironically, the oxygen level in the confined space of an MRI must be monitored because deaths have occurred from asphyxia due to leakage of the liquid helium, used to cool the magnet, into the area around a patient's head.

The symptoms typical of a stroke are not always associated with blockage of a major blood vessel in the brain; symptoms indistinguishable from stroke may affect patients labelled as having multiple sclerosis—only the age of the patient and a history of other symptoms allow it to be distinguished from a stroke. A condition that must be considered in patients with a stroke has already been referred to in relation to multiple sclerosis; it is the disease associated with thrombosis known as the anti-phospholipid syndrome, discovered by Dr. Graham Hughes in the 1980s, often referred to as the Hughes syndrome.[18] When it affects the nervous system it mimics multiple sclerosis and so provides yet more confirmation that the disease underlying the formation of the areas of sclerosis starts in the blood vessels. A hundred years before the anti-phospholipid syndrome was discovered, Harald Ribbert, a German pathologist, had suggested that multiple sclerosis was associated with thrombosis, after he had seen that the earliest damage surrounded veins. Hughes syndrome is one cause of venous thrombosis, although it may also cause arterial thrombosis and embolism. Optic neuritis and paraplegia from damage to the spinal cord may also occur in Hughes syndrome, just as they do in multiple sclerosis, almost certainly from tiny emboli breaking off from an area of thrombosis. It is most important for the diagnosis of Hughes syndrome to be made, because the condition can be treated with aspirin and other drugs to prevent further attacks. However, it is also clear from the localised brain swelling seen on MRI in patients with the anti-phospholipid syndrome, that the attacks are likely to respond to hyperbaric oxygen treatment.

But we now need to consider the sequence of events occurring when an artery is partially or completely blocked reducing, or stopping, blood flow to an area of the brain. If the blockage is short-lived and the symptoms resolve in less than 24 hours, the event is termed a "transient ischaemic attack," or TIA. Again, the word "ischaemic" simply refers to a reduction of blood flow. If the symptoms last longer than 24 hours, then the word *transient* is clearly not appropriate, and the event is then classified as a stroke. The symptoms are very variable and may include brief loss of consciousness, weakness, numbness, vertigo, and even blindness in an eye. The 24-hour limit is entirely arbitrary and certainly not based on any science. This is slowly being recognised and there are calls for a new classification based on symptoms that last less than one hour. Many MRI studies[19–21] have followed events in TIAs, with one patient imaged 11 minutes after displaying symptoms.[22] For many medical professionals, the term TIA implies that, with the resolution of symptoms, no damage has been sustained, but this may not be the case in at least half of affected patients. There is another disturbing aspect; in some patients these short-lived attacks may herald the onset of a major stroke. As in multiple sclerosis patients, leakage from a disturbance of the blood-brain barrier also occurs in stroke, with reduced oxygen availability.[23,24] So there are very good reasons for patients with transient attacks to have oxygen treatment to resolve the symptoms, and for preventive measures to be used to reduce their risk of a stroke.

Strokes are the equivalent in the brain of a heart attack and are sometimes referred to as a "brain attack." Heart attacks may be rapidly fatal and so the need for emergency treatment is all too obvious, and the same urgency needs to be evident in the treatment of stroke. But, because of time constraints, the treatment of stroke will never be entirely satisfactory and, with proven links to high blood pressure and obesity, major public health campaigns aimed at prevention are needed. About a third of patients with stroke die and, sad though it is for the loved ones, this limits the human effort expended and the costs involved to society. A third of patients will eventually make a reasonable recovery and regain their independence. This leaves the remaining third as survivors in need of constant care, often in an institution. Given the treatment currently used, most of these patients will never resume an independent life and the families and carers have to face the heartbreak and hard work caused by their ongoing disability. With medical advances being able to add years to life, but often not life to years, the human and financial costs are truly enormous and, with the population aging, the costs are getting ever greater. The elderly are the group most affected by strokes, although they also occur in younger people. In young stroke patients it is important to investigate if there is a persisting hole in the heart, which allows the trapping normally undertaken by the lungs to be bypassed. Such a hole can now be closed without open heart surgery. Even a baby still in the womb may suffer a stroke leading to cerebral palsy evident after birth, although most strokes in the newborn are the result of a birth injury. If the treatment of stroke could be improved with fewer patients suffering prolonged disability, much suffering could be avoided and enormous savings made, but the record for drug interventions is dismal.

In a 2010 article entitled "The Amazing Brain," Richard Gray, scientific correspondent of the *Daily Telegraph*, quotes from an interview with the distinguished Oxford neuroscientist, Professor Colin Blakemore. Blakemore endorses the conventional view that recovery after a stroke is not due to the formation of new brain cells but to "plasticity." This popular, but curious term, attributes the recovery, for example of the paralysis and loss of speech typical of a stroke, to the function being taken over by other areas of the brain.

> *When we have a stroke, our brain is starved of oxygen, causing the catastrophic death of those nerve cells and leaving us paralysed and unable to speak. Yet within days, the same patients start to regain movement and the ability to speak. This is not a sign of nerves coming back to life, but the brain rebuilding itself, creating new nerve connections and bypassing the damaged areas.*

An indication of the lack of awareness of the importance of oxygen is evident in the superb Harveian Oration, "In Celebration of Cerebration," delivered by Professor Blakemore at the Royal College of Physicians in London on the 18th of October 2005. The details of the structure and function of the brain is extraordinary, but oxygen is mentioned only once. There can be no question, both from animal experiments and from human data, that the mammalian brain can reprogram functions, indeed, so can the spinal cord. For example, experimentally, when half the cord is cut transversely, that is, a "hemi-section" of the cord, a state of spinal shock develops. This lasts for several days, but over the following weeks, spinal cord function slowly recovers, despite the cut area healing with scar tissue. This indicates that the nerve impulses are crossing over to be transmitted on the opposite side of the spinal cord, past the area of scar tissue. This type of recovery may also take place in the brain. However, it is now well established that the adult human brain contains stem cells capable of rebuilding the brain by forming new cells.[25] Also, bone marrow stem cells can migrate into the brain[26] as they can into the heart.[27] However, attributing the *rapid* recovery in some stroke patients to regrowth is problematic because of the time scale involved in new cell formation, which is measured in weeks and months, not hours or days. Rapid recovery seen is therefore due to the recovery of brain tissue containing cells that are not dead, but immobilised, because of lack of sufficient oxygen. As the water content of the tissues reduces when the swelling subsides, the oxygen level rises and function may return. This is where oxygen treatment can make a substantial difference to both the extent of permanent damage, and to the speed of recovery.

In stroke, in contrast to the leakage from veins that characterises areas affected in multiple sclerosis and head injury, blood flow is greatly reduced or even stopped. The implications of this for the delivery of oxygen and for attempts to use drugs in treatment are all too obvious; to reach the affected area agents have to be transported in blood. Nevertheless, the tissue surrounding the critically affected area of the brain cells may have enough oxygen to survive, although not to function. Neurologists have termed this tissue the "ischaemic penumbra" which, translated, means the low blood flow surrounding area.[28] Although some have stated that the time available to rescue this tissue may be only a few hours, this is certainly incorrect;[29] MRI has shown that some patients only deteriorate after a considerable delay.[30] And, as we have seen, imaging has shown the nerve cells in the penumbra may persist and be recoverable for many years.[31]

When material stops in an artery it often provokes the local clotting, known as thrombosis, and this is targeted by the drug treatment called thrombolysis, known in popular jargon as "clot busting." It is obvious that, when an artery is blocked, oxygen delivery is greatly reduced and so some brain cells are likely to die. The key question posed is therefore: When do the nerve cells actually die? This is of paramount importance because it determines the time frame for treatment to benefit, and is often referred to as the "window of opportunity." In fact, the clot busting drugs used for the treatment of stroke must be administered early; they are not effective after a delay of more than about four hours.

Drug companies have spent billions over the last decades trying to find a drug which will provide *neuroprotection*, that is, protection for nerve cells until conditions in the brain improve. They have targeted the changes occurring in strokes down to the molecules in the membranes of nerve cells, but have failed spectacularly. The failure was highlighted in an editorial comment in the *Lancet* in 2006[32] entitled "Neuroprotection: The End of an Era?" It featured a drug developed by Astra Zeneca, code named NXY-059, described as a free-radical trapping agent. The company announced that they were dropping the drug from clinical development. It had shown promise in animal trials, but so had, according to the *Lancet* article, some 114 other compounds which went on to human studies and also failed. Astra Zeneca's drug appeared to show great promise for the treatment of stroke patients in the first clinical trial, but it failed to live up to its promise. The results from a much longer and larger trial, published nine years later,[33] showed that the optimism was ill-founded; the group of patients on the drug actually fared worse than the group given the placebo. The *Lancet* commentary pointed out that NXY-059 was one of over 1,000 compounds that have been tested on animal models, and then added an extraordinary rider; "the stroke community needs to think long and hard about whether these animal models are financially and ethically viable." They are right; after such a tortuous and prolonged effort, the cost of animal testing has been truly enormous. It is difficult to compute a figure, but it must certainly be billions of dollars. But "ethical viability" is a very curious expression and it is difficult to understand just what is meant. Surprisingly, it does not seem to have been noticed by the animal rights activists; there can be no doubt about the suffering involved in these experiments.

The failure of the drug raises an obvious question: What about those patients who worsened after being given one of the many drugs that have been studied in the trials? They would, of course, have needed to give informed consent, but some will have had their lives shortened. Unfortunately, this is by no means a unique event in the pharmaceutical world; as mentioned in Chapter 10, a drug initiative in the treatment of heart failure in the 1980s ended in an even greater disaster. The failure of NXY-059 to gain approval prompted representatives from Wyeth, a division of Pfizer, and Biotrofix Inc., a drug testing company, to demand a change in the assessment of efficacy for drugs developed for the treatment of stroke. In an article published in 2006 in the *Journal of Cerebral Blood Flow and Metabolism*,[34] they appeared to criticise the regulatory authorities for failing to approve the drug and called for more "rational patient selection." So what did the editorial team of the *Lancet* feel is the way forward in stroke treatment after stating that the failure of Astra Zeneca's NXY-059 signalled the end of drug initiatives? They suggested that cooling the head may be valuable, and methods of controlling blood glucose levels should be investigated. But there is still no mention of actually giving patients oxygen; perhaps because the damage in stroke is due to lack of oxygen, it seems just *too* obvious to give more!

By 2001, over 5,000 patients had been included in studies of clot busting agents and it had been shown that they are only effective in a limited number of patients. The risks of these agents are the worsening of neurological deficits, coma, and death. Unfortunately, it is not possible to identify patients who can benefit prior to treatment, nor is it possible to predict those patients who will suffer the dangerous complication of bleeding. The properties required of a successful neuroprotectant[35] have been detailed: "It could extend the period for salvage of potentially reversible ischaemic brain tissue, extend the time window for thrombolytic therapy, and extend the window for thrombolysis in 'reperfusion' injury. Thrombolytic therapy could improve vessel patency and allow larger amounts of a neuroprotectant to reach ischaemic tissue." It is obvious that to produce benefit, any neuroprotective agent needs access to the threatened brain tissue and this requires blood flow. In contrast to the drugs trialled, oxygen is safe, easy to administer, and readily crosses the blood-brain barrier. In a review of the use of high levels of oxygen as a treatment for stroke in 2007, Dr. Aneesh Singal,[36] who is active in researching oxygen treatment, disarmingly states:

> *Hyperoxia is an attractive acute stroke therapeutic option because it has several properties of an "ideal" neuroprotective agent. Unlike most pharmaceutical drugs it easily diffuses across the blood-brain barrier to reach target tissues, is simple to administer, well tolerated, can be delivered in 100% concentrations without significant side effects and theoretically can be combined with other acute stroke treatments such as tissue plasminogen activator, tPA.*

The word "hyperoxia" simply indicates a high level of oxygen but at normal atmospheric pressure, that is, an increased dose of the same molecular oxygen we gain from the air we breathe. It is perfectly obvious that oxygen is the ideal neuroprotective agent, because it operates as such in all of us all of the time, and we know the dire consequences that follow when it is absent. Those in medicine must understand that we have an overriding duty to correct a deficiency of oxygen, just as we do in correcting dehydration or starvation. We know it is necessary to act immediately when breathing ceases, but have simply not recognised that if only a part of the brain suffers deprivation of oxygen, the same responsibility and urgency applies.

To evaluate the use of oxygen in stroke patients it is necessary to return to first principles. Apart from severe trauma, the worst case for the brain occurs when blood flow ceases completely if the heart stops. In effect, cardiac arrest can be viewed as causing a "global" stroke because it, obviously, involves the whole brain. So, therefore, evidence derived from patients who have suffered cardiac arrest can provide an invaluable guide to the factors involved when a small area of the brain is deprived of blood flow. Traditional teaching reproduced in most medical textbooks is that, at normal body temperature, the brain is irreversibly damaged if the stoppage of the heart is longer than about four minutes. This figure dates from carefully controlled experiments in dogs undertaken more than 25 years ago in the University of Pennsylvania. Researchers found that it was not difficult to restart the heart even 14 minutes after it had stopped. If it was restarted in less than five minutes, examination of the brain showed it to be undamaged. The animals were observed for two to six hours after the heart was restarted and normal images of the blood circulation through the brain were obtained. However, if there was a delay of *more* than five minutes in restarting the heart, it was found that blood flow did not return in some areas of the brain, and it was termed the no reflow phenomenon, that is, the *no return of blood flow* phenomenon.[37] When the heart was restarted after 14 minutes and the animals examined after a lapse of four hours, multiple areas were found in the brain where blood flow was reduced, or absent. The currently accepted figure of five minutes of cardiac arrest without brain damage relates to patients who have a normal body temperature; it has been well established that this five minute cut off certainly does not apply in hypothermia, as was clearly demonstrated in the early days of cardiac surgery. Not surprisingly, this is because chilling greatly reduces the demand of the tissues of the brain for oxygen. In 1977, 20 year old Jean Jawbone was revived by a cardiac team at Health Services Center in Winnipeg, Manitoba, after a cardiac arrest lasting three hours forty minutes.

To put this in context, we must return to the astonishing experiments already discussed in Chapter 2 from the research letter published by the *Lancet* in 1998[38] entitled "Recovery of Axonal Transport in Dead Neurons." They showed without question that the nerve cells were still alive after eight hours, and they could be kept functioning for up to 18 hours, *providing* oxygen and glucose were available. At the time the heart stops, there is usually a good deal of oxygen present in the brain. This was demonstrated in a study published in 1996 in which near infrared rays were beamed into the brain at a routine post-mortem examination to allow the oxygen saturation of the haemoglobin present to be measured.[39] Six of eighteen bodies examined had oxygen levels *above the lowest values found in conscious healthy adults.* The studies illustrate why, after a sudden cardiac arrest, cardiac massage alone is as effective, indeed probably more effective if only one person is involved, than when it is combined with mouth to mouth resuscitation. This was shown by a large study in the city of Seattle,[40] which has promoted the responsible policy of training all adults to be competent in cardiopulmonary resuscitation. It is clear that, in the short-term, it is just necessary to keep blood circulating through the brain until the heart can be defibrillated. Thereafter, like head-injured patients, the problem is controlling the brain swelling caused by the lack of oxygen, and this is when hyperbaric oxygen treatment can save lives and brains.

But does the survival of brain cells after cardiac arrest mean that patients can be resuscitated eight hours after clinically verified death? It does NOT and the evidence from the experimental studies published 30 years ago still stands for normal methods of resuscitation. However, it raises the obvious question—why not? The answer is that it relates to a sudden reduction of the level of oxygen and, paradoxically, the brain damage that renders recovery of the brain impossible after eight hours actually occurs when the blood flow that is so desperately needed returns, that is, *reperfusion injury*, translated as "injury due to the turn of blood flow." The seminal research on the return of blood flow to muscle by Dr. Zamboni and his colleagues[41] has already been discussed in detail in Chapter 9. It will be recalled that the damage occurs because of free radical attack by white blood cells, triggered by a sudden fall in the tissue oxygen level. Again, this is a *principle of disease* and is of the greatest importance to any organ, when blood flow is stopped and then restarted. This includes stoppage of blood flow in organs used in transplantation surgery, or restarting the heart after a heart attack, which will be covered in the next chapter.

Trials have now been undertaken to see if the benefit of giving clot-busting drugs can be found when giving them as late as six hours post-onset. Unfortunately, they failed to show any benefit over placebo and haemorrhage remains a significant risk. This highlights the well-recognised statement that in stroke patients "time is brain"; it is alleged that for every minute of blood flow reduction one million brain cells die, although this has not been verified. It is, nevertheless, clear that if it were possible to supplement the benefit of a clot-busting agent with a truly neuroprotective drug, especially one that could reduce the risk of haemorrhage, it would be of enormous value. This defines another Holy Grail for pharmaceutical companies but they have now ended their neuroscience research; there is only one agent with a proven track record in animal and human studies; it is oxygen. Nevertheless, physicians do not give stroke patients more oxygen, even using the standard apparatus available on every hospital ward, and it is clear that most do not think of oxygen as a neuroprotective agent. Raising the dissolved oxygen concentration in the plasma protects blood vessels by reducing the activity of neutrophils and, as a consequence, it lowers the risk of haemorrhage.

Two remarkable studies have confirmed that neutrophils are involved in the tissue damage resulting from a stroke. Fifteen patients who had suffered a stroke affecting the area supplied by a middle cerebral artery were injected with radioactively labelled neutrophils within 24 hours of the onset of symptoms.[42] Single photon computed tomography (SPECT) demonstrated that neutrophils accumulated in the affected area of the brain in nine of the patients. Two patients died and confirmation of the presence of neutrophils was obtained from sections of tissue obtained at post-mortem examination. Further confirmation was produced by the same group using an advanced form of positron emission tomography (PET) in four patients in three time periods up to 30 days post-stroke.[43] They were able to show that neutrophils begin to be attracted to the damaged areas in the first 72 hours and further activity extends to 30 days. However, it is obvious that blood flow is needed for neutrophils to be carried to the site of the damage and reflow may take place at varying times. The authors concluded:

> *Given the ongoing paucity of effective neuroprotective strategies in stroke, the detection of microglial activity at later time when patients present to physicians may provide a target for novel therapeutic agents designed to limit late neuronal damage and improve outcome.*

So what studies have been done to see if giving more oxygen is of value in stroke patients? Unfortunately, the story is the same as it is in most investigations of oxygen treatment, with neither the timing nor the dosage properly regulated. For example, a study in Norway published in 1999[44] looked at the use of supplemental oxygen for stroke patients. The description in brackets in the summary of the paper was "oxygen at 100% *atmospheres*, 3 l/min." Such a simple mistake leaps out of the page for those knowledgeable about the subject, but it is telling that it escaped the notice of the journal referees. In the final paragraph of the paper it also refers to "breathing 100% oxygen through a nasal catheter" as if the patients were actually getting 100% oxygen when, at a flow rate of 3 litres a minute, the actual percentage passing down the airway into the lungs is likely to have been no more than about 26%. In other words, a very small increase over the oxygen percentage we normally breathe. Incredibly, no measurements of oxygen levels were done, either of haemoglobin oxygen saturation, or oxygen levels through the skin which can be measured using a transcutaneous oxygen sensor. This method gives a reasonable guide to the oxygen level in arterial blood. There is also no mention of the prevailing barometric pressure although, as the patients would have been fairly close to sea level, at least altitude would not have been a significant factor. Nevertheless, like Scotland, the barometric pressure at sea level in Norway varies by as much as 10% because of the weather. Haemoglobin saturation is very easy to measure by a simple finger-mounted oximeter (oxygen meter) and would have been a very relevant observation, because it would have at least identified those patients whose oxygen saturation was below 100%. This, of course, correlates with an arterial concentration less than 100 mm Hg. However, following current fashion the authors were not prepared to recommend giving supplemental oxygen to stroke patients unless there is clear evidence that they are lacking oxygen *in the blood* and given the poor methods used and the small number of patients recruited, the study is simply not credible. A similarly defective study in heart attack patients, which was published in 1976, is often cited as a reason not to give them oxygen.[45] No measurements of oxygen levels were taken and the study does not warrant serious consideration; however, it is regularly cited as being a reason not to give supplemental oxygen to patients with heart attacks. Despite all this, and in clear contrast to the stated results of the Norwegian study, it has been clearly shown that continuous supplemental oxygen reduces the amount of brain damage in stroke patients.

A 2005 paper described benefit to stroke patients from oxygen at normal atmospheric pressure, but again the time to treatment is simply recorded as being given "less than 12 hours post-onset" and no details are recorded.[46] Again, with the window of opportunity in acute stroke known to be no more than four hours, the failure to treat within this time frame is a major concern. A facemask was used for the treatment supplied with oxygen at 4 to 5 litres a minute, but blood oxygen levels were measured in only two of the seven patients who were both in the treated group. The values measured were 368 and 420 mm Hg, which is almost a 30% difference in the plasma oxygen concentration and, of course, must influence the outcome. Imagine a study of the performance of a 440 volt electric motor in which a reduction of 52 volts was simply ignored! The MRI scans showed that the higher levels of oxygen were actually associated with less brain damage. Despite this, the authors were very guarded about the value of supplemental oxygen for stroke, citing the flawed Norwegian study discussed above. A very large number of animal models of stroke have also shown benefits from the use of more oxygen, both at normal atmospheric pressure and the benefit of the dose attainable under hyperbaric conditions. Most studies have used rats which, with a brain weight of only 2 grams, represent a "worst case" situation. One of the issues sometimes queried is the use of hyperbaric oxygen treatment when stroke is complicated by haemorrhage following the use of a clot-busting agent. This has been answered: hyperbaric oxygen treatment *is* beneficial.[47,48,49]

Several early studies of hyperbaric oxygen treatment in stroke patients in the 1960s and 70s showed that patients often improved whilst in the chamber breathing oxygen, but, in most cases, the patients had only a single treatment. Not surprisingly, the improvements usually disappeared shortly after the session was completed. There was very limited understanding of the biology of oxygen at the time, and no studies were undertaken using a *course* of oxygen treatment to see if the improvements would persist. There were, however, notable exceptions to this approach. Dr. Edgar End in Milwaukee General Hospital, who rarely published his work, started treating stroke patients in the 1940s and he had seen sustained improvement from courses of treatment. In 1980 he collaborated with Dr. Richard Neubauer to publish the results from the treatment of 122 patients in the journal *Stroke*, using what were regarded at the time as low oxygen pressures, that is from 1.5 atmospheres to 2 atmospheres absolute.[50] This was a critical move away from the much higher pressures used in diving which, as discussed in Chapter 8 may be associated with convulsions. Dr. George B. Hart, a former US Naval officer, who first reported his experience in using repeated treatments for a stroke patient in 1971, continued to treat stroke patients at the Memorial Medical Center in Long Beach California. In 2003, Drs. Hart and Strauss reported that they had treated more than 80 stroke patients.[51]

A key issue is the *dosage* of oxygen used, and here it is necessary to again state the obvious; all patients with stroke already receive oxygen, that is, the dose of oxygen that is delivered in the air they breathe. The early work on organ transplantation showed that free radical damage occurred when blood flow resumed in donor hearts in transplantation experiments. The animals were breathing air and, therefore, this evidence indicates that the oxygen level in air is *not safe*. In the 1970s a neurosurgical group in the University of Bonn under Professor Holbach undertook a detailed study of the optimum level of oxygen in the treatment of the injured brain.[52] Their publication in 1979 was the last in a series and reported that, in patients with chronic brain injury after stroke and head injury, the optimum level of oxygen was 100% at 1.5 ATA. This begs the question; would patients with long-term brain injuries benefit from a course of treatment using 100% oxygen at *normal* atmospheric pressure, for example, from giving them an hour morning and evening for two weeks? The studies certainly need to be done.

The letter "Enhancing Idling Neurons," which was published in the *Lancet* in 1990 by Drs. Neubauer, Gottlieb, and Kagan, was discussed in the last chapter.[31] It described the benefit of a course of hyperbaric oxygen treatment to 60-year-old female patient who had suffered a stroke 14 years previously and regained the ability to live independently. The improvements correlated with remarkable changes evident on SPECT imaging undertaken before and after treatment. The images identified still viable brain tissue in the area surrounding the zone of tissue death. It is telling that the letter did not generate any correspondence, but the concept has been confirmed by further imaging studies.[53]

More studies of the use of hyperbaric oxygen treatment have been published but, unfortunately, no patient was treated in the "window of opportunity," that is, within four hours. In 2007, an issue of the journal *Neurological Research* was dedicated to detailed papers on the use of oxygen treatment in neurological conditions including stroke.[54] With drugs failing to show benefit, the need to focus efforts on oxygen, the only proven neuroprotective agent, is all too apparent. A comprehensive study has recently been completed in the Assaf Harofeh Hyperbaric Centre, which is near Tel Aviv in Israel, and it has now been published.[55] SPECT imaging was used before and after treatment. Figure 20.4 shows the 3-D brain images of a 72-year-old man who still had right-sided weakness 34 months post-stroke. Unable to hold either his right arm or leg against gravity, he had little movement of the fingers of his right hand and could only communicate with single words. A course of 40 sessions of HBOT was undertaken at 100% oxygen by mask at 2 ATA for a total chamber time of 90 minutes five days a week.

After treatment he was able to hold both his arm and leg up against gravity, move his fingers, and complete sentences. The initial baseline 3-D SPECT image of the brain shows a wide area of penumbral brain tissue (green regions) around the stroke area (blue region), involving part of the left motor cortex, correlating with his impairment of right leg and hand function. The left cortex of the frontal lobes, and Broca's area responsible for speech, also shows improved blood flow, as do the areas in the mid-brain known as the basal ganglia. The sessions took a total of 60 hours, that is, less than a week of his life. The use of SPECT imaging provides spectacular evidence (pun intended) of the importance of oxygen in recovering brain tissue that is not dead, but sleeping.

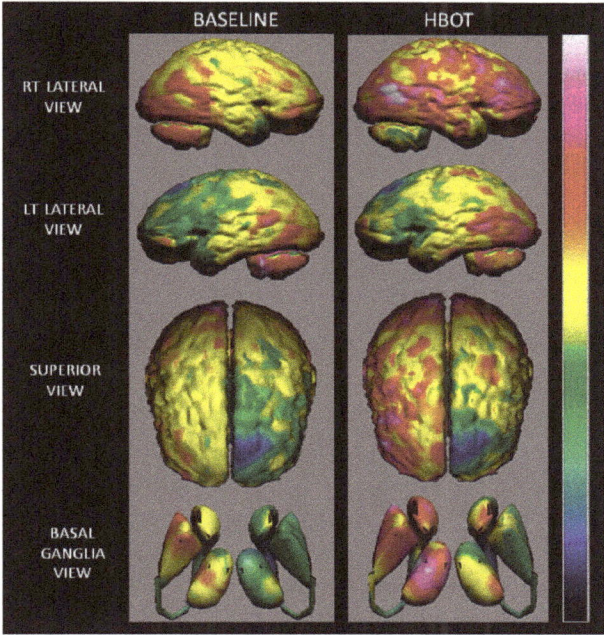

Figure 20.4:
3-D SPECT images of a 72-year-old man shows improved brain blood flow post-40 HBOT sessions. (Courtesy of Dr.Shai Efrati et al. Assaf Harofeh Medical Centre, Israel.)

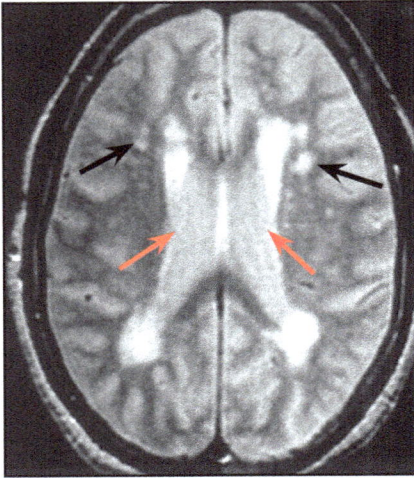

Figure 20.5:
Typical MRI of an elderly patient with dementia showing enlargement of the ventricles (red arrows) and multiple white matter lesions (black arrows).

Most people think of a stroke as a paralysing illness, but the term stroke is also used when there is damage to areas of the brain not associated with the control of arm or leg function. For example, strokes may cause loss of vision or balance, and personality changes, or even slight memory disturbances only obvious to relatives. There may also be damage in the white matter associated with the formation of UBOs on MRI. They are common with advancing years and usually do not cause any signs, or even symptoms. Figure 20.5 shows a typical MRI of an elderly patient with enlargement of the liquid-filled ventricles in each hemisphere and obvious bright areas in the white matter (arrowed). They can only be distinguished from that of advanced multiple sclerosis on the basis of the patient's history. However, there is also some thinning of the grey matter, which is more common in older patients.[56]

Long before the introduction of brain imaging, Dr. Edgar End had found benefit from hyperbaric oxygen treatment in a number of patients with memory disturbances and dementia in the 1960s. A group in the State University of New York at Buffalo became interested and undertook a double-blind, controlled crossover study using a battery of validated psychological tests in 13 patients, with a mean age of 68. They were treated very intensively, receiving two 90-minute sessions a day over 15 days at 2.5 ATA. Elaborate blinding was used and the authors reported that the group receiving the high level of oxygen on completing the treatment course showed uniform and large improvements. The five control patients, who were all pressurised, but given a lower oxygen content gas to produce normal oxygen levels in their blood, did not improve. These patients were then given a course of hyperbaric oxygen treatment and showed the same degrees of improvement. The authors commented that the treatment had allowed the patients to care for themselves, often despite years of institutional care. They also pointed out that their treatment protocol may not have been optimal and that lower pressures may be equally effective. These very positive results merited detailed publication in the *New England Journal of Medicine* in 1969.[57] Given the cost of institutional care, these results desperately need to be translated into practice as many patients will be able to retain their independence. The care in the community model developed for multiple sclerosis patients in the UK can provide an inexpensive way of adding life to the years that medical science has made possible.

In the last few years, many experimental studies on the use of oxygen in stroke have been published, and they have come from prestigious centres. Unfortunately, it is often clear that the principles of treatment are simply not understood. For example, the title of one paper begins: "Hyperbaric Oxygen Reduces Tissue Hypoxia," which translates from the medical jargon simply as "a high level of oxygen can reduce lack of oxygen in the tissues." This is equivalent to stating that giving water reduces dehydration. Nevertheless, the paper has addressed the issue of the dose of oxygen needed in stroke, albeit using a rat model, and the changes induced in gene regulation were followed.[58] Although well-conducted, the study had two important limitations that are common in small animal research; it will be recalled that the human brain weighs 1,350 grams, which is in stark contrast to the 2 grams of a typical rat brain. Nevertheless, this at least means that the results can be a guide to the treatment of the *same weight of tissue* in a human brain. Secondly, most human strokes are suffered by the elderly, whereas the rats used were eight to 10 weeks old and so far from elderly. Although the method used to reduce blood flow is accepted scientifically, it is only because it is a standardised technique; it certainly does not reproduce the events responsible for human stroke; a carotid artery was "obstructed," rather than blocked, for 90 minutes, a 70% reduction of blood flow verified using ultrasound. The symptoms that followed the release of blood flow were studied, and the tissue changes were evaluated by MRI. It was shown that giving oxygen *during the time that blood flow was obstructed* was beneficial. The authors rightly point out the need to understand the "oxygen-sensitive mechanisms" responsible for the brain damage caused by a stroke; this is hardly surprising when the oxygen consumption of the brain is the highest consumption of any organ. But it is truly astonishing that we remain unsure of such basic facts in the twenty-first century, and illustrates the abject failure in medical practice to grasp the unique importance of oxygen to recovery.

The use of clot busting drugs has, not surprisingly, established that a stroke must be treated as an emergency; action is needed in the first few hours, especially when the symptoms are severe. The failure to treat early is the principal reason for the lack of benefit found in the controlled studies of hyperbaric oxygen treatment in patients with acute stroke, as discussed earlier. It is also clear that many researchers, including many in the hyperbaric field, have yet to appreciate the immense complexity of the physiological actions of oxygen. It is astonishing that many disregard a major increase in the concentration of oxygen breathed as, for example, from 2 to 3 atmospheres; both levels are simply referred to as "hyperbaric," despite a vast increase in the number of oxygen molecules dissolved in plasma at the higher pressure. Again, it is important to draw attention to the use of the grammatically incorrect term "hyperbaric oxygen" because it constantly reinforces this absurdity; the correct terms are hyperbaric oxygenation and hyperbaric oxygen treatment.

It may be helpful here to return to the analogy used earlier of a blocked river. Although a large volume of water is clearly necessary to restart flow, it risks damage from debris it carries downstream. Nevertheless, it is obvious that restoring flow slowly with a trickle of water cannot be effective because, without delivering a sufficient volume of water, the dependent ecosystem will die. However, if flow is restored, people and animals can drink and water will be available to irrigate parched fields allowing crops to grow. During the period blood flow is obstructed in stroke patients, affected areas of the brain downstream accumulate an oxygen debt. Tissue swelling associated with the lack of oxygen may prevent clot busting drugs from actually reaching the area, and restricting the passage of red blood cells leaves only the oxygen delivered by plasma to meet the demand. Under hyperbaric conditions a much larger number of oxygen molecules can be carried dissolved in plasma, but a high pressure of oxygen must be breathed, simply because oxygen is poorly soluble in water. This is not a matter of medical opinion; it is dictated by science being defined by the gas laws. However, increasing the availability of oxygen adds another critically important dimension not covered by the simplistic analogy of a blocked river; oxygen is highly active physiologically and this raises a key issue: The trickle of supplementary oxygen referred to in mainstream medicine as "oxygen therapy" will actually cause constriction of blood vessels and reduce blood flow, whilst failing to transport enough dissolved oxygen to meet the need of the tissues. So the lesson is simple; the more severe the deficiency of oxygen, the greater the oxygen pressure, that is, the concentration a patient needs to breathe to correct it. This is just as when a patient is bleeding; the greater the loss of blood, the more units need to be transfused. Moreover, the timing is critical; no one expects a blood transfusion to be postponed for hours when a patient is bleeding to death.

The reader will recall the discussion in Chapter 9 of the research by Dr. William Zamboni and his team,[41] which was prompted by the success of hyperbaric oxygen treatment for Jessica's leg injury. The research provided direct visual confirmation of the events that follow blockage of blood vessels in the living animal, with the blood supply to the thigh muscle of a rat stopped using a ligature, and then released after four hours. To be completely successful hyperbaric oxygen treatment had to be given either during the last hour of the stoppage of the blood flow, or within an hour of the release of the ligature. Both timings were seen to *prevent* the neutrophil accumulation that would have led to blockage of the circulation and death of the muscle. Note that hyperbaric oxygenation was not, as claimed by the authors, *treating* reperfusion injury, it was actually *preventing* it.

Another seminal study of equal significance was published in 1995 from the department of neurology in the Mayo Foundation.[59] It was undertaken by a group headed by Dr. Phillip A. Low, who established a research unit many years ago to investigate diseases of peripheral nerves, that is, disorders of nerves in the limbs. They developed a rat model to study ischaemia of the sciatic nerve in the leg by injecting micro-emboli, with an average diameter of 14 microns into the supplying arteries. (Note, sometimes, emboli of this size may pass through the lung capillaries.) The group investigated all the factors that have been highlighted in the text, from free radical damage and reperfusion injury, to the protection afforded by hypothermia. Three outcomes were found from the injection of the micro spheres which, predictably, depended on the number of emboli injected: There was no damage with the lowest dose of emboli used, an intermediate dose caused degeneration of the nerve fibres, and the largest dose caused irreversible nerve damage.

The researchers decided to see if hyperbaric oxygenation could salvage the sciatic nerves of animals given the *intermediate* dose of emboli, which they referred to as "a moderate ischaemia model." After the injection of the emboli, the animals were studied using sophisticated techniques to assess the benefit of the hyperbaric oxygen treatment, including behavioural observations, measurement of nerve blood flow, and electrical studies of nerve conduction. Finally, nerves were examined microscopically to determine if there were any pathological changes. The authors observed that increasing the oxygen supply under hyperbaric conditions resulted in a *dramatic* improvement. An intensive course of hyperbaric oxygen treatment was given at a pressure of 2.5 ATA for two hours a day over seven days. The benefit was confirmed microscopically; there was little evidence of nerve damage.

It is at this point that the contrast between the experience of the very small number of physicians in the world involved in diving, and the vast majority of doctors in mainstream medicine is all too obvious: The former are familiar with pressure chambers and the technology needed, the latter are not. Thousands of divers have been treated with hyperbaric oxygenation for the neurological symptoms induced by bubbles in the circulation, which are models for the damage associated with multiple sclerosis and stroke. Many of these divers in offshore locations have been treated by their colleagues without most doctors being present. It has been assumed by doctors involved in hyperbaric medicine, despite clear evidence to the contrary, that the increased pressure simply squashes and dissolves bubbles. That this misconception has persisted so long reflects the dominance of military institutions in the development of treatment procedures in diving. Lowest common denominator "one size fits all" instructions obviously have to be issued for military situations, because lay personnel and inexperienced doctors often must take responsibility for emergency treatment. As discussed, the neurological symptoms caused by bubbles in the circulation range from a full-blown stroke, when large bubbles enter blood through a torn lung, to numbness and pins and needles from micro bubbles released from solution on decompression reaching the spinal cord. The CT scan in Figure 20.6 of a 69-year-old patient, who suffered a stroke from air embolism during a medical procedure, shows a

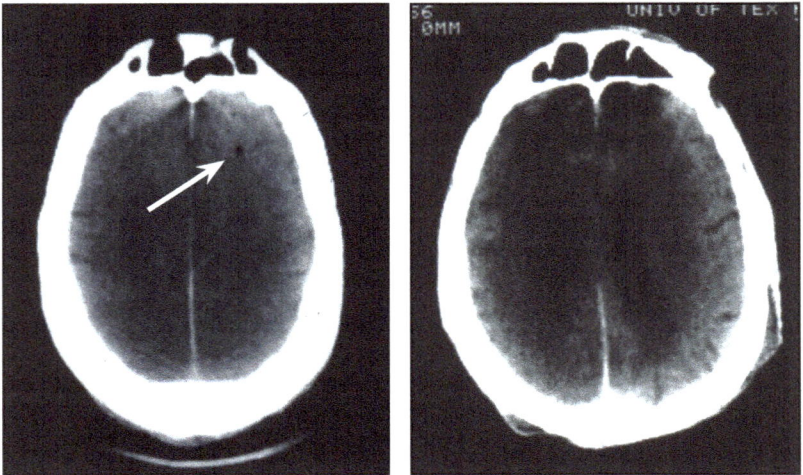

Figure 20.6:
CT of air embolism; bubble in the right middle cerebral artery arrowed and the ischaemic infarct of the right hemisphere. (Courtesy of the late Professor B.A. Hills.)

large bubble in the left middle cerebral artery (arrowed, see also Figure 13.2). Unfortunately, he did not respond to treatment and the second image shows the damage to a large area of the left hemisphere.

Treatment using high oxygen pressures was developed by the US Navy physicians for both air embolism and decompression sickness in the 1960s due to the failure of recompression using air.[60] In the US Navy Treatment Table 6, oxygen is breathed by mask at 2.8 ATA for just 20 minutes before a five minute break breathing air is used to avoid a convulsion. The cycle is then repeated up to four times. The US Air Force has developed similar procedures using the same high pressure oxygen approach for treating aviators with decompression sickness resulting from an ascent, that is, a decompression to altitude.

There can be no question that procedures like the US Navy table 6, which use oxygen at 2.8 ATA, have been largely successful in treating neurological decompression sickness, although there may be subtle residua, detectable only on psychometric testing.[61] Although this is acknowledged in the latest editions of the *US Navy Diving Manual*, the advice given is confusing; the manual states that further treatment should be undertaken either using table 6 or a lower pressure of 2 ATA. However, there is another important problem associated with the high oxygen pressure used in military procedures that is rarely discussed, despite being included in the first *US Navy Diving Manual* to contain the oxygen tables in 1970; a very high level of oxygen may actually cause *deterioration* of neurological symptoms. It will be remembered that this was discussed in Chapter 8, and the reason is because patients respond differently to high levels of oxygen and the effect can be seen simply by looking in the eye; in some patients there is a very marked reduction of the diameter of the arteries of the retina, in others remarkably little. It should not surprise us that differences occur, because when breathing 100% oxygen at 2.8 ATA, the level of oxygen is *14 times* the level breathed by those of us who live at sea level. In fact, it is truly astonishing that the physiology of the body can tolerate such high levels of oxygen. Nevertheless, it is clear that, once an oxygen deficiency has been corrected, the oxygen level should be lowered so that the constriction of the blood vessels does not limit the transport of other agents in blood vital for recovery. This approach is used in US Navy table 6; the sessions of oxygen breathing at 2.8 ATA are interrupted by breathing chamber air because of the risk of a convulsion, and after three or four cycles of oxygen breathing at 2.8 ATA, the oxygen pressure is reduced to 2 ATA. However, in treating divers, there is concern that the gas which triggered the symptoms may still be present, and so the problem may return. This fear is actually unfounded and it is time that the tables are reviewed, especially as the physiology of oxygen is now better understood. Regardless, the timing of oxygen treatment is critical; "time is brain" and neurological symptoms must be viewed as an emergency. In the trials of hyperbaric oxygen treatment in stroke, the delay to treatment has often been many hours and by this time high oxygen pressures are inappropriate. The treatment of patients with multiple sclerosis and mild traumatic brain injury over the last 40 years has confirmed beyond doubt the effectiveness of lower oxygen pressures than used for divers. In general, the longer treatment is delayed the lower the oxygen pressure that should be used and the latest imaging should be used to validate the simplest and easiest intervention; giving 100% oxygen as an emergency measure.

The latest development in the treatment of stroke—the insertion of stents into diseased arteries, is not being pioneered by neurologists, but by radiologists. The technology has transferred from cardiology, where it is used for patients with narrowing of the coronary arteries. However, the arteries of the brain have much thinner walls than those in the heart, which increases the risk of a catastrophic tear with the insertion of a catheter. The use of hyperbaric oxygenation has already been shown to be successful in reducing the complications from the insertion of stents in the coronary arteries[62] and holds the same promise for the use of stents in stroke patients. This will be covered in the next chapter, which discusses the use of hyperbaric oxygen treatment for conditions other than those involving the brain. As will be seen, the same principles apply although, in most cases, without quite the same urgency.

CHAPTER 21

Healing More than the Brain

Data, data everywhere, but no one stops to think.

With apologies to Samuel Taylor Coleridge, 1772–1834

It is common for physicians who use pressure chambers to be asked if patients with a particular disease or injury will benefit from hyperbaric oxygen treatment and to put this question in context, it is necessary to return to first principles. We are a hydraulic machine with our trillions of cells serviced by blood vessels and pumps—the heart being the primary pump, but other muscles also pump blood when they contract. When disease or trauma damages tissue, the capillaries within the tissue are inevitably also affected, reducing blood flow and, inevitably, the delivery of oxygen. However, as we have seen, a modest fall in the tissue oxygen level is needed because it signals the genes involved in three processes involved in recovery. The overall process is called the *inflammatory response* and it underpins tissue repair, both from injury and from infection. For healing to take place, first the damaged cells of the tissue must be deconstructed and the debris removed. This is undertaken by the same white cells, the macrophages which kill infecting microbes, and so involves the immune system. The response to infecting organisms is for them to be identified as *antigens*; the immune system then produces *antibodies*, which are able to attach to microbes—the antigens, and result in their destruction. However, when our own cells are damaged, for example, by trauma, they must also be identified as antigens and the necessary antibodies produced so that they can be removed, or "deconstructed." This is the auto-immune response and is *essential* to healing. Secondly, new capillaries must be created, and, finally, new cells must be produced. This mechanism, clearly vital for tissue repair, has yet to be recognised by immunologists. Indeed, it has been stated[1] that any response to a self-antigen is "inappropriate." However, chronic "auto-immune" disease may follow the deposition of the "immune complexes" which are formed by the union of antigens and antibodies. They are normally removed by phagocytes but when they adhere to the lining endothelium of capillaries and venules in excessive quantities, they reduce oxygen transport, creating a vicious cycle by prolonging inflammation.

As already discussed, a small reduction in the oxygen is inevitable and necessary for the activation of the HIF proteins but, if the reduction of the level of oxygen in a wound is too severe, healing stops. When this happens, not only is there less energy available for repair, the persistence of hypoxia and tissue swelling reduces oxygen transport even further, creating a vicious cycle which continues the inflammation. The "end game" occurs when blood flow stops altogether because, if oxygen cannot diffuse from adjacent areas of tissue, cells will die. Healing then takes place slowly, by the formation of a *scar*, as it does in the plaques of multiple sclerosis or following the death of tissue in a stroke or a heart attack. Sometimes healing actually stops altogether, and a chronic wound develops, as it may do in patients with leg ulcers—the open sore being the ultimate proof that insufficient oxygen has been available to allow normal recovery. Before this happens, it may be possible for healing to be restarted by giving more oxygen as a treatment but, crucially, this depends on blood flow. The discovery of the regulation of the genes involved in creating new blood vessels by oxygen has now completed our understanding of the science involved.[2]

Earlier chapters discussed the importance of these mechanisms to our most vulnerable and sensitive tissues in the brain, but they apply regardless of the organ involved, although, for most, the time scale is less critical. Surprisingly some claim that "normal" wounds will not benefit from hyperbaric oxygen treatment, but wounds, by definition, cannot be regarded as normal, and it is simply impossible to know how low oxygen levels have fallen in damaged tissues without invasive and expensive technology. So, for the most part, we have to rely on the oxygen concentration in air. The question raised is: Does hyperbaric oxygen therapy ensure the *best* healing, even when there are no complications? The answer is a definite no! Although uncomplicated wounds would undoubtedly heal faster, clearly, for most of us, this would not justify using hyperbaric treatment. Highly-paid sportsmen, however, have found that it is worthwhile and top motorcyclists are regularly flown to the Isle of Man Hyperbaric Facility for treatment. The centre, led by technologist David Downie M.B.E., has achieved widespread acceptance in treating patients with problem wounds on the island over the last 25 years. Figure 21.1 shows the direction of changes in the oxygen levels that accompany simple tissue damage. The formation of new capillaries improves oxygen delivery allowing new cells to be formed and a return to the original status quo.

Ironically, this schematic is confirmed by studies of early and late areas of damage in multiple sclerosis by the group in Sydney mentioned in Chapter 14.[3] The damage caused by toxic components of blood entering the brain across a damaged blood-brain barrier triggers inflammation. The tissue damage is then cleared by the macrophages of the immune system prior to the

KEY EVENTS IN INJURY AND REPAIR

NORMAL TISSUE	NORMAL TISSUE
↓	↑
Tissue damage	Stem cells- tissue repair
↓	↑
Reduced blood flow	Increased blood flow
↓	↑
Hypoxia—falling oxygen levels	New capillary formation
↓	↑
Upregulation of HIF Proteins →	**NEUTROPHILS INFLAMMATION** → Tissue Deconstruction

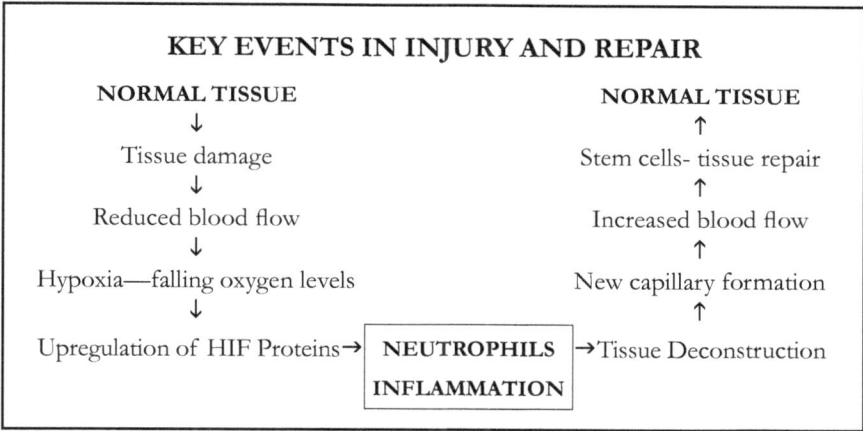

Figure 21.1:
Blood flow and oxygen changes in tissue recovery. Tissue deconstruction is the auto-immune response to damage.

repair—as they state: "Macrophage activity is largely an innate scavenging response to the presence of degenerate or dead myelin."

It will be recalled that when giant insects inhabited our planet the oxygen levels were much higher than they are today, perhaps as high as 35%. Research into wound healing has shown this concentration would have positively influenced both the *rate* at which wounds heal and, for ligaments and tendons, the *strength* of the new connective tissue formed.[4] Many years ago the author failed to interest a physician involved with Olympic athletes in hyperbaric oxygen treatment, but now elite and highly motivated athletes are making their own decisions from information they access on the Internet. They are using both negative and positive pressure changes, sleeping in altitude tents to improve aerobic fitness, and using hyperbaric oxygen treatment for injuries. The author, with colleagues, undertook a study of hyperbaric oxygen treatment at a Scottish football club in the late 1980s.[5] The schedule used was for the player to be in the chamber within one hour of the injury breathing oxygen at 2 ATA for an hour, with two more treatments over the next 24 hours. Each of 20 players estimated the number of days it would take before they would be able to resume full fitness training after sustaining common football injuries such as muscle, tendon, and ligament tears. The club physiotherapist then did an independent assessment and there was close agreement in their estimates.

Figure 21.2 shows the results with the time to returning to full fitness training reduced from an estimated 210 days to 63 days. Despite the enormous cost savings that halving recovery time would make in sports like professional football, attempts by the manufacturers of the equipment to market

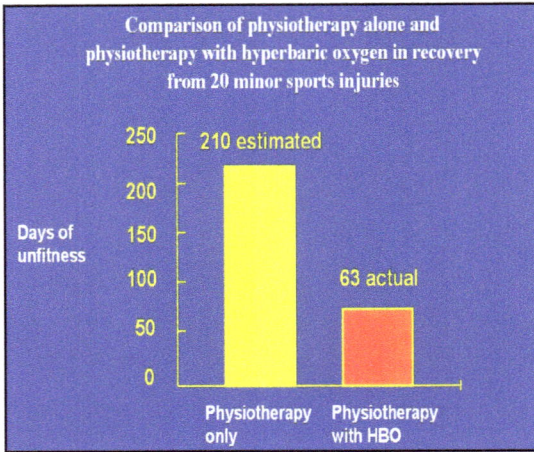

Comparison of physiotherapy alone and physiotherapy with hyperbaric oxygen in recovery from 20 minor sports injuries

Days of unfitness

210 estimated

63 actual

Physiotherapy only | Physiotherapy with HBO

Figure 21.2:
Football injuries: Days of unfitness after treatment with physiotherapy alone and together with hyperbaric oxygenation.

the technology in the 1980s fell on deaf ears. Club managers generally rely on the advice of their medical and paramedical advisors who, not having been taught about hyperbaric oxygen treatment, usually dismiss it out-of-hand. It needs a very robust management to insist that a treatment is used against the advice of medical professionals, especially when they appear to take the moral "high ground" by glibly citing lack of evidence from controlled trials. As discussed in Chapter 10, controlled trials to prove the value of using *more* oxygen to relieve *lack* of oxygen are absurd. To be fully effective in controlling the inflammation associated with reperfusion, the science clearly dictates that oxygen treatment must be used in the first hour after an injury.

The upper line A in Figure 21.3a shows normal healing and line B shows how HBOT can reduce the time taken for a more serious tissue wound to heal. If the damage to the blood supply of a tissue creates a more serious deficiency of oxygen, recovery is further delayed perhaps for years—Figure 21.3b line C but HBOT can still improve healing. However, as shown by line D, healing may fail altogether despite oxygen treatment because it cannot elevate the tissue level above 25 mm Hg. Lesser oxygen availability may trigger a slow secondary repair process over years to form a scar. An example is the fracture of a femur which often tears the arteries supplying the bone: if there is insufficient oxygen at the fracture site, it will not heal with new bone, but with scar tissue. This non union results in a loss of stability and function. So, whilst the mild hypoxia that always accompanies tissue damage is needed to upregulate the necessary genes for healing to occur, anoxia may prevent recovery and cause the death of cells.

Experiments on human volunteers have demonstrated the changes in oxygen levels in the skin of the forearm during inflammation.[6] The injec-

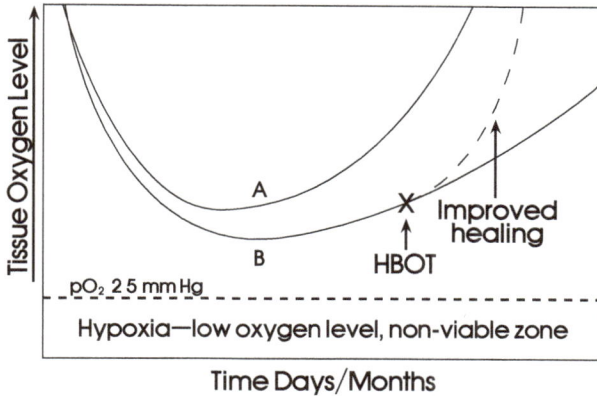

Figure 21.3a:
A- Reduction and recovery of tissue oxygen levels in a mild injury.

B- More severe tissue injury showing benefit from HBOT.

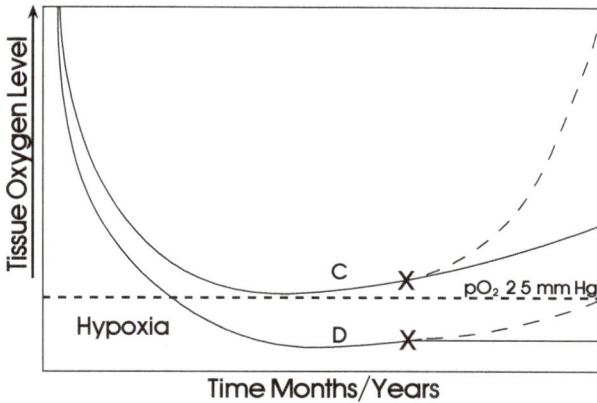

Figure 21.3b:
C- Very delayed healing improved with HBOT.

D- Critical hypoxia—no healing despite HBOT.

tion of tuberculin, which is used to induce immunity to tuberculosis, causes the inflammation shown in Figure 21.4, with the classical signs of redness, heat, and swelling with the volunteer, of course, experiencing the symptom of pain!

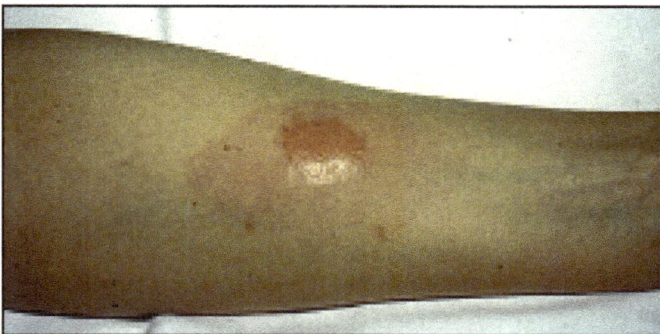

Figure 21.4:
The left forearm after the injection of tuberculin.

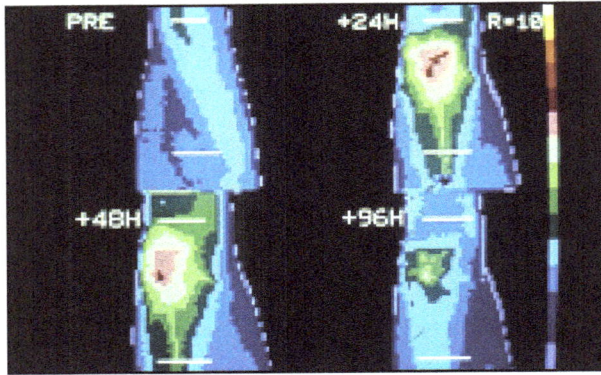

Figure 21.5:
Thermogram of the forearm before (PRE) at 24, 48, and 96 hours after a tuberculin injection. (Courtesy of Dr. VA Spence.)

The area affected is often considerably larger than it appears visually and this can be demonstrated using a heat sensitive camera, known as a thermograph. Figure 21.5 shows four scans of the forearm of another subject, the first before injection of tuberculin (PRE) and then after 24, 48, and 96 hours.

When inflammation is very intense the cells in the centre die and a blackened area forms with the later development of a scar. We now know that this is due to the invasion of neutrophils signalled by the lack of oxygen to act as if the tissue was infected. Figure 21.6 shows that the oxygen level measured through the skin falls to zero after the injection, and it needed the subject to breathe 100% oxygen at 2 ATA to elevate the level in the tissue.

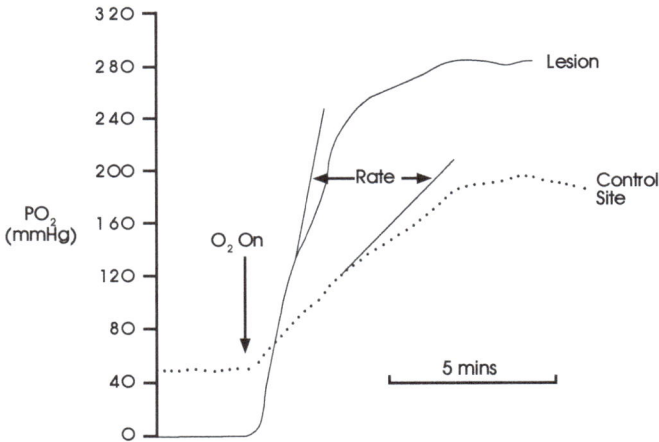

Figure 21.6:
Graph of oxygen values on the injected (solid line) versus the non injected arm (dotted line). (Courtesy of Dr. VA Spence.)

This graph is important because it provides key evidence to support breathing oxygen at an increased ambient pressure. The solid line, which is the oxygen level at the injection site, begins at zero and rapidly rises when 100% oxygen was breathed, peaking at a value of about 280 mm Hg. In contrast, the dotted line shows the base tissue oxygen level in the normal arm at 45 mm Hg rising much more slowly to a peak at less than 200 mm Hg. The value then starts to fall as the blood vessels constrict, because auto-regulation reduces blood flow to normalise the oxygen levels in the tissue. This quotation, from an unknown source, summarises the obvious; wound healing is compromised when there is insufficient oxygen for normal metabolism.

An adequate supply of oxygen is of vital importance for healing wounds since fibroblasts require oxygen for energy production and collagen (connective tissue) cannot be synthesised in the absence of molecular oxygen. Earlier work from this laboratory demonstrated that hyperoxia shifts wound metabolism from anaerobic towards aerobic glycolysis and thereby activates the citric acid cycle.

Nothing has changed, absolutely nothing, we have not found a substitute for oxygen and no one, scientist or physician, can dispute the massive clinical experience that severe tissue oxygen deficiency is associated with delayed or failed recovery of wounds. Equally, in such patients the oxygen gained from breathing air is simply not enough; they are outside the envelope of recovery and we can and must do better. It may be enough to use the equipment pioneered by John Scott Haldane when he treated soldiers gassed at the front in WW1, that is, *baric* oxygen treatment with 100% oxygen administered without a pressure enclosure,[7] and this approach certainly needs to be explored. Nevertheless, there are now probably well in excess of 100,000 papers on the use of hyperbaric oxygen treatment dating back to the nineteenth century, including, for those who still demand them, hundreds of controlled studies.

The first report of the use of oxygen under hyperbaric conditions in treatment "Oxygen as an Antipyretic," was published in the *Lancet* in 1887.[8] It gave details of a young man with both lungs affected by pneumonia, who was successfully treated by Dr. Don Francisco Valenzuela in Madrid using pure oxygen in a chamber at a pressure of 997 mm Hg (1.3 ATA). It is difficult for us today to realise the terror that pneumonia held for people before the introduction of antibiotics, as it was a major killer of young people. The course of the illness was followed by monitoring the temperature and breathing rate of the patient and they often reached very high values. However, if they suddenly reduced it meant that "the crisis" was over and the patient was very likely to survive. Valenzuela watched his young patient steadily improve with the oxygen treatment and the crisis passed. Of course, if he had believed the allegation that oxygen is toxic to the lungs, he would not have used hyperbaric oxygen treatment, and his patient would have died.

Valenzuela had already investigated the effects of oxygen treatment under hyperbaric conditions in rabbits, after deliberately infecting them with bacteria. Astonishingly he used matched control animals treated with oxygen at normal atmospheric pressure; the results of his investigations were unequivocal, the rabbits given hyperbaric oxygen treatment survived, whereas the control animals died. These were almost certainly the first controlled studies in the history of medicine and, although they rank alongside the research of Pasteur, they are almost unknown. In the 1960s, a halcyon era for hyperbaric oxygen treatment, the group in the University of Glasgow showed that the treatment prolonged survival in mice with infection introduced into the blood stream (septicaemia), paving the way for research into the antibiotic actions of oxygen.[9] They also showed that topically applied oxygen using an enclosure, for example of a leg wound, in a chamber was effective. By this time there were many reports of the successful treatment of patients with gas gangrene.[10] The organism responsible for this form of gangrene, *Clostridium perfringens* is *anaerobic* and killed by exposure to oxygen. Its toxin is also neutralised, but, unbelievably, there is no recommendation for this indication in the draft of the latest UK guidelines for hyperbaric oxygen treatment.[11] There are many other case reports of life-saving treatment of patients with other anaerobic infections using hyperbaric oxygenation. Interestingly, none of the post-war reports reference the work of Valenzuela, and it would be nearly a hundred years later, in 1978, that the *New England Journal of Medicine* would invite a scientist, Bernard Babior, to review in two detailed articles the key role of oxygen as the antibiotic of the body.[12,13]

We now know how oxygen controls infection; white blood cells, the neutrophils, are attracted to a site of infection by a local reduction in the level of oxygen and use oxygen to form free radicals to kill bacteria and viruses. The neutrophils' attraction is controlled by the hypoxia-inducible factor proteins. Neutrophils either ingest the infecting agents to kill them inside their cell membrane, or they may create an external web to entrap them.[14] In both cases, the neutrophils produce oxygen free radicals to complete microbial destruction. Oxygen is, of course, essential for the extraordinary mobility of neutrophils which allows them to invade infected tissues. But how many of our medical students are taught that oxygen controls infection? Sadly, it is likely to be very, very few, because their teachers do not know these facts. Faced with growing antibiotic resistance and the reluctance of the drug industry to invest in this area when there are no obvious leads, we are faced with no alternative to using oxygen in treatment, which simply extends the control of infection and the envelope of healing. Hyperbaric oxygen treatment would revolutionise the outcome in sepsis where neutrophil over-activity contributes to tissue damage in multiple organ failure.[15]

Sepsis is the generalised inflammatory response of the body to infection and may lead to the failure not just of tissues, but of whole organs including, eventually, the brain. It is associated with a cascade of events accompanied by a reduction of blood flow together with a reduction of oxygen transfer into the blood in the lungs because they too sustain damage.[16] Despite all the innovations introduced since the introduction of penicillin in WW2, the mortality rate of severe sepsis is still about 35%. The most usual cause of sepsis is bacterial infection and bacterial toxins cause profound effects on the circulation, and even on the heart itself. Specific drugs have been developed to address many components of the cascade, but they have had no effect on survival and often damage the body's own immune response, for example by reducing the number of circulating lymphocytes. The blame has now been firmly placed on neutrophils as the cause of the tissue damage; this is far from a new concept and has been intensively researched.[17] It is not difficult to see why, when neutrophils are able to cause damage to the nervous system of divers, activated by nothing more sinister than tiny circulating bubbles.[18] So, although neutrophils are critical to the control of infection, their actions need to be controlled in sepsis to prevent failure of organs, especially the lungs. Drugs have failed in this quest, but overwhelming evidence of benefit from hyperbaric oxygen treatment has already been provided by its successful use, from decompression sickness, to desperately ill patients with anaerobic bacterial infections suffering from multi-organ failure.

Attempts to use 100% oxygen as a treatment at normal atmospheric pressure were actually made before the turn of the last century, although the oxygen was usually just wafted over the face of the patient—not a great deal different to oxygen administration today. A distinguished physician and contemporary of Haldane working in London, Leonard Hill, described it as "futile."[19] After Haldane's introduction of oxygen apparatus capable of delivering 100% oxygen in the Great War, there was considerable interest in using oxygen treatment at normal atmospheric pressure. Between the war years this was championed by eminent physicians in America, the most notable being Drs. William Stadie[20] and Walter Boothby.[21] Stadie had hospital rooms constructed to maintain oxygen levels at about 50% for patients with pneumonia. There would appear to be only one paper referring to the use of a hyperbaric chamber for oxygen treatment in the inter-war years; in the 1930s, Dr. A.O. de Almeida in Brazil found that high levels of oxygen apparently cured patients suffering from leprosy. The paper was published in a Brasilian journal[22] but, sadly, it is not available on the Internet. Also during the 1930s, Dr. Albert Behnke and colleagues in the US Navy investigated the use of oxygen in decompression sickness and he advocated the use of hyperbaric treatment in general medicine.[23] Another development, actually during WW2 by another great pioneer, Dr. Edgar End, was the introduction of hyperbaric oxygen treatment for carbon monoxide poisoning, after experiments in a chamber located in the basement of the County Emergency Hospital in the centre of Milwaukee.[24] Carbon monoxide poisoning will be discussed in the final chapter. As outlined in Chapter 8, in 1965 Drs. Goodman and Workman in the Experimental Diving Unit of the US Navy in Washington Navy Yard unwittingly laid the foundations for the clinical use of hyperbaric oxygen treatment with the procedures they developed for treating gas embolism and decompression sickness.[25] The physiological science that underpins the success of these hyperbaric oxygen treatment tables has slowly unfolded over the last 40 years, from the constriction of blood vessels, which limits swelling, to the prevention of neutrophils sticking inside blood vessels and causing reperfusion injury.

Clearly the importance of the heart is beyond question as cardiac arrest ends life for us all; an event often devastating for loved ones and it terminates the involvement of those in clinical medicine. Early in the 1920s the importance of oxygen to the function of the heart was beginning to be recognised, although coronary artery heart disease was rare. The chest pain known as angina, induced by exercise, is usually caused by insufficient blood flow in the arteries of the heart. The link to oxygen deficiency was shown in elegant experiments using an exercise treadmill; patients with a history of angina were exercised on a treadmill until they developed chest pain. They were then given a gas to breathe with an increased percentage of oxygen by mask and the pain was relieved. The level of exercise was then increased and when the pain returned it was again relieved by giving more oxygen. Today, angina is regarded as synonymous with restricted blood flow caused by narrowing of the coronary arteries, but few now know that angina can occur when blood flow increases in patients suffering from severe anaemia who exercise. Anaemia occurs when the number of red blood cells in the circulation falls, reducing the ability of blood to carry sufficient oxygen.

The heart as a blood pump requires its own blood flow, which is provided through the left and right coronary arteries, and oxygen is at the top of the list of the substances it needs. In the years following the end of WW2, with the pace of research gaining momentum, there was increasing recognition of the central importance of oxygen to the heart. This culminated in some astonishing experiments by a group based in the department of surgery of the Johns Hopkins Hospital in Baltimore.[26] They were driven by the need to preserve organs out of the body for transplantation and, astonishingly, they used bubbles—bubbles of oxygen. The group, prompted by reports of experiments in which both spinal cords and hearts had been maintained with gaseous oxygen, built an apparatus to allow small bubbles of humidified gas to be passed through the coronary arteries of the heart of dogs. It is truly remarkable that it is, in fact, possible to pass bubbles freely through the coronary arteries, but they succeeded with pressures similar to normal blood pressures. A heart removed from an animal and placed in a bath of salt water will continue to beat for as long as 10 minutes. However in these experiments, instead of the heartbeat stopping in 10 minutes, it continued to beat for several hours—indeed, in one case, for eight hours. In the first hours of the experiments, the contractions of the heart muscle were described as strong, but then gradually faded. What is particularly remarkable is that it is clear that bubbling gaseous oxygen through the heart does not transport any *nutrients* and so the heart muscle must contain remarkable stores of energy. These experiments have long since been forgotten, but the author recalls Professor Sir Roy Calne, a liver transplant surgeon, mentioning in a public lecture at the University of Dundee, that his team had found that bubbling gaseous oxygen through a liver awaiting transplantation increased its survival. He said they did not know why! However, organs including the liver are now being preserved by a smaller version of the complex heart-lung machines developed for cardiac surgery. This is known as extra corporeal membrane oxygenation (ECMO) and has also been used to revive patients after cardiac arrest.[27]

A group in Long Beach, California studied the use of hyperbaric oxygen treatment in heart attacks over a four-year period. Their paper, the "HOT MI Pilot Study" (Hyperbaric Oxygen Treatment of Myocardial Infarction) was publicised by a press release in 1997, after appearing in the *American Heart Journal*.[28] It is difficult to believe that 15 years have now passed without the publication of any follow-up studies. As in stroke, the obstruction to flow in the coronary arteries, whether due to thrombosis or embolism, often involves clot formation and, again, when blood flow is obstructed, then so is oxygen delivery. The injection of a clot-busting agent (recombinant tissue plasminogen activator, rTPA) in heart attacks has been shown to improve survival. Experiments using an animal model had shown the benefit of adding oxygen treatment to clot busting agents which prompted the trial in patients. The researchers found that an enzyme marker of muscle damage was reduced 35% by the use of hyperbaric oxygenation. Also, the time to the resolution of pain, and the resolution of the electrical changes recorded on ECG, was significantly reduced when compared to the control group. There were no side effects and, in contrast to ECMO, hyperbaric oxygenation is simple, safe, and non-invasive.

Few today will be aware of an astonishing paper entitled "Coronary Heart Disease" by Dr. Claude Beck, a surgeon who worked in Cleveland, Ohio. It was published in the *American Journal of Surgery* in 1958,[29] and pre-dated the introduction of closed chest massage for patients in cardiac arrest. From direct observations of the heart in many animal experiments, he states the obvious; a uniformly *pink* heart is electrically stable. But rather less obvious is that a uniformly *blue*, or cyanosed heart is also electrically stable, and he gives the reason; the heart muscle will not have been injured by a modest lowering of the oxygen level. However, he found that the typical changes in the electrocardiogram from a heart attack, the elevation or depression of the "ST" segment of the record, were produced by obstructing blood flow to a small area of muscle; this was producing a juxtaposition of pink and blue areas in the muscle. Beck found that these areas of pink and blue muscle were associated with the disturbance of heart rhythm known as ventricular fibrillation. The muscles quiver, the heart fails to pump blood, and death soon ensues. However, this can usually be reversed by defibrillation, and automatic defibrillators are now being sited in many public places. Readers of a robust disposition should read Beck's remarkable accounts of open chest massage and defibrillation in *conscious* patients. One patient, who was talking to the surgeon, who had his hand in her chest massaging her heart through her open chest, was told that she was to be subjected to an electric shock; she objected, saying that it implied she was suffering from a psychiatric disorder! However, the observation that the development of small areas of blue heart muscle is responsible for electrical instability means that giving more oxygen, to render such blue areas pink, will undoubtedly reduce the threat of fibrillation.

Researchers at Case Western Reserve University, the University Hospitals of Cleveland, and Texas Tech University Health Science Center in Dallas have investigated the use of hyperbaric oxygenation to improve the results from stents inserted to relieve obstructions, which may close the coronary arteries.[30] Most stents are not placed by surgeons or cardiologists, but by an emerging specialist group of radiologists, because they are experts at interpreting the images needed to guide the placement of the catheter. Stents are expandable metal cages encircling a balloon which are inserted into a coronary artery using a catheter, usually passed up the femoral artery. Once in place, the balloon is inflated expanding the metal cage which is left in place when the catheter is withdrawn. It is truly astonishing that so few immediate complications occur using this technology, because the inflation of the catheter balloon actually blocks flow along the coronary artery. Unfortunately, scarring is a late complication resulting from damage to the lining of the coronary artery during the insertion of the catheter, and often causes the artery to close again. If this occurs, it is usually in about eight months after the insertion of the stent. The investigators reasoned that if hyperbaric oxygen treatment could heal the "miniature wound," it would stop the artery from closing again. The study used just three sessions of hyperbaric oxygen treatment in a monoplace chamber compressed with pure oxygen to just 2 ATA. A total of 24 patients received oxygen treatment and 37 patients, who were not treated, served as controls. The results fully justified the reasoning used and the effort expended. The reduction of the risk of death from causes related to the heart in the hyperbaric oxygen treated group was highly significant with just one patient dying in the treated group in contrast to 13 in the control group. Restenosis, that is, the closure of the stented coronary artery, was also less, as was the recurrence of angina pain, all from just three hours in which the patients simply reclined in a simple clear plastic cylinder breathing oxygen. There were no side effects, and the reason for the benefit from breathing oxygen? It is due to a reduction in neutrophils sticking to the lining of the damaged artery, and so we again return to the experiments that followed Jessica falling down the well in Texas. There is, of course, a significant risk associated with the blockage of a coronary artery and it argues for the routine use of hyperbaric oxygenation during the placement of stents. Patients are physically safe in a chamber and protected against fatal abnormalities of heart rhythm breathing a high concentration of oxygen, which has been dramatically demonstrated in newborn babies.

Beginning in the 1950s, many large, pressurised operating theatres were installed in cities in Europe and the US. The first, in Amsterdam,[31] was followed by one in Glasgow, and others in Durham, North Carolina, Boston, Chicago, New Jersey, Seattle, Sydney Australia, Marseille, and Graz in Austria. Many others were built in the Soviet Union, China, and Japan—in the latter a large, mobile operating theatre was even developed for trauma surgery. The clinical experience gained in these facilities amply confirmed the value of hyperbaric oxygenation in a wide variety of conditions, from using oxygen delivered with, when compared to diving, a very modest increase in pressure.

Perhaps the most dramatic experience came from the use of hyperbaric conditions to allow the heart to be arrested to undertake surgery without causing damage to the brain. In Amsterdam and Boston, this included operations on children with congenital heart defects.

Operating on heart defects in children is an enormous challenge to surgeons, not least because of the delicacy required, but also because small changes that would be shrugged off by an adult often prove fatal to very small infants. In the UK, the requirement for surgeons to publish the results of such surgery has just been introduced, otherwise they will be named and shamed. A 1965 paper published by the group in Boston[32] dramatically illustrates the *envelope of safety* given by the additional oxygen possible by using a chamber. The report details results in 107 babies with severe cardiac abnormalities operated on in the chamber in the Children's Hospital Medical Center at Harvard Medical School. Over the period from 1957 to 1962, before the hyperbaric operating theatre was installed, of 130 operations conducted, 26 deaths occurred actually *during* the surgery, which is obviously an extremely distressing event for all concerned. From 1963 to 1965, a total of 70 operations were undertaken in the chamber, with short periods at a pressure of 4 ATA. Deaths during the surgery were completely abolished. Overall, in the period from 1957 to 1962, before the chamber came into use, there was a total of 60 deaths which followed 130 operations, whereas, of the 72 children in the group who had hyperbaric oxygenation in the chamber, only 12 died. The impressive results from Boston were noticed and the lead surgeon, Dr. William Bernhard, was invited to submit an article on hyperbaric oxygenation by the *New England Journal of Medicine*.[33] It was published in a section appropriately headed "Medical Intelligence; Current Concepts." Bernhard highlighted his very positive experience in patients with carbon monoxide poisoning and gas gangrene, in addition to cardiac surgery, stating that; "logic dictates that many pathologic processes characterised by diffuse hypoxia should be benefited by hyperbaric oxygenation."

We now know why abolishing lack of oxygen has many profound effects, not least preventing death, but it is interesting to note the reaction of one cardiac surgeon when the Boston results were presented at the American Association for Thoracic Surgery held in New Orleans in 1965. A surgeon from Chicago, Dr. Thomas G. Baffes, said that they were also "very enthusiastic about hyperbaric oxygenation." However, he then surprisingly stated; "about a year ago we decided to stop." The reason given was that they went back to the laboratory and tried to reduce it to controlled animal experiments. This approach was, unfortunately, also adopted by the group under Sir Charles

Illingworth in Glasgow who, after having had positive clinical experience, studied animal models of both heart attacks and strokes. Inevitably, healthy young animals were used and techniques which certainly do not reproduce the disease processes in man. The surgeon from Chicago revealingly stated; "Nevertheless, the medical implications of hyperbaric oxygenation are such that it is difficult to abandon it." Nevertheless, they *did* abandon it. Dr. Ivan Brown, from the Duke University facility in Durham North Carolina, commented that their results were not as impressive and he gave the reason: "We have used hyperbaric surgery only for those infants that we feel would not survive under normal atmospheric pressure." It is painfully obvious that less severely affected infants would clearly benefit. In the UK, a study of heart attack patients in St. Thomas' Hospital[34] showed, not surprisingly, the same benefit in patients in low cardiac output failure that had been so dramatically shown in the patient treated in the chamber in the back of an ambulance by Drs. Yacoub and Zeitlin in 1964.[35]

Although coronary artery stenting has reduced the need for coronary bypass surgery, bypass surgery is still necessary for some patients. The procedure requires the chest to be opened and the heart must be stopped to allow the vein used as the graft to be stitched across the blocked coronary artery. It is now common for several grafts to be used, often in one operation. The pumping action of the heart and the oxygenation of blood undertaken by the lungs are taken over by a heart-lung machine. Development of these machines began in the 1960s and signalled the end of the use of the large hyperbaric operating theatres for heart surgery. Unfortunately, abandoning hyperbaric treatment was ill advised because, by 1963, it was recognised that open heart surgery was associated with brain damage from embolism.[36,37] Eventually the same ultrasonic technology used to detect bubbles in divers also demonstrated them in patients during cardiac surgery when they were on the heart-lung machine.[38] CT scanning of children after heart surgery showed enlargement of the liquid-filled cavities in the brain hemispheres.[39] It is most likely that this was due to damage to the myelin sheaths which form the bulk of the white matter. However, repeat scans showed that the changes reversed over a period of months which is clear evidence of myelin regeneration in children.

There could not be more compelling proof of the importance of the lungs in filtering the blood, or of the general failure to understand that small emboli may cause brain damage, than the experience which followed the introduction of heart-lung machines. The emboli found have included silicone antifoam agents, p.v.c. from the tubing used in the pump,[40] fat, bone marrow, and, inevitably, bubbles. This problem had very personal implications for the author after finding that his eldest son, Adrian, at just four months old, had a hole in the septum in the heart that divides the atria. Fortunately, it was possible to postpone the heart surgery that was needed until he was 13 years old. The Scottish centre for cardiac surgery was Glasgow Royal Infirmary but, although the chamber installed by Sir Charles Illingworth in the nearby Western Infirmary was still in place, it was no longer in use. The late Dr. Richard Neubauer kindly introduced me to a wonderful surgeon, Dr. Salem Habal, who then operated in Northridge Hospital in Fort Lauderdale, Florida, which had a hyperbaric chamber. At a meeting in his office I explained the research on micro-embolism and the blood-brain barrier undertaken with Professor Brian Hills in the University Health Science Center in Houston,[41] and that I could not allow open heart surgery to be undertaken on my son without a hyperbaric chamber available. He reassured me that he always used double filtration on bypass and, to my surprise, printed out his operating results over the previous three years. The operation was performed on a Tuesday morning in July 1986 by Dr. Habal, with Dr. Rocky Prakash responsible for the anaesthesia. The care from all the staff in Northridge Hospital was superb and we will never be able to repay the kindness of Dr. Habal and Dr. Prakash. Adrian was discharged on Saturday morning. After some hyperbaric oxygen treatment to ensure optimum wound healing, the family was soon on holiday in the Florida Keys. He has not looked back.

With the availability of MRI, it was inevitable that it would be used to study the effects on the brain of patients undergoing heart surgery on bypass and, in 1993, a remarkable report appeared in the *Lancet*.[42] Patients requiring coronary artery bypass surgery were scanned in an MR imager before the operation, and then, astonishingly, rescanned *within 20 minutes* of the operation being completed. Damage was found in central areas of the brain. They were rescanned at three months and it was found that the damage had persisted in some of the patients. The study was soon discontinued. Given the extensive literature on embolism, especially from bubbles, in heart surgery, the use of hyperbaric oxygen treatment should be routine.

Faced with the hostility directed at hyperbaric oxygen treatment from the medical establishment in the 1960s and 70s, many of the doctors involved withdrew to conventional careers rather than confront those in powerful, well-organised, high-earning medical specialities like neurology, neurosurgery, and cardiac surgery. Not surprisingly, most of the hyperbaric community, especially in the US, has retreated to the security of running wound care programmes incorporating oxygen treatment—taking the crumbs from the rich man's table. However, some, like Dr. Paul Cianci, who retired as a Surgeon Captain in the US Navy, continued the development of the treatment and has undertaken a superb review of its cost effectiveness.[43] He has recently published a comprehensive review, with colleagues, of the human and animal evidence supporting the use of hyperbaric oxygen treatment in burns patients.[44] The results can be spectacular, as the images reproduced below show, which are from his hyperbaric unit in San Pablo, across the bay from San Francisco. The patient was Christmas shopping in a mall, and had just handed her young son to Santa to get a present, when a light aircraft crashed on to the roof. A fireball of flaming petroleum and tar cascaded down from the ceiling onto her.

The swelling of her face is all too obvious, but what is *not* obvious is that her air passages will also have been swollen from the inhalation of hot gases and particulate products of combustion. She would also have inhaled carbon monoxide and other toxic gases which would have caused her lung membranes and brain to swell. She regained consciousness with the hyperbaric oxygen treatment, and it clearly reduced the swelling of her facial tissues. After two hyperbaric sessions she was able to open her eyes and to breathe with her mouth closed. Surgery was not needed.

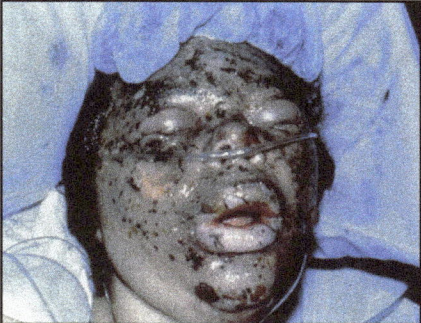

12 hours post-injury.

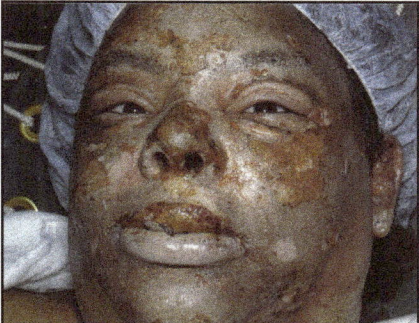

24 hours after two hyperbaric treatments.

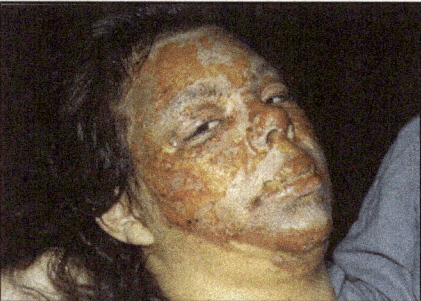

72 hours after six hyperbaric treatments.

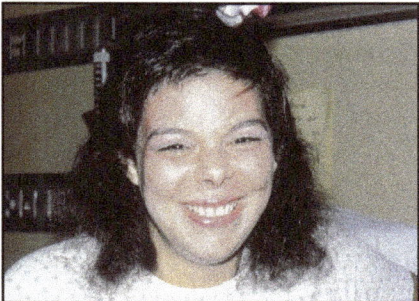

Final results.

Figure 21.7:
(Courtesy of Dr. Paul Cianci.)

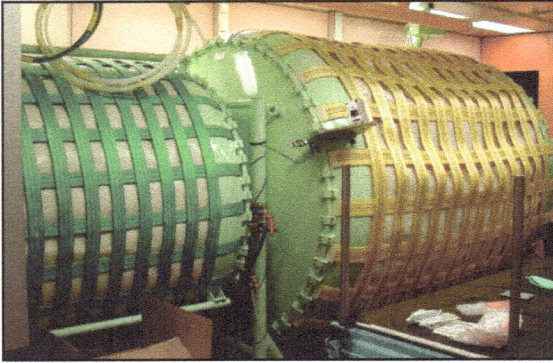

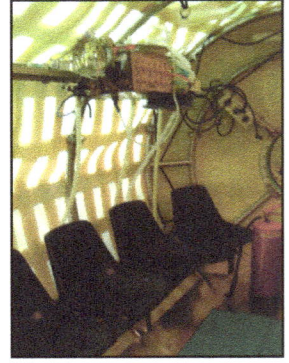

Figure 21.8:
Lightweight chamber in the Vienna General Hospital.

It is fair to ask what would have happened without hyperbaric treatment; she may have recovered without needing surgery, but it would certainly not have taken place over just a few days. Also, studies of psychiatric residua after burns, smoke inhalation, and carbon monoxide poisoning indicate that she may not have been quite the same person. Without oxygen treatment, the tissue damage to her face may have worsened and the burn may have progressed from a second to a third degree, with the skin falling away. It is likely that she would then have faced extended plastic surgery, as did the British soldier, Simon Weston, who suffered severe burns of his head in the Argentine attack on the transport ship, the *Sir Galahad*, in the Falklands War. After the terrorist attack in London on July 7, 2007, the image of one of the victims emerging from the underground with her face covered were beamed around the world.[45] Her treatment involved wearing a facial mask to control the swelling for 18 months. This clearly indicates that those involved in directing her care understand the importance of controlling the swelling of the facial tissues to prevent scarring. There are other developments in Europe; an extraordinary hyperbaric unit has been installed in the burns unit on the sixth floor of the general hospital in the centre of Vienna by Professor Harald Andel. It was necessary to use this novel method of lightweight chamber construction to be able to accommodate it in the hospital lift!

But what about the use of hyperbaric oxygen treatment of more mundane conditions—yet again this illustrates the extraordinary powers of the body to recover when it is given the right conditions and, critically, lack of oxygen in tissues is relieved promptly by using sufficient oxygen. There were many case reports published in the UK from the 1950s to the 70s, for example, about the treatment of bone infections and the salvage of skin grafts. An editorial in the *British Medical Journal* in 1978[46] referred to "established indications," listing burns, carbon monoxide poisoning, decompression sickness, air embolism, and gas gangrene. It also included sickle cell crises, salvage of skin flaps, ulcers, and pressure sores, and referred to the results in heart attacks, head injury, and cognitive function in the elderly as encouraging. By this time many hyperbaric facilities were operating in the US, but in the late 1980s they faced a major problem with the crisis in health care funding. The insurers, Blue Cross and Blue Shield, came very close to denying payment for every indication, including diving disorders. As the cost of an hour of treatment was typically about $400, of which the oxygen cost was, at most, $20, it is not difficult to see why hyperbaric practitioners, already a marginalised group in medicine, were vulnerable. The quantity of oxygen used breathing 100% at 2 ATA for an hour is the same as breathing 100% at 1 ATA for two hours. The field was only saved by the efforts of the late Dr. Richard Neubauer, who enlisted the help of one of his famous patients, the physicist, the late Dr. Edward Teller. Dr. Teller's conviction came from his personal experience of hyperbaric oxygen treatment for the effects of disease affecting the small arteries of the brain. As detailed earlier in Chapter 4, he was, however, even more convinced by the benefits he saw in his wife, Mici, after a Vickers hyperbaric bed had been installed in their home. Suffering from advanced chronic obstructive pulmonary disease (COPD) she had been given just months to live but, with daily hyperbaric treatment, she survived, enjoying life, for another five years.[47] Dr. Teller, who had devised the Star Wars project for the administration of Ronald Reagan, still had powerful connections on Capitol Hill and so, with his help, hyperbaric medicine survived. The author had the privilege of discussing hyperbaric oxygen treatment with Dr. Teller on several occasions, and his grasp of both the physics and medicine involved was formidable.

Dr. James Clark, then president of the Undersea and Hyperbaric Medical Society, and Dr. Leon Greenbaum, the executive director at the time, wrote on January 13, 1994 to thank Dr. Neubauer for his timely intervention in saving the field of hyperbaric oxygen treatment. The end result of this bruising experience for most clinical hyperbaric facilities in the US was a return to the treatment of patients with problem wounds, usually the result of self-referral after an Internet search. This means, almost inevitably, that the treatment is used as a last resort, when "standard" management has failed. The treatment of such patients is very profitable; problem wounds are becoming quite common with the increase in life expectancy in the developed world, and they often require long courses of hyperbaric treatment. The insurers of a disabled patient with a pressure sore were billed for $3,588 for a single 90 minute treatment in a Miami Hospital. Although this figure would be subject to the usual negotiations with the provider, given a typical base cost in a hospital setting of about $50,[48] the use of an eight person chamber, with each patient being billed for the full amount, is very lucrative. Insurers may be prepared to pay, simply because there is no other treatment. This relegates the administration of the appropriate dose of oxygen, which is correctly regarded as an emergency gas, to a last resort medicine.

In 1999, the German federal committee of social insurance companies and their contracted physicians met at the request of the government because the bloated health care system was facing serious financial difficulties. Hyperbaric medicine came under vigorous scrutiny and the committee, which did not include a single physician with experience of the discipline, opted to deny all reimbursement, including use for diving disorders.[49] It is noteworthy that this was not directed at hospital-based facilities, but at private free-standing clinics. After a storm of protest, which included the sport diving fraternity, decompression sickness and air embolism were reinstated. Unfortunately, most centres were forced to close. In the UK, a list of conditions had accumulated in the NHS Specialist Services Definition Set No. 28. A range of conditions for which it was stated that "HBOT is widely accepted as standard care" was included until it was withdrawn in 2007. A commissioned review by a group led by a public health doctor, also with no experience of hyperbaric medicine, was finally published in April 2013,[50] and now recommends only three conditions: decompression illness, air embolism, and carbon monoxide poisoning. The anaerobic infections, including gas gangrene and necrotising fasciitis, previously included, do not appear to have been considered. Despite oxygen levels being easily measured in problem wounds, all the studies, including many controlled trials, were dismissed. It is even stated that there is no "theoretical basis" for giving oxygen to correct the lack of oxygen in tissue damage!

In the 1980s, Dr. Brandon Tamayo, then a medical student, conducted a survey to assess knowledge of this treatment in medical staff of a Scottish teaching hospital. His questionnaire asked if hyperbaric oxygen treatment should be used for the four conditions. The possible answers were yes, no, or not sure. Of a total of 179 questionnaires given out, 127 were returned, which, at 71%, is a robust sample. There were returns from 66 consultants and associate specialists, and 61 from junior medical staff. Not all the questions were answered, which accounts for the small discrepancies in the totals reproduced in Table 21.1.

Table 21.1
Indications For Hyperbaric Oxygen Treatment

	Yes	No	Not Sure	% Yes	Total
Air embolism	57	27	39	46	126
Decompression sickness	112	6	8	89	123
Carbon monoxide poisoning	100	8	11	87	119
Gas gangrene	99	9	11	78	119

It was notable that the head of microbiology was against the use of hyperbaric oxygen treatment for gas gangrene, despite the fact that the organisms of the *Clostridial* species responsible for the infection will not grow in the presence of oxygen—they are anaerobic—and the toxins they produce are also destroyed by oxygen!

The 1978 editorial in the *British Medical Journal* noted that there were 43 single-person pressure chambers in the hospitals of the NHS in the UK.[46] Regional centres had been established and five large walk-in multiplace chambers were in use. It was stated that hyperbaric oxygen treatment has a "firmly established place" in clinical practice. Sadly, this is no longer correct, at least for Great Britain; only two NHS hospitals now have chambers. In contrast, Japan has over 800 in use, with 33 of their medical schools having hyperbaric facilities, and a Scottish company exports chambers to the country. They are baffled by the failure to develop hyperbaric services. Russia was a leader in the 70s and 80s, with over 1,000 chambers, and hosted one of the International Congresses in Moscow in 1981. But the collapse of the Soviet system had disastrous effects on their health care system. Japan has a well-established hyperbaric provision, with engineers and physicians jointly involved. For example, Kyusho Island in southern Japan has 168 single person chambers and

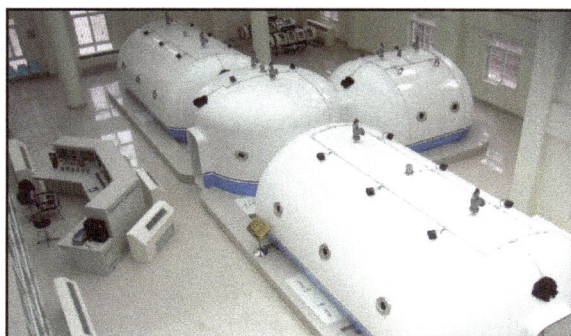

Figure 21.9:
Hyperbaric complex in Beijing China.
(Courtesy of Dr.Gao Chunjin.)

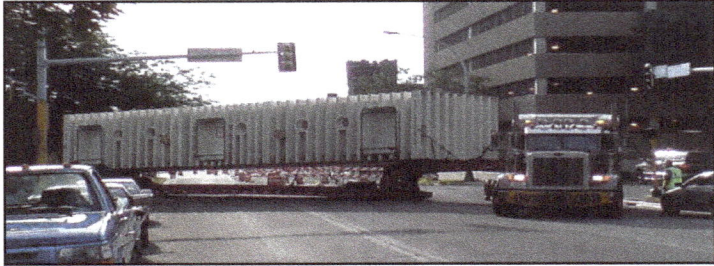

Figure 21.10:
Delivery of the Mayo Clinic chamber.

17 multiplace chambers in use.[51] China also has a well-established network of facilities in every city and over 3,500 chambers in use. The investment in the technology evident from this chamber complex in Beijing, which takes 42 patients, is truly remarkable.

It is difficult to gain a figure for the number of hyperbaric facilities in the US, though it is certain to be several thousand, with by far the largest number being in free-standing clinics. In all these countries, some historical indications for hyperbaric oxygen treatment are well established and, most importantly, government bodies, or insurers, will cover the cost. However, this does not mean that oxygen treatment is in widespread use; it still cannot be regarded as mainstream, nor do the majority of patients with carbon monoxide poisoning receive hyperbaric oxygen treatment—most are treated in intensive care units. The most common use of hyperbaric oxygenation is certainly the highly-profitable treatment of patients with problem wounds.

But things are changing in the US because prestigious organisations are becoming involved; the Mayo Clinic in Rochester, Minnesota recently installed an enormous chamber for wound care patients. It was built in Australia and cost over $1 million.

In contrast to the UK, many new wound healing clinics are opening in America and, given the increase in obesity and diabetes, risk factors for non-healing wounds, many more will undoubtedly be needed. In the 1980s, in absence of any other agency, the US government and insurance companies looked to the UHMS for advice on hyperbaric oxygen treatment. However, the list of recommended indications steadily contracted for many years; only in the last decade have some new conditions been added. Perhaps the most surprising, given the fashionable insistence on an evidence-based approach, has been the inclusion of cerebral abscess, curiously without any supporting evidence from randomised controlled trials.

The first English textbook on hyperbaric oxygen treatment was published by the Undersea Medical Society in 1977, edited by the late Colonel Jefferson Davis and Professor Thomas K. Hunt.[52] At the time, Dr. Davis worked at Brooks Air Force Base in San Antonio, Texas, and he established clinical hyperbaric oxygen treatment in the USAF. Thomas Hunt is professor of surgery at the University of California Medical Center in San Francisco. The author first met Dr. Davis at a meeting in Washington in December 1975, and was invited to dinner with him by Captain "Chuck" Shilling, then CEO of the Undersea Medical Society. The 1977 text covers the subject comprehensively and it is difficult not to feel that, despite the extensive science since added, the field has gone backwards. One case report in the book from the Brooks Air Force facility deserves special mention. The patient featured had suffered from leg ulceration on the inside of the right ankle for *40 years*.

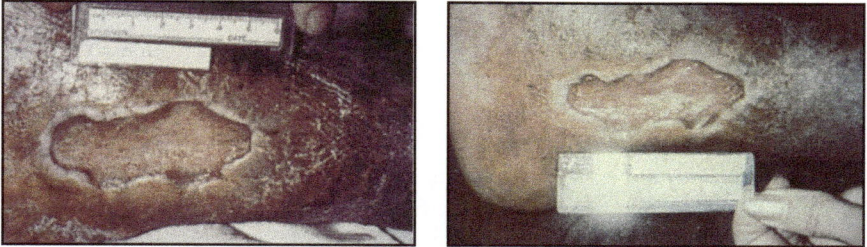

Figure 21.11:
Forty-year duration leg ulcer before and after 25 oxygen treatments.
(Courtesy of the late Col. J.C. Davis M.C.)

It can be seen in the first picture that the margin of the ulcer is white, because it has become *sclerotic*, in other words, over many years, scar tissue has formed and, like the scars of multiple sclerosis in the brain, it cannot be removed by oxygen treatment. The skin had also suffered, becoming grossly thickened. With just 25 sessions of hyperbaric oxygen treatment, the size of the ulcer reduced, new capillaries grew in the bed of the ulcer, and the infection was controlled. However, the ulcer margin still had the boundary of scar tissue. This allows an important principle to be stated, using oxygen

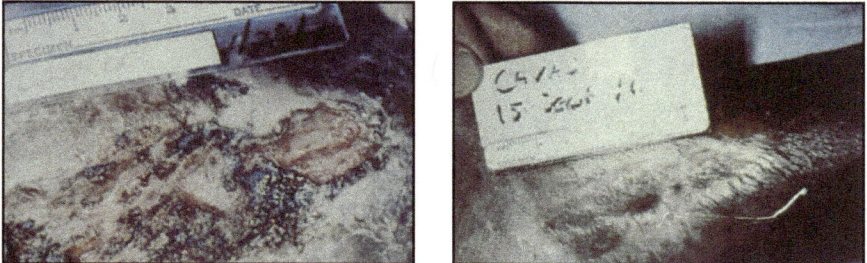

Figure 21.12:
The skin graft and the final result two years post-treatment.
(Courtesy of the late Col. J.C. Davis M.C.)

treatment does *not* mean that other measures are not needed. In this case, the improvement allowed a surgeon to use a skin graft and the final picture shows that the site remained healed after two years. The underlying problem was the presence of varicose veins and they required additional surgery.

Mention must be made of the impressive contribution of Thomas Hunt to the investigation of the role of oxygen in wound healing. Professor Hunt has devoted his life to scientific studies of oxygen measurement in damaged tissue and has influenced many others.[53] Although aware of the need for increased pressure to improve the delivery of oxygen to wounds, he has steadfastly refused to be involved in the use of hyperbaric oxygen treatment. Indeed, Dr. Albert Behnke, who retired from the US Navy as an Admiral after a distinguished career in diving medicine, offered Dr. Hunt one of the chambers used for tunnel workers on the Bay Area Rapid Transit Scheme, but without success.

One of the European pioneers of this treatment, Dr. Per-Oluf Barr, studied the long-term use of oxygen treatment to save limbs in patients facing amputation.[54] Most of the patients were elderly and one almost certainly holds the record for consecutive daily hyperbaric oxygen treatments at 1,241

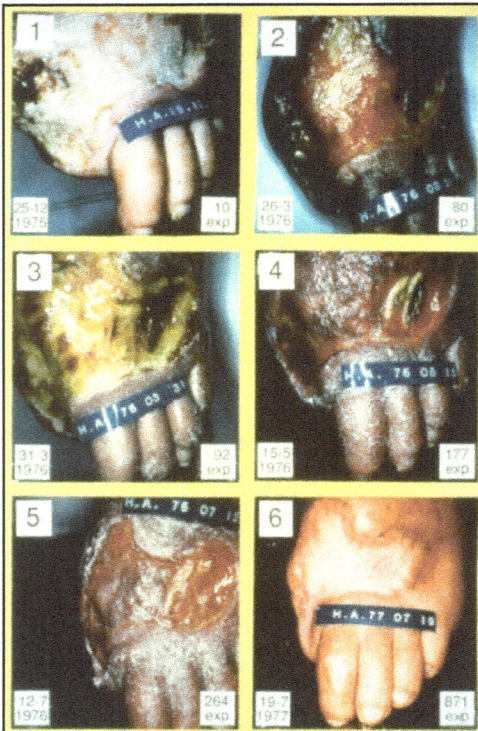

Figure 21.13:
Result of 871 oxygen sessions in a patient aged 72 with severe tissue damage from diabetes and atheroma. (Courtesy of Dr. Per-Oluf Barr, Stockholm.)

sessions! The sequence in Figure 21.13 relates to a 72-year-old patient with diabetes and arterial disease who received 871 sessions. Again, the result, without any intervention other than oxygen treatment, illustrates the astonishing power of the body to recover when given the right conditions.

However one, a 42-year-old man with complications from insulin-dependant diabetes, needs special mention. He was facing amputation of his right leg and it was almost certain that this would have been followed soon after by amputation of his left leg. His treatment was begun on the 12th of July (picture 1, Figure 21.14), and by the 15th of November he had completed 102 one-hour sessions at 2 ATA from Monday to Friday each week.

A major factor encouraging the continuation of treatment in this patient was the use of technology to actually *measure* the oxygen levels in his skin. The skin is normally not permeable to oxygen, but the device used heats the skin allowing oxygen to diffuse through to a sensor, which can measure the oxygen concentration. It is called transcutaneous oximetry.

At first glance the foot appears to be getting worse but, in fact, the most severely affected areas have blackened simply because the skin has died. The measurements, however, show that the oxygen levels in the *viable* skin improved. The treatment was continued with further improvement of the oxygen levels. Dr. Barr continued treatment on the same schedule completing the

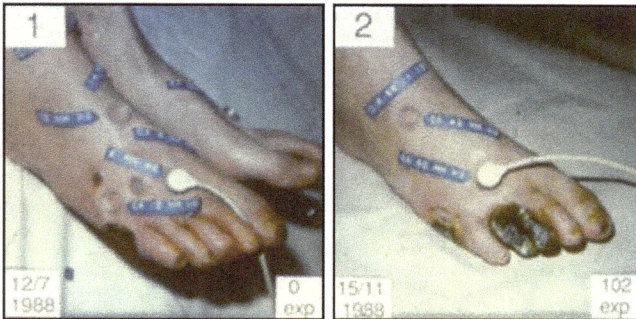

Figure 21.14:
42-year-old diabetic patient before and after 102 hours of treatment. (Courtesy of Dr. Per-Oluf Barr.)

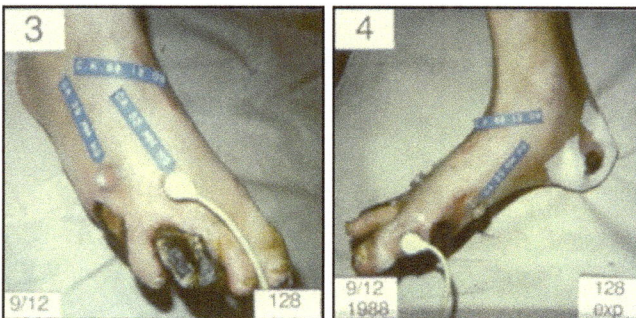

Figure 21.15:
Appearance of the foot after 128 hours of treatment. (Courtesy of Dr. Per-Oluf Barr.)

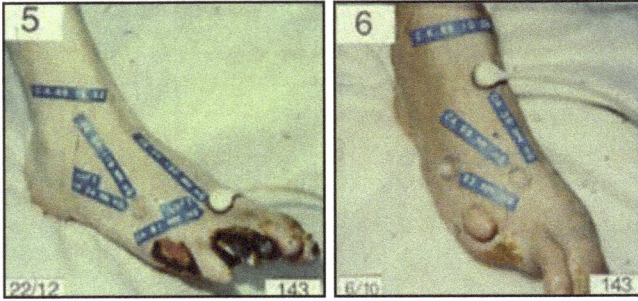

Figure 21.16:
Appearance of the foot on completion of treatment and the final result. (Courtesy of Dr. Per-Oluf Barr.)

course at 143 sessions (picture 5, Figure 21.16) with further improvement of the oxygen levels in the skin. By this time, the dead tissue simply fell away to reveal the area underneath which had healed.

The last photograph (6) was taken at a follow-up outpatient appointment more than a year after the beginning of treatment, when amputation had seemed inevitable. The skin oxygen levels were found to be within the normal range and so the tissues were healthy. It is obvious that without treatment, the patient's left leg would soon have required amputation but, of course, it also benefited from the oxygen treatment! Dr. Barr maintained contact with this patient for many years; he confirmed in 2002 that the patient remained well and with both his legs in place. The experience of just this *one patient* is compelling and illustrates the absurdity of the demands made for controlled trials of hyperbaric oxygen treatment. Evidence is being *debased* by dismissing patient reports of hyperbaric oxygen treatment as "anecdotal." The oxygen levels in this patient were measured before treatment and showed that the skin of the foot was actually dying. Repeated measurements documented the improvement with treatment, although some of the skin and underlying bone and soft tissue could not be salvaged. There are other reports; in 1992, a group in Italy published their 10-year experience of successfully treating patients with diabetic foot ulcers.[55]

The lack of oxygen in diabetic wounds is due to the wall of the capillaries becoming thickened, because glucose combines with the structural proteins. This forms a barrier to the transport of oxygen and it is particularly important in the retina and diabetic retinopathy is a leading cause of blindness in the Western world. There is support to the retina from very high levels of blood flow provided from the "choroidal" circulation directly behind it. This provides a minimal level of oxygen to allow the formation of new blood vessels in the "diabetic" retina with, of course, involves the hypoxia-inducible factor proteins. As with the retinal problems that result from withdrawing oxygen too quickly in the newborn, the overgrowth of new blood vessels in the retina compresses the light receptors, eventually causing blindness. It is no surprise that a superb Russian study has shown that diabetic retinopathy can readily be treated with sessions of hyperbaric oxygenation and there is the added benefit that the treatment reduces the blood glucose level.[56] A study of diabetic patients undergoing hyperbaric oxygen treatment for chronic leg ulceration has shown that the number of circulating stem cells doubles after the sessions.[57,58] Hyperbaric oxygen treatment mobilises bone marrow stem cells by stimulating the release of nitric oxide synthase, which remains elevated in blood for at least 20 hours post-treatment.

Amputation for severe leg ulcers is a convenient solution, at least for the surgeon, because it removes the problem, but it is not for patients. They often suffer psychological trauma and many, like the author's father, experience phantom pains for the rest of their lives. In reality, patient life expectancy may be significantly reduced after amputation and, overall, with prostheses and rehabilitation, it is a very expensive procedure. A report in 2010 in the *Journal of Bone and Joint Surgery*[59] indicated that the lifetime costs for dealing with patients after amputation, were three times higher than for those patients whose limb was salvaged. A US investigation of outcomes after amputation in military personnel, which cost $14 million, has highlighted the dreadful post-traumatic stress disorder that often follows the loss of a limb.[60] Adopting hyperbaric treatment, may avoid amputation in many such patients, improving their quality of life, with a dramatic reduction in the associated health care costs.

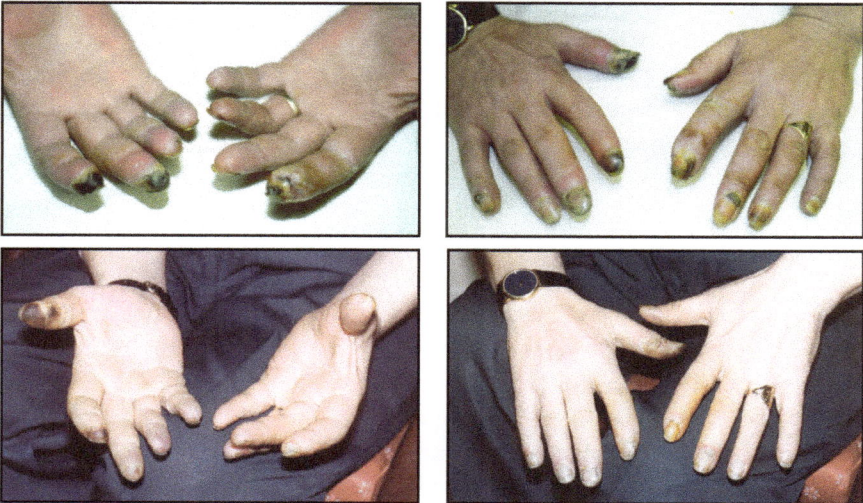

Figure 21.17:
The top photos were taken before hyperbaric treatment of frostbite damage; the bottom photos were taken after 43 sessions of hyperbaric oxygen treatment.
(Courtesy of Paul Feasby.)

A patient suffered severe frostbite after cleaning car windows on an extremely cold morning without gloves and a surgeon was consulted about the amputation of the ends of his fingers. He had a course of hyperbaric treatment in the author's unit which spared him this disabling surgery.

In 1987, the author attended a meeting in Oxford where a remarkable presentation was made by an Indian professor of surgery from Bombay who had treated a Himalayan climber with even more severe frostbite affecting the fingers and thumbs of both hands. He used hyperbaric treatment to salvage the bony infrastructure of the digits and, when the black skin sloughed away, he reconstructed them using skin grafts. The results could not be described as appealing, but the grateful patient regained fully-functional hands. Unfortunately, the author is unable to remember the name of the surgeon to credit him for this pioneering work. Disability after hand amputation can often be devastating, especially when it is necessary to amputate both hands, for example, when patients suffer the blood-borne infection known as meningococcal septicaemia.[61] This infection sometimes affects children even as young as six months which, inevitably, attracts media interest.[62] Sadly, attempts to interest the National Referral Centre at St. Mary's Hospital in London to install a hyperbaric oxygen chamber have been unsuccessful, despite funding being available (personal communication, Mr. Duncan Black PhD, FRCS).

The frustration felt by those of us who have seen the benefits from this remarkable, scientific, and safe intervention often spills over. The journal of the Undersea and Hyperbaric Medicine Society is currently republishing the evidence for each of the indications they support. Unfortunately, most members of this society subscribe to the view that the value of using oxygen to treat lack of oxygen must be questioned for every tissue of the body and subject to controlled trials. A paper by Dr. Michael Strauss, an orthopaedic surgeon now in charge of the hyperbaric facility founded in the 1970s at Long Beach Memorial Hospital by Dr. George Hart—another pioneer in this field— discusses why hyperbaric oxygen treatment may be of value in crush injury and in the muscle problems in the lower limb known as compartment syndrome.[63] Dr. Strauss wrote, after publishing about hyperbaric oxygen treatment for over 30 years, "I am frustrated that my orthopaedic colleagues have not embraced this modality." He wrote that when he confronted his colleagues, " . . . they appear to accept disconcerting complication rates as acceptable for their trauma patients. They always end their caveats (about hyperbaric oxygen treatment) with comments like 'who needs it'; 'there is no evidence to support its use'; 'no randomised control studies are available'; 'our patients are too sick to be moved to a chamber'; and 'even if

we wanted to use hyperbaric oxygen treatment, chambers are not available'."
No one ever states the obvious in this debate; allowing a patient to recover
on their own, sitting in a chamber receiving just a few hundred grams more
oxygen a day, is bad for business.

One orthopaedic condition, destruction of the head of the femur, in
which improvement from hyperbaric oxygen treatment has been followed
by MRI, was not mentioned by Dr. Strauss. Over the last few decades, there
have been several published case reports and series of patients treated with
femoral head damage monitored by MRI. They have usually been of patients
who have opted for hyperbaric oxygen treatment rather than face surgery.[64]
In 2010, a controlled study of hyperbaric oxygen treatment of patients with
this hip problem was published by investigators in Italy and the US.[65] Thirty
sessions were given, with 10 patients breathing oxygen at 2.5 ATA, and nine
control patients given compressed air for an hour. Both groups were, therefore, treated in the chamber and, after completing 30 sessions, significant improvement was recorded in the oxygen group, but not the compressed air
group. At six weeks, the control group was given oxygen treatment and, for
the remainder of the first year, treatment was continued as indicated for residual pain. The MRI images of one of the patients show that the head of the
femur repaired. The patient was re-imaged at seven years and it can be seen
that the bone remained healed.

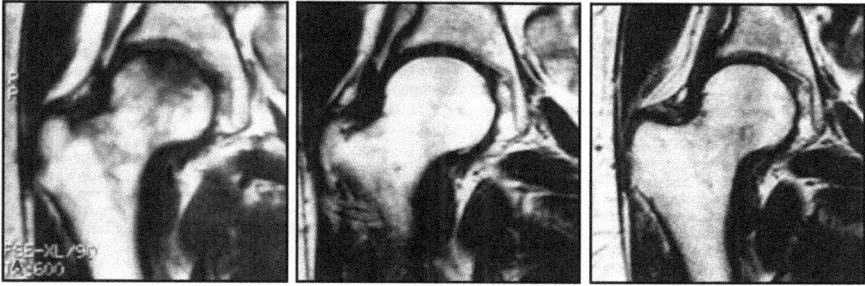

Figure 21.18:
MRI head of a femur before treatment, 12 months after hyperbaric oxygen treatment, and
at seven years after treatment. (Courtesy of Prof G. Vezzani et al.)

Higher oxygen concentrations and longer treatment times are needed
when treating deep tissues like bone, which usually have a poor blood supply.
Figure 21.19, with mean and standard deviations indicated, shows the time to
equilibration from measurements using electrodes in normal muscle tissue. The
readings were taken from eight volunteers in experiments in a laboratory at
Long Beach Memorial Hospital in California.[66]

The first increase in the oxygen level in the muscle, starting at one hour,

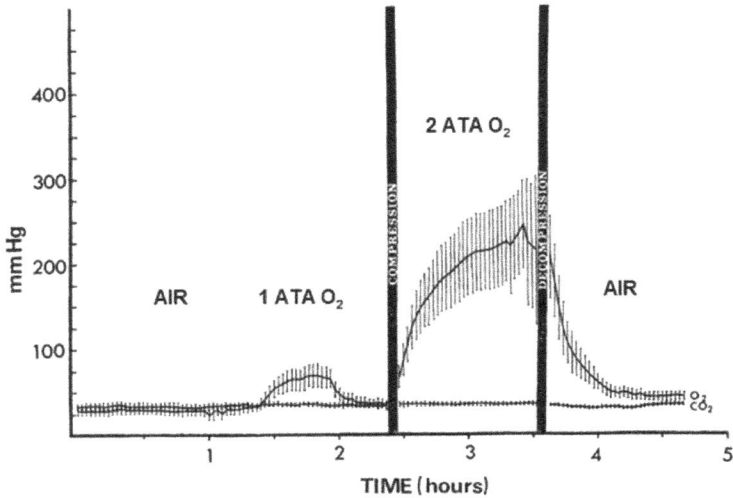

Figure 21.19:
Muscle gas tensions: Eight normal volunteers showing means and standard deviations.
Oxygen upper line, 90 mins breathing air, 1 ATA O_2 for 30 mins, 2 ATA O_2 for 60 mins.
Lower line, CO_2, remains constant.

was produced by the subject breathing 100% oxygen for 30 minutes at normal barometric pressure (1 ATA) with the second, and much larger increase, produced by breathing 100% oxygen at 2 ATA. This clearly shows that for muscle, the time to equilibration is about one hour and, as it is likely that the peak concentration is critical, also shows why treating patients with soft tissue injuries need hourly sessions. In those with damaged bone and soft tissue, equilibration may need longer, however, the time to equilibration for the tissues of the nervous system will be very much shorter. For example, the retina will reach peak values in less than a minute and so with oxygen is acting by regulating gene expression via the HIF proteins it may be possible for treatment times in brain injury to be shortened.

Not surprisingly, many other conditions have been successfully treated with hyperbaric oxygenation when all other interventions have failed. Infections with flesh-eating bacteria, with Streptococcus A, and with MRSA (methicillin-resistant Staphylococcus aureus), often achieve banner headlines in national newspapers but, in the UK, the fact that they can be successfully treated with oxygen is never mentioned. In the US it is a reimbursable indication by insurers. Increased pressure and oxygen can remove gas obstructing the bowel post-surgery and restore bowel function;[67] aspergillosis[68] of the lungs has been successfully treated, avoiding removal of a lung.

No discussion of oxygen is complete without mentioning the importance of lack of oxygen, hypoxia, in the causation of cancer. It is clear that the uncontrolled division of cells that constitutes cancer may be initiated by a vast number of agents from infections, or mechanical factors, such as the irritation of the membrane of the lungs by a single fibre of blue asbestos. What is little known is that cells intermittently lacking oxygen in culture become cancerous.[69] There has to be a common factor and logic dictates that it is *inflammation*.

The cancer story begins with a controversial Nobel laureate working in the Kaiser Wilhelm Institute in Berlin and funded by the Rockefeller Foundation, Otto Heinrich Warburg (1883-1970). Warburg was nominated for the Nobel Prize for three independent discoveries but, despite assisting in the treatment of Adolf Hitler when he developed a precancerous nodule on his vocal chords in 1935, Hitler blocked Warburg's last nomination in 1944 (although he protected him from the attentions of the Gestapo). This association certainly did not help the acceptance of Warburg's research. He had received the Nobel Prize in 1931 for his work on how oxygen is used by cells to produce energy in the production of the molecule central to our lives—adenosine triphosphate (ATP). He found that this very efficient mechanism is damaged in cancer cells, which revert to glycolysis, the breaking down of glucose without using oxygen, which in turn produces lactic acid and is known as fermentation. He was so convinced that he wrote in 1956:[70]

> *The era in which the fermentation of the cancer cells or its importance could be disputed is over, and no one today can doubt that we understand the origin of cancer cells if we know how the damaged respiration and the excessive fermentation (about 200 times greater than normal) of the cancer cells originate.*

It has always been assumed that cells switch to using glycolysis when their oxygen supply fails but it has been discovered that this is not true; cells can switch to using glycolysis when oxygen is present. The switch is controlled by genes regulated by the hypoxia-inducible factor protein system, which also controls the expression of the tumour inhibiting gene p53. Jack Haldane identified the key problem in treating cancer is switching off cell division. Clearly, the full story has yet to unfold but lack of oxygen is the common factor in cancer and, conversely, oxygen inhibits cancer.

This latter point is of great importance because, given the misinformation about oxygen when it used as a treatment, many assume that hyperbaric oxygen treatment may encourage the growth of such cells. In fact, not only does the science discussed above indicate that this is not the case, vast clinical experience around the world has also shown it is not true, because hyperbaric oxygen treatment has been widely used to treat the side effects and complications of radiotherapy, chemotherapy and surgery. The reason is obvious and the principle has already been stated many times; damage to tissues damages the capillaries they contain reducing the supply of oxygen essential to recovery.

Not surprisingly, the list of publications is endless and it is notable that "uncontrolled" studies of conditions where hyperbaric oxygen treatment has been spectacularly successful are sometimes accepted by leading medical journals. Radiation of patients with cancer of pelvic areas may, unfortunately, damage small blood vessels in the bladder, resulting in chronic inflammation and, eventually, scarring. This may lead to bleeding into the urine, which can present after a delay of as long as 21 years. The author can attest to the misery of haematuria, which resulted from a traumatic injury. In 1995, the *Lancet* published an *uncontrolled* study of the use of hyperbaric oxygen treatment for 40 severely affected patients with haemorrhagic cystitis from 56 to 80 years old.[71] After 20 sessions of breathing oxygen for 90 minute at 3 ATA, the bleeding either disappeared completely or improved significantly in 37 of the 40 patients. There were no adverse effects, but oxygen treatment is still not the standard of care. The paper lists the many truly dreadful treatments which have been tried, from instillations of toxic agents, like phenol, to actual removal of the bladder itself. Nevertheless, the authors suggested that hyperbaric oxygen treatment should only be *considered* for patients with *severe* radiation-induced cystitis. What this implies is that there is actually an alternative to oxygen for less severe cases, but if less severe cases do heal, it is only because the oxygen in the air has been sufficient. To a lay person this "last resort" use of oxygen treatment must seem ridiculous—as absurd as giving blood only as a last resort when bleeding renders a patient close to death. Giving more oxygen needs to be the first consideration in treatment, not the last.

CHAPTER 22

The Way Forward

An invasion of armies can be resisted but not an idea whose time has come.

Victor Hugo, 1802–1885

There can be no better example to highlight the need to provide emergency hyperbaric oxygen treatment than for poisoning with the gas carbon monoxide. Chapter 4 covered Haldane's investigation of the deaths that followed an explosion down a mine in a Welsh valley in 1896. Of the 57 miners who died, only four were killed by the blast, with the rest dying from burns and carbon monoxide poisoning. Now the story needs to be completed.

The growth of civilisation began with man discovering how to create and control fire and it allowed human migration, from the rift valleys of Kenya to successively colder climes—the subject of a fascinating book, *Man in a Cold Environment* by Burton and Edholm.[1] Despite the extraordinary benefits fire has brought to mankind there are risks—it may go out of control burning property and killing people. But the least recognised risk occurs when the combustion of hydrocarbons is incomplete, because carbon monoxide is produced. It is the commonest human poison and it is estimated that it kills over 4,000 people a year in the US. The gas simply prevents oxygen from being used by the cells of the body and, not surprisingly, it is the brain that is the first to suffer. Carbon monoxide concentrations of just a few hundred parts per million in air cause headache and fatigue, which, it will be remembered, are also the first symptoms of oxygen lack when climbing to altitude. Death may occur at concentrations of carbon monoxide in air of less than 1,000 parts per million. Because carbon monoxide prevents cells using oxygen causing hypoxia, the mechanisms of poisoning, the symptoms, and the pathology are highly relevant to other conditions associated with lack of oxygen.

Carbon monoxide poisoning is one of four conditions where treatment with oxygen under hyperbaric conditions has generally been accepted, if not used, around the world. Nevertheless, the vast majority of affected patients are still treated with 100% oxygen at the prevailing barometric pressure in conventional intensive care units, sedated, intubated, and on a ventilator. It is also likely that many poisoned patients only receive 30-40% oxygen from ward oxygen delivery equipment. In 1977, a judge in Wayne County, Michigan reviewed the evidence that hyperbaric oxygen treatment should be used for patients with carbon monoxide poisoning,[2] ruling that a 16-year-old victim was treated "with inadequate concentrations of oxygen." The American Medical Association Legal Department circulated the details (Figure 22.1) to all its members on June 6, 1978.

Professional Malpractice
Medical

CARBON MONOXIDE POISONING: FAILURE TO USE HYPERBARIC CHAMBER: HOSPITAL LIABILITY
***Sponenburgh v. County of Wayne*, Mich., Wayne County Circuit Court No. 73254137 CM, Sept. 22, 1977.**

$3,888,000 verdict for 16-year-old victim of carbon monoxide poisoning who was treated with inadequate concentrations of oxygen at defendant hospital.

Plaintiff was discovered in his family car, unconscious and breathing shallowly, apparently a victim of self-induced CO poisoning. He was treated with oxygen and rushed to a local hospital. Emergency room physicians there felt that he needed more intensive treatment, including a hyperbaric chamber, and sent him to defendant hospital, where such equipment was available. There, he was seen by 2 new residents, neither of whom was aware of the hyperbaric chamber and who continued to treat him with 30-40% oxygen instead of the 100% concentration which is the treatment of choice for CO poisoning. Plaintiff suffered severe, irreversible brain damage, including mental retardation, loss of control of his extremities, and ability to talk.

[*SOURCE:* Letter from ATLA Member Samuel Charloos, Detroit, Mich., counsel for plaintiff.]

Figure 22.1: Notification by the AMA of the 1977 case verdict: Failure to use hyperbaric oxygen treatment in carbon monoxide poisoning.

The case came to court because the family realised that instead of receiving intensive care in the first hospital, he was transferred to the second hospital because it had a hyperbaric chamber but it was not used. The residents in the second hospital clearly did not know about the critical importance of hyperbaric oxygen treatment in carbon monoxide poisoning and, in all probability, were unaware of the presence of a pressure chamber in the building. A settlement of $3,888,000 was made after the judge had reviewed the evidence that hyperbaric oxygen treatment should have been used, collated by the lawyer representing the family. This may appear to be a large sum; translated from 1977 values, it probably represents at least $15 million today, but it is likely that it would not cover the cost of caring for a person with profound mental and physical disabilities if they lived to the normal age of 70.

It is common for lesser degrees of carbon monoxide poisoning to be overlooked and the earliest symptoms are, not surprisingly, often mistaken for the onset of influenza. The presentations found have been listed in terms of frequency, but it is important to recognise that considerable variation exists, especially in children.

1. Fatigue	8. Breathlessness
2. Headache	9. Numbness and tingling
3. Trouble thinking	10. Chest pain
4. Dizziness	11. Decreased vision
5. Nausea	12. Diarrhoea
6. Insomnia	13. Strange behavior
7. Palpitations	14. Abdominal pain

It is also not surprising that chronic low-level carbon monoxide poisoning mimics many psychiatric syndromes, because they relate to damage in the so-called "silent" areas in the mid-brain responsible for emotions and memory.[3] This is due to opening of the blood-brain barrier and was investigated by Dr. Tracy Putnam in the 1930s.[4] The failure to recognise this silent killer, and the need for hyperbaric oxygen treatment, was highlighted in the UK in 1998 by an advisory letter to all hospital trusts from the chief medical officer,[5] and it was reinforced in 2002. Not surprisingly, there was no mention of the lack of provision of hyperbaric units in the NHS which, of course, means that patients continue to be admitted to intensive care units and given too little oxygen.

In 1895, Haldane had shown that the effects of carbon monoxide can actually be prevented by giving oxygen under hyperbaric conditions.[6] In a remarkable, but little-known experiment published in the *Journal of Physiology*, he showed that a high level of oxygen prevented the poisoning of a mouse by carbon monoxide. He placed a mouse in a glass cylinder at a total pressure of 2.8 ATA, which was produced by 1.8 atmospheres of oxygen and 1 atmosphere of carbon monoxide. Under these conditions, the four sites normally occupied by oxygen on the haemoglobin molecule would have been taken over by carbon monoxide to form *carboxyhaemoglobin*. The mouse was being kept alive by the oxygen *dissolved* in the blood plasma, as were the pigs in the Amsterdam "Life Without Blood" experiment, after their red blood cells had been removed.[7] Jack Haldane showed, in 1927, that the poisonous effects of the gas are not due to its combination with haemoglobin; it is the combination of carbon monoxide with the enzymes in cells, known as the *cytochromes*, which renders the gas so dangerous.[8] It will be recalled that the cytochromes are responsible for the oxidation of glucose in mitochondria to create energy. Like haemoglobin, they are molecules in which a metal is combined with a protein. Carbon monoxide blocks their action, but Haldane's experiment has shown that this actually can be *prevented* by the presence of a sufficiently high level of oxygen.

Carbon monoxide may not only kill; survivors often suffer damage to structures in the centre of the brain and, just as in head-injured patients, proof of this is difficult to find on clinical examination. The MRI findings are non-specific[9] and, as a consequence, patients often attract the label "psychosomatic." Haldane would profoundly disagree, as is evident in this statement from his book *Respiration*.[10]

> *When an unconscious man is removed from the poisonous air, the CO is very rapidly washed out of his blood; but he may still be unconscious, and in a dying condition, with his blood perfectly free of CO, and the cause of the oxygen want thus completely removed . . . In the light of present knowledge it is childish to believe that as soon as the lack of oxygen is relieved a patient will recover.*

Carbon monoxide combines with the haemoglobin in red blood cells about 200 times more readily than oxygen, and so renders the sites where oxygen normally binds unavailable. The degree of the oxygenation of haemoglobin, which is responsible for the redness of blood, is easily measured and similar instrumentation can measure carboxyhaemoglobin levels. The rate of elimination of carbon monoxide from its binding to haemoglobin can be measured and, breathing air, the half-life is over five hours. When a poisoned patient is given oxygen at 3 ATA, this is reduced to 23 minutes. Although the dynamics of the interaction of carbon monoxide with the cytochromes at the cellular level cannot be measured, there is every reason to believe that the reduction of binding by carbon monoxide is of the same order. Experimentally, blood has been removed from animals and the red blood cells exposed to carbon monoxide outside the body.[11] When the blood was returned to the animals, it produced carboxyhaemoglobin levels normally not compatible with life, but they remained healthy because their cellular cytochrome enzymes were still functioning; they had not been poisoned.

Haldane's discovery early in his career that most deaths in mine explosions are from carbon monoxide poisoning, and not from blast trauma, was tragically confirmed in 2006 by the disaster at the Sago mine in West Virginia,

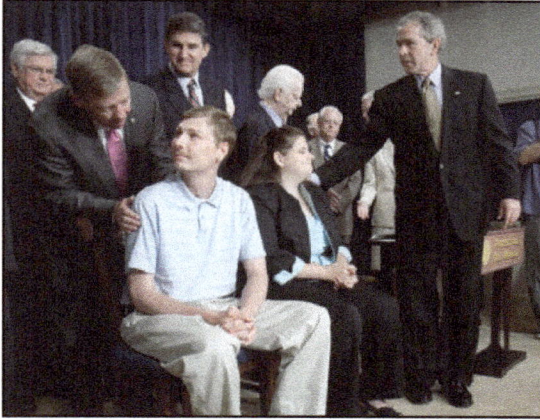

Figure 22.2:
President George W. Bush greets Anna McCloy, wife of miner Randal McCloy, during the signing of S. 2803, the Miner Act, in the Dwight D. Eisenhower Executive Office Building on Thursday, June 15, 2006. Senator Johnny Isakson (R-GA) greets Randal McCloy.
(White House photograph by Eric Draper.)

which was given worldwide coverage. It trapped 13 men 280 feet underground and there was a high carbon monoxide level in their refuge. Only one miner survived; Randy McCloy was rescued 42 hours after the explosion. He was very sick and it must be remembered that carbon monoxide is a generalised poison; there is often damage to the heart and kidneys.[12] He was transported 70 miles to Allegheny General Hospital in Pittsburgh for hyperbaric oxygen treatment.[13] His doctors considered it futile, but they were wrong; he made a remarkable and almost complete recovery. He has made a difference; the Miner Act was signed into force in 2006 to improve safety in mining.

Incredible though it may seem to lay people, giving a large dose of oxygen in a pressure chamber when carbon monoxide has robbed the brain of its oxygen is still regarded as "controversial," and even unproven. Yet giving 100% oxygen is standard practice in such cases, but, as we have seen, it is given without any consideration of barometric pressure, which means that the dose can vary by more than 10%, simply because of the weather. So the rejection of hyperbaric oxygen treatment is really not of oxygen itself, it is of the *equipment* needed to increase the dose. Again the irony is that aircraft capable of supplying the necessary pressure fly over us all the time. The controversies raised can only be resolved by returning to *first principles*, but it must be borne in mind that strong emotions are roused in medicine by duty of care issues, and the reaction of medical professionals sometimes defies logic.

The *first principle* is that the effects of lack of oxygen on the brain depend on the *degree* and *duration* of the hypoxia. This discussion relates to carbon monoxide contaminated air; a carbon monoxide concentration of 2,000 parts per million in air is fatal in minutes, whereas 50 parts per million can be breathed indefinitely, although it usually causes fatigue and headache. If the brain is observed through a hole in the skull in an animal model, high concentrations of carbon monoxide cause immediate swelling and brain tissue may exude through the hole. This links carbon monoxide poisoning to other conditions causing brain swelling discussed earlier, like air embolism and head injury. It is due to the transfer of water from the blood vessels into brain tissue associated with failure of the blood-brain barrier, which requires oxygen to function.[14] As we have seen, tissue swelling and lack of oxygen go hand in hand with the upregulation of inflammation with neutrophil activity regulated by the hypoxia-inducible factor proteins.

The *second principle* relates to the *vulnerability* of the tissues of the body; when tissues are damaged, so are the capillaries they contain. The reduction of blood flow that results causes hypoxia. Because the brain uses the most oxygen it is the first to suffer, whereas lowly skin cells are relatively unaffected. The brain has only a small number of different cell types, but it is far from being a uniform mass and the number of blood vessels for a volume of tissue in different areas varies enormously—the grey matter of the cortex has hundreds of capillaries per cubic millimetre, whereas there are vulnerable zones *without* capillaries in the central white matter. Vulnerability determines the degree of tissue death from a particular insult and this, of course, determines the degree of recovery possible.

The *third principle* is the need to establish the oxygen *dosage*, that is, the concentration and duration needed for the best outcome. Prevention has been proven, and it has been shown that, after oxygen deprivation, cells may be left with sufficient energy to survive, but not to function. This has established the biological plausibility of oxygen treatment, but a key question is how to determine the viability of cells in the brain. Two mechanisms of toxicity have been discussed in carbon monoxide poisoning, and both involve the release of free radicals, either by disturbed metabolism, or by neutrophils attracted to the area. The latter mechanism has now been verified in carbon monoxide poisoning[15,16] and, by implicating neutrophils, links the damage seen in many conditions, including decompression sickness, tetanus toxin, and the first event in multiple sclerosis. Dr. Tracy Putnam had witnessed the immediate effects of carbon monoxide on the blood-brain barrier in his experimental model.[4] A high concentration caused severe swelling of the whole brain, due to disruption of the barrier, but lesser concentrations mainly affected the veins passing through the deep white matter, leading to damage to the most vulnerable cell, responsible for myelin sheaths—the oligodendrocyte. Fifty years after Putnam's ground breaking research, the technology of MRI has demonstrated this damage to the white matter in survivors of carbon monoxide poisoning visible as bright areas in the central areas of the brain.[17] Again, if their cause was *not known* they would, of course, be called unidentified bright objects.

The *fourth principle* is the *timing* of treatment; would anyone seriously disagree that the sooner a lack of oxygen is corrected the better? Clearly, the higher the level of carbon monoxide exposure, the more urgent is the need for treatment. The cascade of events has been studied in great detail experimentally and imaged in acutely ill patients over the last 30 years, using advanced technology costing millions. Studies have correlated the pathology with the areas seen on CT[18] and MRI.[19] MRI has shown the vulnerability of structures in the middle of the brain,[20] with the all-too-familiar pattern of blood-brain barrier failure, inflammation, and developing tissue damage. Clearly this is often *not* controlled by the level of oxygen in air, but may be controlled by using oxygen at a sufficient dose, provided it is given *promptly*. The treatment of a patient with carbon monoxide poisoning is an *emergency*; to delay treatment for investigations risks brain damage, and often death. In the 1960s, when "town" gas, which contains 5% carbon monoxide, was still used in homes in Glasgow, an ambulance equipped with a Vickers hyperbaric chamber was used to treat poisoned patients at the scene.[21]

Despite the truly massive experimental and human evidence supporting the use of hyperbaric oxygen treatment in carbon monoxide poisoning, the lack of acceptance prompted a controlled trial. It was published in the *New England Journal of Medicine* in 2002[22] and graphically illustrates the problem of proper timing. Despite the use of the word "acute," no patient received hyperbaric oxygen treatment in the first six hours. Imagine a wounded patient bleeding almost to the point of death, desperately needing a blood transfusion; would it be acceptable to wait as long as 34 hours to test the benefit of a transfusion? It would obviously be completely unacceptable. Despite the delays introduced, many patients in the 2002 controlled study were shown to benefit. Neurological deterioration from carbon monoxide poisoning may also be seen after a considerable delay,[23,24] and hyperbaric oxygen treatment may still be effective even when 100% oxygen at normal atmospheric pressure has failed.[25] This should not be surprising—it will be recalled that patients with mid-brain damage from Encephalitis lethargica and long-term disabilities improved with the drug dopamine.[26] This has shown conclusively that brain recovery may be possible despite the lapse of many years and the story of Rose in the book *Awakenings* by the neurologist Oliver Sacks[27] (summarised in Appendix 3) is truly a landmark.

The word "encephalitis" in Encephalitis lethargica links the condition to the problems that may follow both virus infections and vaccinations. In 2007, Fox News in the US carried a feature by the journalist Lila Lazarus on the treatment of a little girl who was left disabled after developing encephalitis from chickenpox. Her mother, using the Internet, had found the mother of a child who had recovered from encephalitis using hyperbaric oxygen treatment in Australia. She was determined that her daughter would also have hyperbaric treatment, but the attending neurologist refused to write a prescription. Nevertheless, she was treated by Dr. Stephen Guthrie in the Detroit Medical Center's hyperbaric facility. Despite the lapse of many months, she made an astonishing recovery, improving incrementally with each treatment. Her grateful parents started a hyperbaric facility and now operate three hyperbaric centres in Michigan.[28] There has been a recent epidemic of measles in South Wales which, in most cases, is a mild illness; such patients may also develop encephalitis, which will also respond to hyperbaric oxygen treatment.

Physicians using hyperbaric oxygen treatment have been progressively marginalised over the last 50 years in Europe and this prompted a series of meetings known as the European Consensus Conference on Hyperbaric Medicine to collate the evidence for each condition. The first, held in the northern French town of Lille in September 1994, attracted the usual mix of physicians in the field—from those involved in deep diving research and commercial diving, to those operating clinical hyperbaric units, mainly treating patients with problem wounds. Recommendations were made for the indications to be supported and number VI related to "post-anoxic encephalopathy," which is the pathological state that can follow lack of oxygen in the brain and includes carbon monoxide poisoning. The recommendation stated that "HBO is *optional* for the treatment of cerebral anoxia"; translated, this means that a large dose of oxygen is optional when the brain has been deprived of oxygen. There was no reference whatever to the timing of the administration of the hyperbaric oxygen treatment. To say the least, this is frustrating, especially as the hyperbaric unit in Lille University Medical Centre has extensive experience of treating near-hanging patients, with a remarkable success rate.[29]

One of the first attempts to bring pressure into the treatment of illness was made by the physician Thomas Beddoes who, working with the renowned engineer Humphrey Davy, founded the Pneumatic Institute in Bristol in 1798. It was not supported by the medical profession, and soon closed. In 1857, Dr. Stanley B. Birch drew attention in the *Lancet* to professional ignorance of the use of oxygen in treatment and his perceptive comments are astonishingly relevant today. It is an extraordinary analysis of the psychology involved when physicians are confronted with a fundamental challenge to their knowledge. (The italics have been added by the author.)

ON THE THERAPEUTIC USE OF OXYGEN
by S.B. Birch, M.D.
The Lancet
August 1, 1857

In venturing to call professional attention to the subject of this paper, I may safely premise with the remark, that it is one respecting which there exist great diversity of opinion and *very little practical knowledge*. The therapeutic use of oxygen gas, either alone or as an adjunct, in various intractable diseases, is a subject of vast importance to my professional brethren, enhanced in value as it is by an impartial reflection upon the still very uncertain and unsatisfactory state of our knowledge of medicinal *modus operandi*. Thus far, excepting to a few individuals and to a very limited extent, this gas, although so well known in its physiological relations, *has been practically little better than a "secret" in its therapeutic bearings*.

Notwithstanding that from the time of Dr. Beddoes and Sir Humphrey Davy several practitioners have made successful trial in private practice—notwithstanding that the researches of modern chemistry have made us more scientifically cognisant than formerly of the relations of oxygen to the other elements of the vital organism —notwithstanding that the daily observations of every man who has disease to treat shows him that the patient needs plenty of pure air, more air (in other words more oxygen) than he can possibly obtain under many circumstances and in many diseased states from the atmosphere around him - *the idea seems merely to float through the professional mind, without any resulting general endeavour to make a practical application of it.*

It would not be difficult to show cause why the use of this remedy has been neglected. *It involves some trouble and loss of time* to the practitioner, and consequently the very want of practical knowledge still existing may be justly attributed to the neglect to carry out fair trials on a sufficient scale in practice.

Thus the profession has been led to overlook or ignore oxygen as a medicine, even though chemical science tells us decidedly that it ought to be a most valuable remedial agent. *A single trial, or several trials on several patients, are no evidence, if they fail, against its value; they are only proof either that it was not suited to the case, or that it was not properly exhibited.*

It is difficult to believe that this was written more than 150 years ago! The last comment is so relevant today because the use of oxygen for head-injured patients is currently being examined in an endless and futile series of so-called "controlled" trials in the US. As discussed in Chapter 10, controlled trials are needed to test *efficacy*, but not *dosage*, and this is especially true when the agent is the most critical to life itself. If treatment with additional oxygen fails, it is not because oxygen is ineffective, or not needed, it is simply because it has not been used promptly, at the correct dosage, or the damage has gone *too far* for recovery to take place. However, the sad fact is that today, without *marketing*, publications very rarely change medical practice—they are lost in the fog created by the millions of papers published every year.

The range of symptoms, syndromes, and pathology that can follow carbon monoxide poisoning is very wide and reflects the vulnerability of different areas of the brain to lack of oxygen. Very severe poisoning leads to mental retardation and dementia because of damage to the grey matter of the cortex,[30] whilst lesser degrees produce headache and nausea, easily attributable to food poisoning. Not surprisingly, carbon monoxide-poisoned patients often suffer from depression, and some exhibit violent behaviour, easily mistaken for alcohol intoxication. A connection to the symptoms labelled Parkinson's disease is not widely known,[31,32] and poisoning may cause the development of epilepsy.[33] Older patients exposed to carbon monoxide may develop symptoms which are essentially the same as those of Alzheimer's disease, often after a considerable delay, and "minor" symptoms ranging from fatigue to weakness and changes in skin sensation are easily overlooked.[34] NHS Choices[35] is the online "front door" to the health service in the UK and the advice about carbon monoxide poisoning includes all the misinformation discussed, including reliance on the measurement of the carboxyhaemoglobin level in blood.[36] It states: "Hyperbaric oxygen therapy (HBOT) floods the body with pure oxygen, helping it to overcome the oxygen shortage caused by carbon monoxide poisoning." It then, absurdly, alleges that: "There is currently insufficient evidence regarding the *long-term* effectiveness of HBOT for treating severe cases of carbon monoxide poisoning." Survival from certain death is proof of long-term effectiveness!

The author's experience ranges from treating a patient with mild poisoning after rescuing his dog from a house fire, who said that breathing oxygen in the chamber was "like a curtain being pulled away from his mind," to seeing a patient with dilated pupils and no reflexes wake up in the chamber at 2 ATA before the end of an hour of treatment. Whenever a patient has suffered lack of oxygen, whether it be the whole body, or just a few grams of

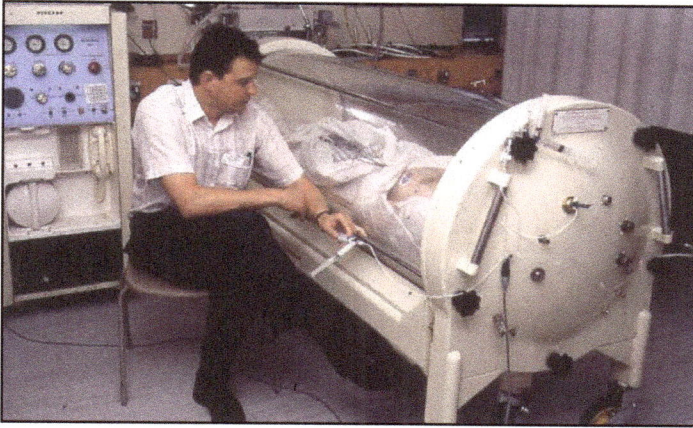

Figure 22.3:
A carbon monoxide-poisoned patient in a Vickers hyperbaric chamber.

tissue in the brain, there is a duty of care to give sufficient oxygen; witness the resuscitation of the canaries used in detecting carbon monoxide in mines in a "normobaric"oxygen chamber (see Figure 4.3), and the brain of a canary weighs just a few milligrams.

However, a sealed enclosure may be needed simply to increase the ambient pressure and Figure 22.3 shows a young man the author treated for carbon monoxide poisoning in the 1990s. A bed was removed from a bay in the intensive care unit and replaced by the Vickers chamber, which was built in 1973. All the beloved electronic surveillance of an ICU has been replaced by the Mark 1 eyeball of the doctor in attendance. It is human to question how long it would take to remove the patient from such a chamber but the patient is in a place of safety—recall that Peter Colat's world breath-hold record after just 10 minutes of oxygen breathing is 19 minutes and 21 seconds. The patient made a full recovery.

As the research that followed Jessica's ordeal demonstrated, a high level of oxygen can prevent the neutrophil attack which follows when blood flow is restarted in ligatured *muscle*, and it has been shown that it can prevent the same events causing damage to the *brain* in patients after carbon monoxide poisoning. But hyperbaric oxygen treatment should be the standard of care for patients who have suffered any other cause of oxygen deprivation to the brain. This is especially the case following cardiac arrest because, again, the stoppage of blood flow paves the way for neutrophil free radical damage when the heart is restarted.

We will always face the problem in a given patient, and with any condition, of not knowing how much benefit is possible from using more oxygen in treatment. This dilemma is far from being unique to the use of oxygen, it also applies to the use of drugs. The answer is simple—it needs professional medical assessment of the response of an individual in order to titrate treatment and monitor the actions of interventions and this is actually the practice of medicine. The reliance on one-size-fits-all protocols for hyperbaric oxygen treatment, and even more so for drug treatment, dictated by reimbursement policy, is unscientific, absurd, and must be resisted. The importance of individualising treatment is now being recognised by the pharmaceutical industry, which is now advocating the use of gene profiling, for example, in drugs used against breast cancer. It must also be remembered that if the monitoring of side effects in trials is not undertaken responsibly, adverse media publicity can result in the failure of drug; with investment in the billions, drug development has become a very risky business. The contrast with hyperbaric oxygen treatment, which simply extends the envelope of *normal* healing, could not be greater, and we all use oxygen in the same way. Properly used, the risk associated with hyperbaric oxygenation is not from the oxygen itself, it is from the minor changes in pressure on the ears. In fact, the risk to the patient is from *not* using it.

Patients struggle to understand rejection of the use of hyperbaric oxygen treatment by otherwise sensible doctors, but it is not taught in our medical schools, and to suggest to a qualified doctor that they neither know about the importance of oxygen in healing, nor how to correct lack of oxygen in their patients, is a full-frontal assault on their competence. Nevertheless, no one can surely disagree that there is not a more justified and scientific action than to *restore normal oxygen* levels in the tissues of the body, especially in the brain? An obvious difficulty is that we cannot separate the quantity of oxygen in the air we breathe that we need to stay alive, from that which we use in recovery from illness or injury. Put more simply: we fail to recognise the *importance of breathing* to recovery and the fact that the dose of oxygen we gain from air may not be sufficient. The most recent official document from the UK NHS[37] illustrates the problem; quite apart from insisting on evidence from controlled trials, it often states that there is no *theoretical basis* for hyperbaric oxygen treatment. Not only, without defining "baric" oxygen treatment, is this scientifically absurd, it ignores that many conditions are treated in other countries and reimbursed by insurers, which is surely the gold standard.

The explosion of scientific evidence supporting the use of oxygen in the last decades from massive funding of animal experiments has been ignored. The use of animal models mirrors drug development, but with one important difference—there is considerable variation in the way drugs are metabolised in other animals. However, there is little difference in the way oxygen is used, or in the hydraulic system of blood vessels needed, the size of red blood cells, and the pumps required for its delivery. Animal data from hyperbaric oxygen studies, therefore, provides a solid and certain basis for human treatment, with the sole proviso that scale is important. A study, often quoted as suggesting that oxygen treatment fails to prevent neurological residua in carbon monoxide poisoning, actually used a mouse model.[38] As Haldane showed in his mouse experiment, hyperbaric oxygen treatment can prevent death, obviously the most profound of neurological residua. A mouse brain typically weighs half a gram—a stark contrast to the 1,350 grams of a human brain. Nevertheless, dismissing the massive evidence supporting hyperbaric oxygen treatment from animal research is a travesty.

A dramatic example of the consequences of the failure to use hyperbaric conditions to give enough oxygen in carbon monoxide poisoning was published in 2005.[39] A 51-year-old man unconscious from severe poisoning was ventilated on 100% oxygen in an ICU and discharged after four days, with no apparent signs or symptoms. He was followed up seven days after discharge, and an MRI showed "bilateral globus pallidus changes and moderate diffuse high intensity of the white matter." In other words he had not recovered—he had the typical swelling and oedema of carbon monoxide poisoning, but, despite this, he was not treated. Three weeks after he had been poisoned, the patient started to deteriorate to the point where, 10 days later, he had regressed to a totally withdrawn state, doubly incontinent. This delayed syndrome after an episode of oxygen deprivation was first described in the journal *Archives of Internal Medicine* over 50 years ago.[40] The symptoms the patient developed during this time reads like a compendium of neurological disease, with MRI charting his deterioration. Finally, he received a course of 35 sessions of hyperbaric oxygen treatment with progressive improvement and returned to "near normalcy" after five months. The authors commented that "the contribution of hyperbaric oxygen treatment to the favourable outcome remains uncertain" and the reason given was that such patients "may improve spontaneously."

These are exciting times and we are just beginning to recognise the immense capability of the body to repair itself, from rebuilding the cartilage of a hip joint to making new nerve cells and connections in the brain. The role of the brain in directing recovery is also now emerging with evidence that supports the power of positive thinking; a healthy brain is needed for a healthy body. Haldane was not aware of the intricacies of the Kreb tricarboxylic acid cycle, of stem cells, or the complexities of DNA and the translation of the information it carries in controlling life. He was, nevertheless, acutely aware of the central role of oxygen in recovery and healing, which applies whether it is spontaneous, induced by the placebo effect, or assisted by drugs. Healing *cannot* take place without sufficient oxygen and, when air is not enough, more needs to be given. Using the very latest technologies, the effects can now be followed by measurements, and, in contrast to drugs, oxygen levels can be measured in the tissues. This is true science, but a way of measuring the concentration of oxygen in arteries without arterial puncture is desperately needed.

There is constant debate in hyperbaric circles about "correct" treatment pressures, for example, in brain injury, when, without measuring the arterial oxygen level, knowing the oxygen concentration being breathed and the chamber pressure can only give an indication of the maximum level possible. Fischer and colleagues showed in the New York University study[41] at a constant chamber pressure of 2 ATA, with a full face mask, the arterial oxygen level varies by a massive 44%—from 1.11 ATA to 1.59 ATA, (850–1,140 mm Hg).

We are spending billions on colliding protons in the Large Hadron Collider to satisfy our curiosity about the universe when, at a fraction of the cost, advanced imaging would allow events in the brain from giving more oxygen to be followed in real time. Worldwide publicity followed when a group in Cambridge used functional MRI to follow brain activation when discussing tennis with a 23-year-old girl in coma.[42] An MR imager can be easily fitted into a Boeing 747 and the aircraft pressurised, so that the effects of giving hyperbaric oxygen treatment can be followed in real time and, as for safety, it will not need to leave the ground! Science fiction?—NASA has already modified a Boeing 747SP it named *Sofia* to fly an infrared astronomical telescope to an altitude of 41,000 feet to reduce the effects of atmospheric contamination. The aircraft has been extensively re-engineered with the telescope which, like an MRI, uses liquid helium cooling, isolated in a rear compartment by a pressure bulkhead.

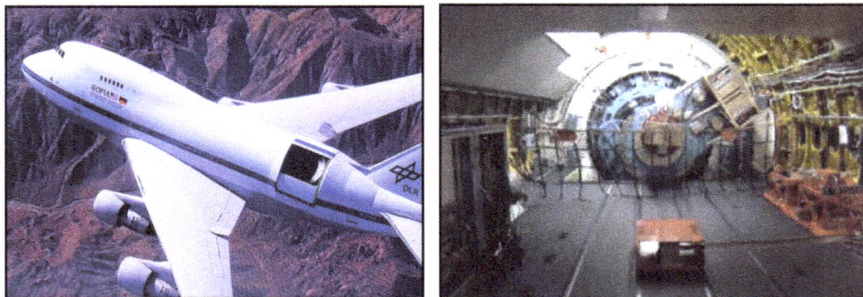

Figure 22.4:
The NASA Boeing 747SP *Sofia* fitted with a liquid helium-cooled telescope.

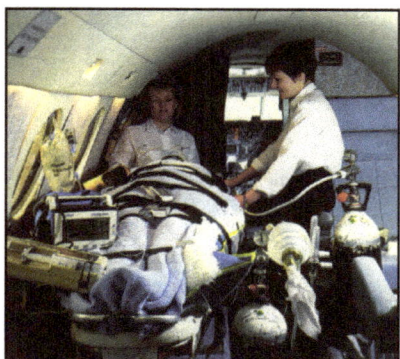

Figure 22.5:
Intensive care in a pressurised aircraft: The windscreens and cockpit instruments are clearly visible.
(Courtesy of the Australian Flying Doctor service.)

Although there has been much discussion in this text of diving and the treatment of bubble-related disease in diving chambers, in fact, clinical hyperbaric treatment is much more closely related to the operation of pressurised aircraft which could bring economies of scale. Unfortunately, this highlights the absurd charges made for clinical hyperbaric treatment, which should be in the tens of dollars per session, rather than thousands.[43] The billing for a single session of hyperbaric oxygen treatment of 90 minutes in a Miami hospital would pay for an eight hour business class flight across the Atlantic! Aircraft have been used to provide intensive care for many years by the flying doctor service in Australia. Ironically, kept on the ground and pressurised, the aircraft used could provide effective hyperbaric oxygen treatment at a pressure as high as 2 ATA.

The irony of spending colossal sums on advanced physics when we do not understand the workings of the brain is being noticed, notably, by President Barack Obama, who has recently unveiled a $100 million dollar project to map the human brain. The stated aim is uncovering new treatments for Alzheimer's disease, Parkinson's disease, and epilepsy. He pointed out that, "As humans, we can identify galaxies light years away, we can study particles smaller than an atom, but we still haven't unlocked the mystery of the three pounds of matter that sits between our ears." The brain has, of course, already been mapped by post-mortem studies and so we will be reinventing the wheel. Other initiatives are even more bizarre: The European community has given an enormous grant to a consortium of universities for a project linking a large number of powerful computers to "simulate" a mouse brain. The stated rationale is also to develop new drugs and, again, Alzheimer's disease features—perhaps electronic drugs can be developed to feed down the power cables. Another billion euros is being sought to build an even larger computer network to simulate the human brain, but it seems that to provide sufficient power it will need its own nuclear power station!

Unfortunately, there can be little doubt that the rejection of hyperbaric oxygen treatment has much to do with fear; fear of the physics involved, the equipment, and even fear of being asked to enter a pressure chamber. This is ironic, since physicians, as a group, are probably among the most frequent users of aircraft and they, of course, *cannot* be made fail-safe. If an aircraft loses pressure at altitude would they demand evidence from controlled trials before donning an oxygen mask? Unlikely—they would be the first to use one, but the "evidence" from controlled trials does not exist nor, indeed, does it exist for the use of a parachute.[44] In fact, hyperbaric oxygen treatment is not, as has been claimed,[45] "high technology," as the experience of the UK MS Therapy Centres has shown over more than 30 years. The equipment is simple and is so safe that it was *deregulated* in the UK by an Act of Parliament in 2008. So, the most powerful agent in medicine can now be controlled by patients! Contrast this with complex medical investigations such as MRI which, costing thousands of dollars, dwarf the cost of providing hyperbaric oxygen treatment but often do not lead to effective treatment. The way forward must be to use oxygen treatment as a first response in brain disorders, with investigations later. Given the huge expenditure we face in providing health care in chronic disease with aging populations, the treatment should be made available at low cost in the community.

In most countries, a government regulatory body dictates the curriculum used by medical schools—in the UK it is the General Medical Council (GMC). The GMC requires students to be taught "oxygen therapy," but without any reference to the importance of barometric pressure. In 2004, the author approached the chairman of the House of Commons Select Committee on Science and Technology, in an attempt to influence the GMC. As a former life scientist, he was convinced by the scientific evidence and, as promised, he wrote to the GMC.[46] The reply, inexplicably, stated that the remit of the council "does not extend to individual treatments and, as a result, the GMC does not have a position on hyperbaric medicine." Nor, by inference, will it have a position on "baric" medicine and so medical students will continue to be taught simply to ensure that blood is red, without any consideration of the need to ensure that tissues have enough oxygen.[47] This gravely mistaken approach is highly relevant to carbon monoxide poisoning where the damage in the brain, initiated by the lack of oxygen, may continue long after the exposure, simply because the lack of oxygen in the tissues of the brain has not been corrected. We will remain in the Dark Ages until *political* action ensures that oxygen treatment is given its rightful place in medicine. Lives continue to be lost every day, when they can easily be saved, and much suffering will go unrelieved at enormous cost—to individuals, their families, and to society as a whole. We simply cannot afford to ignore the value of using oxygen treatment, especially for the brain. As in every situation, the way forward is education. In 1977, Ivan Illich,[48] attacking the epidemic of medically-induced disease in his book *Limits to Medicine: Medical Nemesis* wrote;

> *The layman in medicine, for whom this book is written, will himself have to acquire the competence to evaluate the impact of medicine on health care.*

Unfortunately, this applies to the use of oxygen in treatment but, in contrast to the negativity of Illich's campaign, using oxygen opens a dramatic and exciting new era in medicine. We can now manipulate gene expression safely. So, a *positive* campaign is needed; but it will not be led by medical professionals. Another quote from Ivan Illich is, unfortunately, appropriate:

> *Among all our contemporary experts, physicians are those trained to the highest level of specialised incompetence for this urgently needed pursuit.*

This is not a comfortable assertion, indeed, some may well view it as insulting, but competence only comes with training and knowledge. In fact, much of medical practice is the treatment of hypoxia and medical training must change because it is obvious that there is simply no substitute for oxygen and there never will be.

The two remarkable stories in this book recount the horror of being trapped underground; Jessica was rescued after 58 hours down the well, and Randy McCloy survived 42 hours not only trapped, but poisoned with deadly carbon monoxide in the mine. Both needed a pressure chamber to allow them to breathe a much higher concentration of oxygen than routinely available in most of our hospitals. Without it, Jessica would have lost her leg, Randy his mind and, in all probability, his life. The remarkable success of their treatment highlights a key theme of this book, control of the white blood cells that roam freely in our blood; the neutrophils responsible for the *inflammation*, which are not only central to our resistance to infection, but crucially are also essential for tissue repair by removing non-viable debris, in the process known as auto-immunity.[49] However, if they get out of control, because lack of oxygen persists, neutrophils damage *healthy* tissue. Over the last 70 years, attempts to bring this cell under control using immuno-suppressive drugs have failed spectacularly. With the discoveries that began with the event in Texas, the recognition is finally dawning that, correcting hypoxia with oxygen is the only way that neutrophils can be controlled safely.

Another dramatic development also dates back to Jessica's ordeal; it is called *preconditioning* and it is set to make a radical difference to the practice of medicine. It will be recalled that Dr. Zamboni ligatured the blood supply to muscle for four hours and when the ligature was released, the neutrophils attached to the walls of the veins, eventually blocking blood flow.[50] In one group of animals, the oxygen was given whilst blood flow was obstructed by the ligature and it was successful in stopping the adhesion of neutrophils. In practice, this means that the behaviour of neutrophils can be programmed before potentially adverse events. The timing needs to be researched, but the effect has already been used for patients receiving stents in coronary arteries[51] and prior to cardiac surgery.[52,53]

But there could not be a clearer signal that we desperately need to embrace the simple technology of oxygen treatment than the ending of attempts by pharmaceutical giants to develop drugs to treat the brain. Faced with the rapidly rising costs of care, one thing is certain—we cannot continue to neglect oxygen treatment;[54] adding years to life is pointless without adding life to the years, and the science underpinning the use of oxygen is as certain as life itself. The astonishing developments from biological research over the last decade are finally appearing in the *medical* literature.[55,56] Those who have read and studied this text will now be aware of the unique role of oxygen in healing, but it will come as no surprise to the author if this text is ignored by professional bodies; the phenomenon has been termed "organisational silence."[57] Nevertheless, we must start somewhere; knowledge is power and, as consumers, we must take on the daunting task of changing the world of medicine. President John F. Kennedy, in a speech to Congress in 1962, said:

> *Consumers have the right to safety, the right to be informed, the right to choose, and the right to be heard.*

As patients, we need to assert our rights; each of us must take control of our lives, as the dedicated patients in the UK MS Therapy Centres have done. Over the last 30 years, they have established the safety of oxygen treatment, even to the satisfaction of the UK Parliament. This text with the references provided for each chapter, allows the reader to be informed; the papers have been peer-reviewed and many are available to download from the Internet. It is to be hoped, as Haldane would certainly have wished, that the tide of ignorance that is allowing so much unnecessary suffering to continue, can now be turned. But it will only begin when patients ask for the treatment—for just a few hundred grams more oxygen a day! As Dr. George Mychaskiw, editor of the journal of the Undersea and Hyperbaric Medical Society, has said: The time has come.[58,59]

It would be wrong to end on a negative note when the exciting advances made about oxygen in the biological sciences are beginning to reveal the origins of life—we are spending billions looking for life on other planets, when we do not understand it on our own! Now there is a way to investigate the regulation of our genes safely using the agent central to life, spectacular advances in both managing and preventing disease will surely follow. In contrast to the risks that accompany so many interventions in medical practice—from drug treatment to surgery—the risk of oxygen treatment is of not using it.

John Scott Haldane

Curriculum Vitae

1860	Born in Edinburgh
1870-6	Attended Edinburgh Academy
1876	Entered Edinburgh University
1879	M.A., Edinburgh, Stud. Rer. Nat. Jena
1884	Medical registration with the General Medical Council
1885	M.B. and C.M., Edinburgh
	Began work in chemistry laboratory, University College, Dundee
1886	Worked in Salkowski's laboratory in Berlin
	Member of the Royal College of Physicians of Edinburgh
1887	Work in University Laboratory of Physiology, Oxford
1889	M.D., Edinburgh
1891	Married Louise Kathleen Trotter
1893	Worked on blood gas analysis with Christian Bohr, Copenhagen
1894	Lecturer in Physiology, University of Oxford
1895	Grocers' Company Research Scholar
1896	Matriculated at Oxford as a member of Jesus College
	Fellow of the Royal Society
1901	Elected Fellow of New College, Oxford
	Co-founder and co-editor of the *Journal of Hygiene*, Cambridge
	Received prize with F. G. Meachem for Paper 1.
1899	Appointed a Metropolitan Gas Referee
1904	Awarded, with R.A.Thomas, The Consolidated Gold Fields of South Africa, Ltd. Gold Medal for Paper 3
	Awarded G.C.Greenwell Medal for Paper 1 (of 1903)
1906	Member of the Royal Commission on Mines
1907	Reader in Physiology, University of Oxford
1908	President of the Physiology Section of the British Association for the Advancement of Science

1912	Member of the Royal Commission on Metalliferous Mine and Quarries
	Appointed Director of the Doncaster Coal-Owners' Research Laboratory (Bentley Colliery)
1913	Awarded Baly Medal of the Royal College of Physicians, London
	Resigned from the University of Oxford
1915	Awarded the Gold Medal of the Institution of Mining Engineers
1916	Appointed Silliman Lecturer, Yale University
	Awarded the Royal Medal of the Royal Society
1917	Appointed Member of the Mine Rescue Apparatus Research Committee
1921	Became Gas Referee for the United Kingdom
	Appointed Member of Safety in Mines Research Board
	Elected Honorary Member of the Institution of Mining Engineers Mining Research Laboratory transferred to Birmingham University
1925	Elected President of the Institution of Mining Engineers (and for successive years until 1928)
1926	Awarded Gold Medal of the Royal Society of Medicine
1928	Elected Gifford Lecturer, Glasgow University
1928	Elected Vice-President of the Institution of Mining Engineers Appointed Companion of Honour
1930	Presentation made by the Physiological Society, at Oxford Donnellan Lecturer, Dublin University
1932	Presented with the G. C. Greenwell Gold Medal of the North of England Institute of Mining Engineers
1934	Awarded the Copley Medal of the Royal Society
1935	Honorary Fellow of the Royal Society of Medicine
	Honorary Doctor of Science of Oxford, Cambridge, Dublin, Leeds, and Witwatersrand
	Honorary Doctor of Letters of Edinburgh and Birmingham.
1936	Died in Oxford
	Journal of Hygiene Part 3 of Volume 36 is dedicated to J.S.H. with a photograph as frontispiece.

APPENDIX 2

References to Fat Embolism and Multiple Sclerosis

1. Über Cerebrale Fett - und Luftembolie

Neuburger K. *Klin Woch* 1925;**4**:278-318.

Two lesions: Die Ringblutungen und perivaskuläre Lichtungsbezirke mit rarificierten. Discusses similarity of late lesions of fat embolism to multiple sclerosis and refers to the earlier discussion of myelin damage by Grondahl in 1911.

2. Caisson Disease

Lichtenstein BW, Zeitlin H. Caisson Disease: A histologic study of late lesions. *Arch Path* 1935;**22**:86-98.

Chronic combined degeneration of the cord due to aeropathy (caisson disease) of over 25 years duration is presented. The thoracic portion of the spinal cord is the site of prevalent involvement and of this the white matter is very much more affected than the grey . . . ectodermal and characterised pathologically as anisomorphous gliosis. This condition is best differentiated from multiple sclerosis by detailed study of the areas adjacent to the scars and of those of normal remote regions.

3. Formation of Demyelinated plaques Associated with Cerebral Fat Embolism in Man

Scheinker I.M. *Arch Neurol Psychiat* 1943;**49**:754-64.

"This presentation is concerned with a detailed histopathologic study of the lesions associated with fat embolism. Their analysis revealed certain similarities to the early focal lesions of demyelination occurring in cases of disseminated sclerosis."

". . . again attention should be drawn to their similarity to focal lesions observed in cases of acute multiple sclerosis"

4. Nekrotisierende und Entmarkungsvorgänge bei Cerebraler Gasembolie

Scholtz W, Wechsler W. *Acta Neuropathol* 1961;**1**:85-100.

Tissue changes, due to temporary closure of the vessels occurred chiefly as laminary or as infarction-like elective neuronal necrosis similar in their to-pography to lesions from temporary cerebral ischaemia. Besides these chang-es, spots of pure demyelination, but without any neuronal damage, were present in the cerebral cortex and in the white matter of three cases. Their similarities to and distinctions from foci of multiple sclerosis are discussed.

5. Fat Embolism: A Monograph on the Disease

Sevitt S. Fat Embolism, Butterworths, London 1964.

An important character of the lesions in white matter is shown in preparations for myelin which reveals them as plaques of perivascular de-myelination. In many foci all the myelin sheaths have disappeared centrally, but some are preserved in other lesions giving the appearance of the myelin shadow plaque. Early lesions generally contain more myelin than older ones and are only partly demyelinated; some of the myelin present is swollen or fragmented but many other sheaths appear intact.

It is not impossible that some of the demyelination is only apparent and that the local separation of myelin sheaths may be partly due to focal oedema.

Foci where axons are swollen and free of myelin are a characteristic feature or stage, as shown in the periphery of the lesion. However, in some lesions most of the axis cylinders appear normal suggesting the possibility of recovery.

Scheinker thought that the demyelinated foci were like the early lesions of multiple sclerosis. This is largely true . . .

6. Further Notes on Traumatic Fat Embolism: Comparison of Nervous Lesions with those of Multiple Sclerosis

Courville CB. *Bull Los Ang Neurol Soc* 1964;**29**:143-49.

In addition many of the microscopic features were also similar to those of the plaques of multiple sclerosis. In fact only the obvious freshness of these lesions (6 days) constituted the essential difference.

In this case, fat embolism to all portions of the spinal cord, but especially in the central grey matter, were abundant even after the short survival period of 7.5 hours. It is thus made clear that fat embolisms after trauma are to be found only in locations within the nervous system where plaques of multiple sclerosis have been observed.

7. Pathogenic Mechanisms in the Leucoencephalopathies, in Anoxic Ischaemic Processes in Disorders of the Blood and in Intoxication

Lumsden CE. Chapter 20. In; Vinken PJ, Bruyn GW, eds. Handbook of clinical neurology. Amsterdam, North Holland, 1970;572-663.

The second lesion is one, the frequency of which has only recently been recognised. These characteristic, minor - traumatic lesions can simulate early multiple sclerosis plaques quite remarkably.

The vast numbers of lesions attending classical instances of fat embolism are always very striking and one cannot help feeling that sporadic and clinically silent lesions must commonly be associated with many non-fatal fractures and soft tissue trauma of minor, even trivial degree.

8. Zur Klinik des Dekompressionstraumas bei Tauchunfällen

Gerstenbrand F, Pallua A. Clinical study of Decompression disease caused by diving accidents. In; von Gerstenbrand F, Lorenzoni E, Seemann K. Eds. Tauchmedizin. Schlutersche, Verlagsanstalt und Druckerei GmbH & Co Hannover 1980.

A comparison of decompression sickness and fat embolism, mentioning multiple sclerosis and emphasising the disturbance of the blood-brain barrier and focal oedema in demyelination.

9. A Rarely Reported Multifocal Demyelinating Disease: Pancreatic Encephalopathy

Brucher JM, De Smet Y, Gonsette RE. In; Immunological and clinical aspects of multiple sclerosis. Gonsette RE, Delmotte P eds. MTP Press Ltd., Lancaster, England 1986.

Reporting two cases of pancreatic encephalopathy, the authors emphasise the ability of enzymes to destroy myelin either directly, a hypothesis already suggested by Joseph Balo as far back as 1940 in a case of diffuse sclerosis of the Schilder type or indirectly through released fatty acids, a hypothesis sustained by the evidence for subacute fat embolism as the cause of MS.

10. Evidence for Subacute Fat Embolism as the Cause of Multiple Sclerosis

James PB. *Lancet* 1982;**i**:380-386.

The neurological features of decompression sickness, which is thought to be due to gas embolism, are similar to those of multiple sclerosis (MS). There is also evidence in man that fat may lodge in the microcirculation of the nervous system and cause distal perivenous oedema with loss of myelin from axons. Since acute fat embolism may produce lesions not only in the white matter of the brain, but also in the cord, the retina, the meninges and the skin, and since all these have been described in MS, subacute fat embolism may be the cause of MS.

APPENDIX 3

Anecdotes—The Patients' Stories

It is often claimed that knowledge multiplies so rapidly that nobody can follow it. I believe that this is incorrect. At least in science it is not true. The main purpose of science is simplicity and as we understand more things everything is becoming simpler.

Dr. Edward Teller, 1908–2003

These reports of the benefit experienced by patients from using oxygen under hyperbaric conditions illustrate the unique importance of oxygen to recovery from every injury or illness. No one doubts that breathing is essential to life but, clearly, many fail to recognise that it underpins all healing. Sceptics often claim that patients can get better without the additional oxygen provided in a chamber and they may be correct, but this improvement does not happen without oxygen—it happens because of the oxygen we gain from breathing. However, as we all know, healing may stall, or stop altogether. This often happens because diseases and injuries are associated with prolonged and damaging lack of oxygen which is, most importantly, associated with continuing inflammation. So the naysayers are, in effect, claiming that the dosage of oxygen we gain from breathing air—at whatever the barometric pressure is where we happen to be—is the best dose.

An obvious question raised by hyperbaric oxygen treatment is simply: Why does the lack of oxygen and inflammation return after a session? The answer is simple: It is because the blood vessels in damaged tissue need time to be reformed because when tissues are injured or diseased, the process not only affects the cells of the tissues, it affects their adjacent capillaries. This indicates that a threshold needs to be reached in restoring the microcirculation for normal oxygen levels to finally be re-established. These stories collected over the years reflect the many facets of the clinical use of oxygen treatment from the very young to the very old.

Hyperbaric Treatment of Acute Eczema

A baby boy just 19 weeks old developed eczema and was scratching his scalp and body to the point of bleeding. Every remedy was tried but to no avail, and his distraught parents could only resort to cutting his finger nails

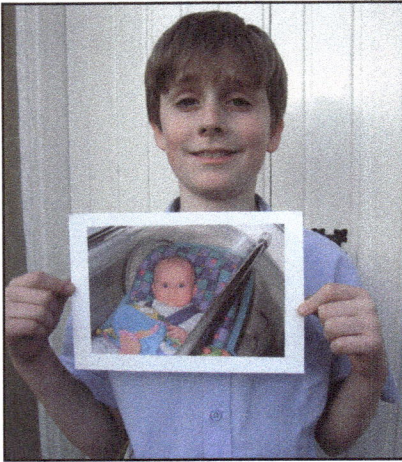

The patient, now a young man, holding the picture of himself as a baby in the Vickers hyperbaric chamber.

and bandaging his hands. Knowing of their distress, a friend who had benefitted from hyperbaric oxygenation who knew it controls inflammation suggested an opinion should be sought at a local teaching hospital hyperbaric unit. Within days, the little boy started daily sessions of an hour treated at 2 ATA in the pure oxygen atmosphere of a Vickers chamber. The benefit was visible after just a few sessions and, after a total of just six, the redness had faded and he stopped scratching altogether. He has not looked back and even a bout of chicken pox a year later did not rekindle his eczema. Clearly, if gene down-regulation can be achieved early they may stay "down-regulated" and avoid years of misery.

A similarly dramatic effect was seen in a 54-year-old man almost suicidal with a bout of the severe eczema he had suffered from since childhood. He reported relief from the pain and intense itch minutes after breathing oxygen at 2 ATA. A course of 12 sessions led to a major reduction in the severity of his eczema which has persisted, without further treatment, for over five years.

Hyperbaric Oxygen Treatment Restores a Patient's Speech

A 39-year-old professor of civil engineering had an upper respiratory virus infection and lost his voice. When about two weeks had passed, his family doctor arranged an appointment with an ear nose and throat specialist who found severe swelling of the vocal chords. Another week passed without resolution; he could only whisper and the sore throat continued. A session of hyperbaric oxygen treatment was undertaken at 2 ATA in a multi-person chamber. Upon removing his mask after just 20 minutes he was able to speak normally, and he completed the session of one hour. The following day his throat discomfort had returned although his voice was normal and two more sessions were undertaken on successive days with complete resolution. A similar episode two years later was treated more promptly again with success.

Problems from Lumbar Puncture Resolved with Hyperbaric Oxygen Treatment

A lady in her mid-forties felt mildly unwell for a couple of days and woke during the early hours of a Friday morning with a severe headache. After she vomited the pain began to subside, and about 30 minutes later she was able to go back to sleep. Over the weekend she felt fine, but her husband, who was working abroad, suggested a consultation with the family doctor and she was admitted to hospital that Monday. During the week she had two CT examinations of her head, the second with an injected dye. A sample of spinal fluid was obtained by lumbar puncture on the third attempt. She finally returned home that Friday evening with a headache and rested on Saturday, experiencing odd transient sensations in the fingertips of her right hand. On Sunday morning she woke with a bad headache, feeling sick and shaky. The symptoms were relieved within 20 minutes in a chamber, breathing oxygen at 2 ATA, and a one-hour session was completed. The patient described the relief as amazing. Some of the mild transient strange sensations persisted. She had additional treatment sessions and they slowly resolved over the subsequent weeks. Although initially stating that this patient had suffered a "mild" brain haemorrhage, the hospital consultant later admitted that there had been contamination of the specimen. The use of 100% oxygen, both to prevent and to treat lumbar puncture headache, was discovered in the 1930s.

Hyperbaric Oxygen Treatment of Rheumatoid Arthritis and Lung Damage

This patient suffered from rheumatoid arthritis for many years but, with frequent hand surgery, was able to continue working until 2001, at the age of 55. He was maintained on steroids and morphine to control his joint pain, and had a course of gold injections. He developed breathlessness and cough which became persistent. In May 2006, he was told that he had end-stage pulmonary fibrosis—lung scarring—and that his life expectancy without a lung transplant, was two months to, at most, two years. The word "hypoxia" had been used frequently and the patient found the website of a hyperbaric unit in a local teaching hospital. Supplementary oxygen had been prescribed for 15 hours a day, and being a physicist, this puzzled him: What about the other nine hours in the day? There is no scientific evidence to support this restriction and he started supplementary oxygen 24 hours a day. He began to feel much better in the mornings with less pain. In 2006, the latest immuno-suppressive drug used for patients after lung transplantation was prescribed by a specialist in London: It made him very ill. He stopped the drug and started a course of treatment in a local hospital hyperbaric unit. After five hourly sessions at 2 ATA, his coughing was dramatically reduced and he was able to walk out of the hospital holding a normal conversation. After further treatment and later sessions in a charity chamber he bought his own unit. His lung function tests in August 2008 had improved by more than 10% and the laboratory scientist commented that he had never seen a patient with this form of lung fibrosis improve. Since 2006, he has not used any immuno-suppressive drugs: It is clear that both his lung and joint disease are due to inflammation, not auto-immunity. The redness and swelling of his hands and the Heberden nodes on his knuckles have long since disappeared: The skin is pearly white. The steroid medication for his arthritis has been greatly reduced and he no longer needs to use morphia. It is ironic that many pulmonary specialists believe that oxygen is toxic to the lungs and would strongly advise patients against hyperbaric oxygen treatment. Now in his seventh year from his diagnosis of terminal lung disease, and despite deteriorating lung func-tion, he has started a new charitable hyperbaric facility for others to benefit. One has been the young lady in the next story diagnosed as having juvenile rheumatoid arthritis.

Rheumatoid Arthritis in a Young Person Controlled by Oxygen Treatment

At the age of 10, this healthy, fit young lady suffered from an unknown virus infection that left her fatigued for months. She continued to suffer fa-tigue on joining high school and was prone to virus infections. In her third year she was complaining of cold, painful hands even on warm days, and by the age of 14, her problems escalated with pains in the joints of her hands and debilitating headaches. After many visits to the family doctor, the label of Raynaud's disease was suggested: It is not usually associated with pain, but by this time the joint pain was affecting her ability to write and even hold a cup of tea. A consultant thought it was most likely that she was developing "auto-immune" disease and prescribed the drug hydroxychloroquine. This caused nausea and the parents discontinued it after researching its side effects. How-ever, their daughter's symptoms worsened and headaches and fatigue kept her off school for several days at a time. Pain developed in almost all of her joints and, at 16, it was a major effort for her to cope with her examinations. The school even suggested that she not return until she was well again. At another hospital review hydroxychloroquine was again prescribed together with gabapentin and celecoxib; they had no effect on her joint pain and headaches and caused constant nausea. Unable to tolerate the unpleasant drug side effects she reverted back to using paracetamol and ibuprofen. At this point, a trial of hyperbaric oxygen treatment was suggested with a course of 20 sessions over four weeks. The parents were told to play down expectations. The day after the first session the patient asked her father if oxygen could help her to sleep: She had just slept through the night for the first time in months. Her parents report that "from that point on she has been full of energy and active in a way we hadn't seen for years." After five sessions she said that, although her fingers were still sore, the pain in all her larger joints had gone. After the eighth treatment session she told her father that she couldn't find a pain anywhere in her body: All the swelling had gone from her fingers and the headaches had stopped.

A year has passed and she continues weekly sessions. This keeps most of her symptoms under control, although if it is missed her symptoms worsen. She still suffers some pain in her hands, which is worse in cold weather. Her father recalls that these symptoms are exacerbated in times of stress, especially during examinations. Nevertheless, with one hour of hyperbaric oxygen treatment—out of the 168 hours of a week—his daughter is living a normal, active teenager's life, rarely affected by headaches and, apart from an occasional paracetamol tablet, takes no medication. She has even taken up athletics and competed in her first national competition. With missing very little school over the past year she has performed well academically and hopes to gain a place at university in the near future.

Hyperbaric Oxygen Treatment for Steroid-Induced Hip Damage

A 40-year-old man, who experienced sudden hearing loss in June 2013, was given steroid treatment. Two months later he developed pain in both hips and MRI showed the typical bone damage to the femoral heads that is occasionally associated with steroid medication. He was referred for hyperbaric oxygen treatment but developed nausea during his first session breathing oxygen at 2 ATA. Unsuccessful attempts were made to reduce this effect by interrupting oxygen breathing with periods breathing air. Measurements made of his blood glucose when breathing oxygen in the chamber at 2 ATA showed a dramatic fall from 120 to less than 50 mg/dl over 20 minutes.

Measurements were also made of the oxygen levels in the skin of his feet breathing 100% oxygen at 2 ATA, which showed the oxygen level fell, paradoxically, to less than 15 mm Hg—typical values breathing air at 1 ATA are over 40 mm Hg. Despite the problems, the patient reported relief of his pain. Investigation of the patient is continuing in order to devise a suitable protocol for continuing his treatment. His response provides confirmation that the so-called toxicity of oxygen affecting the brain is due to the constriction of blood vessels causing a reduction of the availability of glucose, as detailed in Chapter 8. All the symptoms ascribed to oxygen toxicity are typical of a hypoglycaemic attack. Because the patient's blood glucose level was measured in blood from a finger, the constriction of blood flow appears to be affecting the normal control of blood glucose levels. This will obviously reduce the supply available to the brain.

Treating Injured Legs with Oxygen Includes the Brain

In 2009, a 64-year-old professor of theoretical physics in Israel was hit by a car crossing the street near his home in Tel Aviv, sustaining severe injuries to his head and legs. After life-saving surgery he spent several weeks in intensive care in a critical condition. His feet were so badly damaged that amputations seemed inevitable. However, he was even more distraught to find that his ability to think had been severely impaired and his memory almost destroyed. As he slowly recovered, still in hospital, his new book covering a very complex area of science and advanced mathematics arrived from his publishers: He was horrified to find he did not understand a single formula. In fact, he could not even understand why he had written the book. With amputations seeming inevitable, it was decided to send him to the hyperbaric facility in Haifa to try and save his feet, although not, of course, his brain—at least according to the stricture of the medical insurers that reimburse treatment in Israel. His feet soon began to heal and the threat of amputation receded, but what was even more dramatic was that his cognitive ability started to return. Steadily over weeks of hyperbaric oxygen treatment, his book began to make sense and his understanding of his research returned. This astonishing recovery of his faculties was witnessed by visiting friends—professors working in applied mathematics, chemistry, and physics. Soon they were discussing the failure of mainstream medicine to understand the physics of oxygen transport and to use oxygen as a treatment. The first result of their efforts, guided by the treating physician, Dr. Yehuda Melamed, was the publication of a paper in a leading international physico-chemical journal. (See Ref: No. 8, Chapter 12.)

Is the Brain a Soft Tissue? Not when Hyperbaric Oxygen Treatment is Needed!

Over the period that the professor from Tel Aviv was being treated, a bizarre case was being heard in a high court in Israel to decide if the brain is actually a soft tissue. The Israeli Health Ministry had approved the use of hyperbaric oxygen treatment of soft tissue damage from radiotherapy in 1986. However, the Israeli insurers, Kopat Holim, refused to meet a claim for reimbursement after hyperbaric oxygen treatment from a 52-year-old patient who developed progressively failing vision and unsteadiness after radiotherapy for leukaemia. The damage was confirmed by MRI and, after finding information about hyperbaric oxygen treatment on the Internet, the patient contacted the hyperbaric facility in Haifa. He had dramatic benefit from 40 sessions of hyperbaric oxygen treatment at 2 ATA, five days a week, and he was able to return to work. On being refused reimbursement, he enlisted the help of Dr. Melamed and opinions from other experts, including the author. The case came to court and after five hearings over four years, the judge upheld the patient's claim ruling that the brain is indeed a soft tissue!

A Dedicated Wife Proves that the Brain May Not be Dead but Sleeping

This story begins on May 1, 1997, when the patient collapsed at the age of 55 with a brain haemorrhage. Airlifted in coma back to his home city of Dallas, a neurosurgeon reluctantly operated, however the patient remained in coma for six months. After he regained consciousness he spent six months in rehabilitation hospitals unable to converse and fed by naso-gastric tube. His wife had researched treatment and, finding hyperbaric medicine, she spoke to many doctors, including Dr. Richard Neubauer, but it was considered that the patient was too ill to fly to Florida. In fact, three years were to pass before treatment became possible. After eight sessions in August 2000, improvement was obvious and it was ongoing: Following 25 sessions he had major improvements in speech and short term memory, he could walk without assistance, and he regained bladder function. In February 2001, he consolidated the improvement with a second course of 40 sessions. He had further brain haemorrhages in 2005 and 2010, not to mention two heart attacks, a knee implant, and hip surgery after a fall. His wife continued to organise hyperbaric treatment for his problems. She now owns and operates a hyperbaric facility, where he has several sessions a week. Today, 16 years after it was suggested that he should be an organ donor, he still enjoys life. Clearly SPECT imaging would have allowed the sleeping areas of the brain to have been identified with the improvement from the additional oxygen provided under hyperbaric conditions. His wife is a leading figure in the patient movement, the American Association for Hyperbaric Awareness.

Torture by "Diagnosis": A Multiple Sclerosis Patient's Story

In Chapter 14, the nonsense of calling the terms "multiple" and "sclerosis" a diagnosis was discussed. Clearly, neither a patient nor, indeed, a neurologist wants this label applied and it is often years before the nettle is grasped. It is said that multiple sclerosis is more common in the islands around Scotland than mainland UK following epidemiological studies in the 1950s in the Shetlands. This patient, from an island on the west coast of Scotland, had migraines as a teenager and suffered from episodes of vertigo in her 20s. Her father had been told she had multiple sclerosis. At the age of 29 she abruptly lost feeling down the left side of her body and the inside of her mouth, and was examined by the family doctor who at the time thought she was developing multiple sclerosis. The symptoms slowly disappeared over the following year but, when she was 36, she lost the vision in her right eye. This resolved over several months, but again there was no specialist referral. In her 40s she began suffering excessive fatigue and falling without explanation, with one episode leaving her with severe lower back pain and right leg weakness. By this time short courses of steroids were being prescribed by general practitioners and eventually, after waiting a year, she was seen by a neurologist in a hospital on the mainland. An attempt at lumbar puncture failed but, despite MRI revealing four bright areas in her brain and the long history of neurological symptoms, it was not considered that there was enough evidence for a "diagnosis" of multiple sclerosis to be made. With relapses in her 50s several times a year and courses of steroid treatment and hospital admissions, a repeat MRI confirmed the affected areas. She was finally told she did, indeed, have progressive multiple sclerosis, only to have the "diagnosis" questioned months later by another neurologist, who wanted the label changed to "probable multiple sclerosis." And so this dismal story continues.

A "Clinically Isolated Syndrome" After a Bruise – Is it Multiple Sclerosis?

On a Sunday morning, a family of four was having breakfast expecting to go to church, but as they finished the daughter, a young lady of 14, said she did not feel very well. Her mother suggested that she go back to bed but, on attempting to stand up the girls's left leg buckled and she fell to the floor. The bewildered family watched helplessly as, over minutes, both legs became paralysed. The family doctor made an urgent house visit and she was bundled into a car and taken to a well-known hospital in Glasgow. A history was taken, she was examined, and lumbar puncture was done, although no diagnosis was offered to the distraught parents. A day later a steroid treatment was started but by the end of the week the girl was still unable to stand. Her parents were told that the diagnosis was an "'acute transverse myelitis"—a description of damage across the spinal cord, but not a diagnosis, and it was "probably due to a virus." Later it was recalled that she had bruising to a leg two days before collapsing from playing hockey. Is it possible that a simple bruise may cause such a devastating illness? Indeed it can—a simple bruise can be fatal and we have seen that the mechanisms are understood. Her parents discharged her from hospital in order to obtain hyperbaric oxygen treatment and within days she was walking again, although some mild bladder problems persisted.

A Doctor with Multiple Sclerosis Recovers from an Attack Using More Oxygen

This doctor, newly qualified in 1982, self "diagnosed" her multiple sclerosis from neurological signs she found during her training at a Scottish medical school; it was later confirmed by a neurologist. In June of 1982, she had visited the author to discuss the author's *Lancet* publication of February 13th that year "Subacute Fat Embolism as the Cause of Multiple Sclerosis." Her comment was direct: It was the only explanation she had read that made sense. She took up a residency in a seaside town in southwest England and, on a weekend off, went to Bristol to be with friends. On the Saturday evening they went to a local hotel and she had just sat down when she began to feel unwell: The room began spinning round with the onset of acute vertigo. She was violently sick and her friends took her to their lodgings but the oral steroids she carried made no difference. After a couple of days she was taken to the residency of her hospital, then admitted to a ward and given intravenous fluids. Some days later, still feeling ill, she appealed to her family to take her back to Scotland and she was duly driven north a few days later. She had read in the Addendum of the *Lancet* paper the account of a young man successfully treated with hyperbaric oxygenation and her family telephoned to ask if she could also be treated. This required a further journey north and she has daily sessions at 2 ATA for 12 days with dramatic improvement. The vertigo and nausea disappeared after the first treatment with continuing improvement in balance and bladder function over the course of treatment. Over the subsequent years she has had several more attacks successfully treated.

Doctor Reacts to a Patient Reporting Benefit from Hyperbaric Oxygen Treatment

This patient, who has a progressive form of multiple sclerosis, attended her local hospital for a routine six monthly appointment. After having had several months of hyperbaric oxygen treatment she was excited to report the benefit she had experienced and, for once, was accompanied by her husband. The island community of about 70,000 was considered too small for a full-time neurologist to be employed and the role was taken by a general physician, who had seen the patient regularly for over 12 years. The tests showed great improvement in the patient's vision and her nystagmus had disappeared, but the patient saw that the doctor was clearly becoming very annoyed. On further reporting that the improvement in her trigeminal neuralgia had allowed her to discontinue drug therapy, the doctor pushed his chair back and aggressively stated that none of this could be the result of hyperbaric oxygen treatment: It was all in her mind. By this time, the patient said that he was shaking uncontrollably with rage—she had never seen anyone so angry in her life. The clinic nurse was visibly shocked by the doctor's behaviour and concerned for the patient. The doctor barked that she should leave and threw the door open. Her husband found great difficulty controlling his desire to intervene with physical action.

Oxygen Treatment Beneficial 45 Years After Inflammation from a Spinal Injection

This former Merchant Navy officer developed back pain from a disc problem in July 1966 at the age of 27 and early in January 1967 had surgery. He developed further difficulties over the next few months and an X-ray agent called Myodil was injected in an attempt to define the problem. However, his disabilities prevented him from returning to sea and he was eventually employed by a company providing work for the disabled. He had a second injection of Myodil investigating his back problem in 1976 and continued working for a further 19 years, although with much time off sick. By 1987, his mobility had become severely impaired and he had to stop work altogether. Three years later he became aware of the publicity about the problems that derive from retained Myodil after lumbar puncture and a scan confirmed that the dye was still present. It was trapped in the membranes which cover the spinal cord at the bottom of the spine, causing chronic inflammation and pain. Because of his previous back surgery it was decided that another operation to remove the dye posed too much risk. He continued to deteriorate, only able to walk with a slow shuffle, with chronic pain, and he needed modifications to his home to cope. As he thought his disability was rather like multiple sclerosis, in 2012 he discussed hyperbaric oxygen treatment with his family doctor and started sessions in a local charity centre. After 20 one-hour sessions five days a week, he was able to walk properly—without the slow shuffling gait—and he has become much more active in his community. On reducing his treatment to just one session a week he lost a little of the benefit, but remains very much more active and has little pain.

Dr. Oliver Sacks and *Awakenings*—The Stories Neurology has Forgotten

The influenza epidemic that began during WW1 and vanished in 1926 left a legacy known as Encephalitis lethargica. The term relates to persisting symptoms with profound fatigue from the most feared complication of the illness, inflammation of the brain. In his book *Awakenings*, Dr. Sacks, a British neurologist, recounts the story of Miss R., a talented, rich, and privileged young lady of 21, who went to bed in normal health. After a night of dramatic dreams her family found her in a strange contorted state, unable to speak. The family physician diagnosed "catatonia" and said that she would recover in a week. She did not and she remained profoundly disabled in a trance-like state with constant spasms and terrifying crises. She was first looked after at home but, in 1935, she was admitted to Mount Carmel Hospital in New York. Dr. Sacks administered the drug leva dopamine on the June 18, 1969, 43 years after the onset of her illness, with dramatic results. He was astonished to find that by the 6th of July Miss R. had been free of her crises for eight days and was able to walk unaided for 600 yards between hospital buildings. She was elated but after some days, the response to the drug began to fail and new neurological symptoms appeared, together with acute paranoia. By the end of August 1969, the awful symptoms had returned and her face assumed a horrified, tortured expression. Attempts were made over the next three years to improve matters with further courses of leva dopamine at differing dosages but, sadly, they failed. Dr. Sacks recorded many dramatic, although usually fleeting improvements in patients with Encephalitis lethargica, and a film based on the remarkable events at Mount Carmel Hospital, which starred Robert De Niro and Robin Williams, distributed by Columbia Pictures in 1990, has now been virtually forgotten. What the drug demonstrated beyond doubt is that improvement is possible in some apparently intransigent neurological diseases.

Brain Injury: Late Benefit from Hyperbaric Oxygen Treatment Followed by MRI

This patient, now 58 years old, was injured in a motor vehicle accident after colliding with a wall at speed in January 2004. He had a prolonged period of loss of consciousness, was hospitalised in intensive care, and later developed seizures. After months of recovering he began to run his disaster restoration business, but continued to decline and eventually became unable to manage his own affairs. He was diagnosed as suffering from the delayed effects of head injury; the medical term being "chronic traumatic encephalopathy." He was admitted to intensive care in January 2012 with bacterial meningitis, and following successful treatment, he returned home. He was evaluated by a physician on August 8, 2012 who found he was apathetic and emotionally flat. He did not volunteer information and would respond only when prodded and with single words. He was not eating regular meals and said he was frequently lost when driving. An EEG done in August 2012 was abnormal, demonstrating intermittent slowing of activity over the temporal lobes. Initial MR scans of the brain with diffusion tensor imaging (DTI) was also undertaken and showed damage with loss of fibre tracts. He had 40 one-hour sessions of HBOT at 1.5 ATA. On June 3, 2013 he was much more animated than at his initial appointment; indeed he was argumentative, which his doctor records as an obvious improvement! He is now able to drive around town without getting lost. His follow-up brain MRI, again with DTI,

	August 2012	June 2013
No. of nerve fibre tracts	619	791
Nerve fibre tract volume (cu mm)	5,287	5,517

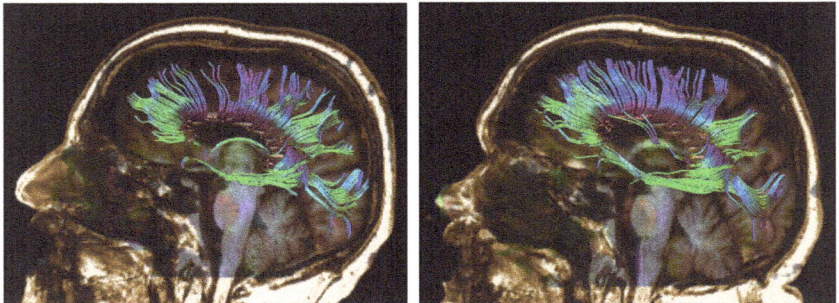

DTI from August 2012 (left) and June 2013 (right). (Courtesy of Dr. Carol Henricks.)

demonstrated improvement of the nerve fibre tracts in the bridge of fibres that connects the hemispheres known as the corpus callosum.

Predictably, some fibre tracts showed mild deterioration despite the improvement recorded in all other values. His physician observes that this is a remarkable recovery nine years post-injury and suggests that we need to continue to pursue research and hyperbaric oxygen treatment protocols. Clearly, as argued in Chapter 19, hyperbaric oxygen treatment should be used in the first hours following injury, not nine years later.

A Veteran Improves from Brain Injury with Hyperbaric Oxygen Treatment

This patient, a US Army soldier deployed to Iraq, was injured in a mortar attack on his position in 2008 at the age of 45 years. After waking from a brief loss of consciousness, he had a headache which proved resistant to treatment and he also had cognitive problems. He was assessed at an army base in Washington state but, in the absence of his medical records and documentation of the blast injury, he was diagnosed with a "conversion disorder"—old fashioned hysteria, implying that there was no "organic" basis for his symptoms. Civilian specialists later diagnosed him with persistent post-concussion syndrome and post-traumatic stress disorder. He was referred for participation in a study of hyperbaric oxygen treatment at the LSU School of Medicine in New Orleans, where his history was reviewed and he received a physical examination and cognitive testing. He had 16 pieces of shrapnel in his left arm visible on X-rays, as well as neurological abnormalities. In July 2009, SPECT brain imaging was undertaken before HBO treatment, after a single HBO treatment, and then after 40 HBO treatments. Improvement was visualised on the pre- and post-SPECT imaging, especially on the blast-injured left side of the brain.

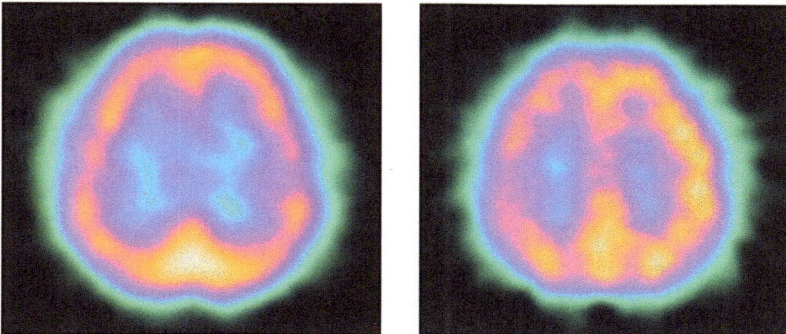

Pre   Post

(Courtesy of Dr. Paul Harch, MD.)

It should be noted that it is difficult to produce sliced images at exactly the same level, but the improvement in blood flow evident from the colour change from red to yellow in the left hemisphere is obvious. All SPECT imaging was performed under identical conditions with expert processing and three-dimensional "thresholding" by Dr. Phillip J. Tranchina. The patient reported that his symptoms had improved and he became less anxious and depressed. However, the post-traumatic checklist—military (PCL-M) did not change with the hyperbaric treatment. Unfortunately, doctors continue to discount the patient's story and constantly look for "objective evidence from tests which often are far more expensive than giving a little more oxygen." As more veterans have committed suicide on returning from Iraq and Afghanistan than have been killed in action and the technology is available to study the benefits in real time, government action is mandatory. It is obviously unscientific to claim that oxygen is a placebo: Breathing underpins all improvement in patients with brain injury!

Hyperbaric Treatment of a Four-Year-Old Boy with Autism

Right-sided SPECT images of brain blood flow of a four-year-old child before and after 10 hyperbaric treatments of one hour at 1.3 ATA. He developed autism aged eighteen months, shortly after vaccination with MMR. Red/yellow areas represent return of normal blood flow. The patient showed striking improvements in behaviour, memory, and cognitive function. He became affectionate, started pointing, verbalising, and began interacting with people. This case report confirms the benefits at 1.3 ATA demonstrated in the UDAAN study discussed in Chapter 12 (reference 23). From: Hyperbaric oxygenation for cerebral palsy and the brain-injured child. Best Publishing Company, 2002. The May 7, 2014 issue of *JAMA*, which is devoted to child health, includes research which reinforces the importance of environmental factors in autism.

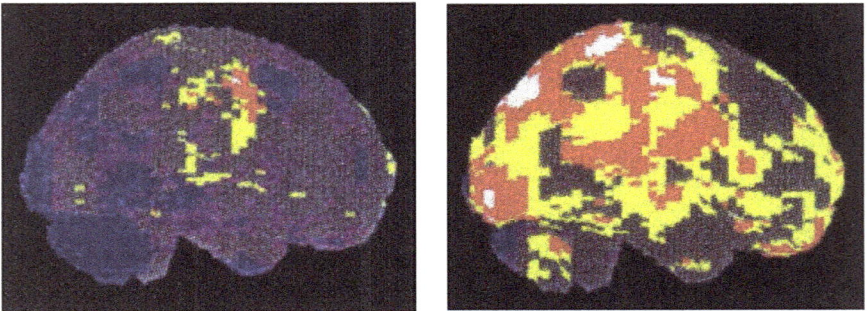

(Courtesy of Drs. Gunnar Heuser and Michael Uszler.)

REFERENCES

Introduction

1. Dai J, Swaab DF, Buijs RM. Recovery of axonal transport in "dead neurons." *Lancet* 1998;**351**:499-500.
2. Astrup J, Siesjo BK, Symon L. Thresholds in cerebral ischemia - the ischemic penumbra. *Stroke* 1981;**12**:723-725.
3. Steindler DA, Pincus DW. Stem cells and neuropoiesis in the adult human brain. *Lancet* 2002;**359**:1047-1054.
4. Bayes-Genis A, Salido M, Ristol FS, et al. Host cell-derived cardiomyocytes in sex-mismatch cardiac allografts. *Cardiovasc Res* 2002;**56**:404-410.
5. Quaini F, Urbanek K, Beltrami AP et al. Chimerism of the transplanted heart. *N Eng J Med* 2002;**346**:5-15.
6. British Thoracic Society Guideline for emergency oxygen use in adult patients. *Thorax* 2008;**63**:Supplement VI.
7. Lane N. Power Sex and Suicide. Oxford University Press, Oxford 2005.
8. Lane N. Life Ascending. Publisher Profile Books, London 2009.
9. Money Report; Pfizer marketing budget for Lipitor by 2002, estimated by Lehman Brothers as $1.3 billion. International Herald Tribune, March 1st 2003.

Chapter 1: Setting the Scene

1. Sagan L. On the origin of mitosing cells. *J Theor Biol* 1967;**14**:225-274.
2. Lee WL, Harrison RE, Grinstein S. Phagocytosis by neutrophils. *Microbes Infect* 2003;**5**:1344.
3. Schneider EM, Flacke S, Liu F, et al. Autophagy and ATP-induced anti-apoptosis in antigen presenting cells (APC) follows the cytokine storm in patients after major trauma. *J Cell Commun Signal* 2011;**5**:145-156.
4. Mitchell P. Coupling of phosphorylation to electron and hydrogen transfer by a chemi-osmotic type of mechanism. *Nature* 1961;**161**:144–148.
5. Lane N. Oxygen: the molecule that made the world. Oxford University Press 2002.
6. de Monchaux N. Spacesuit: fashioning Apollo. MIT Press 2011.
7. Fridovich I. Oxygen is Toxic! *Bioscience* 1977;**27**:462-466.
8. Fridovich I. Hypoxia and oxygen toxicity. *Adv Neurol* 1979;**26**:255-259.
9. Cramer T, Yamanishi Y, Clausen BE, et al. HIF-1alpha is essential for myeloid cell-mediated inflammation. Cell 2003;112:645-657.

10. Bailey-Serres J, Chang R. Sensing and signaling in response to oxygen deprivation in plants and other organisms. *Ann Bot* 2005;**96**:507-518.

11. Kim JW, Tchernyshyov I, Semenza GL, Dang CV. HIF-1-mediated expression of pyruvate dehydrogenase kinase: a metabolic switch required for cellular adaptation to hypoxia. *Cell Metab* 2006;**3**:177-185.

12. Husain J, Juurlink BHJ. Oligodendroglial precursor cell susceptibility to hypoxia is related to poor ability to cope with reactive oxygen species. *Brain Res* 1995;**698**:86-89.

13. Delektorskii VV, Anton'ev AA, Nomnoeva TN, et al. Ultrastructural changes in the mitochondria of patients with scleroderma during treatment with hyperbaric oxygenation. *Vestn Dermatol Venerol* 1987;**11**:20-27.

14. Brierley JB, Cooper JE. Cerebral complications of hypotensive anaesthesia in a healthy adult. *J Neurol* 1962;**25**:24-30.

15. Simpson A. Compressed air as a therapeutic agent in the treatment of consumption, asthma, chronic bronchitis and other diseases. Sutherland and Knox, Edinburgh, 1857.

16. Nunn JF. Applied Respiratory Physiology. Butterworth-Heineman 1993.

17. Kramer MR, Springer C, Berkman N, et al. Rehabilitation of hypoxemic patients with COPD at low altitude at the dead sea, the lowest place on earth. *Chest* 1998;**113**:571-575.

18. Medawar PB. The behaviour of mammalian skin epithelium under strictly anaerobic conditions. *Quart J Micr Sci* 1947;**88**:27-37.

19. Nathan C. Oxygen and the inflammatory cell. *Nature* 2003;**422**:675-676.

20. Ratcliffe PJ. HIF 1 and HIF 2: Working alone or together in hypoxia? *J Clin Invest* 2007;**117**:862-865.

21. Li QF, Wang XR, Yang Yw, Lin H. Hypoxia upregulates hypoxia inducible factor (HIF)-3α in lung epithelial cells: Characterization and comparison with HIF 1-1α. *Cell Res* 2006;**16**:548-558.

22. Forrester RM. Oxygen, cerebral palsy and retrolental fibroplasia. *Develop Med Child Neurol* 1964;**6**:648-650.

23. Jones D. Heal thyself. *New Scientist* 14 August 2010.

24. Singer M, Glynne P. Treating critical illness: The importance of doing no harm. *PLoS Medicine* 2005;**2**:e167.

25. Parnes O. Historical keyword: Inflammation. *Lancet* 2008;**372**:621,

26. Eltzschig HK, Carmeliet P. Hypoxia and inflammation. *N Engl J Med* 2011;**364**:656-665.

27. British National Formulary. British Medical Association, London 2003.

Chapter 2: The Brain: The Ultimate Oxygen Machine

1. Hills BA. Gas transfer in the lung. Cambridge University Press, Cambridge 1974.

2. Groskloss HH. Fat embolism. *Yale J Biol Med.* 1935;**8**:59-91.

3. Scientific tables 7th edition. Eds; Diem K, Lentner C. Geigy SA, Basel 1970.

4. James PB. Multiple sclerosis or blood-brain barrier disease. *Lancet* 1989;**i**:46.

5. Neuwelt EA, Bauer B, Fahika C, et al. Engaging neuroscience to advance translational research in brain barrier biology. *Nat Rev Neurosci* 2011;**12**:169-182.

6. Xie L, Kang H, Xu Q, et al. Sleep drives metabolite clearance from the adult brain. *Science* 2013;**342**:373-377.

7. Iliff JJ, Wang M, Liao Y, et al. A paravascular pathway facilitates CSF low through the brain parenchyma and the clearance of interstitial solutes including amyloid. *Sci Trans Med* 2012;**4**(147):147ra111.

8. Crane RK, Miller D. Bihler I. The restrictions on possible mechanisms of intestinal transport of sugars. In: Membrane Transport and Metabolism. Proceedings of a Symposium held in Prague, August 22–27, 1960. Edited by A. Kleinzeller and A. Kotyk. Czech Academy of Sciences, Prague, 1961, pp. 439-449.

9. Hills BA. The biology of surfactant. Cambridge University Press 1989.

10. Shih AY, Blinder P, Tsai PS, et al. The smallest stroke: occlusion of one penetrating vessel leads to infarction and a cognitive deficit. *Nature Neuroscience* 2013;**16**:55-63.

11. Toole J. Cardiovascular disorders. 5th Edition, Lippincott Williams & Wilkins,1998.

12. Brownell B, Hughes JT. The distribution of plaques in the cerebrum in multiple sclerosis. *J Neurol Neurosurg Psychiatry* 1962;**25**:315-320.

13. Hassler O. Blood supply to human spinal cord: A microangiographic study. *Arch Neurol* 1966;**14**:302-307.

14. Pfeifer RA. Grundlegende Untersuchungen für die Angio-Architektonik des menschlichen Gehirns. Springer, Berlin 1930.

15. Voss HU, Ulug AM, Dyke JP, et al. Possible axonal regrowth in late recovery from the minimally conscious state. *J Clin Invest* 2006;**116**:2005-2011.

16. Dai J, Swaab DF, Buijs RM. Recovery of axonal transport in "dead neurons." *Lancet* 1998;**351**:499-500.

Chapter 3: The Importance of Pressure and Oxygen

1. Glaisher J. Notes of effects experienced during recent balloon ascents. *Lancet* 1862;**ii**:559-60.
2. Molecular mechanisms in general anaesthesia. Eds. Halsey MJ, Millar, RA, Sutton JA. Churchill Livingstone, Edinburgh 1974.
3. McFarland RA, Barach AL. The response of pyschoneurotics to variations in oxygen tension. *Am J Psychiat* 1938;**93**:1315-1341.
4. Markovic D, Kovacevic H. Recompression therapy of mountain sickness. *Arh Hig Rada Toksikol* 2002;**53**:3-6.
5. Lawrence JH, Tobias CR, Lyons WMR, et al. A study of aero medical problems in a Liberator bomber at high altitude. *J Aviat Med* 1945;**16**:286-303.
6. Bert P. La Pression Barométrique: recherches de physiologie experimentale. Masson, Paris 1878.
7. Houston C. Going higher: oxygen, man and mountains. Swan Hill Press, Shrewsbury 1998.
8. Brown HK, Simpson AJ, Murchison JT. The influence of meteorological variables on the development of deep venous thrombosis. *Thromb Haemost* 2009;**102**:676-82.
9. Hitchcock MA, Hitchcock FA. Barometric pressure: researches in experimental physiology by Paul Bert. College Book Company, Columbus, Ohio 1943.
10. Goodman M. Suffer and Survive. Simon & Shuster UK Ltd., London 2007.

Chapter 4: John Scott Haldane: A Giant of Medicine

1. Haldane A. The lives of Robert Haldane of Aithrey and his brother, James Alexander Haldane. Eighth edition. William P. Kennedy, Glasgow 1871.
2. Haldane JBS, Keeping cool and other essays. Chatto & Windus, London 1940.
3. Haldane JS. Respiration, Yale University Press 1922.
4. Haldane, JS, Hamilton FT, Bacon HS, Lees E. Report of a Committee Appointed by the Lords Commissioners of the Admiralty to Consider and Report Upon the Conditions of Deepwater Diving. Parliamentary Paper C.N. 1549/1907. London, HM Stationary Office 1907.
5. Haldane JS. Gases and liquids; a contribution to molecular physics. Oliver & Lloyd, Edinburgh 1928.

6. Haldane JS. The philosophy of a biologist. Clarendon Press, Oxford 1935.

7. James PB, Calder IM. Anoxic asphyxia - a cause of industrial fatalities: a review. *J Roy Soc Med* 1991;**84**:493-495.

8. Haldane JS. The action of carbonic oxide on man. *J Physiol (Lond)* 1895;**12**:430-462.

9. Haldane JS Smith JL. The physiological effects of air vitiated by respiration. *J. Path. Bact* 1893;**1**:168-86.

10. Glaisher J. Notes of effects experienced during recent balloon ascents. *Lancet* 1862;**ii**:559-560.

11. Haldane JS. A new apparatus for accurate blood gas analysis. *J Physiol (Lond)* 1920;**10**:443-450.

12. Saul GB, Lukina WJ, Brakebush SC, et al. Voluntary hyperventilation into a simple mixing chamber relieves high altitude hypoxia. *Aviat Space Environ Med* 2002;**73**:404-407.

13. Schneider EC, Truesdell D. The circulatory responses of man to a sudden and extreme anoxemia. *Am J Physiol* 1923;**65**:379-385.

14. Janocha AJ, Koch CD, Tiso M, et al. Nitric oxide during altitude acclimatization. *N Eng J Med* 2011;**365**:1942-1944.

15. Gorka A-A, Beall CM, Witonsky DB, et al. The genetic architecture of adaptations to high altitude in Ethiopia. *PLoS Genetics*, 2012; **8**:e1003110 doi:10.1371/journal.pgen.1003110.

16. Yi Y, Liang E, Huerta-Sanchez X, et al. Sequencing of 50 human exomes reveals adaptation to high altitude. *Science* 2010;**329**:75-78.

17. Stamler JS, Jia L, Eu JP, et al. Blood flow regulation by S-nitrosohemoglobin in the physiological oxygen gradient. *Science* 1997;**276**:2034-2037.

18. Campbell EJM. The relation between oxygen concentrations of inspired air and arterial blood. *Lancet* 1960;**ii**:10-12.

19. Campbell EJM. A method of controlled oxygen administration which reduces the risk of carbon-dioxide retention. *Lancet* 1960;**ii**:12-14.

20. British Thoracic Society Guideline for emergency oxygen use in adult patients. *Thorax* 2008;**63**:Supplement VI.

21. Fitzgerald JM, Baynham R, Powles ACP. Use of oxygen therapy for adult patients outside the critical care areas of a University Hospital. *Lancet* 1988;**333**:981-983.

22. Einarsson S, Stenqvist O, Bengtsson A, et al. Nitrous oxide elimination and diffusion hypoxia during normo and hypoventilation. *Br J Anaesth* 1993;**71**:189-193.

23. Aubier M, Murciano D, Fournier M et al. Central respiratory drive in acute respiratory failure of patients with chronic obstructive pulmonary disease. *Am Rev Respir Dis* 1980;**122**:191-199.

24. Aubier M, Murciano D, Millic-Emili J, et al. Effects of the administration of O_2 on ventilation and blood gases in patients with chronic obstructive pulmonary disease during acute respiratory failure. *Am Rev Respir Dis* 1980;**122**:747-754.

25. Schmidt GA, Hall JBH. Oxygen therapy and hypoxic drive to breathe: is there danger in the patient with COPD? *Crit Care Med* 1989;**8**:52-53.

26. Hoyt JW. Debunking myths of chronic obstructive lung disease. *Crit Care Med* 1997;**25**:1450-1451.

27. Teller E. On hyperbaric oxygenation. *J Am Phys Surg* 2003;**8**:97.

28. Sridhar MK. Why do patients with emphysema lose weight. *Lancet* 1995;**345**:1190-1191.

29. Monge CC, Whittembury J. Chronic mountain sickness. *Johns Hopkins Med J* 1976;**139**: Suppl:87-89.

30. Bruera E, de Stoutz N, Velasco-Leiva A, et al. Effects of oxygen on dyspnoea in hypoxaemic terminal cancer patients. *Lancet* 1993;**342**:13-14.

31. Massie RK. Dreadnought: Britain, Germany and the coming of the Great War. Valentine Books, New York 1992.

Chapter 5: Oxygen Treatment: When Air is Not Enough

1. Haldane JBS. Possible Worlds. Evergreen Books, London 1940.

2. Haldane JS. The therapeutic administration of oxygen. *Br Med J* 1917;**i**:181-183.

3. Hill L. The administration of oxygen. *Br Med J* 1912;i:71-72.

4. Hills BA. The biology of surfactants. Cambridge University Press, Cambridge 1988.

5. Haldane JS. Discussion on the therapeutic administration of oxygen and carbon dioxide. *Proc Roy Soc Med* 1932;**25**: Part I, 621-622.

6. Fitzgerald JM, Baynham R, Powles ACP. Use of oxygen therapy for adult patients outside the critical care areas of a University Hospital. *Lancet* 1988;**333**:981-983.

7. Thiel M, Chouker A. Ohta A, et al. Oxygenation inhibits the physiological tissue-protecting mechanism and thereby exacerbates acute lung injury. *PLoS Biology* 2005;**3**:1088-1100.

8. Meyhoff CS, Stehr AK, Rasmussen LS. Rational use of oxygen in medical disease and anesthesia. *Curr Opin Anesthesiol.* 2012;**25**:363-365.

9. Valenzula DF. Oxygen as an antipyretic. *Lancet* 1887;**ii**: 1144-1145

10. Comroe JH, Dripps RD, Dumke PR, Deming M. Oxygen toxicity: The effect of inhalation of high concentrations of oxygen for twenty-four hours on normal men at sea level and at a simulated altitude of 18,000 feet. *JAMA* 1945;**128**:710-717.

11. British Thoracic Society Guideline for emergency oxygen use in adult patients. *Thorax* 2008;**63**:Supplement VI.

12. Singer MM, Wright F, Stanley LK, et al. Oxygen toxicity in man: A prospective study in patients after open heart surgery. *N Engl J Med* 1970;**283**:1473-1478.

13. Barber RE, Lee J, Hamilton WK. Oxygen toxicity: A prospective study in patients with irreversible brain damage. *N Engl J Med* 1970;**283**:1478-1484.

14. Hedenstierna G, Rothen HU. Atelectasis formation during anesthesia: causes and measures to prevent it. *J Clin Monit Comput* 2000;**16**:329-335.

15. Adawi A, Zhang Y, Baggs R, et al. Disruption of the CD40-CD40 ligand system prevents an oxygen-induced respiratory distress syndrome. *Am J Path* 1998;**152**:651-657.

16. Nunn JF, Coleman AJ, Sachithanandan T, et al. Hypoxaemia and atelectasis produced by forced inspiration. *Br J Anaesth* 1965;**37**:3-11.

17. Nunn JF, Williams IP, Jones JG, et al. Detection and reversal of pulmonary absorption collapse. *Br J Anaesth* 1978;**50**:91-94.

18. Clark JM. Pulmonary tolerance in man to continuous oxygen exposure at 3.0, 2.5, 2.0 and 1.5 ATA. Summary progress report for predictive studies V; definition of tolerance of human organs and systems to continuous hyperoxia. University of Pennsylvania 1986.

19. Till GO, Johnson KJ, Kunkell R, Ward PA. Intravascular activation of complement and acute lung injury; dependency on neutrophils and toxic oxygen metabolites. *J Clin Invest* 1982;**69**:1126-1135.

20. Shasby DM, Fox RB, Harada RN, et al. Reduction of the edema of acute hyperoxic lung injury by granulocyte (neutrophil) depletion. *J Appl Physiol: Respirat Environ Exercise Physiol* 1982;**52**:1237-1244.

21. Sugiura M, McCulloch PR, Wren S, et al. Ventilator pattern influences neutrophil influx and activation in atelectasis prone rabbit lung. *J Appl Physiol* 1994;**77**:1355-1365.

22. Fridovich I. Hypoxia and oxygen toxicity. *Adv Neurol* 1979;**26**:255-259.

23. Wright WB. Use of the University of Pennsylvania Institute for Environmental Medicine procedure for calculation of cumulative pulmonary oxygen toxicity. US Naval Experimental Diving Unit Report

no. 000000309, January 1971.

24. James PB. Hyperbaric oxygen in the treatment of carbon monoxide poisoning and smoke inhalation injury: a review. *Intensive Care World* 1989;**6**:135-138.

25. Jones D. Darwinian medicine: Does intensive care kill or cure? *New Scientist* 19 August 2010.

26. Singer M. Glynne P. Treating critical illness: The importance of first doing no harm. *PLoS* 2005;**2**:e167.

27. Babior BM. Oxygen-dependent microbial killing by phagocytes Part 1. *N Engl J Med* 1978;**298**:659-668.

28. Babior BM. Oxygen dependent microbial killing of phagocytes Part 2. *N Engl J Med* 1978;**298**:721-725.

29. Carvalho CRR, Schettino GP, Maranhao B, Bethlem EP. Hyperoxia and lung disease. *Cur Opin Pulm Med* 1998;**4**:300-304.

30. Pinhu L, Whitehead T, Evans T, Griffiths M. Ventilator–associated lung injury. *Lancet* 2005;**361**:332-340.

Chapter 6: Taking to the Air

1. Bert P. La Pression Barométrique: recherches de physiologie experimentale. Masson, Paris 1878.

2. Glaisher J. Notes of effects experienced during recent balloon ascents. *Lancet* 1862;**ii**:559-560.

3. Schneider EC, Lutz BR. Circulatory responses to low oxygen tension. Air service medical. Washington Gov't Printing Office 1920;**1**:86-98.

4. Kallenberg K, Bailey DM, Christ S, et al. Magnetic resonance imaging evidence of cytotoxic cerebal edema in acute mountain sickness. *J Cereb Blood Flow & Metab* 2007;**27**:1064-1071.

5. Schoonman GG, Sandor PS, Nirkko AC, et al. Hypoxia-induced acute mountain sickness is associated with intracellular cerebral edema: a 3 T magnetic resonance imaging study. *J Cereb Blood Flow & Metab* 2008;**28**:198-206.

6. Bailey DM, Tandorf S, Berg RMG, et al. Increased cerebral output of free radicals during hypoxia: implications for acute mountain sickness. *J Cereb Blood Flow & Metab* 2009;**297**:R1283-1292.

7. Bailey DM, Evans KA, James PE, et al. Altered free radical metabolism in acute mountain sickness: implications for dynamic cerebral autoregulation and blood-brain barrier function. *J Physiol* 2009;**587**:73-85.

8. Davis RH. Deep diving and submarine operations; a manual for deep sea

divers and compressed-air workers. The Saint Catherine Press, London 1951.

9. Armstrong HG. The principles and practice of aviation medicine. Williams and Wilkins, Baltimore 1939.

10. Milne J. The Concorde healing chamber. http://www.dundee.ac.uk/ pressreleases/prnov02/concorde.html

11. Armstrong JA, Fryer DI, Stewart WK, Whittingham HE. Interpretation of injuries in the Comet aircraft disasters: an experimental approach. *Lancet* 1955;**i**:1135-1143.

12. O'Donnell PO, Buxton PJ, Pitkin A, Jarvis LJ. The magnetic resonance appearances of the brain in acute carbon monoxide poisoning. *Clin Radiol* 2000;**55**:273-280.

13. Magalhaes J, Ascensao A, Viscor G, et al. Oxidative stress in humans during and after 4 hours of hypoxia at a simulated altitude of 5500m. *Aviat Space Environ Med* 2004;**75**:16-22.

14. Fridovich I. Hypoxia and oxygen toxicity. *Adv Neurol* 1979;**26**:255-259.

15. Stamler JS, Jia L, Eu JP, et al. Blood flow regulation by S-nitrosohemoglobin in the physiological oxygen gradient. *Science* 1997;**276**:2034-2037.

16. Douglas CG, Haldane JS, Henderson Y, Schneider EC. The physiological effects of low atmospheric pressures, as observed on Pike's Peak, Colorado (preliminary communication). *Proc Roy Soc Biol* 1912;**85**:65-67.

17. Harik SI, Behmand RA, LaManna JC. Hypoxia increases glucose transport at blood-brain barrier. *J Appl Physiol* 1994;**77**:896-901.

18. Fryer DI. Subatmospheric decompression sickness in man. NATO AGARDograph No. 125, Technivision Services, Slough 1969.

19. Lawrence JH, Tobias CR, Lyons WMR, et al. A study of aero medical problems in a Liberator bomber at high altitude. *Aviat Med* 1945;**16**:286-303.

20. Behnke AR. Decompression sickness incident to deep sea diving and high altitude ascent. *Medicine* 1945;**24**:381-402.

21. Davis JC, Sheffield PJ, Schuknecht L, et al. Altitude decompression sickness: hyperbaric therapy results in 145 cases. *Aviat Space Environ Med* 1977;**48**:722-730.

22. Boycott AE, Damant GCC, Haldane JS. The prevention of compressed-air illness. *J Hyg (Camb.)*1908;**8**:342-443.

Chapter 7: Bubbles, "the Bends," and the Lungs

1. Bevan J. The infernal diver. Submex Books, London 1996.

2. Pol B, Watelle TJJ, Mémoire sur les effets de la compression de l'air appliquée au creusement des puits a houille. *Ann Hyg Publique* 1854;**Sér 2,1**:242-279.

3. Charcot JM. Lectures on diseases of the nervous system. The New Sydenham Society, London 1867.

4. Bert P. La Pression Barométrique: recherches de physiologie experimentale. Masson, Paris 1878.

5. Fryer DI. Subatmospheric decompression sickness in man. NATO AGARDograph No. 125. Technivision Services, Slough 1969.

6. Haldane, JS, Hamilton FT, Bacon HS, Lees E. Report of a Committee Appointed by the Lords Commissioners of the Admiralty to Consider and Report Upon the Conditions of Deepwater Diving. Parliamentary Paper C.N. 1549/1907. London, HM Stationary Office 1907.

7. Hills BA. A thermodynamic and kinetic approach to decompression sickness. Libraries Board of South Australia, Adelaide, 1966.

8. Haldane JS. Respiration. Yale University Press, New Haven, Connecticut 1922.

9. Brown H, Simpson AJ, Murchison JT. The influence of meterological variables on the development of deep venous thrombosis. *Throm Haemost* 2009;**102**:676-682.

10. Groskloss HH. Fat embolism. *Yale J Biol Med* 1936;**59**:310-314.

11. Setzer M, Beck J, Hermann E, et al. The influence of barometric pressure changes and standard meteorological variables on the occurrence and clinical features of subarachnoid hemorrhage. *Surg Neurol* 2007;**67**:264-272.

12. Kapronczay K. Semmelweis Akaprint Nyomdaipari Kft, Budapest 2004.

13. Rappaport H. Conspirator: Lenin in exile. Hutchinson 2010.

14. Fieldsteel AH, Cox DL, Moeckli RA. Cultivation of virulent Treponema pallidum in tissue culture. *Infect Immunol* 1981;**32**:908-915.

15. Fitzgerald TJ, Johnson RC, Sykes JA, Miller JN. Interaction of Treponema Pallidum (Nichols strain) with cultured mammalian cells: effects of oxygen, reducing agents, serum supplements, and different cell types. *Infection and Immunity* 1976;**15**:444-452.

16. Dorowini-Zis K, Schmidt K, Huynh H, et al. The neuropathology of fatal cerebral malaria in Malawian children. *Am J Pathol* 2011;**178**:2146-2188.

17. Cordoliani Y-S, Sarrazin J-L, Felten D et al. MRI of cerebral malaria. *Am J Neuroradiol* 1998;**19**:871-874.

18. Boycott AE, Damant GCC, Haldane JS. The prevention of compressed-air illness. *J Hyg (Camb.)* 1908;**8**:342-443.

19. Kaufman RM, Airo R, Pollace S, et al. Origin of pulmonary megakarycytes. *Blood* 1965;**25**:767-775.

20. Swank RL, Hain RF. The effect of different sized emboli on the vascular system and parenchyma of the brain. *J Neuropathol Exp Neurol* 1952;**11**:280-299.

21. Cramer T, Yamanishi Y, Clausen BE, et al. HIF 1α is essential for myeloid cell-mediated inflammation. *Cell* 2003;**112**:645-657.

22. Hills BA, James PB. Microbubble damage to the blood-brain barrier: relevance to decompression sickness. *Undersea Biomed Res* 1991;**18**:111-116.

23. Kihara M, McManis PG, Schmelzer JD, et al. Experimental ischemic neuropathy: salvage with hyperbaric oxygenation. *Ann Neurol* 1995;**37**:89-94.

24. Till GO, Johnson KJ, Kunkel R, Ward PA. Intravascular activation of complement and acute lung injury. *J Clin Invest* 1982;**69**:1126-1135.

25. Gao GK, Wu D, Yang T, et al. Cerebral magnetic resonance imaging of compressed air divers in diving accidents. *Undersea Hyperb Med* 2009;**36**:33-41.

26. Thompson AJ, Kermode AG, MacManus DG, et al. Patterns of disease activity in multiple sclerosis: clinical and magnetic resonance imaging study. *Br Med J* 1990;**300**:631-634.

27. Hallenbeck JM, Bove AA, Elliott DH. Mechanisms underlying spinal cord damage in decompression sickness. *Neurology* 1975;**25**:308-316.

28. Palmer AC, Calder IM, McCallum RI, Mastaglia FL. Spinal cord degeneration in a case of 'recovered' spinal decompression sickness. *Br Med J* 1981;**283**:888.

29. Fuerecdi GA, Czarnecki DJ, Kindwall EP. MR findings in the brains of compressed-air tunnel workers; relationship to psychometric results. *Am J Roentgen* 1991;**12**:67-70.

30. Ebers G. MRI: measure of efficacy? *Brain* 2000;**123**:2187-2188.

31. McGuire S, Sherman P, Profenna L, et al. White matter hyperintensities on MRI in high altitude U2 pilots. *Neurology* 2013;**81**:729-735.

32. Thom S, Yang M, Bhopale VM, et al. Microparticles initiate decompression-induced neutrophil activation and subsequent vascular injuries. *J Appl Physiol* 2011;**110**:340-351.

33. Martin JD, Thom SR. Vascular leukocyte sequestration in decompression sickness and prophylactic hyperbaric oxygen therapy in rats. *Aviat Space Environ Med* 2002;**73**:565-569.

Chapter 8: Oxygen: Diving, Flying, and Medicine

1. James PB, Calder IM. Anoxic asphyxia - a cause of industrial fatalities: a review. *J Roy Soc Med* 1991;**84**:493-495.

2. Bert P. La Pression Barométrique: recherches de physiologie experimentale. Masson, Paris 1878.

3. Donald KW. Oxygen and the diver. The Self Publishing Association Ltd, Hanley Swan 1992.

4. Lane N. Oxygen: The molecule that made the world. Oxford University Press, Oxford 2002.

5. Stamler JS, Jia L, Eu JP, et al. Blood flow regulation by S-nitrosohemoglobin in the physiological oxygen gradient. *Science* 1997;**276**:2034-2037.

6. Demchenko IT, Boso AE, Bennett PB, et al. Hyperbaric oxygen reduces cerebral blood flow by inactivating nitric oxide. *Nitric Oxide* 2000;**4**:597-608.

7. Holbach KH, Caroli A, Wassmann H. Cerebral energy metabolism in patients with brain lesions at normo and hyperbaric oxygen pressures. *J Neurol* 1977;**217**:17-30.

8. Macey PM, Woo MA, Harper RM. Hyperoxic brain effects are normalized by addition of CO_2 *PLoS Med* 2007;**4**:0828-0835.

9. Nichols CW, Lambertsen CJ, Clark JM. Transient unilateral loss of vision associated with oxygen at high pressure. *Arch Ophthalmol* 1969;**81**:548-552.

10. Connelly A. Proton Magnetic Resonance (MRS) in epilepsy. *Epilepsia* 1997;**38** (Suppl 10):33-38.

11. Juhasz C, Scheidl E, Szirmai I. Reversible focal MRI abnormalities due to status epilepticus. An EEG single photon emission computed tomography transcranial Doppler follow-up study. *Electroenceph Clin Neurophysiol* 1998;**107**:402-407.

12. Leitch DR, Hallenbeck JM. Oxygen in the treatment of spinal cord decompression sickness. *Undersea Biomed Res* 1985;**12**:269-289.

13. Gorman DF, Browning DM. Cerebral vasoreactivity and arterial gas embolism. *Undersea Biomed Res* 1986;**13**:317-335.

14. Diving Safety Memorandum, No. 4, Dept of Energy Inspectorate 1985.

15. Triger AG. Lettre à M. Arago. Séanc Acad Sci, Paris 1845.

16. Rivera JC. Decompression sickness among divers: An analysis of 935 cases. *Milit Med* 1964;**129**:314-334.

17. Goodman MW, Workman RD. Minimal recompression oxygen breathing approach to the treatment of decompression sickness in divers and aviators. Research report, 5-6, US Navy Experimental Diving Unit 1965.

18. Fischer BH, Marks M, Reich T. Hyperbaric-oxygen treatment of multiple sclerosis: a randomized, placebo-controlled, double-blind study. *N Engl J Med* 1983;**308**:181-186.

19. James PB, Arnoux GA, Imbere J-P. Comex Medical Book, Comex SA, Marseille 1986.

20. Hyldegaard O, Madsen J. Effect of hypobaric air, oxygen, heliox (50:50) or heliox (80:20) breathing on air bubbles in adipose tissue. *J Appl Physiol* 2007;**103**:757-762.

21. Hills BA, James PB. Microbubble damage to the blood-brain barrier: relevance to decompression sickness. *Undersea Biomed Res* 1991;**18**:111-116.

22. Hallenbeck JM, Bove AA, Elliott DH. Mechanisms underlying spinal cord damage in decompression sickness. *Neurology* 1975;**25**:308-316.

23. Kelly DL Jr, Lassiter KRL, Vongsvivut A, Smith JM. Effects of hyperbaric oxygenation and tissue oxygen studies in experimental paraplegia. *Neurosurgery* 1972;**36**:425-429.

24. Yeo JD. Treatment of paraplegic sheep with hyperbaric oxygenation. *Med J Austr* 1976;**1**:538-540.

25. Sukoff MH. Use of hyperbaric oxygen therapy for spinal cord injury. *Neurochirurgia* 1982;**24**:19-21.

26. Gelderd JB, Fife WP, Bowers DE, et al. Spinal cord transection in rats: the therapeutic effects of dimethyl sulfoxide and hyperbaric oxygen. *Ann NY Acad Sci* 1983;**911**:218-233.

27. Martin JD, Thom SR. Vascular leukocyte sequestration in decompression sickness and prophylactic hyperbaric oxygen therapy in rats. *Aviat Space Environ Med* 2002;**73**:565-569.

28. James PB. HBO in fluid microembolism. *Neurol Res* 2007;**29**:156-161.

Chapter 9: Jessica in the Well

1. Benke PJ. Jessica in the well: ischemia and reperfusion injury. *JAMA* 1988;**259**:1326.

2. Perrins DJD. Influence of hyperbaric oxygen on the survival of split skin grafts. *Lancet* 1967;**289**:868-871.

3. Hearse DJ, Humphrey SM, Chain EB. Abrupt reoxygenation of the anoxic potassium-arrested perused rat heart; a study of myocardial enzyme release. *J Mol Cell Cardiol* 1973;**5**:395-427.

4. Parks DA, Bulkley GB, Granger DN. Role of oxygen free radicals in ischaemia and organ preservation. *Surgery* 1983;**94**:428-432.

5. Hearse DJ, Humphrey SM. Enzyme release during myocardial anoxia. *J*

Mol Cell Cardiol 1973;**5**:463-482.

6. Viney S. Jessica in the well: Ischemia and reperfusion injury. *JAMA* 1988;**259**:3559.

7. Davis JC. Jessica in the well: Ischemia and reperfusion injury. *JAMA* 1988;**259**:3558.

8. Zamboni WA, Roth AC, Russell RC, et al. The effect of acute hyperbaric oxygen therapy on axial pattern skin flap survival when administered during and after total ischemia. *J Reconstruct Microsurg* 1989;**5**:343-342.

9. Zamboni WA, Roth AC, Russell RC, et al. Morphologic analysis of the microcirculation during reperfusion of ischemic skeletal muscle and the effect of hyperbaric oxygen. *Plast Reconstr Surg* 1993;**91**:1110-1123.

10. Clark ER, Clark EL. Observations on changes in blood vascular endothelium in the living animal. *Am J Anat* 1935;**67**:385-438.

11. Lee WL, Grinstein S. The tangled web that neutrophils weave. *Science* 2004;**303**:1477-1478.

12. Buras JA, Stahl GL, Svoboda KKH, Reenstra WR. Hyperbaric oxygen downregulates ICAN-1 expression induced by hypoxia and hypoglycemia: the role of NOS. *Am J Physiol* 2000;**278**:C292-C302.

13. Buras JA, Reenstra WR. Endothelial-neutrophil interactions during ischemia and reperfusion injury: basic mechanisms of hyperbaric oxygen. *Neurol Res* 2007;**29**:127-131.

14. Jones SR, Carpin KM, Woodward SM et al. Hyperbaric oxygen inhibits ischemia-reperfusion induced neutrophil CD18 polarization by a nitric oxide mechanism. *Plast Reconstr Surg* 2010; **126**: 402-411.

15. Cramer T, Yamanishi Y, Clausen BE, et al. HIF 1α is essential for myeloid cell-mediated inflammation. *Cell* 2003;**112**:645-657.

Chapter 10: Anecdotes, Evidence, and Uncontrolled Double-Blindness

1. Fischer BH, Marks M, Reich T. Hyperbaric-oxygen treatment of multiple sclerosis: a randomized, placebo-controlled, double-blind study. *N Engl J Med* 1983;**308**:181-186.

2. Borgstein J. The end of the clinical anecdote. *Lancet* 1999;**354**:2151-2152.

3. Abbot NC, Beck JS, Carnochan FMT, et al. Effect of hyperoxia at 1 and 2 ATA on hypoxia and hypercapnia in human skin during experimental inflammation. *J Appl Physiol* 1994;**77**:767-773.

4. Rawlings M. The Harveian Oration at the Royal College of Physicians, October 2008.

5. Beecher HK. The powerful placebo. *JAMA* 1955;**159**:1602-1606.

6. Summerskill W. Evidence-based practice and the individual. *Lancet* 2005;**365**:13-14.

7. Kaptchuk TJ, Elizabeth Friedlander E, Kelley JM, et al. Placebos without deception: a randomized controlled trial in irritable bowel syndrome. *PLoS* 2010;**5**:e15591.

8. Rothwell PM. Treating individuals 1. External validity of randomised conrolled trials: "To whom do the results of this trial apply?" *Lancet* 2005;**365**:82-91.

9. Stuebe AM. Level IV evidence-adverse anecdote and clinical practice. *N Eng J Med* 2011;**365**:9-9.

10. Niebauer J, Coats AJS. Treating chronic heart failure: time to take stock. *Lancet* 1997;**349**:966-967.

11. Sridhar MK. Why do patients with emphysema lose weight? *Lancet* 1995;**345**:1190-1191.

12. Evidence-based care: 2. Setting guidelines: How should we manage this problem? *Can Med Assoc J* 1994;**150**:1417-1423.

13. Glasziou P, Chalmers I, Rawlins M, McCulloch P. When are randomized trials unnecessary? Picking signals from noise. *Br Med J* 2007;**334**:349-351

14. Hill AB. The environment and disease: association or causation. *Proc R Soc Med* 1965;**58**:295-300.

15. Ramachandran VS, Blakeslee S. Phantoms in the brain: probing the mysteries of the human mind. Harper Perennial, London 1999.

16. British Thoracic Society Guideline for emergency oxygen use in adult patients. *Thorax* 2008;**63**:Supplement VI.

17. Avorn J, Chen M, Hartley R. Scientific versus commercial sources of influence on the prescribing behaviour of physicians. *JAMA* 1982;**73**:4-8.

18. Harris DNF, Bailey SM, Smith PLC, et al. Brain swelling in the first hour after coronary artery bypass surgery. *Lancet* 1993;**342**:586-587.

19. Yacoub MH, Zeitlin GL. Hyperbaric oxygen in the treatment of the postoperative low-cardiac-output syndrome. *Lancet* 1965;**i**:581-83.

20. Editorial: Oxygen under pressure. *Lancet* 1965;**i**:1257-1258.

21. Jacobson I, Harper AM, McDowall DG. Effects of oxygen under pressure on cerebral blood-flow and cerebral venous oxygen tension. *Lancet* 1963;**i**:549.

22. Tsang V, Yacoub M, Sridharan S, et al. Late donor cardiectomy after paediatric heterotopic cardiac transplantation. *Lancet* 2009;**374**:387-392.

23. Ledingham IM, McBride TI, Jennett WB, et al. Fatal brain damage

associated with cardiomyopathy of pregnancy, with notes on caesarian section in a hyperbaric chamber. *Br Med J* 1968;**2**:285-287.

24. Steiner PE, Lushbaugh CC. Maternal pulmonary embolism by amniotic fluid as a cause of obstetric shock and unexpected deaths in obstetrics. *JAMA* 1941;**117**:1340-1345.

25. Nicolaides KH, Campbell S, Bradley RJ, et al. Maternal oxygen therapy for intrauterine growth retardation. *Lancet* 1987;**i**:942-945.

26. Shuster S. Single dose treatment of fungal nail disease. *Lancet* 1992;**339**:1066.

Chapter 11: Suffer the Little Children

1. Nicolaides KH, Campbell S, Bradley RJ, et al. Maternal oxygen therapy for intrauterine growth retardation. *Lancet* 1987;**i**:942-945.

2. Prystowsky H. Fetal blood studies, X1: The effect of prophylactic oxygen on the oxygen pressure gradient between the maternal and fetal bloods of the human in normal and abnormal pregnancy. *Am J Obstet Gynecol* 1959;**10**:483-488.

3. Herpin P, Hulia JC, Le Dividich J,Fillant M. Effect of oxygen inhalation at birth on the reduction of early postnatal mortality. *J Anim Sci* 2001;**79**:5-10.

4. Ledingham IM, McBride TI, Jennett WB, et al. Fatal brain damage associated with cardiomyopathy of pregnancy, with notes on caesarian section in a hyperbaric chamber. *Br Med J* 1968;**2**:285-287.

5. Nelson K, Leviton A. How much of neonatal encephalopathy is due to birth asphyxia? *Am J Dis Child* 1991;**145**:1325 -31.

6. Soothill PW, Nicolaides KH, Todeck CH, Gamsu H. Blood gases and acid-base status of the human second-trimester fetus. *Obstet Gynecol* 1986;**179**:507-513.

7. Malin GL, Morris RK, Khan KS. Strength of association between umbilical cord pH and perinatal and long term outcomes: systematic review and meta-analysis. *Br Med J* 2010;**340**:c1471.

8. Zamboni WA, Roth AC, Russell RC, e al. Morphologic analysis of the microcirculation during reperfusion of ischemic skeletal muscle and the effect of hyperbaric oxygen. *Plast Reconstr Surg* 1993;**91**:1110-1123.

9. Brownell B, Hughes JT. The distribution of plaques in the cerebrum in multiple sclerosis. *J Neurol Neurosurg Psychiatry* 1962;**25**:315-320.

10. Takashima S, Tanaka K. Development of cerebrovascular architecture and its relationship to periventricular leukomalacia. *Arch Neurol* 1978;**35**:11-16.

11. Burke RE, Fahn S, Gold AP. Delayed-onset dystonia in patients with "static" encephalopathy. *J Neurol Neurosurg Psychiatry* 1980;**43**:789-797.

12. St Hilaire M-H, Burke RE, Bressman SB et al. Delayed-onset dystonia due to perinatal or early childhood asphyxia. *Neurology* 1991;**41**:216-222

13. Morley GM. Birth brain injury: etiology and prevention - Part I: Hypoxic-ischemic encephalopathy and cerebral palsy. *Med Veritas* 2005;**2**:500-506.

14. MacLennan A. A template for defining a causal relation between acute intrapartum events and cerebral palsy: international consensus statement. *Br Med J* 1999;**319**:1054-1059.

15. Nelson KB, Grether JK. Potentially asphyxiating conditions and spastic cerebral palsy in infants of normal birth weight. *Am J Obstet Gynecol* 1998;**179**:507-512.

16. Cowan F, Rutherford M, Groenendaal F, Eken P, et al. Origin and timing of brain lesions in term infants with neonatal encephalopathy. *Lancet* 2003;**361**:736-742.

17. Gilbert WM, Jacoby BN, Xing G, Danielsen B, Smith LH. Adverse obstetric events are associated with significant risk of cerebral palsy. *Am J Obstet Gynecol.* 2010;**203**:328:328 e 1-5.

18. Martin E, Buchli R, Ritter S et al. Diagnostic and prognostic value of cerebral Magnetic Resonance Spectroscopy in neonates with perinatal asphyxia. *Pediatr Res.* 1996;**40**:749-758.

19. Apgar V. A proposal for a new method of evaluation of the newborn infant. *Curr. Res Anesth Analg* 1953;**32**:260–267.

20. Hutchison JH. Practical paediatric problems. Year Book Medical Publishers, Chicago 1975.

21. Wyatt JS, and study group. Head cooling in neonatal hypoxic-ischaemic encephalopathy. *Lancet* 2005;**365**:632-670.

22. Shankaran S, Pappas A, Scott A, et al. Childhood outcomes after hypothermia for neonatal encephalopathy. *N Engl J Med* 2012;**366**:2085-2092.

23. Hanrahan JD, Cox IJ, Azzopardi D, et al. Relation between proton magnetic resonance spectroscopy within 18 hours of birth asphyxia and neurodevelopment at 1 year of age. *Develop Med Child Neurol* 1999;**41**:76-82.

24. Groenendaal F, Veenhoven RH, van der Grond J, et al. Cerebral lactate and N-acetyl-aspartate/choline ratios in asphyxiated full-term neonates demonstrated in vivo using proton magnetic resonance spectroscopy. *Pediatr Res* 1994;**35**:148-151.

25. Ashwal S, Holshouser BA, Tomasi LG, et al. ^{1}H magnetic resonance

spectroscopy-determined cerebral lactate and poor neurological outcomes in children with central nervous system disease. *Ann Neurol* 1997;**41**:470-481.

26. Kinsey VE. Retrolental fibroplasias.Cooperative study of retrolental fibroplasias and the use of oxygen. *Arch Ophthalmol* 1955;**59**:481-542.

27. Nathan C. Oxygen and the inflammatory cell. *Nature* 2003;**422**:675-676.

28. Szewczyk TS. Retrolental fibroplasia: etiology and prophylaxis. *Amer J Ophthalmol* 1951;**34**:1649-1650.

29. Bedrossian RH, Carmichael P, Ritter J. Retinopathy of prematurity (retrolental fibroplasia) and oxygen. *Am J Ophthalmol* 1954;**37**:78.

30. Forrester RM, Jefferson E, Naunton WJ. Oxygen and retrolental fibroplasia; a seven-year survey. Lancet 1954;**ii**:258-260.

31. Forrester RM. Oxygen cerebral palsy and retrolental fibroplasia. *Dev Med Child Neurol* 1964;**6**:648-650.

32. Pugh CW, Ratcliffe PJ. Regulation of angiogenesis by hypoxia: role of the HIF system. *Nature (Med)* 2003;**9**:677-684.

33. Lewis G, Mervin K, Valter K, et al. Limiting the proliferation and reactivity of retinal Mueller cells during experimental retinal detachment: The value of oxygen supplementation. *Am J Ophthalmol* 1999;**128**:165-172.

34. James PB. Retinopathy of the newborn is due to hypoxia not oxygen toxicity. Proc 3rd EPNS Congress European Paediatric Neurology Society, Nice, France. Monduzzi Edition S.p.A. Bologna, 1999; pp. 41-44.

35. Hyperbaric oxygenation for cerebral palsy and the brain-injured child. Ed, Joiner JT. Best Publishing Company, Flagstaff, Arizona 2002.

36. McDonald AD. Oxygen Treatment of Premature Babies and Cerebral Palsy. *Dev Med Child Neurol* 1964;**6**:313-314.

37. Carlo WA, Finer NM, Walsh MC, et al. Target ranges of oxygen saturation in extremely premature infants. *N Eng J Med* 2010;**362**:1959-1969.

38. Saugstad OD. Oxygen toxicity in the neonatal period. *Acta Paediatr Scand* 1990;**79**:881-892.

39. Hutchison JH, Kerr MM, Williams KG, et al. Hyperbaric oxygen in the resuscitation of the newborn. *Lancet* 1963;**ii**:1020-1022.

40. Barrie H. Hyperbaric oxygen in resuscitation of the newborn. *Lancet* 1963;**ii**:1223-1224.

41. Hutchison JH, Kerr MM, Williams KG, Hopkinson WI. Hyperbaric oxygen in the resuscitation of the newborn. *Lancet* 1964;**i**:225.

42. Hutchison JH, Kerr MM, Inall JA, Shanks RA. Controlled trials of hyperbaric oxygen and tracheal intubation in asphyxia neonatorum.

Lancet 1966;**i**:935-939.

43. Bernhard WF, Tank ES. Effect of oxygen inhalation at 3.0 to 3.6 atmospheres absolute upon infants with cyanotic congenital heart disease. *Surgery* 1963;**54**:203-215.

44. Bernhard WF. Hyperbaric oxygenation. *N Engl J Med* 1964;**271**:562-564.

45. Calvert JW, Zhang JH. Oxygen treatment restores energy status following experimental neonatal hypoxia-ischemia. *Pediatr Crit Care Med* 2007;**8**:165-173.

46. Palzur E, Zaaroor M, Vlodavsky E, et al. Neuroprotective effect of hyperbaric oxygen therapy in brain injury is mediated by preservation of mitochondrial membrane properties. *Brain Res* 2008;**122**:126-133.

47. Yang Z, Covey MV, Bizel CL, et al. Sustained neocortical neurogenesis after neonatal hypoxic/ischemic injury. *Ann Neurol* 2007;**61**:199-208.

Chapter 12: Cerebral Palsy and Oxygen Treatment: A Tale of Trials

1. Illingworth RS. Cerebral Palsy in children and its treatment. *Develop Med Child Neurol* 1964;**6**:88-96.

2. Machado JJ. Clinically observed reduction of spasticity in patients with neurological diseases and in children with cerebral palsy from hyperbaric oxygen therapy. Presented at the American College of Hyperbaric Medicine, Orlando, Fla, 1989.

3. Qibia W, Hongjun W, Linzheng C, Cuiyun Z. Treatment of Children's Epilepsy by Hyperbaric Oxygenation: Analysis of 100 Cases. Proc 11th International Congress on Hyperbaric Medicine, Fuzhou, China. Best Publishing Company, Flagstaff, Arizona 1993.

4. Montgomery D, Goldberg J, Amar M, et al. Effects of hyperbaric oxygen therapy on children with spastic diplegic cerebral palsy: a pilot project. *Undersea Hyperb Med* 1999;**26**:235-242.

5. Collet JP, Vanasse M, Marois P, et al. Hyperbaric oxygen for children with cerebral palsy: a randomised multicentre trial. *Lancet* 2001;**357**:582-586.

6. Kramer MR, Springer C, Berkman N, et al. Rehabilitation of hypoxemic patients with COPD at low altitude at the dead sea, the lowest place on earth. *Chest* 1998;**113**:571-575.

7. Hills BA. A role for oxygen-induced osmosis in hyperbaric oxygen therapy. *Med Hypotheses* 1999;**52**:259-263.

8. Babchin A, Levich E, Melamed Y, Sivashinsky G. Osmotic phenomena in application of hyperbaric oxygen treatment. *Colloids Surf B Biointerfaces*

2010;**83**:128-132.

9. Editorial; Hyperbaric oxygen: hype or hope? *Lancet* 2001;**357**:10.

10. Neubauer RA. Hyperbaric oxygenation for cerebral palsy. *Lancet* 2001;**357**:2052.

11. James PB. Hyperbaric oxygenation for cerebral palsy. *Lancet* 2001;**357**:2052-2053.

12. Golding FC, Griffiths P, Hempleman HV, et al. Decompression sickness during construction of the Dartford Tunnel. *Br J Ind Med* 1960;**17**:167-180.

13. Austin D. Gamow bag for acute mountain sickness. *Lancet* 1998;**351**:1815.

14. Heuser G, Uszler JM. Hyperbaric oxygenation for cerebral palsy. *Lancet* 2001;**357**:2053-2054.

15. Marois P, Vanasse M. Hyperbaric oxygen therapy and cerebral palsy. *Develop Med Child Neurol* 2003;**45**:646-648.

16. Essex C. Hyperbaric oxygen and cerebral palsy: no proven benefit and potentially harmful. *Develop Med Child Neurol* 2003;**45**:213-215.

17. Waalkes P, Fitzpatrick DT, Stankus S, Topolski R. Adjunctive HBO treatment of children with cerebral anoxic injury. *Army Med Dep Journ* 2003;April-June:13-21.

18. Packard M. Cornell University study of hyperbaric oxygenation in cerebral palsy. International conference on hyperbaric medicine University of Graz November 2000.

19. Orient JM. Salvage therapy for a neurologically devastated child: Whose decision is it? *J Am Coll Phys Surg* 2003;**8**:117-120.

20. Hardy P, Collet JP, Goldberg J, et al. Neuropsychological effects of hyperbaric oxygen therapy in cerebral palsy. *Dev Med Child Neurol* 2002;**44**:436-446.

21. Senechal C, Larivee S, Engelbert R, Marois P. Hyperbaric oxygenation therapy in the treatment of cerebral palsy: a review and comparison to currently accepted therapies. *J Am Coll Phys Surg* 2007;**12**:109-113.

22. Agency for Healthcare Research and Quality (AHRQ). Systems to rate the strength of scientific evidence. Evidence Report/Technology Assessment no.47. Rockville, Md, AHRQ; 2003.

23. Muhkerjee A, Raison M, Sahani T, et al. Intensive rehabilitation combined with HBO_2 therapy in children with cerebral palsy: A longitudinal study. *Undersea Hyperb Med* 2014;**41**:77-83.

24. Lawrence JH, Tobias CR, Lyons WMR, et al, A study of aero medical problems in a liberator bomber at high altitude. *Aviat Med* 1945;**16**:286-303.

25. Markovic D, Kovacevic H. Recompression therapy of mountain sickness. *Arh Hig Rada Toksikol* 2002;**53**:3-6.

26. Degirmenci B, Miral S, Kaya GC, et al. Technitium-99m HMPAO brain SPECT in autistic children and their families. *Pyschiat Res Neuroimag* 2008;**162**:236-243.

27. Rossignol DA, Frye RE. Mitochondrial dysfunction in autism spectrum disorders: a systematic review and meta-analysis. *Mol Psychiatry* 2011;**17**:290-314.

28. Rossignol DA, Frye RE. A review of research trends in physiological abnormalities in autism spectrum disorders: immune dysregulation, inflammation, oxidative stress, mitochondrial dysfunction and environmental toxicant exposures. *Mol Psychiatry* 2011;**17**:389-401.

29. Poser CM, Roman G, Emery ES. Recurrent disseminated vasculomyelinopathy. *Arch Neurol* 1978;**35**:166-170.

30. www.uscfc.uscourts.gov/sites/default/files/campbell-smith.mojabi-proffer.12.13.2012.pdf

31. Rossignol DA, Rossignol LW, Smith S, et al. Hyperbaric treatment for children with autism: a multicentre, randomized, double-blind, controlled trial. *BMC Paediatrics* 2009;**9**:21. doi:10.1186/1471-2431-9-21.

Chapter 13: An Anecdote: A Policeman's Story in the High Courts

1. Gonsette R, Andre-Balisaux G. La premeabilite des vaisseaux cerebraux. V Action des substances tensioactives sur la barriere hemato-encephalique. *Acta Neurol Psychiatr Belg* 1965;**4**:260-279.

2. Gonsette R, Andre-Balisaux G. La permeabilite des vaisseaux cerebraux. IV Etude des lesions de la barriere hemato-encephalique dans la sclerose en plaques. *Acta Neurol Psychiatr Belg* 1965;**1**:19-34

3. Schumacher GA. Critique of experimental trials of therapy in multiple sclerosis. *Neurology* 1974;**24**:1010-1014.

4. Ebers GC. Optic neuritis and multiple sclerosis. *Arch Neurol* 1984;**42**:702-704.

5. Kurtzke JF. Optic neuritis and multiple sclerosis. *Arch Neurol* 1984;**42**:704-710.

6. Levy DE. Transient CNS deficits: a common, benign syndrome in young adults. *Neurology* 1988;**38**:831-836.

7. Espir MLE, Watkins SM, Smith HV. Paroxysmal dysarthria and other transient neurological disturbances in disseminated sclerosis. *J Neurol Neurosurg Psychiatry* 1966;**29**:323-330.

8. Harrison M, McGill JI. Transient neurological disturbances in disseminated sclerosis: a case report. *J Neurol Neurosurg Psychiatry* 1969;**32**:230-232.

9. McDonald WI, Compston A, Edan G, et al. Recommended diagnostic criteria for multiple sclerosis: guidelines from the International Panel on the diagnosis of multiple sclerosis. *Ann Neurol* 2001;**50**:121-127.

10. Miller H. Trauma and multiple sclerosis. *Lancet* 1964;**i**:848-850.

11. Rindfleisch E. Histologische detail zu der degeneration von gehirn und ruckenmarks. *Virchows Arch (Pathol Anat)*1863;**26**:474-483.

12. Charcot JM. Lectures on diseases of the nervous system. The New Sydenham Society, London 1867.

13. Dencker SJ, Broennestam R, Swahn B. Demonstration of large blood proteins in cerebrospinal fluid. *Neurology* 1961;**11**:441-444.

14. McLean BN, Zeman AZJ, Barnes D, Thompson EJ. Patterns of blood-brain barrier impairment and clinical features in multiple sclerosis. *J Neurol Neurosurg Psychiatry* 1993;**56**:356-360.

15. Corcoran M. An unhappy coincidence between multiple sclerosis and trauma? *Lancet* 2002;**359**:726.

16. Naiman JL, Donohue WL, Prichard JS. Fatal nucleus pulposus embolism of spinal cord after trauma. *Neurology* 1961;**11**:83-87.

17. Klawans HL. Trials of an Expert Witness. Little Brown and Company, Boston 1991.

18. Jeffrey M, Wells GAH. Multifocal ischaemic encephalomyelopathy associated with fibrocartilaginous emboli in the lamb. *Neuropathol Appl Neurobiol* 1986;**12**:415-424.

19. McFadden KD, Taylor JR. End-plate lesions of the lumbar spine. *Spine* 1989;**14**:867-869.

20. Toro-Gonzales G, Navarro-Roman L, Roman GC, et al. Acute ischemic stroke from fibrocartilagenous embolism to the middle cerebral artery. *Stroke* 1993;**24**:738-740.

21. Housman AE. Sudden death in young athletes. *N Engl J Med* 2003;**349**:1064-1075.

22. Scully RE, Mark EJ, McNeely WF, McNeely BU. Case records of the Massachusetts General Hospital: weekly clinicopathological exercises - Case 5. A 61-yr old woman with an abrupt onset of paralysis of the legs and impairment of the bladder and bowel function. *N Engl J Med* 1991;**324**:322-332.

23. Beer S, Kesselring J. Fibrocartilagenous embolisation of the spinal cord in a 7 year old girl. *J Neurol* 2002;**249**:936-937.

24. Rugilo CA, Uribe Roca MC, Zurrú MC, et al. Acute reversible paraparesis secondary to probable fibrocartilaginous embolism. *Neurologia* 2003;**18**:166-169.

25. Duprez TP, Danvoye L, Hernalsteen D, et al. Fibrocartilaginous embolization to the spinal cord: serial MR imaging monitoring and pathologic study. *Am J Neuroradiol* 2005;**26**:496-501.

Chapter 14: The Final Appeal to the House of Lords

1. http://www.publications.parliament.uk/pa/ld199900/ldjudgmt/jd000309/dingle-1.htm

2. Husain J, Juurlink BHJ. Hypoxia and oligodendrocyte precursors. *Prog Brain Res* 2001;**132**:131-147.

3. Juurlink BHJ. Response of glial cells to ischemia: roles of reactive oxygen species and glutathione. *Neuroscience Biobehavioral Rev* 1997;**21**:151-166.

4. Volpe JJ, Kinney HC, Jensen FE, Rosenberg PA. The developing oligodendrocyte: key cellular target in brain injury in the premature infant. *Int J Dev Neurosci* 2011;**29**:423-440.

5. Charcot JM. Lectures on diseases of the nervous system. The New Sydenham Society, London 1867.

6. Putnam TJ, Alexander L. Loss of axis-cylinders in sclerotic plaques and similar lesions. *Arch Neurol Psychiatry* 1947;**57**:661-672.

7. Trapp BD, Peterson J, Ransohoff RM, et al. Axonal transection in the lesions of multiple sclerosis. *N Engl J Med* 1998;**338**:278-285.

8. Narayana PA, Doyle TJ, Dejian L, Wolinsky JS. Serial proton magnetic resonance spectroscopic imaging, contrast-enhanced magnetic resonance imaging and quantitative lesion volumetry in multiple sclerosis. *Ann Neurol* 1998;**43**:56-71.

9. Oppenheimer DR. In; Greenfield's Neuropathology 3rd edition. Eds: Blackwood W, Corsellis JAN. Edward Arnold, London 1976.

10. Poser CM. The role of trauma in the pathogenesis of multiple sclerosis: a review. *Clin Neurosurg* 1994;**96**:103-110.

11. Poser CM. Trauma to the central nervous system may result in formation or enlargement of multiple sclerosis plaques. *Arch Neurol* 2000;**57**:1074-1076.

12. Nerup J, Mandrup-Poulsen T, Helqvist S, et al. On the pathogenesis of IDDM. *Diabetologia* 1994;**37**:S82-S89.

13. Ebers G. Commentary: Outcome measures were flawed. *Br Med J* 2010;**340**:c2693.

14. Lumsden CE. Cyanide leucoencephalopathy in rats and observations on the vascular and ferment hypotheses of demyelinating diseases. *J Neurol Neurosurg* 1950;**13**:1-15.

15. Woolf AL. Experimentally produced cerebral venous obstruction. *J Pathol Bacteriol* 1954;**67**:1-16.

16. Freund J. The mode of action of immunologic adjuvants. *Adv Tuberc Res* 1956;**7**:130-148.

17. Cruickshank B, Thomas MJ. Mineral oil (follicular) lipidosis: II. Histologic studies of spleen, liver, lymph nodes, and bone marrow. *Hum Pathol* 1984;**15**:731-737.

18. Jones G. Accidental self inoculation with oil-based veterinary vaccines. *NZ Med J* 1996;**109**:363-365.

19. Chapel HM, August PJ. Report of nine cases of accidental injury to man with Freund's complete adjuvant. *Clin Exp Immunol* 1976;**24**:538-541.

20. Stewart WA, Alvord EC, Hruby S, et al. Early detection of experimental allergic encephalomyelitis by magnetic resonance imaging. *Lancet* 1985;**ii**:898.

21. Karlik SJ, Strejan G, Gilbert JJ, Noseworthy JH. NMR studies in experimental allergic encephalomyelitis (EAE); normalisation of T1 and T2 with parenchymal cellular infiltration. *Neurology* 1986;**36**:1112-1114.

22. Kermode AG, Thompson AJ, Tofts P, et al. Breakdown of the blood-brain barrier precedes symptoms and other MRI signs of new lesions in multiple sclerosis. *Brain* 1990;**115**:1477-1489.

23. Sears ES, Tindall RSA, Zaenow H. Active multiple sclerosis. *Arch Neurol* 1978;**35**:42-34.

24. Levine S, Sowoinski R, Gruenewald R, Kies MW. Experimental allergic encephalomyelitis. Production by myelin basic protein adsorbed on particulate adjuvants. *Immunology* 1972;**23**:609-614.

25. James PB. Oxygen and multiple sclerosis. *Lancet* 1983;**i**:1161.

26. Sriram S, Steiner I. Experimental allergic encephalomyelitis: a misleading model of multiple sclerosis. *Ann Neurol* 2005;**58**:939-945.

27. Wuerfel J, Bellmann-Strobl J, Brunecker P, et al. Changes in cerebral perfusion precede plaque formation in multiple sclerosis: a longitudinal perfusion MRI study. *Brain* 2004;**127**:111-119.

28. Trapp BD, Nave K-A. Multiple sclerosis: an immune or neurodegenerative disorder? *Ann Rev Neurosci* 2008;**31**:247-269.

29. Kostulas VK, Link H. Agarose isoelectric focussing of cerebrospinal fluid and serum evaluated on 998 neurological patients. *Acta Neurol Scand*

1982;**65**(suppl):266-267.

30. Wang WZ, Olsson T, Kostulas V, et al. Myelin antigen reactive T cells in cerebrovascular diseases. *Clin Exp Immunol* 1992;**88**:157-162.

31. Dow RS, Berglund G. Vascular patterns of lesions of multiple sclerosis. *Arch Neurol Psychiat* 1942;**47**:1-18.

32. James PB. Multiple sclerosis or blood-brain barrier disease. *Lancet* 1989;**i**:46.

33. Ge Y, Zohrabian VM, Grossman RI. Seven-Tesla magnetic resonance imaging: a new vision of microvascular abnormalities in multiple sclerosis. *Arch Neurol* 2008;**65**:812-816.

34. Poser CM, Paty DW, Scheinberg L, et al. New diagnostic criteria for multiple sclerosis: guidelines for research protocols. *Ann Neurol* 1983;**13**:227-231.

35. Lumsden CE. The neuropathology of multiple sclerosis. In: Vinken PJ, Bruyn GW, eds. Handbook of clinical neurology: Vol IV. Amsterdam: North Holland, 1970:217-300.

36. Wolfson C, Talbot P. Bacterial infection as a cause of multiple sclerosis. *Lancet* 2002;**360**:352-353.

37. Berger JR, Sheremata WA. Persistent neurological deficit precipitated by hot bath test in multiple sclerosis. *JAMA* 1983;**249**:1751-1753.

38. Barnett MH, Prineas JW. Relapsing and remitting multiple sclerosis: pathology of the newly forming lesion. *Ann Neurol* 2004;**55**:458-468.

39. Prineas JW, Parratt JDE. Oligodendrocytes and the early multiple sclerosis lesion. *Ann Neurol* 2012;**72**:18-31.

40. Juurlink BHJ. The evidence for hypoperfusion as a factor in MS lesion development. www.Lindaur.com/journals/msi/2013/598093

Chapter 15: Evidence Overlooked, but "The Eyes Have It"

1. Brain's Diseases of the nervous system. 8th Edition Ed. Walton JN. Oxford University Press, Oxford 1977.

2. Optic neuritis. Eds. Hess RF, Plant GT. Cambridge University Press, Cambridge 1986.

3. Galligo G, Orue A. Unilateral neurosensory hearing loss as a manifestation of multiple sclerosis. *Acta Oto Esp* 1999;**50**:147-149.

4. Ozunlu A, Mus N, Gulhan M. Multiple sclerosis: A cause of sudden hearing loss. *Audiology* 1998;**37**:52-58.

5. Yamasoba T, Sakai K, Sakurai M. Role of acute cochlear neuritis in sudden hearing loss in multiple sclerosis. *J Neurol Sci* 1997;**146**:179-181.

6. Arenberg IK, Allen GW, DeBoer A. Sudden deafness immediately

following cardiopulmonary bypass. *J Laryngol Otol* 1972;**86**:73-77.

7. Samarasekera S, Doman P. Case report: The case of the forgotten address. *Lancet* 2005;**367**:1290.

8. Bach-y-Rita P. Sensory Plasticity. *Acta Neurologica Scandinavica* 1967;**43**:417-426.

9. Russell WR. Observations on the retinal blood-vessels in monocular blindness. *Lancet* 1961;**ii**:1422-1428.

10. Miller DH, Thompson AJ, Morrissey SP, et al. High dose steroids in acute relapses of multiple sclerosis: MRI evidence for a possible mechanism of therapeutic effect. *J Neurol Neurosurg Psychiatry* 1992;**55**:450-453.

11. Jaafar J, Wan Hitam WH, Noor RAM. Bilateral atypical optic neuritis associated with tuberculosis in an immuno-compromised patient. *Asian Pacific Journal of Tropical Biomedicine* 2012;**2**:586-588.

12. Weinstein JM, Lexow SS, Ho P, Spickards A. Acute syphilitic optic neuritis. *Arch Ophthalmol* 1981;**99**:1392-1395.

13. Ferry AP, Font RL. Carcinoma metastatic to the eye and orbit. *Arch Ophthalmol* 1974;**92**:276-286.

14. Hayreh SS, Blodi FC, Silbermann NN, Summers TB, Potter PH. Unilateral optic nerve head and choroidal metastases from a bronchial carcinoma. *Ophthalmologica* 1982;**185**:232-241.

15. Takahashi T, Oda Y, Isayama Y. Leukemic optic neuropathy. *Ophthalmologica* 1982;**185**:37-45.

16. Butler FK. Decompression sickness presenting as optic neuropathy. *Aviat Space Environ Med* 1991;**62**:346-350.

17. Sweeney PJ, Breuer AC, Selhorst JB, et al. Ischemic optic neuropathy: A complication of cardiopulmonary bypass surgery. *Neurology* 1982;**32**:560-562.

18. Blauth C, Arnold J, Kohner EM, Taylor KM. Retinal microembolism during cardiopulmonary bypass demonstrated by fluorescein angiography. *Lancet* 1986;**ii**:837-839.

19. Plasse HM, Mittleman M, Frost JO. Unilateral sudden hearing loss after open heart surgery: a detailed study of seven cases. *Laryngoscope* 1981;**91**:101-109.

20. Harris DNF, Bailey SM, Smith PLC, et al. Brain swelling in first hour after coronary artery bypass surgery. *Lancet* 1993;**342**:586-587.

21. Muraoka R, Yokota M, Aoshima M, et al. Subclinical changes in brain morphology following cardiac operations as reflected by computed tomographic scans of the brain. *J Thorac Cardiovasc Surg* 1981;**81**:364-369.

22. Gunning AJ, Pickering GW, Robb-Smith AHT, Russell WR. Mural

thrombosis of the internal carotid artery and subsequent embolism. *Q J Med* 1964;**129**:155-195.

23. Field EJ, Foster JB. Periphlebitis retinae and multiple sclerosis. *J Neurol Neurosurg Psychiatry* 1962;**25**:269-270.

24. Arnold AC, Pepose JS, Hepler RS, Foos RY. Retinal periphlebitis and retinitis in multiple sclerosis. 1. Pathologic characteristics. *Ophthalmology* 1984;**91**:255-262.

25. Haining WM. Film: Retinal emboli. *Trans Ophthalmol Soc UK* 1969;**89**:415-416.

26. Franklin CR, Brickner RM. Vasospasm associated with multiple sclerosis. *Arch Neurol Psychiatry* 1947;**58**:125-163.

27. Brickner RM. The significance of localized vasoconstrictions in multiple sclerosis. *Proc Assoc Res Nerv Ment Dis* 1950;**28**:236-244.

28. Putnam TJ. The pathogenesis of multiple sclerosis: a possible vascular factor. *N Engl J Med* 1933;**209**:786-790.

29. Wagener HP. Lesions of the retina and optic nerve secondary to distant trauma. *Am J Med Sc* 1954;**228**:226-235.

Chapter 16: Trauma *May* Cause Multiple Sclerosis

1. Jenkins A, Teasdale, Hadley MDM, et al. Brain lesions detected by magnetic resonance imaging in mild and severe head injuries. *Lancet* 1986;**ii**:445-446.

2. Autti T, Sipila L, Autti, H, Salonen O. Brain lesions in players of contact sports, *Lancet* 1997;**349**:1144.

3. Beer S, Kesselring J. Fibrocartilagenous embolisation of the spinal cord in a 7 year old girl. *J Neurol* 2002;**249**:936-937.

4. Rugilo CA, Uribe Roca MC, Zurrú MC, et al. Acute reversible paraparesis secondary to probable fibrocartilaginous embolism. *Neurologia* 2003;**18**:166-169.

5. Nijsten MWN, Hamer JPN, Ten Duis HJ, Posma JL. Fat embolism and patent foramen ovale. *Lancet* 1989;**i**:1271.

6. Pell ACH, Hughes D, Keating J, et al. Brief report: fulminating fat embolism syndrome caused by paradoxical embolism through a patent foramen ovale. *N Engl J Med* 1993;**329**:926-929.

7. Varma JS. Sub-acute pulmonary hypertension and systemic tumour embolism from cervical cancer. *Scott Med J* 1982;**27**:336-340.

8. Deland FH, Bennett WA. Death due to bone-marrow and tumor embolization in the absence of fracture. *Arch Pathol* 1957;**63**:13-16.

9. Fryer DI. Subatmospheric decompression sickness in man. NATO AGARDograph No. 125. Technivision Services, Slough 1969.

10. Samarasekera S, Dorman PJ. Case report: The case of the forgotten address. *Lancet* 2006;**367**:1290.

11. Peltier LF. Fat embolism. III. The toxic properties of neutral fat and free fatty acids. *Surgery* 1956;**40**:665-670.

12. McTaggart DM, Neubuerger KT. Cerebral fat embolism: pathologic changes in the brain after survival of 7 years. *Acta Neuropathol (Berl)* 1970;**15**:183-187.

13. Cammermeyer J. Subacute cerebral fat embolism complicated by juxtaembolic thrombosis of fibrin. *Arch Pathol* 1953;**56**:254-261.

14. Scheinker M. Formation of demyelinated plaques associated with cerebral fat embolism in man. *Arch Neurol Psychiatry* 1943;**49**:754-64.

15. Park Y-H, Kim KS. Blindness after fat injections. *N Eng J Med* 2011;**365**:2220.

16. Bierre AR, Koelmeyer TD. Pulmonary fat and bone marrow embolism in aircraft accident victims. *Pathology* 1983;**15**:13-35.

17. Pell AC, Christie J, Keating JF, Sutherland GR. The detection of fat embolism by transoesophageal echocardiography during reamed intramedullary nailing. *J Bone Joint Surg* 1993;**75**:921-925.

18. Lessells AM. Fatal fat embolism after minor trauma. *Br Med J* 1981;**282**:1586.

19. Levy DE. Transient CNS deficits: a common, benign syndrome in young adults. *Neurology* 1988;**38**:83-836.

20. Gerard G, Weisberg LA. MRI periventricular lesions in adults. *Neurology* 1986;**36**:998-1001.

21. Bradley WG, Waluch V, Brant-Zawadzki M, et al. Patchy, periventricular white matter lesions in the elderly: A common observation during NMR imaging. *N Med Imaging* 1984;**11**:35-41.

22. Kivipelto M, Solomon A. Cerebral embolism and Alzheimer's disease. *Br Med J* 2006;**332**:1104-1105.

23. Purandare N, Burns A, Daly KJ, Hardicre J, et al. Cerebral emboli as a potential cause of Alzheimer's disease and vascular dementia: case-control study. *Br Med J* 2006;**332**:1119-1124.

24. Bowman GL, Kaye JA, Moore M, et al. Blood-brain barrier impairment in Alzheimer disease. *Neurology* 2007;**68**:1809-1814.

25. Jacobson DM, Terrence CF, Reinmuth OM. The neurologic manifestations of fat embolism. *Neurology* 1986;**36**:847-851.

26. Kawano Y, Ochi M, Hayashi K, Morikawa M, Kimura S. Magnetic resonance imaging of cerebral fat embolism. *Neuroradiology* 1991;**33**:72-74.

27. Chrysikopoulos H, Maniatis V, Pappas J, et al. Case report: Post-traumatic cerebral fat embolism: CT and MR findings: Report of two cases and review of literature. *Clin Radiol* 1996;**51**:728-732.

28. Finlay ME, Benson MD. Case report: magnetic resonance imaging in cerebral fat embolism. *Clin Radiol* 1996;**51**:445-446.

29. Fuerecdi Ga, Czarnecki DJ, Kindwall EP. MR findings in the brains of compressed-air tunnel workers; relationship to psychometric results. *AJR* 1991;**12**:67-70.

30. Sevitt S. Fat embolism. Butterworths, London 1962.

31. James PB, Evidence for subacute fat embolism as the cause of multiple sclerosis. *Lancet* 1982;**i**:380-386.

32. Putnam TJ, McKenna JB, Morrison LR. Studies in multiple sclerosis. I. The histogenesis of experimental sclerotic plaques and their relation to multiple sclerosis. *JAMA* 1931;**97**:1591-1596.

33. Swank RL, Hain RF. The effect of different sized emboli on the vascular system and parenchyma of the brain. *J Neuropathol Exp Neurol* 1952;**11**:280-299.

34. Woolf AL. Experimentally produced cerebral venous obstruction. *J Path Bact* 1954;**67**:1-16.

35. Adams CWM, High OB. Embolism and multiple sclerosis. *Lancet* 1982;**i**:621.

36. James PB. Fat embolism in multiple sclerosis. *Lancet* 1982;**i**:1356.

37. Simon AD,Ulmer JL, Strottman JM. Contrast-enhanced MR imaging of cerebral fat embolism: case report and review of the literature. *AJNR* 2003;**24**:97-101.

38. Leeb CH, Kima HJ, Hae G, et al. Reversible MR Changes in the cat brain after cerebral fat embolism induced by triolein emulsion. *AJNR* 2004;**25**:958-963.

39. Zulch KJ, Tzonos T. Transudation phenomena at the deep veins after blockage of arterioles and capillaries by micro-emboli. *Bibl Anat* 1965;**7**:279-284.

40. Lumsden CE. Pathogenetic mechanisms in the leucoencephalopathies in anoxic ischaemic processes; in disorders of the blood and in intoxications. Chapter 20. In; Vinken PJ, Bruyn GW, eds. Handbook of clinical neurology. Amsterdam, North Holland, 1970; pp. 572-663.

41. Poser CM. The pathogenesis of multiple sclerosis. *J Neurol Sci* 1993;**115**

(Suppl):S3-S15.

42. Poser CM. Trauma to the central nervous system may result in formation or enlargement of multiple sclerosis plaques. *Arch Neurol* 2000;**57**:1074-1076.

43. Ormerod IEC, McDonald WI, Du Boulay GH, et al. Disseminated lesions at presentation in patients with optic neuritis. *J Neurol Neurosurg Psychiatry* 1986;**49**:124-127.

44. McDonald WI, in: Optic neuritis. Eds. Hess RF, Plant GT. Cambridge University Press, Cambridge 1986.

45. Albers, GW, Avalos, SM, Weinrich M. Left ventricular tumor masquerading as multiple sclerosis. *Arch Neurol* 1987;**44**:779-780.

46. Zamboni P. The big idea: Iron-dependent inflammation in venous disease and proposed parallels in multiple sclerosis. *J R Soc Med* 2006;**99**:589-593.

47. Hughes syndrome: Anti-phospholipid syndrome. Ed, Khamashta MA. Springer-Verlag, London 2000.

48. Courville CB. Further notes on traumatic fat embolism: comparison of distribution of nervous lesions with those of multiple sclerosis. *Bull Los Angeles Neurol Soc* 1964;**29**:143-140.

49. Bouaggad A, Harti A, Barrou H, Zryouil B, Benaguida M. Tetraplegie au cours de l'embolie graisseuse. *Ann Fr Anesth Reanim* 1994;**13**:730-733.

50. Allen IV. The pathology of multiple sclerosis - fact, fiction and hypothesis. *Neuropathol Appl Neurobiol* 1981;**7**:169-182.

51. Dow RS, Berglund G. Vascular patterns of lesions of multiple sclerosis. *Arch Neurol Psychiat* 1942;**47**:1-18.

52. Charcot JM. Lectures on diseases of the nervous system. The New Sydenham Society, London 1867.

53. Nicholson M, McLaughlin C. Social constructionism and medical sociology: a study of the vascular theory of multiple sclerosis. *Sociology Health & Illness* 1988;**10**:234-261.

54. Boggild M, Palace J, Barton P, et al. Multiple sclerosis risk sharing scheme: two year results of clinical cohort with a historical comparator. *Br Med J* 2009;**339**:b4677.

55. Ross Russell RW. The origin and effects of cerebral emboli. In: Williams DJ, Feiling A. Modern trends in neurology. London: Butterworths, 1970.

56. Peltier LF. Fat embolism: a pulmonary disease. *Surgery* 1967;**62**:756-758.

57. US Navy Diving Manual, Table 5. Navsea 0994-LP-00l-9010.

58. Prockop LD, Grasso RJ. Ameliorating effects of hyperbaric oxygenation on experimental allergic encephalomyelitis. *Brain Res Bull* 1978;**3**:221-225.

59. Warren J, Sacksteder MR, Thuning CA. Oxygen immunosuppression: modification of experimental allergic encephalomyelitis in rodents. *J Immunol* 1978;**121**:315-320.

60. Neubauer RA. Exposure of multiple sclerosis patients to hyperbaric oxygen at 1·5-2 ATA; a preliminary report. *J Fla Med Assoc* 1980;**67**:498-504.

61. Aita JF, Bennett DR, Anderson RE, Ziter F. Cranial CT appearance of acute multiple sclerosis. *Neurology* 1978;**28**:251-255.

72. Fischer BH, Marks M, Reich T. Hyperbaric-oxygen treatment of multiple sclerosis: a randomized, placebo-controlled, double-blind study. *N Engl J Med* 1983;**308**:181-186.

Chapter 17: A Tale of Trials and the New England Journal of Medicine

1. Schumacher GA. Critique of experimental trials of therapy in multiple sclerosis. *Neurology* 1974;**24**:1010-1014.

2. Haldane JBS. Possible Worlds No 9. Evergreen books, William Heinemann Ltd, London 1940.

3. Simons DJ. Note on effect of heat and of cold upon certain symptoms of multiple sclerosis. *Bull Neurol Soc NY* 1937;**6**:385-386.

4. Berger JR, Sheremata WA. Persistent neurological deficit precipitated by hot bath test in multiple sclerosis. *JAMA* 1983;**249**:1751-1753.

5. Layton DD, Mackay RP. Office management of multiple sclerosis. *Med Clin North Am* 1958;**42**:103-110.

6. Fischer BH, Marks M, Reich T. Hyperbaric-oxygen treatment of multiple sclerosis a randomized, placebo-controlled, double-blind study. *N Eng J Med* 1983;**308**:181-186.

7. Boschetty V, Cernoch J. Aplikace Kysliku za pfetlaku u nekterych neurologickych onemocnenf. *Bratisl Lek Listy* 1970;**53**:298-302.

8. Neubauer RA. Treatment of multiple sclerosis with monoplace hyperbaric oxygenation. *J Fla Med Assoc* 1978;**65**:101.

9. Formai C, Sereni G, Zannini D. L'ossigenoterapia iperbarica nel trattamento della Sclerosi Multipla. Presented at the 4th Congresso Nazionale di Medicina Subacquea ed Iperbarica, Naples, Italy, October 24-26, 1980.

10. Pallotta R, Anceschi S, Costagliola N, et al. Prospettive di terapia iperbarica della Sclerosi a Placche. *Ann Med Navale* 1980;**85**:57-62.

11. Baixe JH. Bilan de onze annees d'activite en medicine hyperbare. *Med Aer*

Spatiale Med Subaquatique Hyperbare 1978;**17**:90-92.

12. Warren JM, Sacksteder MR, Thuning CA. Modification of allergic encephalomyelitis in the guinea pig by oxygen therapy. *Fed Proc* 1977;**36**:1298.

13. Warren J, Sacksteder MR, Thuning CA, Jacobs BB. Suppression of cell mediated immune responses by hyperbaric oxygen. *Fed Proc.* 1978;**37**:560.

14. Warren J, Sacksteder MR, Thuning CA. Oxygen immuno-suppression: modification of experimental allergic encephalomyelitis in rodents. *J Immunol* 1978;**121**:315-320.

15. Prockop LD, Grasso RJ. Ameliorating effects of hyperbaric oxygenation on experimental allergic encephalomyelitis. *Brain Res Bull* 1978;**3**:221-225.

16. Hansbrough JF, Piacentine JG, Eiseman B. Immuno-suppression by hyperbaric oxygen. *Surgery* 1980;**87**:662-667.

17. Neubauer RA. Exposure of multiple sclerosis patients to hyperbaric oxygen at 1.5-2 ATA: a preliminary report. *J Fla Med Assoc* 1980;**67**:498-504.

18. Gottlieb SF. The Naked Mind. Best Publishing Company, Flagstaff, Arizona 2003.

19. Hauser SL, Dawson DM, Lehrich JR, et al. Intensive immunosuppression in progressive multiple sclerosis. A randomized, three-arm study of high-dose intravenous cyclophosphamide, plasma exchange, and ACTH. *N Engl J Med* 1983;**308**:173-180.

20. McFarlin DE. Treatment of Multiple Sclerosis. *N Engl J Med* 1983;**308**:215.

21. Angell M. Multiple Sclerosis and the Ingelfinger Rule. *N Engl J Med* 1983;**308**:215.

22. Bevers RFM, Bakker DJ, Kurth KH. Hyperbaric oxygen treatment for haemorrhagic radiation cystitis. *Lancet* 1995;**346**:803-805.

23. Goodkin DE, Plencner S, Palmer-Saxerud J, et al. Cyclophosphamide in chronic multiple sclerosis. *Arch Neurol* 1987;**44**:823-827.

24. Mertin J, Knight SC, Rudge P, Thompson EJ, et al. Double-blind, controlled trial of immuno-suppression in treatment of multiple sclerosis: Preliminary communication. *Lancet* 1980;**ii**:949-951.

25. Mertin J, Rudge P, Kremer M, et al. Double-blind controlled trial of immuno-suppression in the treatment of multiple sclerosis: Final report. *Lancet* 1982;**ii**:351-353.

26. Wiles CM, Clarke CRA, Irwin HP, et al. Hyperbaric oxygen in multiple sclerosis: a double blind trial. *Br Med J* 1986;**292**:367-371.

27. Appell RA, Goodman JR, Deutsch JS, Van Meter K. The effects of hyperbaric oxygen on the neurogenic vesico-urethral dysfunction of

multiple sclerosis. Proc. 6th Annual Symposium of the Urodynamics Society. New Orleans 1984:53.

28. Barnes MP, Bates D, Cartlidge NEF, et al. Hyperbaric oxygen and multiple sclerosis: Short-term results of a placebo-controlled, double-blind trial. *Lancet* 1985;**i**:297-300.

29. Barnes MP, Bates D, Cartlidge NEF, et al. Hyperbaric oxygen and multiple sclerosis: Final results of a placebo-controlled, double-blind trial. *J Neurol Neurosurg Psychiatry* 1987;**50**:1402-1406.

30. Martin JD, Thom SR. Vascular leukocyte sequestration in decompression sickness and prophylactic hyperbaric oxygen therapy in rats. *Aviat Space Environ Med* 2002;**73**:565-569.

31. Jacobson I, Harper AM, McDowall DG. Effects of oxygen under pressure on cerebral blood-flow and cerebral venous oxygen tension. *Lancet* 1963;**i**:549.

32. Webster C, McIver C, Allen S, James PB. Long-term hyperbaric oxygen therapy for multiple sclerosis patients. ARMS Education report, Dartmouth St., London 1987.

Chapter 18: The UK Multiple Sclerosis Therapy Centres: Self-Help in Action

1. Neubauer RA. Treatment of multiple sclerosis with monoplace hyperbaric oxygenation. *J Fla Med Assoc* 1978;**65**:101.

2. Neubauer RA. Exposure of multiple sclerosis patients to hyperbaric oxygen at 1.5-2 ATA: a preliminary report. *J Fla Med Assoc* 1980;**67**:498-504.

3. Davidson DLW. Hyperbaric oxygen treatment for multiple sclerosis. *Practitioner* 1984;**228**:903-905.

4. Fischer BH, Marks M, Reich T. Hyperbaric-oxygen treatment of multiple sclerosis a randomized, placebo-controlled, double-blind study. *N Eng J Med* 1983;**308**:181-186.

5. Hauser SL, Dawson DM, Lehrich JR, et al. Intensive immunosuppression in progressive multiple sclerosis. A randomized, three-arm study of high-dose intravenous cyclophosphamide, plasma exchange, and ACTH. *N Engl J Med* 1983;**308**:173-180.

6. Wiles CM, Clarke CRA, Irwin HP, et al. Hyperbaric oxygen in multiple sclerosis: a double blind trial. *Br Med J* 1986;**292**:367-371.

7. Barnes MP, Bates D, Cartlidge NEF, et al. Hyperbaric oxygen and multiple sclerosis: Short-term results of a placebo-controlled, double-blind trial. *Lancet* 1985;**i**:297-300.

8. James PB. Hyperbaric oxygen and multiple sclerosis. *Lancet* 1985;**i**:572.

9. Barnes MP, Bates D, Cartlidge NEF, et al. Hyperbaric oxygen and multiple sclerosis: Final results of a placebo-controlled, double-blind trial. *J Neurol Neurosurg Psychiatry* 1987;**50**:1402-1406.

10. Oriani G, Barbieri S, Cislaghi G, et al. Long term hyperbaric oxygen in multiple sclerosis; a placebo controlled, double-blind study with evoked potential studies. *J Hyp Med* 1990;**5**:237-245.

11. Appell RA, Goodman JR, Deutsch JS, Van Meter K. The effects of hyperbaric oxygen therapy on the neurogenic vesico-urethral dysfunction of multiple sclerosis. Proceedings, 6th Annual Symposium, Urodynamics Society, Louisana, May 5th 1984.

12. James PB, Webster CJ. Long-term results of hyperbaric oxygen therapy in multiple sclerosis. *Lancet* 1989;**ii**:327.

13. Webster C, McIver C, Allen S, James PB. Long-term hyperbaric oxygen therapy for multiple sclerosis patients; two year results in 128 patients. ARMS, 11 Dartmouth Street, London 1989.

14. Mertin J, Knight SC, Rudge P, Thompson EJ, et al. Double-blind, controlled trial of immunosuppression in treatment of multiple sclerosis. (Preliminary communication) *Lancet* 1980;**ii**:949-951.

15. Hauser SL, Dawson DM, Lehrich JR, et al. Intensive immunosuppression in progressive multiple sclerosis. A randomized, three-arm study of high-dose intravenous cyclophosphamide, plasma exchange, and ACTH. *N Engl J Med* 1983;**308**:173-180.

16. McFarlin DE. Treatment of Multiple Sclerosis. *N Engl J Med* 1983;**308**:215.

17. Kleijnen J, Knipschild P. Hyperbaric oxygen for multiple sclerosis. *Acta Neurol Scand* 1995;**91**:330-334.

18. INFB MS study group. Interferon beta 1b is effective in relapsing remitting multiple sclerosis: 1 Clinical results of a multicentre randomised trial. *Neurology* 1993;**42**:655-661.

19. Warlow C. Not such a bright idea: the risk sharing scheme for beta interferon and glatimer acetate in multiple sclerosis. *Pract Neurol* 2003;**3**:194-195.

20. James PB. Hyperbaric oxygen for multiple sclerosis. World Medicine 1983;18:33.

21. Tremlett H, Paty D, Devonshire V. Disability progression in multiple sclerosis is slower than previously reported. *Neurology* 2006;**66**:172-177.

22. Ebers G. Commentary: Outcome measures were flawed. *Br Med J* 2010;**340**:c2693.

23. Compston A. Commentary: Scheme has benefited patients. *Br Med J* 2010;**340**:c2707.

24. Hawker K, O'Connor P, Freedman MS, et al. Rituximab in patients with primary progressive multiple sclerosis: Results of a randomized double-blind placebo-controlled multicenter trial. *Ann Neurol* 2009;**66**:460-471.

25. Downie DP, James PB. Code of Construction and Working Practice for Low-Pressure Barochambers, June 2003. Obtainable from; MS National Therapy Centres, PO Box 2199. Buckingham MK18 8AR.

26. Perrins DJD, James PB. Long-term hyperbaric oxygenation retards progression in multiple sclerosis patients. *IJNN* 2005;**2**:45-48.

27. Pallotta R, Anceschi S, Costilgliola N, et al. Prospecttive di terapia iperbarica nella sclerosi a placce. *Ann Med Nav* 1980;**85**:57-62.

28. Smith T. Editorial: Taming high technology. *Br Med J* 1984;**289**:393-394.

29. Treweek S, James PB. A cost analysis of monoplace hyperbaric oxygen treatment with and without recirculation. *J Wound Care* 2006;**5**:1-4.

30. http://www.fda.gov/Fdac/features/2002/602_air.html

Chapter 19: Head Injuries – the Curse of Life in the Fast Lane

1. Voss HU, Ulug AM, Dyke JP, et al. Possible axonal regrowth in late recovery from the minimally conscious state. *J Clin Invest* 2005;**116**:2005-2011.

2. Shin SS, Verstynen T, Pathak S, et al. High-definition fiber tracking for assessment of neurological deficit in a case of traumatic brain injury: finding, visualizing, and interpreting small sites of damage. *J Neurosurg* 2012;**116**:1062-1069.

3. Ghajar J. Traumatic brain injury. *Lancet* 2000;**356**:923–929.

4. http://www.ncbi.nlm.nih.gov/pmc/articles/PMC2542895/

5. Diringer MN. Hyperoxia-good or bad for the injured brain. *Curr Opin Crit Care* 2008;**14**:167–171.

6. Sukoff MH, Ragatz RE. Hyperbaric oxygenation for the treatment of acute cerebral edema. *Neurosurgery* 1982;**10**:29-38.

7. Stamler JS, Jia L, Eu JP, et al. Blood flow regulation by S-nitrosohemoglobin in the physiological oxygen gradient. *Science* 1997;**276**:2034-2037.

8. Cramer T, Yamanishi Y, Clausen BE, et al. HIF 1α is essential for myeloid dell-mediated inflammation. *Cell* 2003;**112**:645-657.

9. Dai J, Swaab DF, Buijs RM. Recovery of axonal transport in "dead neurons." *Lancet* 1998;**351**:499-500.

10. Zamboni WA, Roth AC, Russell RC, e al. Morphologic analysis of the

microcirculation during reperfusion of ischemic skeletal muscle and the effect of hyperbaric oxygen. *Plast Reconstr Surg* 1993;**91**:1110-1123.

11. Gandy SE, Snow RB, Zimmerman RD, Deck MDF. Cranial nuclear magnetic resonance imaging in head trauma. *Ann Neurol* 1984;**16**:254-257.

12. Faden AI. Neuroprotection and traumatic brain injury: The search continues. *Arch Neurol* 2001;**58**:1553-1555.

13. Autti, T, Sipila L, Autti, H, Salonen O. Brain lesions in players of contact sports, *Lancet* 1997;**349**:1144.

14. Jones D. Heal thyself. *New Scientist* 14 August 2010.

15. Singer M. Treating critical illness: The importance of first doing no harm. *PLoS Medicine* 2005;**2**:e167.

16. Pintu L, Whitehead T, Evans T, Griffiths M. Ventilator-associated lung injury. *Lancet* 2003;**361**:332-340.

17. Sukoff MH, Hollin SA, Espinosa OE, Jacobson JH. The protective effect of hyperbaric oxygenation in experimental cerebral edema. *J Neurosurg* 1968;**29**:236-241.

18. Holbach KH, Caroli A, Wassmann H. Cerebral energy metabolism in patients with brain lesions at normo and hyperbaric oxygen pressures. *J Neurol* 1977;**217**:17-30.

19. Ingevar DH, Lassen NA. Treatment of focal cerebral ischemia with hyperbaric oxygen: report of 4 cases. *Acta Neurol Scand* 1965;**41**;92-95.

20. Kelly DL Jr, Lassiter KRL, Vongsvivut A, Smith JM. Effects of hyperbaric oxygenation and tissue oxygen studies in experimental paraplegia. *Neurosurgery* 1972;**36**:425-429.

21. Jacobson I, Harper AM, McDowall DG. Effects of oxygen under pressure on cerebral blood-flow and cerebral venous oxygen tension. *Lancet* 1963;**i**:549.

22. Haldane JS. The therapeutic administration of oxygen. *Br Med J* 1917;**1**:181-183.

23. Nunn JF. 100% oxygen at normal pressure is an alternative. *Br Med J* 1994;**309**:124.

24. Rockswold GL, Ford SE. Preliminary results of a prospective randomized trial for treatment of severely brain-injured patients with hyperbaric oxygen. *Min Med* 1985;**68**:533-535.

25. Rockswold GL, Ford SE, Anderson DC, Bergman TA, Sherman RE. Results of a prospective randomised trial for treatment of severely brain-injured patients with hyperbaric oxygen. *J Neurosurg* 1992;**76**:929-934.

26. Oddo M, Levine JM, Mackenzie L, et al. Brain hypoxia is associated

with short-term outcome after severe head injury independently of intracranial hypertension and low cerebral perfusion pressure. *Neurosurg* 2011;**69**:1037-1045.

27. Spiotta AM, Stiefel MF, Gracias VH, et al. Brain tissue oxygen-directed management and outcome in patients with severe traumatic brain injury. *J Neurosurg* 2010;**113**:571-580.

28. Tolias CM, Reinert M, Seiler R, et al. Normobaric hyperoxia—induced improvement in cerebral metabolism and reduction in intracranial pressure in patients with severe head injury: a prospective historical cohort-matched study. *J Neurosurg* 2004;**101**:435-444.

29. Bardt TF, Unterberg AW, Hartl R, et el. Monitoring of brain tissue PO_2 in traumatic brain injury: effect of cerebral hypoxia on outcome. *Acta Neurochir* 1998;**71**(Suppl):153–156.

30. Neubauer RA, Gottlieb SF, Kagan RL, Enhancing "idling" neurons. *Lancet* 1990;**335**:542.

31. Peters BH, Levin HS, Kelly PJ. Neurologic and psychologic manifestations of decompression illness in divers. *Neurology* 1977;**27**:125-127.

32. Curley MD, Schwartz HJC, Zwingelberg KM. Neuropsychologic assessment of cerebral decompression sickness and gas embolism. *Undersea Biomed Res* 1988;**15**:223-236.

33. Courville CB, Kimball TS. Histologic observations in a case of old gunshot wound of the brain. *Am J Pathol* 1934;**17**:10-21.

34. Harch PG, Fogarty EF, Staabl PK, Van Meter K. Low pressure hyperbaric oxygen therapy and SPECT brain imaging in the treatment of blast-induced chronic traumatic brain injury (post-concussion syndrome) and post traumatic stress disorder: a case report. *Cases Journal* 2009;**2**:6538. (http://www.casesjournal.com/content/2/1/6538)

35. Harch PG, Kriedt C, Van Meter KW, Sutherland RJ. Hyperbaric oxygen therapy improves spatial learning and memory in a rat model of chronic traumatic brain injury. *Brain Res* 2007;**1174**:120-129.

36. Mychaskiw G. How many deaths will it take till they know? Monkeys, madmen and the standard of evidence: an editorial perspective. *Undersea Hyperb Med* 2012;**39**:795-797.

37. Wright JK, Zant E, Groom K., et al. Case report: Treatment of mild traumatic brain injury with hyperbaric oxygen. *Undersea Hyperb Med* 2009;**36**:391-399.

38. Wolf G, Cifu D, Baugh L, Carne W, Profenna L. The effect of hyperbaric oxygen on symptoms following mild traumatic brain injury. *J Neurotrauma*

2012; **29**: 2606-2612.

39. Collet JP, Vanasse M, Marois P, et al. HBO-CP research group. Hyperbaric oxygen for children with cerebral palsy: a randomised multicentre trial. *Lancet* 2001;**357**:582-586.

40. Babchin A, Levich E, Melamed Y, Sivashinsky G. Osmotic phenomena in application of hyperbaric oxygen treatment. *Colloids Surf B Biointerfaces* 2010;**83**:128-132.

41. Lawrence JH, Tobias CR, Lyons WMR, et al. A study of aero medical problems in a Liberator bomber at high altitude. *J Aviat Med* 1945;**16**:286-303.

42. Astrup J, Siesjo BK, Symon L. Thresholds in cerebral ischemia - the ischemic penumbra. *Stroke* 1981;**12**:723-725.

43. Ewing, R, McCarthy D, Gronwall D, Wrightson,. Persisting effects of minor head injury observable during hypoxic stress. *J Clin Exp Neuropsychol* 1980;**2**:147-155.

44. Lin KC, Niu KC, Tsai KJ, et al. Attenuating inflammation but stimulating both angiogenesis and neurogenesis using hyperbaric oxygen in rats with traumatic brain injury. *J Trauma Acute Care Surg* 2012;**72**:650-659.

45. Saunders RL, Harbaugh RE. The second impact in catastrophic contact-sports head trauma. *JAMA* 1984;**252**:538-539.

46. Weinstein E, Turner M, Kuzma BB, Feuer H. Second impact syndrome in football: new imaging and insights into a rare and devastating condition. *J Neurosurg: Pediatrics* 2013;**11**;331-334.

47. Menzel M, Doppenberg MR, Zauner A, et al. Increased inspired oxygen concentration as a factor in improved brain tissue oxygenation and tissue lactate levels after severe human head injury. *J Neurosurg* 1999;**91**:1-10.

48. Johnston AJ, Steiner LA, Gupta AK, Menon DK. Cerebral oxygen vasoreactivity and cerebral tissue oxygen reactivity. *Br J Anaesth* 2003;**90**:774-786.

49. Erecinska M, Silver IA. Tissue oxygen tension and brain sensitivity to hypoxia. *Resp Physiol* 2001;**128**:263–276.

50. MacDonald CL, Johnson AM, Cooper D, et al. Detection of blast-related traumatic brain injury in US military personnel. *N Engl J Med* 2011;**364:**2091–2100.

51. Boussi-Gross R, Golan H, Fishlev G, et al. Hyperbaric oxygen therapy can improve post concussive syndrome years after mild traumatic brain injury - randomized prospective trial. *PLoS ONE* 2013;**8**(11): e79995. doi:10.1371/journal.pone.0079995

Chapter 20: Stroke and Hyperbaric Oxygen Treatment

1. Ostrowski RP, Colohan ART, Zhang JH. Mechanisms of hyperbaric-oxygen induced neuroprotection in a rat model of subarachnoid hemorrhage. J Cereb Blood Flow Metab 2005.

2. Lim J, Lim WK, Yeo TT, Low SE. Management of haemorrhagic stroke with hyperbaric oxygen therapy-a case report. *Singapore Med J* 2001;42:220-223.

3. Nishida N, Chiba T, Ohtani M, Yoshioka N. Selective obstruction of lateral striate capsular arteries due to small cardiogenic embolus as a cause of acute cerebral infarction limited to unilateral putamen. *Eur J Neurol* 2006;**13**:e1-e2.

4. Imakita S, Nishimura T, Naito H, et al. Magnetic resonance imaging of human cerebral infarction: enhancement with Gd-DTPA. *Neuroradiology* 1987;**29**:422-429.

5. Latour LI, Kang D-W, Ezzeddine MA, et al. Early blood-brain barrier disruption in human focal brain ischemia. *Ann Neurol* 2004;**56**:468-477.

6. Stewart PA, Hayakawa K, Akers MA, Vinters HV. A morphometric study of the blood-brain barrier in Alzheimer's disease. *Lab Invest* 1992;**67**:734-742.

7. Wardlaw JM, Sandercock PAG, Dennis MS, Starr J. Is breakdown of the blood-brain barrier responsible for lacunar stroke, leukoaraiosis and dementia? *Stroke* 2003;**34**:806-812.

8. Russell RWR. The origin and effects of cerebral emboli. Chapter 10 in: Modern trends in neurology. Ed, Williams D, Butterworths, London 1970:178-188.

9. Russell RWR, Bharucha N. Recognition and prevention of border zone cerebral ischaemia during cardiac surgery. *Q J Med* 1978;**187**:303-323.

10. Moor GF, Fuson RL, Margolis G, et al. An evaluation of the protective effect of hyperbaric oxygenation on the central nervous system during circulatory arrest. *J Cardiovasc Surg* 1966;**52**:618-628.

11. Toro-Gonzales G, Navarro-Roman L, Roman GC, et al. Acute ischemic stroke from fibrocartilagenous embolism to the middle cerebral artery. *Stroke* 1993;**24**:738-740.

12. Sudo K, Kishimoto R, Tajima Y, et al. A paralysed thumb. *Lancet* 2004;**363**:1364.

13. Whisnant JP. Multiple particles injected may all go to the same cerebral artery branch. *Stroke* 1982;**13**:720.

14. Toole JF. Cerebrovascular disorders. 5th Edition Lippincott Williams and Wilkins Philadelphia 1999.

15. Rodan LH, Aviv RI, Sahlas DJ, et al. Seizures during stroke thrombolysis heralding dramatic neurologic recovery. *Neurology* 2006;**67**:2048-2049.

16. Hankey GJ. New drugs,or new trials of current drugs for the treatment of acute ischaemic stroke. *Lancet* 2001;**358**:683.

17. Department of Health; Reducing brain damage: faster access to better stroke care. National audit office, London 2005.

18. Hughes GRV. The anticardiolipin syndrome. *Clin Exp Rheumatol* 1985;**3**:285.

19. Fazekas F, Fazekas G, Schmidt R, et al. Magnetic resonance imaging correlates of transient cerebral ischemic attacks. *Stroke* 1996;**27**:607-611.

20. Yoneda Y, Tokui K, Hanihara T, et al. Diffusion-weighted magnetic resonance imaging: Detection of ischemic injury 39 minutes after onset in a stroke patient. *Ann Neurol* 1999;**45**:794-797.

21. Coutts SB, Simon JE, Eliasziw M, et al. Triaging transient ischemic attack and minor stroke patients using acute magnetic resonance imaging. *Ann Neurol* 2005;**57**:848-854.

22. Hjort N, Christensen S, Solling C, et al. Ischemic injury detected by diffusion imaging 11 minutes after stroke. *Ann Neurol* 2005;**58**:462-465.

23. Lee JM, Vo KD, An H, et al. Magnetic resonance cerebral metabolic rate of oxygen utilization in hyperacute stroke patients. *Ann Neurol* 2003;**53**:227-232.

24. Heiss WD, Sobesky J, Hesselmann V. Identifying thresholds for penumbra and irreversible tissue damage. *Stroke* 2004;**35**(Suppl I):2671-2674.

25. Finkel E. Stem cells in brain have regenerative potential. *Lancet* 1996;**347**:751.

26. Steindler DA, Pincus DW. Stem cells and neuropoiesis in the adult human brain. *Lancet* 2002;**359**:1047-1054.

27. Bayes-Genis A, Salido M, Ristol FS, et al. Host cell-derived cardiomyocytes in sex-mismatch cardiac allografts. *Cardiovasc Res* 2002;**56**:404-410.

28. Astrup J, Siesjo BK, Symon L. Thresholds in cerebral ischemia - the ischemic penumbra. *Stroke* 1981;**12**:723-725.

29. Marchal G, Beaudouin V, Rioux P, et al. Prolonged persistence of substantial volumes of potentially viable brain tissue after stroke. A correlative PET-CT study with voxel-based data analysis. *Stroke* 1996;**27**:599-606.

30. Fujioka M, Taoko T, Matsuo Y, et al. Magnetic resonance imaging shows delayed ischemic striatal neurodegeneration. *Ann Neurol* 2003;**54**:732-747.

31. Neubauer RA, Gottlieb SF, Kagan RL. Enhancing "idling" neurons.

Lancet 1990;**335**:542.

32. Editorial. Neuroprotection: the end of an era? *Lancet* 2006;**368**:1548.

33. Lees KR, Zivin JA, Ashwood T, et al NXY-059 for acute ischemic stroke. *N Eng J Med* 2006;**354**:588-600.

34. Feurstein GZ, Zaleska MM, Krams M, et el. Missing steps in the STAIR case: a translational medicine perspective on the development of NXY-059 for treatment of acute stroke. *J Cereb Blood Flow Metab* 2006;**28**:217-219.

35. Gorelick PB. Neuroprotection in acute ischaemic stroke: A tale of for whom the bell tolls? *Lancet* 2000;**355**:1925.

36. Singhal AB. A review of oxygen therapy in ischemic stroke. *Neurol Res* 2007;**29**:173-183.

37. Majno G, Ames A, Chiang J, et al. No reflow after cerebral ischaemia. *Lancet* 1967;**ii**:569-570.

38. Dai J, Swaab DF, Buijs RM. Recovery of axonal transport in "dead" neurons. *Lancet* 1998;**351**:499-500.

39. Schwarz G, Litscher G, Kleinert R, Jobstmann R. Cerebral oximetry in dead subjects. *J Neurosurg Anesth* 1996;**8**:189-193.

40. Hallstrom A, Cobb L, Johnson E, et al. Cardiopulmonary resuscitation by chest compression alone or with mouth-to-mouth ventilation. *N Engl J Med* 2000;**342**:1546-1553.

41. Zamboni WA, Roth AC, Russell RC, et al. Morphologic analysis of the microcirculation during reperfusion of ischemic skeletal muscle and the effect of hyperbaric oxygen. *Plast Reconstr Surg* 1993;**91**:1110-1123.

42. Raynaud C, Rancurel G, Samson Y, et al. Pathophysiologic study of chronic infarcts with I-123 isopropyl iodo-amphetamine (IMP): the importance of peri-infarct area. *Stroke* 1987;**18**:21-29.

43. Defer G, Moretti J-L, Cesaro P, et al. Early and delayed SPECT using N-isopropyl p-iodoamphetamine iodine 123 in cerebral ischemia: a prognostic index for clinical recovery. *Arch Neurol* 1987;**44**:715-718.

44. Ronning OM, Guldvog B. Should stroke victims routinely receive supplemental oxygen? A quasi-randomized controlled trial. *Stroke* 1999;**30**:2033-2037.

45. Rawles JM, Kenmure ACF. Controlled trial of oxygen in uncomplicated myocardial infarction. *Br Med J* 1976;**1**:1121-1123.

46. Singhal AB, Benner T, Roccatagliata L, et al. A pilot study of normobaric oxygen therapy in acute ischemic stroke. *Stroke* 2005;**36**:797-802.

47. Eschenfelder CC, Krug R, Yuofi AF, et al. Neuroprotection by oxygen in acute transient focal cerebral ischaemia is dose dependent and shows

superiority of hyperbaric oxygenation. *Cerebrovasc Dis* 2008;**25**:193-201.

48. Sun L, Zhou W, Mueller C, et al. Oxygen therapy reduces secondary hemorrhage after thrombolysis in thromboembolic cerebral ischemia. *J Cereb Blood Flow Metab* 2010;**30**:1651–1660.

49. Matchett GA, Martin RD, Zhang JH. Hyperbaric oxygen therapy and cerebral ischemia: neuroprotective mechanisms. *Neurol Res* 2009;**31**:114–121.

50. Neubauer RA, End E. Hyperbaric oxygenation as an adjunct therapy in strokes due to thrombosis: a review of 122 patients. *Stroke* 1980;**11**:297-300.

51. Hart GP, Strauss MB. Oxygen therapy in ischemic stroke. *Stroke* 2003;**34**:1-4.

52. Holbach KH, Caroli A, Wassmann H. Cerebral energy metabolism in patients with brain lesions at normo and hyperbaric oxygen pressures. *J Neurol* 977;**217**:17-30.

53. Kaufmann AM, Firlik AD, Fukui MB, et al. Ischemic core and penumbra in human stroke. *Stroke* 1999;**30**:93-99.

54. Singhal AB. A review of oxygen therapy in ischemic stroke. *Neurol Res* 2007;**29**:173-183.

55. Efrati S, Fishlev G, Bechor Y, et al. Hyperbaric oxygen induces late neuroplasticity in post stroke patients - randomized prospective trial. *PLoS ONE* 2013;**8**:1-10.

56. Bradley WG, Waluch V, Brant-Zawadzki M, et al. Patchy periventricular white matter lesions in the elderly: A common observation during NMR imaging. *N Med Imaging* 1984;**1**:35-41.

57. Jacobs EA, Winter PM, Alvis HJ, Mouchly-Small S. Hyperoxygenation effect on cognitive functioning in the aged. *N Engl J Med* 1969;**280**:753-757.

58. Sun L, Marti HH, Veltkamp R. Hyperbaric oxygen reduces tissue hypoxia and hypoxia-inducible factor 1-alpha expression in focal cerebral ischemia. *Stroke* 2008;**39**:1000-1006.

59. Kihara M, McManis PG, Schmelzer JD, et al. Experimental ischemic neuropathy: salvage with hyperbaric oxygenation. *Ann Neurol* 1995;**37**:89-94.

60. Goodman MW, Workman RD. Minimal recompression oxygen breathing approach to the treatment of decompression sickness in divers and aviators. Research report, 5-6, US Navy Experimental Diving Unit 1965.

61. Curley MD, Schwartz HJC, Zwingelberg KM. Neuropsychologic assessment of cerebral decompression sickness and gas embolism. *Undersea Biomed Res* 1988;**15**:223-236.

62. Sharifi M, Fares W, Abdel-Karim I, et al. Usefulness of hyperbaric oxygen therapy to inhibit restenosis after percutaneous coronary intervention for acute myocardial infarction or unstable angina pectoris. *Am J Cardiol* 2004;**93**:1533-1535.

Chapter 21: Healing More than the Brain

1. Male D. Immunology: an illustrated guide. Mosby Yearbook Europe Ltd., London 1993.

2. Cramer T, Clausen BE, Pawlinki R, et al. HIF-1α is essential for myeloid cell-mediated inflammation. *Cell* 2003;**112**:645–657.

3. Henderson APD, Barnett MH, Parratt JDE, Prineas JW. Multiple sclerosis: distribution of inflammatory cells in newly forming lesions. *Ann Neurol* 2009;**66**:739-753.

4. Mehm WJ, Pimsler M, Becker RL. Effect of oxygen on in vitro fibroblast cell proliferation and collagen biosynthesis. *J Hyp Med* 1988;**3**:227-234.

5. James PB Allen MW, Scott B. Hyperbaric oxygen therapy in sports injuries. *Physiotherapy* 1993;**79**:571-572.

6. Abbot NC, Beck JS, Carnochan FMT, et al. Effect of hyperoxia at 1 and 2 ATA on hypoxia and hypercapnia in human skin during experimental inflammation. *J Appl Physiol* 1994;**77**:767-773.

7. Haldane JS. The therapeutic administration of oxygen. *Br Med J* 1917;**1**:181-183.

8. Valenzuela DF. Oxygen as an antipyretic. *Lancet* 1887;**129**:1144-1145.

9. Ross RM, Mcallister TA. Protective effect of hyperbaric oxygen in mice with pneumococcal septicaemia. *Lancet* 1965;**285**:579-581.

10. Hart GB, Strauss MB. Gas gangrene - clostridial myonecrosis: a review. *J Hyperbar Med* 1990;**5**:125-144. (Available from http://rubicon-foundation.org)

11. Specialist services definition set no. 28. NHS East Midlands Specialised Commissioning Group 2008.

12. Babior BM. Oxygen-dependent microbial killing by phagocytes. Part 1. *N Engl J Med* 1978;**298**:659-668.

13. Babior BM. Oxygen dependent microbial killing by phagocytes. Part 2. *N Engl J Med* 1978;**298**:721-725.

14. Lee WL, Grinstein S. The tangled webs that neutrophils weave. *Science* 2004;**303**:1477-1478.

15. Brown KA, Pearson SD, Edgeworth JD, et al. Neutrophils in development of multiple organ failure in sepsis. *Lancet* 2006;**368**:157-169.

16. Till GO, Johnson KJ, Kunkel R, Ward PA. Intravascular activation of complement and acute lung injury. *J Clin Invest* 1982;**69**:1126-1135.

17. Weiss SJ. Tissue destruction by neutrophils. *N Eng J Med* 1989;**320**:365-376.

18. Martin JD, Thom SR. Vascular leukocyte sequestration in decompression sickness and prophylactic hyperbaric oxygen therapy in rats. *Aviat Space Environ Med* 2002;**73**:565-569.

19. Hill L. The administration of oxygen. *Br Med J* 1912;**1**:71-72.

20. Stadie WC. The treatment of anoxemia in pneumonia in an oxygen chamber. *J Exp Med* 1922;**35**:337-360.

21. Boothby WM, Mayo CW, Lovelace WR. One hundred per cent oxygen: indications for its use and methods of its administration. *JAMA* 1939;**113**:477-482.

22. Almeida AO, Costa HM. Treatment of leprosy by oxygen under high pressure associated with methylene blue. *Revista Brasileira do Leprologia* 1938;**6**(Suppl):237-265.

23. Behnke AR. High atmospheric pressures; physiological effects of increased and decreased pressure; application of these findings to clinical medicine. *Ann Intern Med* 1940;**13**:2217-2228.

24. End E, Long CW. Oxygen under pressure in carbon monoxide poisoning: Effect on dogs and guinea pigs. *J Ind Hyg Toxicol* 1942;**24**:302-306.

25. Goodman MW, Workman RD. Minimal recompression oxygen breathing approach to the treatment of decompression sickness in divers and aviators. Research report, 5-6, US Navy Experimental Diving Unit 1965.

26. Sabiston DC, Talbert JL, Riley LH, Blalock A. Maintenance of the heartbeat by perfusion of the coronary circulation with gaseous oxygen. *Ann Surg* 1959;**150**:361-370.

27. Leake J. Heart machine brings patients "back from the dead." The Sunday Times, London 10th March 2013.

28. Shandling AH, Ellestad MH, Hart GB, et al. Hyperbaric oxygen and thrombolysis in myocardial infarction: the HOT MI pilot study. *Am Heart J* 1997;**134**:544-550.

29. Beck CS. Coronary heart disease: three dominant causes of death. *Am J Surg* 1958;**95**:743-751.

30. Sharifi M, Fares W, Abdel-Karim I, et al. Usefulness of hyperbaric oxygen therapy to inhibit restenosis after percutaneous coronary intervention for acute myocardial infarction or unstable angina pectoris. *Am J Cardiol* 2004;**93**:1533-1535.

31. Boerema I, Brummelkamp WH, Meijne NG. Clinical applications of

hyperbaric oxygen. Elsevier Publishing Company, Amsterdam 1964.

32. Bernhard WF, Danis R, Gross RE. Metabolic alterations noted in cyanotic and acyanotic infants during operation under hyperbaric conditions. *J Thorac Cardiovasc Surg* 1965;**50**:374-390.

33. Bernhard WF. Hyperbaric oxygenation. *N Engl J Med* 1964;**271**:562-564.

34. Thurston JGB, Greenwood TW, Bending MR, et al. A controlled investigation into the effects of hyperbaric oxygen on mortality following acute myocardial infarction. *Q J Med* 1973;**42**:751-770.

35. Yacoub MH, Zeitlin GL. Hyperbaric oxygen in the treatment of the postoperative low-cardiac-output syndrome. *Lancet* 1965;**i**:581-583.

36. Brierley JB. Neuropathological findings in patients dying after open-heart surgery. *Thorax* 1963;**18**:291-304.

37. Gilman S. Neurological complications of open heart surgery. *Ann Neurol* 1990;**28**:475-476.

38. Gallagher EG, Pearson DT. Ultrasonic identification of sources of gaseous microemboli during open heart surgery. *Thorax* 1973;**28**:295-305.

39. Muaroka R, Yokota M, Aoshima M, et al. Subclinical changes in brain morphology following cardiac operations as reflected by computed tomographic scans of the brain. *J Thorac Cardiovasc Surg* 1981;**81**:364-369.

40. Orenstein M, Sato N, Aaron B, et al. Microemboli observed in deaths following cardiopulmonary bypass surgery: silicone antifoam agents and polyvinyl chloride tubing as sources of emboli. *Hum Pathol* 1982;**13**:1082-1090.

41. Hills BA, James PB. Microbubble damage to the blood-brain barrier: relevance to decompression sickness. *Undersea Biomed Res* 1991;**18**:111-116.

42. Harris DNF, Bailey SM, Smith PLC, et al. Brain swelling in first hour after coronary artery bypass surgery. *Lancet* 1993;**342**:586-587.

43. Cianci P, Williams C, Lueders H, et al. Adjunctive hyperbaric oxygen in the treatment of thermal burns - an economic analysis. *J Burn Care Rehabil* 1990;**11**:140-143.

44. Cianci P, Slade JB, Sato JB, Faulkner J. Adjunctive hyperbaric oxygen therapy in the treatment of thermal burns. *Undersea Hyperb Med* 2013;**40**:89-108.

45. http://www.dailymail.co.uk/news/article-1292533/London-7-7-bombings-Victim-Davinia-Douglasss-miraculous-recovery.html

46. Editorial: Hyperbaric oxygen. *Br Med J* 1978;**1**:1012.

47. Teller E. On hyperbaric oxygenation. *J Am Phys Surg* 2003;**8**:97.

48. Treweek S, James PB. A cost analysis of monoplace hyperbaric oxygen

treatment with and without recirculation. *J Wound Care* 2006;**15**:1-4.

49. Welslau W, van Laak U. Disapproval of HBO by German Health Care System. XXVI annual scientific meeting of the EUBS September 2000.

50. NHS Clinical Commissioning Policy: The Use of Hyperbaric Oxygen Therapy, April 2013. NHSCB/D11/P/a.

51. Mitani M. Brain: implications for HBO_2. *Undersea Hyperb Med* 2004;**31**:163-166.

52. Davis JC, Hunt TK. Hyperbaric oxygen therapy. Undersea Medical Society Inc, Bethesda, Maryland 1977.

53. Davis JC, Hunt TK. Problem wounds; the role of oxygen. Elsevier, Amsterdam 1978.

54. Barr P-O, Enfors W, Eriksson G. Hyperbaric oxygen therapy in dermatology. *Br J Dermatol* 1972;**86**:631-635.

55. Oriani G, Michael M, Meazza D, et al. Diabetic foot ad hyperbaric oxygen therapy: A ten year experience. *J Hyp Med* 1992;**7**:213-220. Available from rubicon-foundation.org

56. Efuni SE, Kakhnovsy IM, Rodionov VV. HBO in the metabolic control of insulin-dependent diabetes mellitus: A controlled study. Proc 7th International Congress on Hyperbaric Medicine, Moscow 1981.

57. Gallagher KA, Goldstein LJ, Thom SR, Velazquez OC. Hyperbaric oxygen and bone marrow-derived endothelial progenitor cells in diabetic wound healing. *Vascular* 2006;**14**:328-337.

58. Thom SR, Milovanova TN, Yang M, et al. Vasculogenic stem cell mobilization and wound recruitment in diabetic patients: increased cell number and intracellular regulatory protein content associated with hyperbaric oxygen therapy. *Wound Repair Regen* 2011;**19**:149-161.

59. Tintle SM, Keeling JJ, Shawen SB, et al. Traumatic and trauma-related amputations: Part I: general principles and lower-extremity amputations. *J Bone Joint Surg Am* 2010;**92**:2852-2868.

60. Pinzur MS. The dark side of amputation rehabilitation. *J Bone Joint Surg Am* 2013;**95**:e12.

61. Canavese F, Krajbich JI, LaFleur BJ. Orthopaedic sequelae of childhood meningococcemia: management considerations and outcome. *J Bone Joint Surg Am* 2010;**92**:2196-2203.

62. Baby goes home after meningitis battle. The Times 29th March 2012.

63. Strauss M. Why hyperbaric oxygen therapy may be useful in treating crush injuries and skeletal muscle compartment syndrome. *Undersea Hyperb Med* 2012;**39**:799-855.

64. Reis ND, Schwartz O, Militianu D, et al. Hyperbaric oxygen therapy as a treatment for stage-I avascular necrosis of the femoral head. *J Bone Joint Surg Br* 2003;**85**:371-375.

65. Camporesi E, Vezzani G, Bosco G, et al. Hyperbaric Oxygen Therapy in Femoral Head Necrosis. *J Arthroplasty* 2010;**25**:118-123.

66. Wells CH, Goodpasture JE, Horrigan DJ, Hart GB. Tissue gas measurements during hyperbaric oxygen exposure. Proc. 6th International Congress on Hyperbaric Medicine, Aberdeen University Press, Aberdeen 1979.

67. Cross FS. Effect of increased atmospheric pressures and the inhalation of 95% oxygen and helium-oxygen mixtures on the viability of the bowel wall and the absorption of gas in closed-loop obstructions. *Recent Adv Surg* 1954;**10**:1001-1005.

68. Garcia-Covarrubias L, Barratt DM, Bartlett R, et al. Invasive aspergillosis treated with adjunctive hyperbaric oxygenation: a retrospective clinical series at a single institution. *South Med J* 2002;95:450-456.

69. Goldblatt H, Cameron G. Induced malignancy in cells from rat myocardium subjected to intermittent anaerobiosis during long propagation in vitro. *J Exp Med Biol* 1958;97:525-552.

70. Warburg O. On the origin of cancer cells. *Science* 1956;**123**:309-314.

71. Bevers RFM, Bakker DJ, Kurth KH. Hyperbaric oxygen treatment for haemorrhagic radiation cystitis. *Lancet* 1995;**346**:803-805.

Chapter 22: The Way Forward

1. Burton AC, Edholm OE. Man in a cold environment. Edward Arnold, London 1955.

2. Carbon monoxide poisoning: failure to use hyperbaric chamber: hospital liability. AMA Legal Department 6/6/78.

3. LaBar KS, Cabezza R. Cognitive neuroscience of emotional memory. *Nat Rev Neurosci* 2006;**7**:54-64.

4. Putnam TJ, McKenna JB, Morrison LR. Studies in multiple sclerosis. I. The histogenesis of experimental sclerotic plaques and their relation to multiple sclerosis. *JAMA* 1931;**97**:1591-1596.

5. Calman KC, Moores Y. Carbon monoxide the forgotten killer. Letter from the Department of Health 1998.

6. Haldane JS. The action of carbonic oxide on man. *J Physiol (Lond)* 1895;**12**:430-462.

7. Boerema I, Meijne NG, Brummelkamp WK, et al. Life without blood; a

study of the influence of high atmospheric pressure and hypothermia on dilution of the blood. *J Cardiovasc Surg* 1960;**1**:133-146.

8. Haldane JBS. CXLII. Carbon monoxide as a tissue poison. *Biochem J* 1927;21:1068-1075.

9. Parkinson RB, Hopkins RO, Cleavinger HB, et al. White matter hyperintensities and neuropsychological outcome following carbon monoxide poisoning. *Neurology* 2002;**58**:1525-1532.

10. Haldane JS. Respiration. Yale University Press, Yale 1922.

11. Goldbaum LR, Ramirez RG, Absalon KB. What is the mechanism of carbon monoxide toxicity? *Aviat Space Environ Med* 1975;**46**:1289-1291.

12. Abdul-Ghaffar N, Farghaly MM, Swamy ASK. Acute renal failure, compartment syndrome, and systematic capillary leak syndrome complicating carbon monoxide poisoning. *Clin Toxicol* 1996;**34**:713-719.

13. Singh AC, Badalyan G, Carlin B, Zikos A. Survival after 42 hours of carbon monoxide exposure from a mining accident with hyperbaric oxygen therapy. *Chest* 2006;**130**:317S.

14. Olesen, S-P. Rapid increase in blood-brain barrier permeability during severe hypoxia and metabolic inhibition. *Brain Res* 1986;**368**:24-29.

15. Thom SR, Fisher D, Manevich Y. Roles for platelet activating factor and nitric oxide-derived oxidants causing neutrophil adherence after CO poisoning. *Am J Physiol Heart Circ Physiol* 2001;**28**:H923-930.

16. Thom SR, Bhopale VM, Han ST, et al. Intravascular neutrophil activation due to carbon monoxide poisoning. *Am J Respir Crit Care Med* 2006;**174**:1239-1248.

17. Horowitz AL, Kaplan R, Sarpel G. Carbon monoxide toxicity: MR imaging of the brain. *Radiology* 1987;**162**:787-788.

18. Sawada Y, Sakamoto T, Nishide K, et al. Correlation of pathological findings with computed tomographic findings after acute carbon monoxide poisoning. *N Engl J Med* 1983;**308**:1296.

19. Fazekas F, Kleinert R, Offenbacher H, Schmidt R, Kleinert G, Payer F, Radner H, Lechner H. Pathologic correlates of incidental MRI white matter signal hyperintensities. *Neurology* 1993;**43**:1683-1689.

20. Kawanami T, Kato T, Kurita K, Sasaki H. The pallidoreticular pattern of brain damage on MRI in a patient with carbon monoxide poisoning. *J Neurol Neurosurg Psychiatry* 1998;**64**:282.

21. Smith G, Ledingham IM, Sharp GR, et al. Treatment of coal-gas poisoning with oxygen at 2 atmospheres pressure. *Lancet* 1962;**i**:816-819.

22. Weaver LK, Hopkins RO, Chan KJ, et al. Hyperbaric oxygen for acute

carbon monoxide poisoning. *N Engl J Med* 2002;**347**:1057-1067.

23. Vila JF, Melf FJ, Serqueira OE, et al. Diffusion tensor magnetic resonance imaging: A promising technique to characterize and track delayed encephalopathy after acute carbon monoxide poisoning. *Undersea Hyperb Med* 2005;**32**:151-156.

24. Murata T, Itoh S, Koshino Y, et al. Serial proton magnetic resonance spectroscopy in a patient with the interval form of carbon monoxide poisoning. *J Neurol Neurosurg Psychiatry* 1995;**58**:100-103.

25. Ziser A, Shupak A, Halpern P, et al. Delayed hyperbaric oxygen treatment for acute carbon monoxide poisoning. *Br Med J* 1984;**289**:960.

26. Verschueren H, Crols R. Bilateral substantia nigra lesions on magnetic resonance imaging in a patient with encephalitis lethargica. *J Neurol Neurosurg Psychiatry* 2001;**71**:275.

27. Sacks O. Awakenings. Harper Perennial, New York 1990.

28. http://oxfordhbot.com/our-facility/

29. Mathieu D, Wattel F, Gosselin et al. Hyperbaric oxygen in the treatment of posthanging cerebral anoxia. *J Hyp Med* 1987;**2**:63-67. (Available at http://rubicon-foundation.org)

30. Kim J-h, Chang K-H, Song IC, et al. Delayed encephalopathy of acute carbon monoxide intoxication: diffusivity of cerebral white matter lesions. *Am J Neuroradiology* 2003;**24**:1592-1597.

31. Gillespie ND, G Hallhead G, B Mutch, et al. Severe Parkinsonism secondary to carbon monoxide poisoning. *J R Soc Med* 1999;**92**:529-530.

32. Sohn YH, Jeong Y, Kim HS, et al. The brain lesion responsible for Parkinsonism after carbon monoxide poisoning. *Arch Neurol* 2000;**57**:1214-1218.

33. Thyagarajan MS, Gunawardena WJ, Coutinho CMA. Seizures and unilateral cystic lesion of the basal ganglia: an unusual clinical and radiological manifestation of chronic non-fatal carbon monoxide (CO) poisoning. *Clin Radiol* 2003;**58**:38-41.

34. Kirkpatrick JN. Occult carbon monoxide poisoning. *West J Med* 1987;**146**:52-56.

35. www.nhs.uk/Conditions/Pages/hub.aspx

36. www.nhs.uk/Conditions/Carbon-monoxide-poisoning/Pages/Treatment.aspx

37. NHS Clinical Commissioning Policy: The Use of Hyperbaric Oxygen Therapy, April 2013. NHSCB/D11/P/a.

38. Gilmer B, Killkenny J, Tomasweski C, Watts JA. Hyperbaric oxygen

does not prevent neurologic sequelae after carbon monoxide poisoning. *Academ Emerg Med* 2002;**9**:1-8.

39. Vila JF, Melf FJ, Serqueira OE, et al. Diffusion tensor magnetic resonance imaging: A promising technique to characterize and track delayed encephalopathy after acute carbon monoxide poisoning. *Undersea Hyperb Med* 2005;**32**:151-156.

40. Plum F, Posner JB, Hain RF. Delayed neurological deterioration after anoxia. *Arch Intern Med* 1962;**110**:56-63.

41. Fischer BH, Marks M, Reich T. Hyperbaric-oxygen treatment of multiple sclerosis: a randomized, placebo-controlled, double-blind study. *N Engl J Med* 1983;**308**:181-186.

42. Cornwall J. The Sunday Times Magazine, December 9th 2007.

43. Treweek S, James PB. A cost analysis of monoplace hyperbaric oxygen treatment with and without recirculation. *J Wound Care* 2006;**15**:1-4.

44. Smith GCS, Pell JP. Parachute use to prevent death and major trauma related to gravitational challenge: systematic review of randomised controlled trials. *Br Med J* 2003;**327**:1459.

45. Jennet B. High technology; medicine and burdens. Rock-Carling Fellowship 1983, London: Nuffield Provincial Hospitals Trust, 1984.

46. Gibson I. Letter to the General Medical Council, March 2004.

47. British Thoracic Society Guideline for emergency oxygen use in adult patients. *Thorax* 2008;**63**:Supplement VI.

48. Illich I. Limits to medicine, medical nemesis: the expropriation of health. Pelican books, Harmondsworth 1977.

49. Kyritsis N, Kizil C, Zocher S, et al. Acute inflammation initiates the regenerative response in the adult zebrafish brain. *Science* 2012;**338**:1353-1356.

50. Zamboni WA, Roth AC, Russell RC, et al. Morphologic analysis of the microcirculation during reperfusion of ischemic skeletal muscle and the effect of hyperbaric oxygen. *Plast Reconstr Surg* 1993;**91**:1110-1123.

51. Sharifi M, Fares W, Abdel-Karim I, et al. Usefulness of hyperbaric oxygen therapy to inhibit restenosis after percutaneous coronary intervention for acute myocardial infarction or unstable angina pectoris. *Am J Cardiol* 2004;**93**:1533-1535.

52. Alex J, Laden G, Cale ARJ, et al. Pretreatment with hyperbaric oxygen and its effect on neuropsychometric dysfunction and systemic inflammatory response after cardiopulmonary bypass: a prospective randomized double-blind trial. *J Thorac Cardiovasc Surg* 2005;**130**:1623-1630.

53. Yogaratnam JZ, Laden G, Madden LA, et al. Hyperbaric oxygen preconditioning safely improves myocardial function, promotes pulmonary vascular flow, and protects the endothelium from ischemic reperfusion injury. *Cardiovasc Revascul Med* 2007;**8**:148-151.

54. Arciniegas DB. Hypoxic-ischemic brain injury: Addressing the disconnect the disconnect between pathophysiology and public policy. *Neuro Rehabilitation* 2010;**26**:1-4.

55. Eltzschig HK. Hypoxia and inflammation. *N Eng J Med* 2011;**364**:656-664.

56. Semenza G. Oxygen sensing homeostasis and disease. *N Eng J Med* 2011;**365**:537-547.

57. Morrison EW, Milliken F. Organizational silence: A barrier to change and development in a pluralistic world. *Acad Management Rev* 2000;**25**:706-725.

58. Mychaskiw G. Hyperbaric oxygen therapy and neurologic disease: the time has come. *Undersea Hyperb Med* 2010;**37**:xi–xiii.

59. Mychaskiw G. Neurologic applications of hyperbaric oxygen: a sad slow story. *Undersea Hyp Med* 2011;**38**:305-306.

INDEX

168, 341

experimental allergic encephalomyelitis (EAE) 244–6, 248, 256, 284, 304

extra corporeal membrane oxygenation (ECMO) 393, 394

F

fermentation 413

fetal distress 175, 176, 180, 183, 184

fetal growth retardation 176, 179

fibrocartilagenous embolism 228–30, 233–5, 270, 272, 283, 358

Fiennes, Sir Ranulph 56

Fischer, Boguslav 287, 293–7, 300–3, 307, 309, 310, 312, 322, 428

Food and Drug Administration (FDA) 324

football injuries 234, 269, 354, 385, 386

foramen magnum 34, 334

foramen ovale 232, 271

Forrester, R.M. "Sam" 193, 194

Franz, Anselm 108

free radical(s) 6–9, 38, 85–9, 91, 99, 105, 106, 122, 125, 129, 133, 142, 149–54, 186, 334, 338, 357–9, 371, 374, 379, 390, 420, 425

Freund's adjuvant 244, 245

Fridovich, Irwin 6, 7, 9, 90, 105

frostbite 409, 410

Fryer, Commander David 107–9

fungal infection 177

G

Gamow bag 45, 46, 209

Gamow, Igor 45, 215

gas gangrene 173, 390, 396, 401–3

gas-induced osmosis 353

gene p53 413

Ghajar, Jamshid 329, 332

Glaisher, James 41–6, 54, 65, 67, 93, 99, 104, 106

Glaxo Smith Kline xv

GLUT proteins 32

glycolysis 8, 9, 389, 413

Goodman, Maurice W. 139, 140, 392

Gottlieb, Sheldon 296

gravity 3, 375

H

Habal, Salem 398

Habeler, Peter 54, 104

haemoglobin xvi, 14, 20, 25–7, 38, 55, 62, 68, 69, 74, 75, 83, 106, 124, 134, 168, 305, 334, 337, 346, 358, 370, 372, 417, 418

haemorrhagic cystitis 414

haemorrhagic stroke 358

Haining, William 267, 268

Haldane, John B.S. "Jack" 59–61 291, 413, 417

Haldane, John Scott 56– 67, 70, 71, 75, 77, 78, 81, 82, 86, 91, 93, 98, 100, 101, 104, 106, 109, 111, 114–6, 118, 123–6, 128, 129, 132, 138, 141, 145, 169, 199, 205, 228, 245, 268, 271, 307, 340, 389, 391, 415, 417, 418, 427, 432, 435

Harch, Paul 347–51, 453

Hart, George B. 374, 410

Heberden nodes 444

Helios plane crash 51, 52

helium 15, 48, 49, 62, 71, 79, 85, 133, 136, 140, 364, 428

hemiplegia 175, 358

hemisphere(s), of the brain 29–5, 126, 204, 258–60, 263, 272, 278, 358, 360, 361, 376, 381, 397, 453, 454

Henderson, Yandell 65–7

Hengist 60, 129

Henry's law 6, 25, 138

Henry, William 6

Heuser, Gunnar 209

Hillary, Edmund 53, 104

Hill, Leonard 78, 115, 391

Hills, Brian 23, 79, 80, 90, 118, 206, 398

Himalayas 106

Hindenburg disaster 97

Hitler, Adolf 102, 121, 413

H.M.S. *Royal George* 111

hot bath test 253, 254, 292

HOT MI pilot study 393

Hounsell, John 172

House of Lords 235, 237

Houston Everest expedition 99

Houston Post 310

Myodil 450

N

natalizumab (Tysabri) 319
National Football League (NFL) 269
National Health Service 314, 362
National Institute of Health and Clinical
    Excellence (NICE) 162, 314–7,
    319, 320
National MS Society of America 243, 244,
    293, 294, 301, 302
Nerup, Jens 241, 242
Neubauer, Richard 73, 74, 200, 201, 208,
    292, 293, 301–3, 307, 312, 347, 348,
    350, 374, 398, 401, 447
Neurosurgery 143, 338, 341, 344
neutrophils 1, 83, 86–90, 129, 142, 146,
    151–4, 181, 241, 247, 255, 334, 357,
    371, 372, 388, 390–2, 395, 420, 431,
    432
Newcastle study 302, 308–12
New England Journal of Medicine (*NEJM*) 84,
    92, 169, 233, 287, 292, 295–8, 301,
    302, 308, 310, 322, 377, 390, 396,
    421
New Scientist 92, 336, 456, 462, 490
New York Times 243
New York University study 287, 292, 293,
    295, 301, 307, 317, 321, 428
New Zealand study 354
NHS Choices 424
NHS Specialist Services Definition Set No.
    28 402
1907 Admiralty Report on Deep Water
    Diving 115, 118, 123
nitric oxide 30, 68, 69, 106, 134, 409
nitric oxide synthase 409
nitrogen 5, 24, 48, 62, 68, 83, 85–8, 115–8,
    138–40, 293, 353
nodes of Ranvier 239
no reflow phenomenon 370
Norgay, Tenzing 53, 104
North Sea 15, 71, 85, 129, 133, 307
NSAIDs 159–61
nucleus pulposus 228
NXY-059 367, 368
nystagmus 226, 299, 450

O

oedema 278, 335, 347, 427, 438, 439
    pulmonary 45, 46, 80, 89, 91, 215
oligoclonal bands 247
oligodendrocyte(s) 9, 32, 239, 256, 420
ophthalmic artery 258, 260, 261, 264, 265,
    286
optic disc 135, 136, 258
optic neuritis 135, 136, 240, 252, 255, 258,
    261–3, 265, 266, 282, 298, 360
    ischaemic 263
organelles 2
Osler, Sir William 169, 199
osmosis 205, 336, 353
    gas-induced 353
oxidation 2, 3, 7, 8, 62, 418
oxygen threshold 38
oxyhaemoglobin xvi, 26–8

P

Pallotta, Raphael 322, 323
Palm Beach Post 290
papillitis 261
paraplegia 36, 109, 204, 233, 234, 254, 283,
    364
parasthesia 226
Parkinson's disease 121, 424, 429
Pascal, Blaise 47
Pasley, Colonel Charles W. 111, 112
penicillin xiii, 168, 294, 391
periphlebitis 261, 266, 267
perivenous syndrome 278
periventricular lesions 249, 482
Perrins, David 131
petechial haemorrhages 277, 286
Pfizer xv, 368
phagocytes 1, 256, 383
phantom pains 409
Pike's Peak 66, 68, 75, 106
Pilâtre de Rozier, Jean-François 41
placebo 155, 157–9, 162–5, 167, 205, 207,
    208, 210, 215, 292–4, 297–9, 309,
    319, 353, 367, 371, 428, 454
placenta 17, 18, 174, 176, 177, 179, 182, 185
Plasmodium 122
platelets 125, 282, 360
pneumothorax 93

Index ~ 513